Pain
A Source Book for Nurses
and Other Health Professionals

PAIN

A Source Book for Nurses and Other Health Professionals

Edited by

Ada K. Jacox, R.N., Ph.D.

Associate Dean and Professor, School of Nursing,
The University of Colorado, Denver

Foreword by Jeanne Q. Benoliel, R.N., D.N.Sc.
Professor of Nursing, Department of Community Health Care Systems,
School of Nursing, University of Washington, Seattle

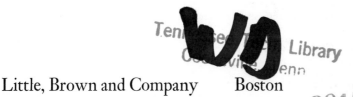

Little, Brown and Company   Boston

Contents

Foreword

Pain has always been part of the human condition. It has been described again and again, in myth and song, in story and verse, in legend and fable, throughout man's brief residence on earth. The agony of pain has been movingly portrayed in such diverse artworks as the ancient Greek drama *Medea*, the etchings of Goya, and the poignant writings of Sylvia Plath.

The advent of science brought a new approach to pain, that of seeking to understand its origins and outcomes in a rigorous way and of identifying systematic methods for alleviating the misery associated with it. People have used potions and pain-relieving remedies for centuries, but the search for treatment based on scientific investigation is a recent development. The scientists' search for answers to the problem of pain has provided nurses and other health professionals with a wealth of information to use in assisting people to cope with pain in positive ways. Yet much remains to be learned about pain, and to date science has provided no neat and tidy solution to the problem of its relief.

The complexity of pain as a phenomenon to be understood and the diversified nature of pain-related clinical problems come through clearly in this book. To provide nurses and other health professionals with "a comprehensive overview of the many dimensions of pain," the focus is on *clinical pain* as a subject worthy of concentrated investigation and as a problem of singular importance to practitioners providing services to patients with pain-producing illnesses and injuries.

Drawing on the work of a variety of people in a variety of scientific and professional disciplines, the book points to the problematic nature of studying pain when different disciplines are brought together. As I read through the book, I could not help but be reminded that knowledge about pain exists at many levels and the meaning ascribed to pain depends on the vantage point and basic assumptions of the discipline being represented. It follows rather easily that interdisciplinary communication about pain and its meaning is difficult to achieve due to differences in primary definitions and levels of analysis and to the "specialized languages" employed for describing and explaining pain. These same differences also interfere with communication between patients and providers of health care.

Given the historical development of the scientific study of pain into neurophysiological, psychological, social, and cultural components, the slow development of theories that integrate varying concepts of pain is readily understood. Yet nurses and other direct care providers need an integrated approach, for their work requires an involvement with persons and not only with "psyche" or "soma" in isolation from the totality.

The publication of this book answers the need for an integrated perspective to assist providers and consumers in understanding the intricate nature of clinical pain and to guide them in their choices and decisions about its alleviation. As a resource, the book is designed to bridge the present gap between theory and practice by bringing together these interrelated areas of knowledge which provide essential background for examining pain in a holistic rather than a partitioned sense. As a human phenomenon to be understood and treated, the psychoneurophysiological experience of clinical pain does not exist in isolation from the social and cultural milieu in which it occurs.

The first part of the book presents the work of basic scientists in several disciplines and offers a general introduction to pain as a neurophysiological phenomenon showing complex and still incompletely understood interrelationships between the individual and sociocultural and psychological influences from the environment. The first four chapters present theoretical discussions of pain, each focusing on a separate set of factors affecting pain responses and experiences. Together they provide a complementary set of perspectives about the causes of pain and the conditions that bring pain into being and influence its effects and interpretations. Two further chapters round out this introductory section, one a thoughtful description of research methods and procedures for measuring clinical pain, and the other an insightful discussion of pain assessment in clinical practice.

The second part of the book is concerned with currently accepted modalities of treatment for pain and draws on the work of practitioners as well as clinical investigators. Each chapter presents a major treatment modality, considers the rationale underlying its use, and describes its limits as well as its values. In addition to chapters dealing with the more traditional methods of pain relief, such as surgery and medication, this section includes discussions of the use of acupuncture, biofeedback techniques, hypnosis, operant conditioning, and combinations of novel and traditional therapies. Those interested in a general review of pain treatment will find this section of considerable interest. Persons interested in ethical issues in health care may also be interested to note the strong psychological influence shown in the newer treatment modalities.

Of particular interest to nurses may be the chapters that deal with pain as it occurs in association with different disease entities or clinical problems. This part of the book draws heavily on the work of clinical specialists in nursing and provides analyses of major pain-producing problems encountered by nurses in practice. In each instance the presentation incorporates discussion of the physiological origins of pain, its typical and atypical characteristics, methods of clinical assessment, and preferred methods of treatment and pain alleviation.

The clinical categories chosen for presentation include some in which the pain tends to be short-lived or temporary in nature, as following general surgery or during labor and delivery. Others focus on chronic pain, which requires long-term adaptation to its demands. The chapters that deal with pain associated with neurological conditions, arthritis and rheumatic disorders, other orthopaedic conditions (including low back pain), and cancer, are all concerned with the assessment and treatment of pain on a long-term rather than short-term basis. Characterized by both immediate and long-term pain, burns and cardiovascular diseases pose special sets of clinical problems. Nurses offering services for such problems must have finely developed assessment skills and psychological/technical abilities. A very thoughtful chapter in this part is devoted to the special problems of pain in children and considers the kinds of assessment and processing tools needed by nurses to offer effective services when children are hospitalized for pain.

The final part of the book is a full, annotated bibliography of the literature on pain with particular emphasis on the last six years. As a reference source, this bibliography offers an excellent starting point for anyone interested in the range of problems falling into the general class of clinical pain.

Appearing at this time, a book that attempts to tie together theoretical discussions of pain and pragmatic problems of clinical practice aims to remedy a deficit in the current literature. The effort is commendable, and the result should help investigators with a special interest in clinical pain and practitioners whose daily work brings them into frequent contact with pain and its problems.

Patients in pain have always posed a special challenge to the art of nursing practice. The rising number of people living with long-term diseases and chronic disabilities suggests that chronic pain will gain importance as a clinical problem. It is clear that services to assist these people in adapting to the multiple consequences of their pain requires more than an understanding of pain as a neurophysiological mechanism. Integrated theory to guide nurses and other health professionals toward the assessment and alleviation of pain in a holistic sense requires an understanding of pain as a mode of personal and interpersonal adaptation to acute or chronic stress. Science is only beginning to focus on this complex phenomenon.

Viewed in historical perspective, this book makes an important contribution to knowledge about pain. It reminds us of the past. It sets the stage for the future. For nurses, the opportunities are endless to participate in building an integrated body of knowledge about a human problem that affects the lives of many.

Jeanne Q. Benoliel

Preface

The study of pain has occupied scientists perhaps as much as any other phenomenon in experience. In spite of a vast body of knowledge of pain, many puzzles remain. Conflicting theories compete in their explanation, and the alleviation of pain continues to be a pervasive and profound problem for clinicians and patients.

The concept of pain has been the focus of study in many scientific disciplines. Physiologists have studied the neurophysiology of pain, considering such problems as the kinds and amount of noxious stimuli necessary to create a response in nerve endings. Psychologists have investigated the relationship of personality characteristics to pain threshold and tolerance, and a few sociologists and anthropologists have studied sociocultural factors related to pain. This research has produced a great deal of knowledge about pain, considered from each theoretical perspective, but the various perspectives have generally not been integrated into a form useful to health professionals.

Health professionals seldom use knowledge from only one basic science. Much nursing practice, for example, is based on the assumption that a person is simultaneously a biological, psychological, and sociocultural being. This assumption should give rise to the development of theories to integrate these levels of analysis, but such conceptualization has been slow to develop. It has been slow not only in nursing but in science generally, since to use a holistic approach in the analysis of behavior is more complex and difficult than to consider each level of analysis largely in isolation from the others. There have been attempts, however, to deal theoretically with various levels of analysis, as evidenced by the emergence of such fields as psychophysiology and social psychology. The need for practitioners to use knowledge gained from several sciences further stimulates the development of unified theories of behavior.

While this book does not present a single unified approach to the study and relief of pain, its contents provide nurses and other health professionals with a comprehensive overview of the many dimensions of pain. In general, the authors of this book view pain as encompassing interrelated biological and psychosocial dimensions, although some chapters emphasize one aspect more than the other. The book should be useful to health professionals interested

in learning more about clinical pain in particular—the assessment and alleviation of pain, the measurement of clinical pain for research purposes, and the
experience of pain with specific groups of patients.

The book is divided into four parts. Part I is a general consideration of
pain, beginning with a discussion of the gate control theory first proposed
by Melzack and Wall a decade ago. While these authors focus primarily on
the neurophysiological basis of pain, they provide a theoretical explanation
of how psychological factors can influence pain perception and response.
The chapter by Fidler and Whidden is a basic discussion of how pain is perceived and communicated at the cellular level, with the material in this chapter complementary to Melzack and Wall's chapter. Following the chapters
on the anatomical and physiological basis of pain is a chapter by Jacox in
which she discusses the influence of sociocultural and psychological factors
on the experience of pain. These factors include analyses of pain threshold
and tolerance, the assessment of pain by health professionals, and methods of
pain relief based on cognitive measures of control. The chapter by Merskey
summarizes some current psychiatric approaches to the explanation and
treatment of pain. In Chapter 5, Stewart describes and analyzes several methods by which clinical pain can be measured for research purposes. Johnson's
chapter deals with the evaluation of clinical pain by clinicians. The six chapters in this first part are intended to provide the reader with a general theoretical understanding of pain and how it is measured or assessed.

Part II comprises seven chapters, each dealing with a major approach to
pain relief. The first two chapters in this part focus on interrupting the pain
sensation mechanically and electrically. The first is a discussion of the major
surgical and electrical stimulation methods for relieving pain. In this chapter,
McDonnell discusses factors to be considered in choosing one procedure
over another. Chapter 8 by Armstrong presents a description and explanation of acupuncture as it has been and is currently practiced, as well as a
discussion of some recent criticisms of acupuncture. In Chapter 9, Gebhardt
considers the merits of various narcotic and nonnarcotic analgesics for relieving pain of different type and origin. The next four chapters in this part
assume that cognitive control of pain is possible. Crasilneck and Hall discuss
clinical hypnosis as a method of relieving pain. The chapter by Fordyce on
operant conditioning is a clear explanation of recent attempts to use this approach in the treatment of chronic pain. Another relatively recent approach
to pain relief is the use of biofeedback procedures to monitor the body's activities. Budzynski, in Chapter 12, presents a theoretical discussion of biofeedback and summarizes some of the research using this method to relieve
various painful conditions. The final chapter in this part is a discussion by
Greenhoot and Sternbach of how traditional methods are combined with
some of the newer cognitively-based interventions and used in the treatment
of chronic pain for patients hospitalized on a "pain unit." Taken together,
the chapters in this part represent a good overview of current methods of
pain relief.

Part III deals with pain associated with particular conditions or groups of patients. The nine chapters in this part discuss the most common kinds of pain with which health professionals must deal, and outline specific nursing and medical approaches for the relief of pain in each condition. Chapter 14 by Sweeney, Johnson, and Eland deals with pain associated with various neurological conditions, including pain of central origin, phantom limb pain, and headache. A special feature of this chapter is a section dealing with nursing care of patients who are using bioelectrical stimulators, including those that are implanted. Chapter 15 is a discussion by Sweeney of some of the neurophysiological and chemical bases for pain associated with surgery, and gives some suggestions on how to deal with this kind of pain. Chapter 16 by O'Dell focuses on pain associated with rheumatic disorders. Rheumatoid and degenerative arthritis, two of the most common forms of arthritis, receive particular attention in this chapter. In the chapter on cancer, Shawver outlines the various mechanisms that produce pain associated with cancer, and suggests approaches to use in helping patients deal with this pain associated with cancer. Chapter 18 by Wagner discusses pain and treatment associated with thermal accidents. In Chapter 19, Houser discusses the physiological basis for pain accompanying various cardiovascular diseases, and gives suggestions for the reduction of pain. Chapter 20 by Field describes the relief of pain for women in labor. Chapter 21 by Buckwalter and Buckwalter is an overview of the most common sources of orthopaedic pain, together with a brief discussion of the treatment and nursing care related to the pain. The final chapter in this part is a discussion by Eland and Anderson on how pain is experienced by children. While the nine chapters in this part do not deal with every possible kind of pain, they do discuss those diseases and conditions with which pain is most commonly associated.

Part IV is an annotated bibliography of the literature on pain. It includes literature primarily from the last six years, although some classic articles and books on pain published earlier are included. The bibliography is organized by section, with cross-referencing between sections.

Appreciation is expressed to the authors whose works in this book originally appeared elsewhere, and their publishers. I would like to acknowledge the valuable assistance of Dr. Jane Anderson in editing some of the copy for this book, and to thank Margie Landuyt for her industriousness and persistence in typing the many drafts of the manuscript.

A. K. J.

Contributing Authors

Jane E. Anderson, Ph.D.
Clinical Psychologist, The University of Iowa, Iowa City

Margaret E. Armstrong, R.N., M.S.
Assistant Professor of Nursing and Neurology, University of Rochester School of Medicine and Dentistry, Rochester

Joseph A. Buckwalter, M.D.
Resident in Orthopaedic Surgery, University of Iowa Hospitals and Clinics, Iowa City

Kathleen C. Buckwalter, R.N., M.A.
Research Assistant, College of Nursing, The University of Iowa, Iowa City

Thomas H. Budzynski, Ph.D.
Assistant Professor of Psychiatry, University of Colorado School of Medicine, Denver

Harold B. Crasilneck, M.A., Ph.D.
Clinical Associate Professor of Anesthesiology and Psychology, The University of Texas Health Science Center at Dallas Southwestern Medical School; Consultant, Parkland Memorial Hospital and Children's Medical Center, Dallas

Jessie S. Daniels, R.N., M.A.
Research Assistant, College of Nursing, The University of Iowa, Iowa City

Joann M. Eland, B.S.N., M.A.
Assistant Professor, College of Nursing, The University of Iowa, Iowa City

Sister Mary Rebecca Fidler, Ph.D.
Associate Professor, College of Nursing, The University of Iowa, Iowa City

Peggy-Anne Field, R.N., M.N.
Associate Professor, School of Nursing, University of Alberta, Edmonton, Alberta, Canada

Wilbert E. Fordyce, Ph.D.
Professor of Psychology, Department of Rehabilitation Medicine, University of Washington School of Medicine, Seattle

Gerald F. Gebhart, Ph.D.
Assistant Professor of Pharmacology, The University of Iowa College of Medicine, Iowa City

Jerry H. Greenhoot, M.D.
Charlotte Neurological Associates, Charlotte, North Carolina

J. A. Hall, M.D.
Assistant Professor of Psychiatry in Obstetrics and Gynecology, and Clinical Assistant Professor of Psychology, The University of Texas Health Science Center at Dallas Southwestern Medical School; Staff Psychiatrist, Baylor Hospital, Dallas

Doris Houser, R.N., M.A.
Clinical Nurse Specialist, University Hospital, The University of Iowa, Iowa City

Ada K. Jacox, R.N., Ph.D.
Professor, School of Nursing, The University of Colorado, Denver

Marion Johnson, R.N., M.S.
Clinical Nurse Specialist, University Hospital, The University of Iowa, Iowa City

Dennis McDonnell, M.D.
Assistant Professor of Surgery, Division of Neurosurgery, Department of Surgery, The University of Iowa College of Medicine, Iowa City

Ronald Melzack, Ph.D.
Professor of Psychology, McGill University, Montreal, Quebec, Canada

H. Merskey, M.A., D.M., D.P.M.
Physician, Psychological Medicine, National Hospital for Nervous Diseases, London, England

Ardis J. O'Dell, R.N., M.A.
Director, St. Luke's Methodist School of Nursing, Cedar Rapids, Iowa

Joanne W. Rains, R.N., M.A.
Research Assistant, College of Nursing, The University of Iowa, Iowa City

Martha M. Shawver, R.N., M.A.
Assistant Professor, School of Nursing, Wichita State University, Wichita, Kansas

Richard A. Sternbach, Ph.D.
Associate Professor of Psychology, University of California, San Diego, School of Medicine, La Jolla; Veterans Administration Hospital, San Diego

Mary L. Stewart, R.N., M.A.
Research Associate, Medical Care and Research Foundation, Denver

Sandra S. Sweeney, R.N., M.A.
Assistant Professor, College of Nursing, The University of Iowa, Iowa City

Mary Wagner, R.N., M.S.N.
Clinical Specialist, Trauma Center, Medical University of South Carolina, Charleston

Patrick D. Wall, Ph.D.
Professor of Psychology, McGill University, Montreal, Canada

Ann Whidden, R.N., M.S.
Associate Professor, College of Nursing, The University of Iowa, Iowa City

I

General Considerations of Pain and Pain Assessment

1

Psychophysiology of Pain

Ronald Melzack and Patrick D. Wall

Evolution of Pain Theories

Theories of pain mechanisms, since the beginning of the century, have undergone evolutionary changes based partly on the accumulation of new experimental evidence and partly on imaginative assumptions derived from clinical and psychological observations. New biological-medical theories, like theories in the physical sciences [4], are accepted reluctantly; old theories are dogmatically maintained in the face of contrary evidence until a new theory supersedes them that can account for both the older and newer facts. In this process of evolution there is usually a characteristic swing of the pendulum between two major theoretical concepts (such as the phlogiston versus oxygen theories of combustion), until one of them eventually dominates. Another feature of this evolution in science [4] is that a theory may be conceptually correct although the particular explanatory *mechanism* that is postulated may well be wrong in one or more details. The theoretical concept thus often awaits widespread acceptance until a satisfactory mechanistic explanation is proposed.

Overriding all these features of the scientific process is the bitter controversy generated between opposing schools of thought. The problems of cutaneous mechanisms in general, and pain in particular, have given rise to vituperation that, according to Dallenbach [5], is unparalleled in the biological sciences. The early three-cornered fight involving von Frey, Goldscheider, and Marshall (whose emotion—or quale—theory of pain was soon pushed out of the ring, despite Sherrington's [42] sympathy with Marshall's view) marks the beginning of a controversy that has continued throughout this century.

Part of the reason for the bitterness engendered by the battle may be the obvious clinical implications that derive from any theoretical advance. The practice of medicine, because it deals with human lives, is generally conservative, so that old ideas that have worked (even imperfectly) are cherished and newer ideas are viewed with suspicion and often antipathy. It is in

Reprinted from *International Anesthesiology Clinics: Anesthesiology and Neurophysiology* 8(1):3, 1970, by permission.

the light of this understanding of scientific processes that we shall here review two major theoretical concepts of pain—the specificity and pattern theories—that are the basis of much of the bitter controversy on pain mechanisms in this century, and describe a third theory—gate control theory—that
we have proposed as an alternative to both.

Specificity Theory

Specificity theory proposes that a mosaic of specific pain receptors in body
tissue projects to a pain center in the brain. It maintains [44] that free nerve
endings are pain receptors and generate pain impulses that are carried by A
delta and C fibers in peripheral nerves and by the lateral spinothalamic tract
in the spinal cord to a pain center in the thalamus. Despite its apparent sim-
plicity, the theory contains an explicit statement of physiological specialization and an implicitly psychological assumption [20, 31, 32]. Consider the
proposition that the skin contains pain receptors. To say that a receptor responds only to intense, noxious stimulation of the skin is a physiological
statement of fact; it says that the receptor is specialized to respond to a particular kind of stimulus. To call a receptor a *pain* receptor, however, is a
psychological assumption; it implies a direct connection from the receptor
to a brain center where pain is felt (Figs. 1-1, 1-2A, and 1-3A), so that stimulation of the receptor must always elicit pain and only the sensation of pain.
The facts of physiological specialization provide the power of specificity
theory; its psychological assumption is its weakness [31, 32].

There can no longer be any doubt that the receptors and fibers of the skin
sensory system exhibit a high degree of specialization of function. There is
no convincing evidence, however, to substantiate the view that there is a
special class of receptor-fiber units that comprise an exclusive pain modality.
In the search for peripheral fibers that respond exclusively to high intensity
stimulation, Burgess and Perl [3] have recently discovered a specialized class
of A delta small-diameter myelinated fibers with slow conduction velocity.
They are attached to true nociceptors, since they transmit impulses only
when the skin is actually damaged. It is reasonable to assume that these fibers
carry impulses which contribute to pain processes, but they cannot be considered as modality-specific "pain fibers" because: (1) pain may be triggered by stimuli (particularly in neuralgic patients) that are inadequate to
fire these fibers, (2) noxious heat, cold, and bradykinin (a noxious chemical)
do not fire them, (3) they adapt fairly rapidly, and (4) there is no afterdischarge. We see, then, that while these fibers may, on occasion, contribute to
the afferent barrage which triggers pain, they do not have the required
properties of explaining all cutaneous pains or the variable relationship between stimulus and response.

These data suggest that a small number of specialized fibers may exist that
respond only to intense stimulation, but this does not mean that they are
"pain fibers"—that they must always produce pain, and only pain, when they
are stimulated. It is more likely that they represent the extreme of a continu-

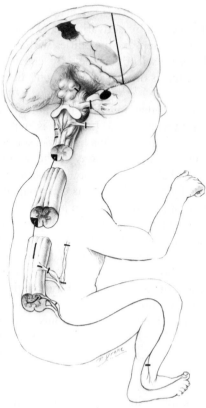

Figure 1-1   MacCarty and Drake's schematic diagram of the pain pathway, illustrating various surgical procedures designed to alleviate pain: 1: Gyrectomy.
2: Prefrontal lobotomy. 3: Thalamotomy. 4: Mesencephalic tractotomy. 5:
Hypophysectomy. 6: Fifth-nerve rhizotomy. 7: Ninth-nerve neurectomy. 8:
Medullary tractotomy. 9: Trigeminal tractotomy. 10: Cervical cordotomy.
11: Thoracic cordotomy. 12: Sympathectomy. 13: Myelotomy. 14: Lissauer
tractotomy. 15: Posterior rhizotomy. 16: Neurectomy [23].

ous distribution of receptor-fiber thresholds rather than a special category.
The transduction properties of receptor-fiber units are a function of many
physiological variables: (1) threshold to mechanical distortion, (2) threshold
to negative and positive temperature change, (3) peak sensitivity to temperature change, (4) threshold to chemical change, (5) stimulus strength-
response curve, (6) rate of adaptation, and (7) afterdischarge. Each
receptor-fiber unit must be specified accurately in terms of its coordinates
with respect to these variables instead of being forced into a preconceived,
oversimplified, psychological modality class. Similarly, experiments that appear to correlate loss of pain sensation with selective block of C fibers by
pharmacological agents are usually interpreted to mean that C fibers are pain

fibers. However, there is an alternative interpretation: that pain results when the total integral of the afferent barrage in all fibers exceeds a critical preset level and that the only way to exceed the level is by activation of C fibers. Indeed, all experiments that attempt to correlate sensory modalities with particular groups of nerve fibers on the basis of selective block by cocaine, ischemia, and the like, can be interpreted in terms of interaction among fiber groups rather than of specific modalities.

This distinction between physiological specialization and psychological assumption also applies to central projection systems [31]. There is, without question, evidence that central nervous system pathways have specialized functions that play a role in pain mechanisms. Surgical lesions of the lateral spinothalamic tract [44] or portions of the thalamus [25] may on occasion abolish pain of pathological origin. But the fact that these areas carry signals related to pain does not mean that they comprise a specific pain system. The lesions have multiple effects: They reduce the total number of responding neurons; they change the temporal and spatial relationships among all ascending systems; and they affect the descending feedback that controls transmission from peripheral fibers to dorsal horn cells. Moreover, pain frequently recurs after apparently successful cordotomy [37]. Physiological specialization is a fact that can be recognized without acceptance of the psychological assumption that pain is determined entirely by impulses in a straight-through transmission system from the skin to a pain center in the brain.

Pattern Theory

As a reaction against the psychological assumption in specificity theory, new theories have been proposed which can be grouped under the general heading of *pattern theory*. Goldscheider [10] was the first to propose that stimulus intensity and central summation are the critical determinants of pain. Goldscheider (Fig. 1-2B) proposed that the large cutaneous fibers comprise a specific touch system, while the smaller fibers converge on dorsal horn cells which summate their input and transmit the pattern to the brain where it is perceived as pain. Other theories have been proposed, within the framework of Goldscheider's concept, which stress central summation mechanisms. Livingston [20] was the first to suggest neural mechanisms to account for the remarkable summation phenomena in clinical pain syndromes. He proposed that intense, pathological stimulation of the body sets up reverberating circuits (central circuit incorporated into Fig. 1-2B) in spinal internuncial pools that can then be triggered by normally nonnoxious inputs and generate abnormal volleys that are interpreted centrally as pain.

Related to theories of central summation is the theory that a specialized input-controlling system normally prevents summation from occurring, and that destruction of this system leads to pathological pain states. Basically, this theory proposes the existence of a rapidly conducting fiber system which inhibits synaptic transmission in a more slowly conducting system that carries the signal for pain [51]. These two systems are identified as the epicritic and protopathic [13], fast and slow [18], phylogenetically new and old [2], and myelinated and unmyelinated [38] fiber systems. Under pathological conditions, the slow system establishes dominance over the fast, and the result is protopathic sensation [13], slow pain [18], diffuse burning pain [2], or hyperalgesia [38]. It is important to note the transition from specificity theory to the pattern concept: Noordenbos [38] does not associate psychological quality with each system but attributes to the rapidly conducting system the ability to modify the input pattern transmitted through the slowly conducting, multisynaptic system in the spinal cord (Fig. 1-2C).

The concepts of central summation and input control have shown remarkable power in their ability to explain many of the clinical phenomena of pain. They lack unity, and no single theory so far proposed is capable of integrating the diverse theoretical mechanisms.

A recent variant of pattern theory has been proposed by Weddell [50] and Sinclair [43] based on the earlier suggestion by Nafe [36] that all cutaneous qualities are produced by spatiotemporal patterns of nerve impulses rather than by separate modality-specific transmission routes. The theory proposes that all fiber endings (apart from those that innervate hair cells) are alike, so that the pattern for pain is produced by intense stimulation of nonspecific receptors. The physiological evidence, however, reveals [31] a high degree of receptor-fiber specialization. The pattern theory proposed by Weddell and Sinclair, then, fails as a satisfactory theory of pain because it ignores the facts of physiological specialization. It is more reasonable to assume that the specialized physiological properties of each receptor-fiber unit, such as response ranges, adaptation rates, and thresholds to different stimulus intensities, play an important role in determining the characteristics of the temporal patterns that are generated when a stimulus is applied to the skin.

SUMMARY In summary, we believe that the specific modality and pattern theories of pain, although they appear to be mutually exclusive, both contain valuable concepts that supplement one another. Recognition of receptor specialization for the transduction of particular kinds and ranges of cutaneous stimulation does not preclude acceptance of the concept that the information generated by skin receptors is coded in the form of patterns of nerve impulses. The law of the adequate stimulus can be retained without also accepting a narrow, fixed relationship between receptor specialization and perceptual and behavioral response. Similarly, the original hopes for a monopolization of a particular modality by a specific fiber-diameter group have not materialized. The evidence permits only a loose association of function with fiber diameter. Moreover, the evidence suggests that central projection pathways are specialized for the transmission of particular kinds of

8

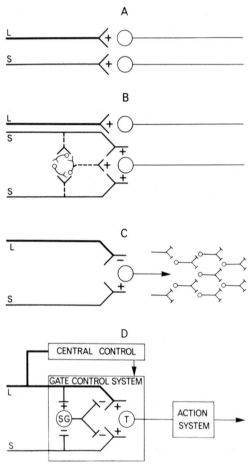

Figure 1-2 Schematic representation of conceptual models of pain mechanisms. A. Specificity theory. Large (L) and small (S) fibers are assumed to transmit touch and pain impulses respectively, in separate, specific, straight-through pathways to touch and pain centers in the brain. B. Summation theory, showing convergence of small fibers onto a dorsal horn cell. The central network projecting to the central cell represents Livingston's conceptual model of reverberatory circuits underlying pathological pain states [20]. Touch is assumed to be carried by large fibers. C. Sensory interaction theory, in which large (L) fibers inhibit (−) and small (S) fibers excite (+) central transmission neurons. The output projects to spinal cord neurons which are conceived by Noordenbos [38] to comprise a multisynaptic afferent system. D. Gate control theory. The large (L) and small (S) fibers project to the substantia gelatinosa (SG) and first central transmission (T) cells. The central control trigger is represented by a line running from the large fiber system to central control mechanisms, which in turn project back to the gate control system. The T cells project to the entry cells of the action system. + = excitation; − = inhibition. (From Melzack and Wall [32].)

information, but there is no evidence that allows us, even at this central level, to assume a one-to-one relationship between physiological specialization and psychological events.

There can no longer be any doubt that temporal and spatial patterns of nerve impulses provide the basis of our sensory perceptions. The coding of information in the form of nerve impulse patterns is a fundamental concept in contemporary neurophysiology and psychology. Yet pattern theory, because of its vagueness, fails to provide an adequate account of somesthesis. The inadequacies of specificity and pattern theories of pain have therefore necessitated the formulation of alternative conceptions. Indeed, the fact that so many forms of pain still resist pharmacological or surgical control demands exploration of new approaches and new concepts.

Gate Control Theory

We have recently proposed a new theory of pain in which a gate control system modulates sensory input from the skin before it evokes pain perception and response [32]. Stimulation of skin evokes nerve impulses that are transmitted to three spinal cord systems (Fig. 1-2D): the cells of the substantia gelatinosa in the dorsal horn, the dorsal column fibers that project toward the brain, and the central transmission (T) cells in the dorsal horn. We proposed that (1) the substantia gelatinosa functions as a gate control mechanism that modulates the afferent patterns before they influence the T cells; (2) the afferent patterns in the dorsal column system act, in part at least, as a central control trigger which activates selective brain processes that then influence, by way of descending fibers, the modulating properties of the gate control system; and (3) the T cells activate neural mechanisms which comprise the action system responsible for perception and response. The theory suggests that pain phenomena are determined by interactions among these three systems.

Figure 1-2D shows the factors involved in the transmission of impulses from peripheral nerve to T cells in the cord. We proposed that the control over transmission is affected by two factors: by the afferent impulses acting on a gating mechanism, and by impulses descending from the brain. Impulses in large-diameter fibers were assumed to decrease the effectiveness of afferent volleys, while small afferents increased it. The substantia gelatinosa was suggested as the actual control mechanism and the presynaptic terminals of afferent fibers as the site of action. Thus, in the model (Fig. 1-2D), volleys in large fibers are effective initially in firing the T cells, but their later effect is reduced by the presynaptic inhibitory gating mechanism. In contrast, volleys in fine fibers reduce the presynaptic inhibition and thereby exaggerate the effect of arriving impulses. Figure 1-2D shows only presynaptic control, but postsynaptic control mechanisms are also presumed to contribute to the observed input-output function. Furthermore, descending impulses from the brain control the presynaptic mechanism, so that the ease with which impulses penetrate the cord cells is determined both by the afferent activity and by central control processes originating in the brain. The output of the T cells, then, is determined by the number of active fibers and their rate of firing, by the balance of large- and small-fiber activity in the afferent barrage, and by the activity of central structures.

We proposed [32] that the signal which triggers the action system responsible for pain perception and response occurs when the output of the T cells reaches or exceeds a critical level. That is, there is a temporal summation or integration of the arriving barrage by central cells which finally results in pain perception and response when the integral exceeds a preset level. The clinical and pharmacological implications of the theory will be discussed after it is first evaluated in the light of recent evidence.

Gate Control Theory: Recent Evidence

Recent physiological evidence necessitates a revision of gate control theory. The laminar organization of the dorsal horns is now better understood and, moreover, indicates a convergence of visceral afferent impulses onto the T cells. In addition, new questions are raised on the actual mechanisms underlying gate control; although the concept of the balance of large-fiber versus small-fiber activity appears to be valid, the actual explanatory *mechanism* still needs to be determined unequivocally.

Spinal Cord Mechanisms and Control of Entering Impulses

Since the gate control theory of pain was proposed in 1965, further research has been done on the dorsal horns, and a much more specific but still highly speculative picture of the process of reception and transmission can be presented. The reason for the necessity for speculation is that it is not yet possible to collect the crucial evidence. The anatomical gaps are produced by the difficulty in staining substantia gelatinosa cells, the extreme complexity of the interconnections, uncertainty about the morphology of functional synapses, and ignorance of the ultimate destination of projecting axons. The physiological ignorance comes from the fact that recordings can be made only from outside a minority of cells and from inside an even smaller number. It is not even certain that the small cells of substantia gelatinosa generate nerve impulses. Under these circumstances, it is not surprising that important details are unknown about the passage of impulses from afferent fibers to central transmitting cells. A final serious problem is the assessment of the significance of the powerful descending influences from the brain on the dorsal horn. We know from physiological experiments that these pathways exist but we cannot know under what circumstances they actually work until they have been studied during behavior. In spite of these difficulties a lot of important results have been generated in the last few years and we can again attempt a summary in the form of an extension of our earlier gate control theory.

ANATOMY   Cutaneous afferent fibers terminate in the dorsal two-thirds of the dorsal horn (Fig. 1-3). These fibers end on cells which are arranged in a series of laminae. The most dorsal of these is the thin scattered layer of marginal cells whose significance remains unknown. Next is the substantia gelatinosa, lamina II, which contains three components: the terminals of afferent fibers, the dendrites of deeper cells, and the small cells and their interconnections. The fibers which terminate in this lamina must be of a special variety since their terminals degenerate within 48 hours of root section [14]. Golgi staining suggests that these are fine afferents which project directly into the dorsal gray from the dorsal roots by way of the medial part of the Lissauer tract [8, 45]. The dendrites rise up from the large deeper cells. These dendrites form broad fans which run rostrocaudally and subdivide the lamina into compartments [39]. The small cells interconnect with each other by short axons and by longer axons running in the lateral part of the Lissauer tract. The region contains large numbers of axoaxonic contacts and many of the receiving axons are presumed to be peripheral afferents

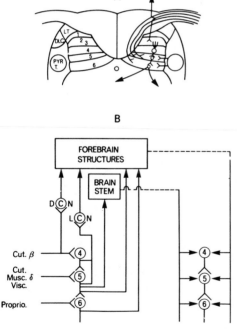

Figure 1-3   (A) Representation of the laminar organization and some of the connections and projections in the dorsal spinal cord. (B) Schematic representation of major connections and projections of the somatic sensory system. 4, 5, 6 represent the dorsal horn laminae (shown in [A]). DLC = dorsolateral column; PYR T. = pyramidal tract; LT = Lissauer's tract; DCN = dorsal column nuclei; LCN = lateral cervical nucleus. Cutaneous, muscular, visceral, and proprioceptive inputs are indicated.

[45]. The small cells receive contacts from each other, probably from afferents, and probably from a special type of small cell in lamina III.

The third lamina contains the same three component types as the second, but the afferents ending here are known to be in part the large myelinated cutaneous afferents which follow a curved course bending back on themselves to project dense fans of terminal arbors intermeshed with the fanshaped dendrites of the deeper cells. The small cells, some of which are pyramidal in shape, receive primary afferents and project their axons into lamina II. Below this layer, there is a layer of cells (lamina IV) with large cell bodies; their dendrites project into laminae II and III and some of their axons travel in the ipsilateral dorsolateral tract, at least in the lower mammals. In the cat these axons project to the lateral cervical nucleus and from there to thalamus and cortex. It is debatable if an analogous nucleus exists in the primates.

Finally, in the narrowest part of the dorsal horn there is lamina V, which receives afferent fibers and projects in a number of directions. A small number of these cells send their axons in the dorsolateral white matter on the same side. Some may project by way of the dorsal columns to unknown end stations in the brain and some may project to thalamus by way of the ventral crossed spinothalamic tract [7]. All five laminae receive axons descending from the brain, including some by way of the pyramidal tract.

PHYSIOLOGY OF CHANGES IN TERMINALS   The original gate control theory was based on the fact that changes are produced in the membrane potential of terminal axons following the arrival of impulses from the periphery. Impulses arriving in large-diameter cutaneous afferents produce a large, prolonged depolarization of the terminals of the active fibers and their passive neighbors. Schmidt, Senges, and Zimmermann [40] have suggested that this depolarizing interaction is particularly strongly produced by certain specific types of afferents. Mendell and Wall [34] believed that the smaller afferents (A delta and C fibers), in contrast to the large fibers, produce a hyperpolarization of terminals so that the actual membrane potential is determined by the balance of large versus small fibers active in the afferent volley. The reported effect of C fibers, however, has recently been challenged.

Whatever the outcome may be, it is clear that the membrane potential of the terminals is controlled by some central mechanism which is in turn controlled by the rival effects of certain large versus certain small afferents. The mechanism is still believed to involve cells in laminae II and III. The membrane potential of the terminal arborization was thought to determine the postsynaptic effectiveness of the arriving impulses, either by a block of impulses in the fine terminal filaments or by controlling the amount of transmitter released. Now, however, it is not at all certain that these purely presynaptic mechanisms exist in isolation. The presynaptic membrane potential control exists but it may be coupled with a simultaneous change in the postsynaptic membrane.

Physiology of the Transmitting Cells

While poor progress has been made in unravelling the details of synaptic transmission from cutaneous afferents to transmitting cells, a great deal more is now known about the input and output functions of these cells. The cells in lamina IV are poor candidates as the transmitters of impulses likely to trigger pain reactions, because they fail to respond to intense cutaneous-pressure stimuli or to electrical stimuli of peripheral nerves involving A delta and C afferents. In contrast, the lamina V cells are the best candidates so far discovered as the first central transmission cells in a pain-signalling pathway because their properties fulfill a number of requirements needed to explain actual phenomena. While summarizing present knowledge and suggesting a pain mechanism, it is essential to remember that the data are based on a partial survey of cell types because present techniques do not permit recording from smaller cells.

There are five laminae in the dorsal horn containing cells which receive cutaneous afferents (Fig. 1-3). We believe that the cells of lamina V are the most likely transmitter cells concerned with triggering pain reactions. The cells of lamina I are very few in number, have large receptive fields with a multiple convergence from skin and muscle, and are not known to be concerned with projection in the crucial contralateral ventral white matter. The cells of laminae II and III have an unknown physiology but their anatomy suggests that they modulate the flow of impulses from the afferents to the larger cells. The cells of lamina IV have small cutaneous receptive fields and project to the ipsilateral white matter and probably to lamina V cells. They respond to light-pressure stimuli and to A beta afferent volleys, but they fail to increase their response to A delta or C volleys. In contrast, the cells of lamina V have somewhat larger cutaneous receptive fields, respond to all types of cutaneous stimuli, and are also involved in the reception of impulses from deep and visceral structures.

The cutaneous receptive fields of lamina V cells have three components. In the center there is a region where low-pressure stimuli and hair movements excite the cell. Very low-level electrical stimuli sufficient to excite A beta afferents excite the cell, probably by way of the lamina IV cells. This region is superimposed on top of a wider area of skin from which the cell is excited by intense electrical or mechanical stimuli. The excitation produced by small fibers is followed by a very prolonged period of afterdischarge. Finally, these two regions are superimposed on top of an even larger region from which low-threshold fibers produce inhibition. This combination of convergences produces a three-zoned receptive field: In the center the cell is excited by the full range of mechanical stimuli, but inhibition follows after light stimuli and facilitation follows heavy stimuli; the firing rate increases with increasing intensity of stimulation, and intense stimulation produces very prolonged repetitive discharges. Around this zone is a region where light stimuli or large-fiber stimulation produces inhibition while heavy stimuli or small-fiber stimulation produces excitation and some facilitation. The two excitatory fields are surrounded by an even larger zone in which no natural stimuli excite but, instead, produce inhibition. The mechanism of the inhibition produced by the large fibers and the facilitation produced by the small fibers is unknown, but it may involve both postsynaptic and presynaptic changes and the small cells of laminae II and III. Certain components of the facilitatory mechanism must be sensitive to barbiturate, since Hillman and Wall [15] never observed prolonged facilitation in the presence of barbiturate anesthesia, confirming Mendell and Wall [35].

In the decerebrate or barbiturate-anesthetized cat, powerful tonic descending impulses from the brainstem arrive in the cord and excite the local inhibitory mechanism (Fig. 1-3B). This means that the number of impulses leaving a lamina V cell after stimulation is controlled by brain structures.

The organization of convergence with associated inhibitory and facilitatory mechanisms allows the cells to operate in several modes. For light stimuli or large-diameter afferents there is a small receptive field with inhibitory surround. For heavy mechanical stimuli, there is a larger receptive field and a facilitatory mechanism which competes with the inhibition. The intensity of inhibition is controlled by the brainstem. For a particular cell, the small-fiber influence may come from one of three sources: the cutaneous delta afferents, the small muscle afferents, or the small visceral afferents. All cells are excited by small afferents, whatever their origin, and inhibited by large-diameter afferents of cutaneous origin. We propose that if the frequency of nerve impulses leaving any of these cells ever rises above some critical level, then pain reactions will be triggered. The presence of convergence, interaction, and control at the entry point helps to explain many pain phenomena, particularly those associated with diseases of peripheral nerves.

Beyond the Gate

We assume that the gating of the input at the dorsal horn level of the spinal cord marks the beginning of repeated modulation, filtering, and abstraction of the input as it ascends toward and into the brain. It is obvious that barbiturates and other analgesics act on the action system as well as gate mechanisms in the spinal cord. Melzack and Casey [26] have noted (Figs. 1-4, 1-5B) that the output of the dorsal horn T cells is transmitted toward the brain by fibers in the anterolateral spinal cord and is projected into two major brain systems: via neospinothalamic fibers into the ventrobasal and posterolateral thalamus and the somatosensory cortex, and via medially coursing fibers, that comprise a paramedial ascending system, into the reticular formation and medial intralaminar thalamus and the limbic system (Fig. 1-4). Electrical stimulation of the tooth at noxious intensities evokes activity in both projection systems, and discrete lesions in each may strikingly diminish pain perception and response [16, 30]. Moreover, analgesic doses of nitrous oxide produce a striking reduction of the amplitude of potentials evoked by tooth stimulation in both systems [12]. Barbiturates and ether are

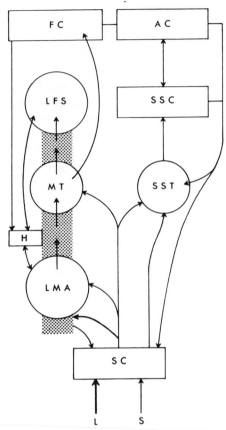

Figure 1-4 Schematic diagram of the anatomical foundation of proposed pain model in Figure 1-5B. (Right) Thalamic and neocortical structures subserving discriminative capacity. (Left) Reticular and limbic systems subserving motivational-affective functions. Ascending pathways from the spinal cord (SC) are: (1) dorsal column–lemniscal and dorsolateral tracts (right ascending arrow) projecting to the somatosensory thalamus (SST) and cortex (SSC), and (2) anterolateral pathway (left ascending arrow) to somatosensory thalamus via neospinothalamic tract, and to reticular formation (stippled area), limbic midbrain area (LMA), and medial thalamus (MT) via paramedial ascending system. Descending pathways to spinal cord originate in somatosensory and associated cortical areas (AC) and in the reticular formation. Polysynaptic and reciprocal relationships in limbic and reticular systems are indicated. Other abbreviations: FC = frontal cortex; LFS = limbic forebrain structures (hippocampus, septum, amygdala, and associated cortex); H = hypothalamus. (From Melzack and Casey [26].)

also known to reduce potentials in the reticular formation [9]. The connections and functional properties of the spinal cord and brain projection and relay systems are complex and still controversial. Since this literature is reviewed in detail elsewhere in this issue, we will here only sketch the major central pathways and their interactions.

Recent behavioral and physiological studies have led Melzack and Casey [26] to propose (Fig. 1-5B) that (1) the selection and modulation of the sensory input through the neospinothalamic projection system provides, in part at least, the neurological basis of the sensory-discriminative dimension of pain [41]; (2) activation of reticular and limbic structures through the paramedial ascending system underlies the powerful motivational drive and unpleasant affect that trigger the organism into action; and (3) neocortical

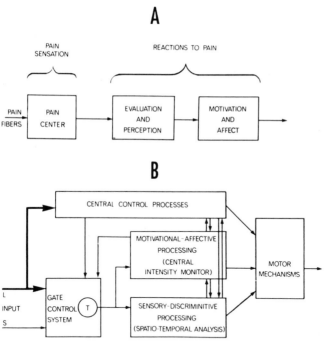

Figure 1-5 (A) Conceptual model of the basis of pain experience according to specificity theory. (B) Conceptual model of the sensory, motivational, and central control determinants of pain. The output of T cells of the gate control system projects to the sensory-discriminative system (via neospinothalamic fibers) and the motivational-affective system (via the paramedial ascending system). The central control trigger (comprising the dorsal column and dorsolateral projection systems) is represented by a line running from the large-fiber system to central control processes; these, in turn, project back to the gate control system, and to the sensory-discriminative and motivational-affective systems. All three systems interact with one another and project to the motor system. (From Melzack and Casey [26].)

or higher central nervous system processes, such as evaluation of the input in terms of past experience, exert control over activity in both the discriminative and motivational systems. It is assumed that these three categories of activity interact with one another to provide perceptual information regarding the location, magnitude, and spatiotemporal properties of the noxious stimulus, motivational tendency toward escape or attack, and cognitive information based on analysis of multimodal information, past experience, and probability of outcome of different response strategies. All three forms of activity could then influence motor mechanisms responsible for the complex pattern of overt responses that characterize pain.

There is now a convincing body of evidence that stimulation of reticular and limbic system structures produces strong aversive drive and behavior typical of responses to naturally occurring painful stimuli. These data together with related evidence (reviewed by Melzack and Casey [26]) on the effects of ablation indicate that limbic structures, although they play a role in many other functions, provide a neural basis for the aversive drive and affect that comprise the motivational dimension of pain. Melzack and Casey propose that the reticular and limbic systems function as a central intensity monitor; that their activities are determined, in part at least, by the intensity of the T cell output (the total number of active fibers and their rate of firing) after it has undergone modulation by the gate control system in the dorsal horns. They suggest that the output of the T cells, beyond a critical intensity level, activates those areas underlying negative affect and aversive drive. Signals from these structures to motor mechanisms set the stage for response patterns that are aimed at dealing with the input on the basis of both sensory information and cognitive processes.

It is now firmly established that stimulation of the brain activates descending efferent fibers [22] which can influence afferent conduction at the earliest synaptic levels of the somesthetic system. Thus it is possible for central nervous system activities subserving attention, emotion, and memories of prior experience to exert control over the sensory input. There is evidence [11, 47] to suggest that these central influences are mediated through the gate control system. While some central activities, such as anxiety or excitement, may open or close the gate for all inputs at any site of the body, others obviously involve selective, localized gate activity. For example, men wounded in battle may feel little or no pain from the wound (because it signifies that they survived the battle) but may complain bitterly about an inept vein puncture [1]. The signals, then, must be identified, evaluated in terms of prior experience, localized, and inhibited before the action system responsible for pain perception and response is activated. We propose, therefore, that there exists in the nervous system a mechanism, which we call the *central control trigger*, that activates the particular, selective brain processes that exert control over the sensory input (Fig. 1-2D).

We have already noted [32] that the dorsal column–medial lemniscal and dorsolateral systems could fulfill the functions of the central control trigger.

They carry precise information about the nature and location of the stimulus, and they conduct so rapidly that they may not only set the receptivity of cortical neurons for subsequent afferent volleys but may, by way of central control efferent fibers, also act on the gate control system. At least part of their function, then, could be to activate selective brain processes that influence information which is still arriving over slowly conducting fibers or is being transmitted up more slowly conducting pathways.

Implications of the Model for Pain Control

We have already noted [32] that gate control theory is able to account for many pain phenomena. If, for example, there is a selective destruction of large peripheral nerve fibers (leaving the smaller fibers relatively intact), as in diabetic or alcoholic neuropathy, the normal presynaptic and postsynaptic inhibition of the input by the gate control system does not occur. Thus the input arriving over the remaining smaller fibers is transmitted through the unchecked, open gate produced by the C fiber input and provides the basis for intense, pathological pain. Moreover, since the total number of peripheral fibers is reduced, it may take a considerable time before the T cells can be wound up to the discharge level necessary to trigger pain, which would account for the delays often observed in pathological pain states [38].

Similar mechanisms may account for neuralgic pains: Kerr and Miller [17] have recently demonstrated that the trigeminal ganglia and adjacent posterior rootlets in patients with trigeminal neuralgia show marked proliferative-degenerative changes in the myelin sheaths of the large fibers. Comparable experimental demyelination [24] produces a striking reduction of conduction velocities in formerly rapidly conducting fibers. This relative decrease in the large-fiber input provides a possible mechanism for the pain of anesthesia dolorosa and the spontaneous pains which develop in these syndromes. Spatial summation would also occur easily under such conditions. The phenomena of referred pain, spread of pain, and trigger points at some distance from the original site of body damage point toward summation mechanisms which can be understood in terms of the model, since the substantia gelatinosa at any level receives inputs from both sides of the body and (by way of Lissauer's tract) from the substantia gelatinosa in neighboring body segments.

In addition to the sensory influences on the gate control system, there is a tonic input to the system from the brain which exerts an inhibitory effect on the sensory input [47]. Thus, any lesion that impairs the normal downflow of impulses to the gate control system would open the gate. Central nervous system lesions associated with hyperalgesia and spontaneous pain could have this effect. On the other hand, any central nervous system condition that increases the flow of descending impulses would tend to close the gate. The model also suggests that psychological factors such as past experience, attention, and emotion influence pain response and perception by acting on the gate control system. The balance between sensory facilitation and central inhibition of the input after peripheral-nerve lesion could account for the variability of pain even in cases of severe nerve injury.

The recent discovery that the small visceral afferents project directly or indirectly into lamina V cells provides gate control theory with still further power in explaining referred pain. It is evident that the phenomenon of referred pain is not simply a mislocation of the origin of a visceral afferent barrage. Somewhere in the nervous system there must be a convergence and summation of nerve impulses from the diseased viscera and from the area of skin to which the pain is referred. The pain is exaggerated if skin is touched in the area where the pain is located. Local anesthesia of skin to which pain is referred abolishes or diminishes the pain. Many theories have suggested possible locations for the convergence between cutaneous and visceral afferents. Lamina V cells exhibit this convergence and are monosynaptically connected to visceral afferents. They are therefore good candidates for explaining the phenomenon of referred pain as well as pain of direct cutaneous origin. Both inhibitory and excitatory interactions exist between the converging visceral and cutaneous inputs, which would account for both inhibitory and excitatory interactions at the clinical perceptual level, although the particular conditions necessary for each is not yet clear.

The role of the autonomic nervous system in pain is also comprehensible in terms of gate control theory. There are obvious signs in a number of severe pain syndromes such as causalgia and Raynaud's disease that the sympathetic system plays a role in pain and, indeed, sympathectomy may abolish the pain [20].

There are three possible mechanisms of autonomic action. (1) Neurohumoral substances released by autonomic efferent activity may change the sensitivity of afferent nerve endings. In the frog there is good evidence that this is the case. In mammalian skin we have indirect evidence that the effect, if present, must be small because sensitivities of particular endings have been shown to be stable over long periods of time and in the presence of various anesthetics which would be expected to vary the sympathetic outflow. (2) The removal of normal pain-producing metabolites such as bradykinin, which are associated with tissue breakdown, is controlled by local circulation which in turn is affected by the autonomic nervous system. Thus, part of the analgesic effect of sympathectomy in such conditions as intermittent claudication and Raynaud's disease may be the consequence of the vasodilation produced by the abolition of sympathetic activity. (3) Somatic afferents pass through the sympathetic ganglia. When sympathetic ganglia are surgically removed or blocked by local anesthesia, an important group of small myelinated and unmyelinated afferent fibers is destroyed in addition to the efferent fibers. Chemical sympathectomy affects only the efferents. Where pains are not relieved by chemical sympathectomy but are relieved by surgical sympathectomy, it seems reasonable to conclude that the pain was produced by the afferents passing through the ganglia and not by any efferent control of peripheral sensitivity. All three of these possibilities imply changes in the *number* of impulses per unit time that impinge on lamina V cells. Thus, the autonomic nervous system may act directly or indirectly on receptor-fiber sensitivity and central cell activity levels. In either case the tendency to summation and facilitation are increased, with an attendant increased probability that the critical level necessary to trigger pain will be exceeded.

Gate control theory has important implications for pain control. Neurosurgery represents only one method of pain control, and not necessarily the best one. Noordenbos [38] has noted that neurosurgical section of so-called pain pathways in the spinal cord produces a high proportion of failures, particularly in attempts to control the neuralgias, causalgia, and phantom limb pain. He has specifically labeled the phenomenon *the leak* and has proposed that the diffuse multisynaptic connections of the anterolateral pathways (Fig. 1-2C) are such that the leak is almost inevitable. To be sure, surgical section of the anterolateral pathway cuts down the number of centrally conducting fibers, which would decrease the summation of inputs at brainstem or higher levels. Control of pain from cancer, however, while often effective, frequently fails. Nathan [37] notes that bilateral or unilateral cordotomy (astonishingly, the former is not more effective than the latter) produces good relief of pain in about 50 percent of patients and only fair relief in 25 percent. A full 25 percent of patients are not significantly helped. Even more important, however, is the frequency of undesired side effects, such as loss of urinary control, dysesthesias, and so on. Nathan notes that these are sufficiently frequent and unpleasant that they should induce the neurosurgeon to try all other possibilities before proceeding with surgical intervention. There is, therefore, a need for other approaches, and gate control theory has implications for pharmacological, sensory, and psychological control of pain.

Pharmacological Control of Pain

Pharmacological agents may act at a variety of levels in the nervous system. They may act at the receptor level, at the level of the dorsal horn, or at higher levels such as the brainstem. A given drug may possibly act at all three sites.

Analgesics that act at peripheral receptors would presumably have the effect of decreasing the amount of their output. Inflammation is associated with tissue breakdown, swelling, vasodilation, and pain. Neither the swelling nor the vasodilation seems to be sufficient to cause the pain. Active research is now in progress to detect and analyze tissue and serum breakdown products which cause pain [19]. Aspirin and phenylbutazone appear to antagonize the action of one of these compounds—bradykinin (which produces pain when injected into the body)—at the receptors [19]. It is not known how this interaction occurs but it may be that the accumulation of the substance is prevented rather than that there is a direct interaction at receptor sites. Similarly the analgesic effect of cortisone occurs presumably because it prevents the appearance or the accumulation of the compounds. Knowledge of the actual nature of the compounds will become particularly important because it will offer the possibility of preventing their synthesis by the body or of flooding the region with a competitive blocking agent which would occupy the receptor sites without producing nerve impulses. Such compounds would be true peripheral analgesics, as would be drugs which speeded the destruction of pain-producing substances.

Drugs may also affect the transmission of input at the spinal cord level. The gate control model suggests that a better understanding of the substantia gelatinosa may lead to new ways of controlling pain. The resistance of the substantia gelatinosa to nerve cell stains suggests that its chemistry differs from that of other neural tissue. Drugs affecting excitation or inhibition of substantia gelatinosa activity may be of particular importance in future attempts to control pain. There is already some evidence on the effects of pharmacological agents on gate control mechanisms. There are three ways in which anesthetics might be acting at the level of the dorsal horns: (1) by decreasing the excitatory effect of individual impulses, (2) by increasing the inhibitory effect of individual impulses, or (3) by disorganizing the spatial and temporal pattern of bombardment. These are not alternative modes of action; all three may be found to occur simultaneously. Recently, Mendell and Wall [34] have demonstrated that the purely positive dorsal root potential evoked by C fibers is completely abolished by light anesthetic doses of barbiturate. Thus, the positive effect exerted by the C fibers via the substantia gelatinosa, which normally facilitates the transmission of input from peripheral fibers to T cells, is abolished, permitting maximal presynaptic and postsynaptic inhibition and a reduction of the afferent barrage below the critical level necessary for pain. De Jong and Wagman [6] have also reported that halothane produces a marked suppression of activity in cells in the dorsal horns.

The effects of anesthetics and analgesics on transmission in the reticular formation are well documented. Nitrous oxide, at analgesic levels, strikingly diminishes the amplitude of potentials evoked in the midbrain reticular formation by supramaximal stimulation of the tooth pulp [12]. The powerful effects of barbiturates and other anesthetics at this level have been described and evaluated by French et al. [9]. At least part of the effects on pain may be the prevention of summation of sensory inputs so that the critical level necessary to trigger pain reactions is not exceeded.

Sensory Control of Pain

Interactions between sensory inputs have long been used as a method to control pain. Scratching to relieve itch, application of mustard plasters to decrease chest pain, and acupuncture fall into this category. The gate control model suggests that control of pain may be achieved by selectively enhancing the large-fiber input. Thus, Livingston [21] found that causalgia could be effectively cured by therapy such as bathing the limb in gently moving water, followed by massage, which would increase the input in the large-fiber system. Similarly, Trent [46] reports a case of pain of central nervous system origin which could be brought under control when the patient tapped his fingers on a hard surface.

The control of itch by scratching or vibration provides further evidence of these effects. Vibration, like scratching, decreases the perceived intensity of mild or moderate itch, but may turn severe itch into frank pain [29, 48]. Melzack, Wall, and Weisz [33] also examined the interaction between a single brief pressure stimulus and a single brief electric shock. It was found that the pressure pulse raised the threshold for the detection of the occurrence of the electric shock and for the level at which the shock produced a sharp pricking sensation. However, if the strength of the electric shock was further raised so that it produced severe pain, then the pressure stimulus increased the severity of the pain. It is therefore apparent that there is a complex interaction between pressure stimuli and painful electrical stimuli. The inhibitory effect of the pressure stimulus was the same if it preceded or if it followed the electrical stimulus by 50 milliseconds. This phenomenon, which is called *metacontrast*, shows that the decision to trigger pain reactions is not made by an instantaneous reading of the arriving information but must involve a prolonged analysis of the incoming signals. The extent to which spatial summation mechanisms are involved is indicated by the fact that vibration of the wrist of one hand decreases itch intensity experienced at the wrist of the other hand [29].

These interactions between sensory inputs also help make sense of the puzzling phenomena produced by stimulation of the skin with very small-diameter tactile or thermal probes. Touching the skin, particularly the lip, with a von Frey hair frequently sets off a tingling or afterglow sensation that may persist for several minutes [27]. The afterglow sometimes spreads beyond the site of stimulation, and occasionally the mirror area on the other side of the lip may begin to tingle. There is characteristically a delay in the onset of the afterglow. These effects are even more pronounced when a small-diameter warm probe stimulates the skin. The afterglow appears after a delay, wells up into a sharp stinging pain, and persists long after stimulation. Stimulation of a larger area of skin with a probe of the same temperature produces only reports of warmth sensation. These effects are not found uniformly across the skin, but only in particular regions, which may vary in location from one testing period to the next [28]. The tendency for these effects to occur is diminished if the skin is vibrated immediately before stimulation with the probes.

These effects of delay, spread, aftersensations, and unusual, unpleasant sensory qualities are reminiscent of the properties of the neuralgias, and it is interesting to speculate that the underlying mechanisms may be essentially alike. Lamina V cells receive, directly or indirectly, inputs from the A delta as well as the A beta fibers (Fig. 1-5B). These connections provide the large triple receptive field previously described. It is possible, then, that from time to time a small-diameter stimulus would activate the predominantly excitatory center of the three superimposed fields with minimal stimulation of the inhibitory peripheral region. As we have already noted in the foregoing discussion of neuralgia, the decreased inhibitory influence would tend to open the dorsal horn "gate," which would be the basis for delayed, long-lasting, hyperesthetic sensations.

One of the most exciting applications of the principle of sensory interaction is Wall and Sweet's [49] investigation of the effect of electrical stimulation of large-diameter nerve fibers originating from a painful region. The stimulation, which is just above threshold and causes a mild tingling sensation, interferes with the perception of pain. In patients with peripheral nerve lesions, the effect of 10 minutes of stimulation may last for a half-hour or more. In patients with carcinoma, the pain blocked but returned shortly after stimulation. This method, we believe, holds great promise as an effective tool for the control of pain.

Psychological Control of Pain

Finally, it is important to recognize the role of cognitive or "higher central nervous system" activities such as anxiety, attention, and suggestion in pain processes. The model suggests that psychological factors such as past experience, attention, and emotion influence pain response and perception by acting on the gate control system. The degree of central control, however, would be determined, in part at least, by the temporal-spatial properties of the input patterns. Some of the most unbearable pains, such as cardiac pain, rise so rapidly in intensity that the patient is unable to achieve any control over them. On the other hand, more slowly rising temporal patterns are susceptible to central control and may allow the patient to "think about something else" or use other stratagems to keep the pain under control.

It is clear that the surgical and pharmacological attacks on pain might well profit by redirecting thinking toward the neglected and almost forgotten contributions of motivational and cognitive processes. Pain can be treated not only by trying to cut down the sensory input by anesthetic block, surgical intervention, and the like, but also by influencing the motivational-affective and cognitive factors as well. Relaxants, tranquilizers, sedatives, suggestion, placebos, and hypnosis are known to exert a profound influence on pain [1], but the historical emphasis on sensory mechanisms and the relative neglect of the motivational and cognitive contributions to pain have made these forms of therapy suspect, seemingly fraudulent, almost a sideshow in the mainstream of pain treatment. Yet, if we can recover from historical accident, these methods deserve more attention than they have received.

References

1. Beecher, H. K. *Measurement of Subjective Responses*. New York: Oxford University Press, 1959.

2. Bishop, G. H.   The relation between nerve fiber size and sensory modality: Phylogenetic implications of the afferent innervation of cortex. *J. Nerv. Ment. Dis.* 128:39, 1959.

3. Burgess, P. R., and Perl, E. R.   Myelinated afferent fibres responding specifically to noxious stimulation of the skin. *J. Physiol.* (London) 190:541, 1967.

4. Conant, J. B.   *On Understanding Science.* New York: Mentor Books, 1951.

5. Dallenbach, K. M.   Pain: History and present status. *Am. J. Psychol.* 52:331, 1939.

6. de Jong, R. H., and Wagman, I. H.   Block of afferent impulses in the dorsal horn of monkey: A possible mechanism of anesthesia. *Exp. Neurol.* 20:352, 1968.

7. Dilly, P. N., Wall, P. D., and Webster, K. E.   Cells of origin of the spinothalamic tract in cat or rat. *Exp. Neurol.* 21:550, 1968.

8. Earle, K. M.   Tract of Lissauer and its possible relation to the pain pathway. *J. Comp. Neurol.* 96:93, 1952.

9. French, J. D., Verzeano, M., and Magoun, W. H.   Neural basis of anesthetic state. *A.M.A. Arch. Neurol. Psychiat.* 69:519, 1953.

10. Goldscheider, A.   *Ueber den Schmerz in Physiologischer und Klinischer Hinsicht.* Berlin: Hirschwald, 1894.

11. Hagbarth, K. E., and Kerr, D. I. B.   Central influences on spinal afferent conduction. *J. Neurophysiol.* 17:295, 1954.

12. Haugen, F. P., and Melzack, R.   Effects of nitrous oxide on responses evoked in the brainstem by tooth stimulation. *Anesthesiology* 18:183, 1957.

13. Head, H.   *Studies in Neurology.* London: Kegan Paul, 1920.

14. Heimer, L., and Wall, P. D.   Dorsal root distribution to the substantia gelatinosa in the rat with a note on the distribution in the cat. *Exp. Brain Res.* 6:89, 1968.

15. Hillman, P., and Wall, P. D.   Inhibitory and excitatory factors influencing the receptive fields of lamina 5 spinal cord cells. *Exp. Brain Res.*

16. Kerr, D. I. B., Haugen, F. P., and Melzack, R.   Responses evoked in the brainstem by tooth stimulation. *Am. J. Psychol.* 183:253, 1955.

17. Kerr, F. W. L., and Miller, R. H.   The ultrastructural pathology of trigeminal neuralgia. *Arch. Neurol.* (Chicago) 15:308, 1966.

18. Lewis, T.   *Pain.* New York: Macmillan, Inc., 1942.

19. Lim, R. K. S.   Neuropharmacology of pain and analgesia. In Lim, R. K. S., Armstrong, D., and Pardo, E. G., eds., *Pharmacology of Pain.* London: Pergamon Press, Inc., 1968.

20. Livingston, W. K.   *Pain Mechanisms.* New York: Macmillan, 1943.

21. Livingston, W. K.   The vicious circle in causalgia. *Ann. N.Y. Acad. Sci.* 50:247, 1948.

22. Lundberg, A.   Supraspinal control of transmission in reflex paths to motoneurons and primary afferents. *Prog. Brain Res.* 12:197, 1964.

23. MacCarty, C. S., and Drake, R. L.   Neurosurgical procedures for the control of pain. *Mayo Clin. Proc.* 31:208, 1956.

24. McDonald, W. I.   The effects of experimental demyelination on conduction in peripheral nerve: A histological and electrophysiological study. II. Electrophysiological observations. *Brain* 86:501, 1963.

25. Mark, V. H., Ervin, F. R., and Yakovlev, P. I.   Stereotactic thalamotomy. *Arch. Neurol.* (Chicago) 8:528, 1963.

26. Melzack, R., and Casey, K. L.   Sensory, motivational, and central control determinants of pain: A new conceptual model. In Kenshalo, D., ed., *The Skin Senses.* Springfield, Ill.: Charles C Thomas, Publisher, 1968.

27. Melzack, R., and Eisenberg, H.   Skin sensory afterglows. *Science* 159:445, 1968.

28. Melzack, R., Rose, G., and McGinty, D.   Skin sensitivity to thermal stimuli. *Exp. Neurol.* 6:300, 1962.
29. Melzack, R., and Schecter, B.   Itch and vibration. *Science* 147:1047, 1965.
30. Melzack, R., Stotler, W. A., and Livingston, W. K.   Effects of discrete brainstem lesions in cats on perception of noxious stimulation. *J. Neurophysiol.* 21:353, 1958.
31. Melzack, R., and Wall, P. D.   On the nature of cutaneous sensory mechanisms. *Brain* 85:331, 1962.
32. Melzack, R., and Wall, P. D.   Pain mechanisms: A new theory. *Science* 150: 971, 1965.
33. Melzack, R., Wall, P. D., and Weisz, A. Z.   Masking and metacontrast phenomena in the skin sensory system. *Exp. Neurol.* 8:35, 1963.
34. Mendell, L. M., and Wall, P. D.   Presynaptic hyperpolarization: A role for fine afferent fibers. *J. Physiol.* (London) 172:274, 1964.
35. Mendell, L. M., and Wall, P. D.   Response of single dorsal cord cells to peripheral cutaneous unmyelinated fibers. *Nature* (London) 206:97, 1965.
36. Nafe, J. P.   The pressure, pain, and temperature senses. In Murchison, C., ed., *Handbook of General Experimental Psychology*. Worcester: Clark University Press, 1934.
37. Nathan, P. W.   Results of anterolateral cordotomy for pain in cancer. *J. Neurol. Neurosurg. Psychiatry* 26:353, 1963.
38. Noordenbos, W.   *Pain*. Amsterdam: Elsevier, 1959.
39. Scheibel, M. E., and Scheibel, A. B.   Terminal axon patterns in cat spinal cord. II. Dorsal horn. *Brain Res.* 9:32, 1968.
40. Schmidt, R. F., Senges, J., and Zimmermann, M.   Presynaptic depolarization of cutaneous mechanoreceptor afferents after mechanical skin stimulation. *Exp. Brain Res.* 3:234, 1967.
41. Semmes, J., and Mishkin, M.   Somatosensory loss in monkeys after ipsilateral cortical ablation. *J. Neurophysiol.* 28:473, 1965.
42. Sherrington, C. S.   Cutaneous sensations. In Schafer, E. A., ed., *Textbook of Physiology*. Edinburgh: Pentland, 1900.
43. Sinclair, D. C.   Cutaneous sensation and the doctrine of specific nerve energy. *Brain* 78:584, 1955.
44. Sweet, W.   Pain. In Field, J., Magoun, H. W., and Hall, V. E., eds., *Handbook of Physiology*. Sect. 1, Vol. 1, Chap. 19, pp. 459–506. Washington, D.C.: American Physiological Society, 1959.
45. Szentagothai, J.   Neuronal and synaptic arrangement in the substantia gelatinosa rolandi. *J. Comp. Neurol.* 122:219, 1964.
46. Trent, S. E.   Peripheral sensory inhibition of pain with a parietal lobe lesion. *J. Nerv. Ment. Dis.* 123:356, 1956.
47. Wall, P. D.   The laminar organization of dorsal horn and effects of descending impulses. *J. Physiol.* (London) 188:403, 1967.
48. Wall, P. D., and Cronly-Dillon, J. R.   Pain, itch and vibration. *Arch. Neurol.* (Chicago) 2:365, 1960.
49. Wall, P. D., and Sweet, W. H.   Temporary abolition of pain in man. *Science* 155:108, 1967.
50. Weddell, G.   Somesthesis and the chemical senses. *Annu. Rev. Psychol.* 6:119, 1955.
51. Zotterman, Y.   Touch, pain and tickling: An electrophysiological investigation on cutaneous sensory nerves. *J. Physiol.* (London) 95:1, 1939.

2

Pathophysiology of Pain

Ann Whidden and Sister Mary Rebecca Fidler

If we believe that all pathology begins in the cell [83], we can postulate that when pain is first experienced it signals a change in the immediate environment of the cell and may or may not be antecedent to subsequent pathology. All illnesses appear to be expressions of cellular alterations of molecular structure and function. Pain experienced in this basic unit, the single cell, even though neither grossly visible nor audible, is in reality a situation in which "cells cry, too." Indeed, single cells microscopically observed in tissue culture when subjected to harmful chemical or mechanical changes actually weep portions of their cytoplasm [26]. Although this is not analogous to pain, it does represent a change in the environment that results in adaptive changes directed toward cell survival and ultimately the survival of the total organism. This allows us to correctly assume, then, that when cells experience pain so does the total person.

The *Puzzle of Pain* by Melzack [61] presents a complex mechanism integrating physiological, anatomical, and psychological aspects as a basis for understanding pain. That Melzack and Wall should come to this type of integration is not surprising if one approaches the problem from the cellular aspect. However, it must be admitted that sensory discrimination is in some way based on cellular communication and integration or we risk negating the very object of our study—man himself as he experiences pain. It is true that anatomical and physiological explanations of pain pathways and sensory specificities as historically described are not sufficient to explain the reality of pain. This inadequacy perhaps represents man's ignorance of cellular communication as viewed in the various pathways or circuitry of the nervous system—an ignorance that results from man's insistence on looking for answers about an isolated system or even an isolated part of a system in such a complex organism as man. It seems useful, then, to review the simplest unit of structure and function, the single cell, to study how it communicates, integrates, and responds to changes in the total organism.

The essential function of the nervous system is "communication, which depends on special signalling properties of the nerve cells and their long processes" [10]. These properties are, of course, irritability and conductivity. In reception of information from the environment, various forms of the message are converted to an electrical impulse by specialized cellular structures, the receptors. These impulses are transmitted from the receptor to specific central nuclei where they synapse and evoke the same message in other cells that ultimately results in appropriate responses. It is by this communication and integration that man is able to react to environmental changes of the world in which he lives, and thus to survive. The nervous system also provides the structural and chemical basis of conscious experience and so furnishes the mechanism for behavior—regulation of behavior and sustained unity of personality [10]. Iggo [42] more succinctly stated neural function as "several distinct steps in the chain of events that intervene between the stimulus and the percepts. These events are receptor mechanisms, conduction/transmission mechanisms and interactive perceptual mechanisms."

Cellular communication, then, when integrated, must be the basis for understanding the behavior of man. The neuron must through its structural and functional aspects indicate the way in which messages are created, transmitted, and received. Therefore, the neuron forms the knowledge base for understanding changes that occur in cellular communication, be it pain or pleasure.

If health professionals can understand how cells function, why communication among cells is necessary for man to adapt, why cells cry, then it can be believed that these practitioners will begin to understand human responses to pain. Indeed, interventions at the cellular level should be a reality and may well make a difference in man's basic needs at any level and, if achieved, can minimize structural and functional changes when injury has occurred or is about to occur.

What kind of a background then, must one have in order to understand pain? It must, of course, be a holistic understanding. But, to do this, it seems imperative that the nurse and others understand the anatomical and physiological bases of pain as a foundation upon which to place the psychological perception, and the behavioral as well as the cultural and environmental influences of the man who is experiencing the pain. Thus, the intent of this chapter is to help the nurse and others in the health field to understand cellular communication, cellular perception, and cellular response as a basis for understanding pain.

The Structural Unit of Pain

The human cell exists in an environment of intercellular fluid and ground substance which is, homeostatically, a closely guarded physiological and biochemical situation. Oxygen and carbon dioxide gases are regulated by diffusion based on gradients of partial pressure. The pH can vary in an extremely narrow range of approximately one unit, and if this range is exceeded, the enzymatic processes will stop and subsequently cellular function will cease. Ions such as sodium, calcium, and potassium are regulated by active and passive transport mechanisms, some of which depend on adequate amounts of cellular energy—adenosine triphosphate (ATP)—which requires an adequate and consistent oxygen supply and normal pH. Thus the integrity of the cell depends on many things, but the cell membrane is of utmost importance if the cell is to survive. This membrane, a lipid protein, pore-studded structure surrounding the cell, selectively permits passage into and out of the cells of those things that it needs to obtain or get rid of. Cells, then, are in a continual dynamic state trying to maintain intracellular homeostasis, which depends on maintaining the constancy of the extracellular environment both systemically and locally. Changes in these environments must be communicated between cells of the nervous system and, subsequently, to all systems of the organism to ensure adequate adaptation.

The capacity to communicate is a feature of all living cells. Stent [90] so aptly indicated that there really are three types of communication—or information—that can be identified among cells. First is a genetic, the second is a metabolic, and the third is a nervous type of communication. Genetic information, of course, is that which is handed down from parent to offspring and is incorporated in the DNA molecules of the chromosomes. Cellular communication of the metabolic type is found in chemical molecules, which are often termed hormones, and which receive instructions on how and when to differentiate, or when to produce a certain enzyme, or when to become involved in a particular type of metabolism. This metabolic communication, slow and sustained, is extremely important in homeostatic mechanisms of the human body. The neural type of communication is fast, short-lived, and accomplished by electrical impulse transmission in the cells that are called neurons. Survival is the aim of neural communication.

Historically, anatomists have divided the nervous system into a peripheral portion and a central portion. However, it seems more appropriate to think of it as being three integrated parts: an input (afferent) part that informs about the internal and external environment, a second part (central or internuncial) connecting the input to a third part, which is the output (effector portion) of the nervous system. Without a doubt, the most complicated part is the internuncial or the central circuitry of the nervous system. This central part demands abstraction as a prerequisite to conceptual formation and then, finally, synthesis that results in some form of observable behavior [10, 90].

The neuron allows information to be communicated and integrated in a rapid manner aimed at survival. The concept of the neuron as a distinct cell was confirmed by Deiters (1834–1863) and brought to fame by Cajal (1852–1934). It was given the name neuron by Waldeyer (1836–1921) in 1891. This neuron doctrine is undergoing considerable renovation at the present time [87].

All cells communicate, but the specialized cell of communication and integration is the neuron. Examination of this particular cell as to how it accomplishes this function seems in order.

The nerve cell has a cell body (soma) consisting of a nucleus (karyon) and its surrounding cytoplasm (the perikaryon). Most neurons extend their cytoplasm into many short processes called dendrites and one long process called the axis cylinder or axon. The axon may be very long indeed and often gives off collaterals along its path and finally terminally branches out into many fine ramifications. This basic structure varies from neuron to neuron with respect to size, shape, and length of its processes (Fig. 2-1).

Nerve cells never actually touch one another, but are brought together in functional proximity in an area called the synapse, a term first used by Sherrington in 1926 [29].

Neurophysiologists classically designate the synapse as the area where control of information occurs. When a message (action potential) arrives at a synapse, several possibilities as to its fate exist. The impulse may terminate or be inhibited from passing to the next neuron. It may pass on to the next neuron in a facilitated manner. It may be facilitated by summation or be influenced by convergence or divergence. Lastly, it may be blocked or facili-

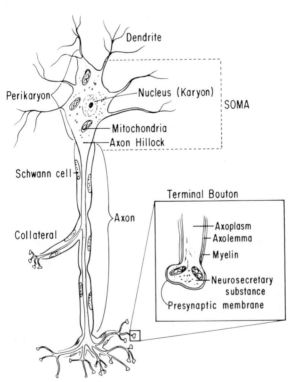

Figure 2-1 The neuron.

tated by therapeutic drugs or chemicals. Nevertheless, it is the sum of all influences impinging upon the synapse that finally determines if transmission of the message will occur. Thus, even though the neuron is the *basic* unit of structure for the nervous system, the *functional* unit of the system is a chain of neurons interrelated at the synapse.

The nerve cell presents itself anatomically as a large protein factory. The perikaryon is crowded around a centrally placed nucleus with organelles arranged concentrically. These organelles include neurofibrils, Nissl substance, Golgi apparatus, mitochondria, a centrosome, and various inclusions. Neurofibrils are slender interlacing structures extending through the cytoplasm from dendrite to dendrite to axon. They are found in all neuronal processes in which they usually run parallel to their long axis. The electron microscope reveals them as composed of neurofilaments or minute tubules with a dense wall and a clear center. Neurotubules are also found in arcs around the nucleus and extending into the various processes. Their function is not known, but is thought to be associated with fast transport (axoplasmic flow) from cell body to the axonal nerve terminal. Microtubules are also thought to confer mechanical strength and rigidity to the long, slender neuronal processes [72].

The cytoplasm of the perikaryon is rich in granular and agranular endoplasmic reticulum; the latter often forms large aggregations of RNA called Nissl substance or chromatin bodies. Functionally this allows for efficient synthesis of large amounts of protein and lipids needed for repair and maintenance of structural integrity as well as rapid transmission of information. Many different classes of proteins and other compounds are synthesized by neurons. Some are necessary for the secretory functions of the neuron and include transmitters, hormones, surface membrane receptors, and enzymes. These are transported into the neuronal processes and thus it can be seen that the cell body is necessary for the life of the neuron and the maintenance of its processes.

Mitochondria (the energy-producing organelles) are variables in size, shape, and number. They are found in the perikaryon, in the cell processes, and, as would be expected, in great abundance at synaptic terminals.

Axoplasmic flow of neurons is a continual process. In tissue culture one can observe cytoplasmic movements of particulate matter and vesicles along axons in both directions [103]. The transport from cell body to the terminals, however, is a net transport, i.e., more transport occurs toward the axon than toward the cell body.

Two types of axoplasmic transport have been demonstrated—one slow and one fast. The slow type is a bulk flow of axoplasm including mitochondria, lysosomes, and vesicles at a rate of 1 to 3 mm per day. The rapid transport carries selected substances at a rate of 100 mm per day and when transporting neurosecretory substance an approximate rate of 2,800 mm per day can be achieved. Neurotubules have been associated with the latter, fast transport system [48].

32

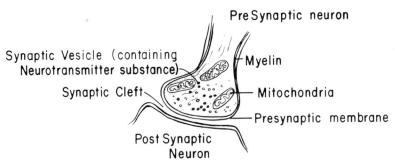

Figure 2-2   The synapse.

The cellular apparatus of microtubules and microfilaments whose origin is from the centriole extends throughout the length of all dendrites and axons. The cytoplasm of dendrites is anatomically very similar to that found in the cell body (soma). Axons are also similar except that they normally do not contain ribosomes.

The morphology of the synapse (Fig. 2-2) is very important in controlling communication. It is at the synapse that a delay in the impulse is found, where either excitation, inhibition, or facilitation occurs and where theories of summation, convergence, and divergence are operable.

It must be recalled that neural impulse conduction is unidirectional at the synapse due to the anatomical features of the presynaptic terminal bouton. Although impulses can travel toward the cell body (antidromic) as well as toward the axonal terminal (orthodromic), it is only the axonal terminal that contains the energy and synaptic vessels to transmit the message to the next neuron.

Synapses are most commonly axodendritic or axosomatic and less commonly, but occasionally, axoaxonic, dendrosomatic, dendroaxonic, dendrodendritic, and somatodendritic. Functionally, synapses are inhibitory type I or excitatory type II [31], depending on the type of neurosecretory substance released from their respective presynaptic membranes [96]. Therefore, the type of messenger RNA produced will determine the type of transmitter substance produced and thus the type of functional neuron (i.e., inhibitory or facilitatory) observed. Neurochemical transmitters, then, are produced in the area of the soma, transported via axoplasmic flow to the presynaptic area of the axon where they are released by the arrival of an electric impulse into the synaptic cleft. The neurotransmitter released then either depolarizes (excites) or hyperpolarizes (inhibits) the postsynaptic membrane.

Cell fractionation and autoradiographic techniques have allowed the study and identification of neurochemical transmitter substances (Table 2-1). The monoamines (biogenic amines—catecholamine, dopamine, and serotonin) are thought to act in a facilitatory manner at the synapse [106]. The precursor

Table 2-1   Neurochemical transmitter substances

Neurotransmitter	Local area of synthesis
Acetylcholine	Motor neurons
	Postganglionic parasympathetic neurons
	Striated interneurons
Norepinephrine	Lateral portions of reticular formations of
	brainstem, especially the locus ceruleus
	Brainstem
	Spinal cord
Dopamine	Hypothalamus
	Substantia nigra
	Midbrain
	Limbic-midbrain system
Glycine	Spinal cord interneurons
Epinephrine	Adrenal medulla
	Sympathetic postganglionic
Serotonin	Brainstem
	Spinal cord
GABA	Deiters' nuclei
	Globus pallidus
	Hypocampus
	Retinal neurons

Source: modified from Gardner and Williams [29].

of catecholamine synthesis is the amino acid tyrosine. The endolamine, serotonin, an excitatory transmitter substance, is implicated in contraction of smooth muscle, and in regulation of sleep and body temperature [106]. Certain amino acids, i.e., gamma-aminobutyric acid (GABA) and glycine, have been shown to be present at inhibitory type II synapses [79]. Other amino acids such as L-glutamic acid and L-aspartic acid are thought to be excitatory. These transmitters, especially the monoamines, have significance in behavioral states of consciousness and mental disorders [84]. The dopamines are involved in the extrapyramidal motor systems of the basal nuclei. Norepinephrine projection to the hypothalamus and dopamine neurons in the hypothalamus are important in neuroendocrinology. Norepinephrine-synthesizing cells in the midbrain are probably important in the reticular activating system (RAS). Depletions of the biogenic amine can precipitate profound depression and serious behavioral changes, as can the pharmaceutical blocking of their actions [30, 52, 58]. This chemical type of transmission is the ordinary situation. At the synapse, electrical transmission, however, does occur (especially in cardiac and occasionally smooth muscle). Electrical synapses are generally more rapid than chemical synapses.

The identified neurotransmitters probably represent only a fraction of the actual existing ones. It is hypothesized that many more are unknown than are known. Many of the suspected transmitters may be precursors of, or breakdown products of, the real transmitters yet unidentified. Dale's theory [20] that each neuron synthesizes only one transmitter substance has been accepted for peripheral neurons, but central neurons have on occasion demonstrated two or more types of synaptic vesicles in the same axonal terminal, thus adding to the complexity. The importance of these biochemical substances in pain has been established. Sicuteri [89] studied the effect of denervation on biochemical components. He demonstrated a loss of serotonin, noradrenaline, and acetylcholine with denervation. These amines are important in the modulation and inhibition of pain, particularly at central levels. Drugs have been used to effect the turnover and uptake of these monamines at synaptic levels which Sicuteri believes can be operative any place in the nervous system. Taub [93] also gives support to the importance of biogenic animes in pain. He suggested that a state of depression and pain may be simultaneous results of a biochemical defect.

Although the basic structure of the neuron and its synapses are usually quite consistent, functionally they present great variance. Individual neurons seem to differ from one another more than cells of other tissues do. The orderly development of the neural circuits depends on the differentiation of cells with specific chemical properties at particular locations and on the formation of spatially ordered connections between selected cells [47]. For example, an optic neuron would never be functional connecting or transmitting to the cochlear cells, nor is the converse true. Therefore, in order for the neuron to become operative, the functional aspects of the neuron must be understood.

The Functional Unit of Pain

With recent knowledge of synaptic types and interneuronal activity, the neuron doctrine seems no longer valid [87]. To see the neuron as a basic morpholgical unit is somewhat suspect in the light of present data. For Cajal and Sherrington studying peripheral nerves it seemed adequate, but inconsistencies in this doctrine became evident as the central neuronal circuitry began to be outlined. Thus the functional unit is not equivalent to the structural unit, since similar structures may, in fact, support different functions. The converse is also true.

The functional unit, then, is interneuronal and lies within the context of impulse transmission and control in specifically designated neuronal chains. In discussing the functional unit of pain, concepts to be reviewed are: how the message of pain is created (i.e., reception or nociception), then how the message is transmitted or communicated, and, finally, how the transmission is controlled or modified.

How is the message created in man? How does man receive sensory information? This has long been a disputed area among neurophysiologists. Johann Müller [68] proposed that a specific sense was communicated from specific receptors in the skin to a specific central area in the brain; this was called the theory of specific nerve energies. To Müller, the quality of the experience was somehow determined by the receptor or the sensory nerve.

Max Von Frey (1894) expanded Müller's theory to include theories of skin spots and cutaneous receptors. Information regarding local areas of these specific skin spots and anatomical evidence of specialized structures (receptors) were found and described.

The study of pain arises from clinical evidence that the functioning of the nervous system has been disturbed. At a point, or at various points, the integrative and communicative abilities fail.

Cultural, sociological, anthropological, and psychological aspects of the pain experience are being explored as vigorously as the anatomical and physiological. However, as Abraham [1] states, "Variability of pain thresholds and the ability to suppress the sensation of pain, must, like the mechanisms of pain itself, be sought within the framework of the physiology of the nervous system."

Noxious stimuli, nociceptors, and nociception are terms introduced by Sherrington [88]. Noxious stimuli, he observed, "threaten or actually do damage to the tissue to which they are applied" [88]. Nerves which respond to noxious stimuli are nociceptive nerves, but there is generally a "lack of specificity of nerve endings or receptors for pain."

Early studies of reception or receptors by Adrian [2, 3] and Adrian and Zotterman [4, 5] revealed that nociception was elusive in terms of both receptor organ and response to noxious stimulators. Adrian did confirm, however, that pain was not produced by the increase or frequency of stimulation, as was commonly held. Zotterman [110], expanding Adrian's work, began to relate fiber type rather than receptor specificity as the basis for nociception. More recently, Iggo [42] has listed nociceptors as a separate class of receptors (high-intensity receptors) distinguished from mechanical and thermal receptors (low-intensity receptors). Noordenbos [74], however, takes an opposing view of nociception and sees pain as quantitative rather than qualitative; it is believed by him to be experienced via any available pathway when stimuli, whatever their nature, exceed certain limits.

Whether pain is a modality similar to touch or temperature remains an unanswered question despite the abundance of research conducted in both clinical and laboratory settings. Still, it is commonly held that cellular or tissue injury, from whatever cause, activates specific pain receptors either by direct damage or by release of chemical mediators of pain. However, it is equally clear that other receptors are often involved.

Weddell et al [102] studied peripheral nerve endings extensively. Throughout the skin and also in deeper structures, free nerve endings are found in abundance. Through their studies it was found that these free nerve endings arose chiefly from nonmyelinated or thinly myelinated axons. These free nerve endings (without conclusive evidence) are often described as the nociceptors. This is a bit disconcerting if one recalls that the human cornea contains only free nerve endings, yet temperature, pain, and touch are still distinguishable [53]. The manner in which the nerve endings are stimulated has also been studied. Keele [49] investigated the action of chemicals on nerve endings. Further, Lim [54] in his study of sterile inflammation in the rat concluded that pain was associated with electrophilic attraction, i.e., the receptor site was electron efficient and thus negatively charged, and analgesics were electron deficient or positively charged. His studies led him to postulate chemoreception rather than nociception as a basis for the creation of the pain message. A wide variety of chemical substances are known to elicit pain, including acids, alkalis, increased concentration of sodium and potassium ions, histamine, serotonin, acetylcholine, polypeptides (bradykinins), and hydrogen ions. According to Lim [54, 55] the pain experience is abrogated by analgesics which block the generation of impulses at the chemoreceptor. Peripherally this is accomplished by aspirin or nonnarcotic analgesics. Morphine and narcotic analgesics probably block synaptic transmission in the central pain pathways and amphetamines and other nonnarcotic anorectic analgesics inhibit perception centrally. Lindahl [56] supports a hypothesis of hydrogen ion as the variable in pain production. Werle [104] appears to support this hypothesis, but considers potassium ions as equally important when cell breakdown is involved, since intracellular substances are usually compartmentally separated from the sensory nerve endings, only coming into play when cell injury has occurred. Werle [104], Sicuteri [89], and Keele and Armstrong [50], among others, also recognize that kinins may be very important in initiating the pain impulse. Kinins are in the plasma and are released into extracellular spaces as a result of inflammatory exudation. Bradykinin has been implicated in the initiation of the pain associated with myocardial infarction [22] and migraine headaches [28]. Besson et al [11] utilizing intra-arterial bradykinin administration demonstrated inhibitory effects of midbrain descending paths on transmission of impulses coming into lamina V of the spinal cord, which resulted in pain. Despite all this, pain receptors still remain a conundrum.

In the face of much investigation and few answers, researchers began to look beyond the receptor to the peripheral-nerve fiber size and conduction speed for a pattern or code for pain conduction. It was discovered that, due to differences in structure, different classes of neurons conduct at different rates. In 1930 Erlanger and Gasser [23] classified the neuronal fibers according to size, action potentials, and conduction rates into 3 classes: classes A, B, and C. These investigators believed that the speed of impulse transmission was dependent on fiber diameter and the myelin arrangement. Their theory was never seriously challenged until Bishop [12] presented the possibility that the size of the fiber may be more important for effective carrying of "essential metabolites from cell-body to synaptic-transmitting terminal" than for its relation to conduction rate. Erlanger and Gasser's [23] letter classification still holds prominence in the literature. Class A fibers are large, myelinated, fast-conducting fibers that are further divided into sub-class A types alpha, beta, gamma, and delta. Class B fibers are smaller, myelinated, slower-conducting fibers. Class C fibers are nonmyelinated, small, and slowest-conducting. The pain literature and research is often confusing as to fiber class in that class A sensory fibers have often been described by a numerical subclassification, while muscular motor fibers retained the letter classification of Erlanger and Gasser. See Table 2-2 for the relationship between and clarification of these two subclassifications. In any case, it is the sensory class A alpha and delta plus the class C dorsal root fibers that figure prominently in the study of pain.

The class A alpha fibers are thought to be important in modification and inhibition of pain transmission in substantia gelatinosa. Delta fibers of class A are usually associated with clear localized "first" pain of the specific pain pathway. Class C fibers are usually associated with vague, dull, generalized pain related to the nonspecific second pain pathway [15, 23, 35, 111]. Many investigators have studied the class A and class C fibers in relation to pain from a peripheral [12, 18, 51, 111] as well as from a central consideration.

After the impulse is created, it is conducted along the afferent process to the cell body located in the peripheral ganglion (i.e., the dorsal root ganglia or cranial nerve ganglia) and passes to the axon. These afferent axons are divided into a medial and a lateral division before entering the spinal cord [81]. See Figure 2-3.

The fibers forming the medial division enter the posterior funiculus and divide into long ascending and shorter descending branches, while fibers of the lateral division are small and unmyelinated and enter the dorsolateral fasciculus of Lissauer and ascend one or two segments, giving off collaterals to the posterior gray column, or descend a shorter distance connecting in a similar manner.

The impulse, as can be seen, is transmitted from the periphery to the spinal cord via the dorsal root cells. It is in the spinal cord or medulla that the impulse created synapses with the second or next order neuron located in the dorsal horn gray or various other nuclei. The arrangement of the neurons in the spinal cord gray were described and ordered by the early investigators primarily according to the anatomical location of cell bodies. A laminar concept as proposed by Rexed [82], studying cats, identified 10 layers or laminae of the spinal cord gray. This greatly modified earlier nuclei descriptions, for Rexed's laminae were based on the interconnections or synaptic (functional) designations of the dorsal horn cells. Thus, this laminar pattern has helped establish a more precise description and understanding of functional rather than structural components of the spinal cord.

Figure 2-3 is a schematic drawing visualizing the laminae and the specifically identified older-described nuclei of the spinal cord gray matter. Figure 2-4 is an attempt to adapt and correlate the various anatomical positions of the laminae and the nuclei and, also, to indicate various terms used in the pain literature to designate each part since the two modes of description are not mutually exclusive.

The tract of Lissauer and the substantia gelatinosa may be significant in the transmission of pain [81] (Fig. 2-5). Swanson et al [91] found a complete lack of the tract of Lissauer in a child who had exhibited insensitivity

Table 2-2 Nerve fiber types

Fiber class	Myelin morphology	Functional type	Subgroup letter	Subgroup number	Fiber size (μ)	Conduction speed M/sec	Receptor class
Class A	Myelinated	Somatic afferents	Alpha α	Ia	12–20	70–120 fast	Muscle spindle
			Alpha α	Ib	12–20	70–120 fast	Golgi tendon
			Beta β	II	5–15	20–90 slower	Mechanoreceptors
			Gamma γ	II	2–10	10–45 slow	Flower-spray ending
			Delta δ	III	2–5	12–30 slow	Pain & temp.
Class B	Myelinated	Visceral efferents			<3	5–15	Visceral preganglionic sympathetic
Class C	Unmyelinated	Visceral and somatic afferents	Dorsal root c	IV	0.2–1.5	0.3–1.6 slowest	Pain
			Postganglionic sympathetic		0.3–1.3	0.7–2.3	Visceral postganglionic efferents

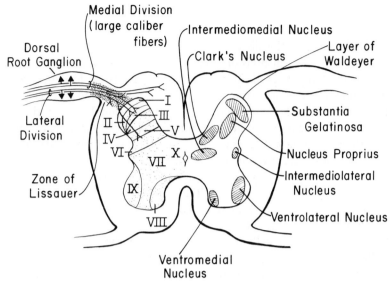

Figure 2-3 A schematic cross section of cervical spinal cord and its roots: The structural designations of Rexed's laminae are on the left portion of the spinal gray. The nuclei are on the right. The left dorsal root shows anatomical location of the medial and lateral divisions of afferent axons. (Adapted from various texts.)

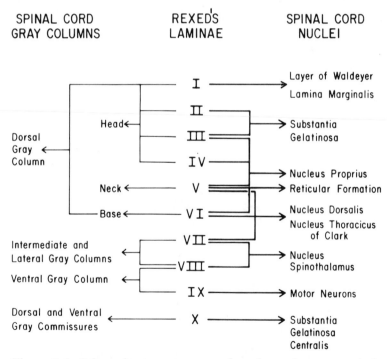

Figure 2-4 Schematic attempt to correlate the various anatomical positions of Rexed's laminae and older descriptive nuclei and also to indicate various terms used in the pain literature to describe each. Note the two groups of laminae versus nuclei are not mutually exclusive.

to pain. In this clinical case the fibers of the dorsal root medial division were intact, but those of the lateral division were not found. Conversely, Pearson [78] found that large myelinated fibers in the dorsal roots could degenerate without corresponding degeneration of the small unmyelinated fibers. Further, Cassinari and Pagni [16] showed a direct association between the A delta fibers of the lateral division and the neospinothalamic tract that sends collaterals to the substantia gelatinosa. This is in contrast to the fibers that go directly to the substantia gelatinosa.

There are two major types of neurons in the gray matter of the spinal cord: Golgi type I and Golgi type II. The Golgi type II are small and their axons do not leave the gray matter. They may, however, pass to another gray column on the same side (ipsilateral) or cross to the opposite side (contralateral). Golgi type I cells occur in all parts of the gray matter and are large cells forming the long tracts of the spinal cord. Their axons enter the white matter to ascend or descend for varying distances. They may be intrasegmental (reenter the gray matter of the same segment), intersegmental (reenter the gray matter of another segment), or suprasegmental (ascend to brain). Any of the above can be ipsilateral or contralateral [46].

Lamina I, at the marginal edge of the dorsal horn, curves in a dorsal and lateral direction. Entry by way of the tract of Lissauer (Fig. 2-5) of the many fibers from the lateral division of the dorsal root gives this lamina a spongy appearance. Little is known about the function of the cells in this layer. However, the large cells in lamina I have been associated with high threshold reception and pain [17]. Taub [93], among others, has identified

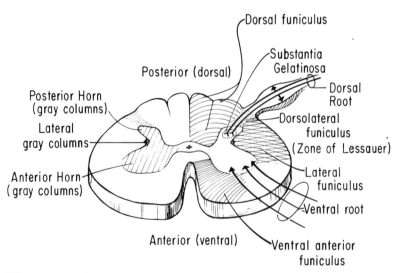

Figure 2-5 Schematic cross section of cervical spinal cord showing anatomical locations of the gray columns and the funiculi. (Adapted from various texts.)

decreased sensitivity of lamina I cells to drugs in comparison to cells of the other layers.

The substantia gelatinosa of Rolandi is contained in lamina II [82] and also in lamina III [64]. Activity in cells of the substantia gelatinosa is an integral part of the gate control theory of pain [63]. Pearson's [78] study of the substantia gelatinosa is a basic reference for pain research. Microscopic examination reveals these laminae to contain a large number of Golgi type II cells, a lesser number of scattered larger cells called pericornual, and a large number of finely myelinated and unmyelinated axons. Some of the axons in this layer make synaptic connections with the pericornual cells and others with cells of the nucleus proprii whose dendrites extend into the substantia gelatinosa. These short interneuronal Golgi type II activities create a delay in the impulse transmission that is apparently important in pain. The larger fibers are not involved in these short-fiber relays, but may go through the substantia gelatinosa or around it to synapse with the pericornual cells or with the cells of the nucleus proprii [45, 78], or with both. Heavner [40] states, "anatomically lamina II and III cells relate closely the arriving cutaneous afferent fibers with dendrites of deeper lying cells. The intimate association of cells in lamina II and III with afferent terminals and dendrites from deeper layers hints at extensive presynaptic control over afferent impulses." The substantia gelatinosa is also seen as a storehouse for pain memory.

Mehta states, without citing sources, "Some neurophysiologists maintain that painful experiences are recorded in much the same way that a photographic film registers visual events, but the images gradually fade with the passage of time; provided the original injury is not reactivated. These memory traces, which are stored in the substantia gelatinosa, are revived by a peripheral irritant focus, sometimes far removed from the damaged part, and once pain is re-established it is extraordinarily difficult to treat" [60]. Further support is given to this idea by Noordenbos who indicates, in his discussion of referred pain, that prior trauma may have influence on the mechanism of referred pain because of "habit reference" [73]. Evans, in 1974, supported this concept and referred to false localization of pain being related to habit reference. The example given is that of pain from visceral disease being referred not to an expected site, but to a scar from previous surgery. He goes on to cite Reynolds et al, who conducted a study of pilots flying at high altitudes. These subjects developed pain in different parts of the head. Expansion of air entrapped in the maxillary sinuses produced facial pain in some pilots. Other pilots, particularly those who had had dental work, experienced pain in the teeth. The conclusion was that "the painful stimulus had left some permanent trace within the central nervous system that localized subsequent pains arising from that region to the site of the previous pain" [24].

Lamina IV contains, among other neurons, the nucleus proprii, and recent studies [80, 98] show that these cells respond to stimulation of the skin via large myelinated afferents. Previously, Rexed [82] described the cells of laminae II to IV as being related primarily to exteroceptive functions and Wilson [108] indicated a modification of activities of lamina IV cells by descending pathways. "Lamina IV contains mysterious large neurons with branching dendrites which ramify in the substantia gelatinosa" and have the relationships previously indicated above [46].

The Pain Pathways (Second-Order Neurons)

After the impulse is created, it is communicated to the spinal cord gray laminar cells. These second-order afferent neurons project to higher levels of the central nervous system and are organized in many ways. However, only three systems need to be considered in this chapter. (See Figure 2-6.)

The first of these is the spinothalamic system [25, 98]. In 1957 Keele [49] identified the anterolateral quadrant of the spinal cord white matter as important in the pain pathway. Cassinari and Pagni [16] described this sys-

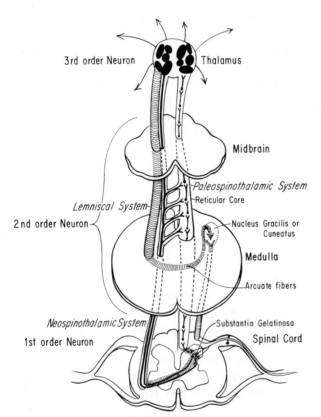

Figure 2-6 Schematic drawing of the three major pain pathways. (Adapted from various texts.)

tem as arising from Rexed's laminae IV to VI, crossing to the opposite side to ascend in the ventral and lateral funiculi. Touch, pain, and temperature will activate this system. Pain and temperature information become the lateral spinothalamic tract, while touch impulses comprise the anterior spinothalamic tract. Sensory discrimination seems to be one function of this system. It enables the individual to relate the stimulus to the peripheral area being stimulated. Although lamina V is usually considered the primary source of the fibers of the spinothalamic system, more recent evidence places their origin in laminae I, IV, V, VI, VII, and VIII, and even the pericornual cells have been suggested. Pomeranz [80] identified small afferent visceral fibers converging on lamina V cells which further supports the role of lamina V cells in the pain pathway. This relationship suggested to Wilson [108] that the small-fiber afferent input may be the basis for referred pain. Studies of this system have revealed that only part of the pain information is carried in this described spinothalamic system. Subsequently, two subpathways (neospinothalamic and paleospinothalamic systems) have been described (Fig. 2-6). The neospinothalamic system terminates in the posterior and ventrobasal nuclei of the thalamus. This tract is best developed in phylogenetically more recent (neo) animals such as the ape and man. The paleospinothalamic system extends into the reticular formation of the medulla and midbrain, also to the dorsolateral nuclei of central gray of midbrain, and terminates in the intralaminar nuclei of the thalamus. This system, however, is found in phylogenetically primitive (paleo) animals. Other terminology is used to identify these two systems. (See Table 2-3.)

The neospinothalamic system [59] is usually associated with long fibers, few synapses, and rapid transmission of the message (Fig. 2-6). Thus, Class

Table 2-3 Terminologies related to the neo- and paleospinothalamic systems

Investigator	Neospinothalamic system	Paleospinothalamic system
*Rosenbach (1884) *Goldscheider (1926) *Thunburg (1902)	First pain	Second pain
Head (1905)	Epicritic sensation	Protopathic sensation
Mehler (1957)	Neospinothalamic	Paleospinothalamic
Bowsher (1957)	Spinothalamocortical system	Medial spinoreticulothalamic system
Herrick and Bishop (1958)	Specific pain pathway	Nonspecific pain pathway
Noordenbos (1959)	Spinothalamocortical (fast system)	Multisynaptic afferent system MAS (slow system)
Hassler (1960)		Trunkothalamische
Cassineri and Pagni (1969)	Paucisynaptic system	Polysynaptic system

* As quoted by Hassler, R. Afferent Systems. In R. Jansen, W. Keidel, A. Herz, C. Steichele, eds., *Pain: Basic Principles—Pharmacology—Therapy*. Baltimore: The Williams & Wilkins Company, 1972.

A alpha fibers are involved. Cassineri and Pagni [16] describe it as clear localized pain with only three neurons involved in the transmission. However, this system sends numerous collaterals to the older paleospinothalamic system which ascends medially to it. In the cat the paleospinothalamic system has its origin from laminae VII and VIII [7, 100]. This other system is associated with short fibers, frequent synapses, and slow transmission. It is also associated with primitive disagreeable deep diffuse sensation. Class A delta and C fibers are associated with this tract. It includes the reticular core, the limbic midbrain, the thalamus, and the limbic forebrain, which gives support for a structural relationship between this pathway and the psychological aspects or quality of pain. The integration of this older system is accomplished by convergent input and synaptic delay of both slow-myelinated and unmyelinated afferent fibers. It has been suggested by Cassinari and Pagni [16] that interference of the neospinothalamic system allows this phylogenetically older system to dominate in the pain experience.

Utilizing cats and monkeys as subjects, Albe-Fessard et al [7] used antidromic (impulse traveling backward) technique to locate the origin of the cells of the neospinothalamic and paleospinothalamic tracts. Stimulation was accomplished by placing electrodes "in the thalamus, lemniscus lateralis, or central gray at the mesencephalic level, as well as the bulbar reticular formation." Trevino et al [95] similarly stimulated the spinothalamic tracts. Cells of origin, using central stimulation, were located in different layers, i.e., laminae V, VII, and VIII, than had been identified by stimulating peripherally, i.e., laminae V and VI. These findings suggest that modifications may occur beyond the dorsal horn. Albe-Fessard concluded that in monkeys an important pathway connects lamina V with the ventral posterior nucleus of the thalamus and, moreover, that this corresponds to the neospinothalamic tract described by Mehler [59] and that such a tract does not exist in the cat, although it probably does exist in man.

It seems clear from these studies that this afferent system differs with the species being studied and points to the caution that must be exercised in applying these facts to the study of pain in man.

A second projection system of importance in pain is the lemniscal system (Fig. 2-6). It originates from large class A alpha fibers of the medial root division which enter the dorsal funiculi (dorsal columns) and ascend to the medulla to synapse with the second-order neurons of the nucleus gracilis or cuneatus. After synapsing in these nuclei, the message is carried by these second-order neurons to the opposite side to ascend in the medial lemniscus projection system. These axons terminate by synapsing with the third-order neurons of the ventral and medial thalamus, which subsequently take the message via the internal capsule and corona radiata to the sensory cortex. This system includes fast-conducting fibers of touch, pressure, vibration, and movement (propriosensation). Information received through this system is thought to initiate and program a search of both the state of the external world and the information arriving over afferent pathways [99]. Dorsal column pathways, then, are essential for stimuli where activity is required for analysis. The stimuli must be actively explored by motor movement before discrimination is possible. Wall and others believe that dorsal columns initiate and carry sensory information produced by an exploration (motor) of the stimulus object.

This pathway has recently become important in the study of pain [8, 36, 69, 86, 97]. Wagman and McMillan [97] indicated that dorsal column activity in some way inhibited dorsal horn cells (laminae II, III, IV, V, etc.) and thus modified or inhibited the pain impulses of the spinothalamic system. They further suggested dorsal column stimulation could become important in alleviation of pain. Melzack and Wall postulate central control via the dorsal columns, which partially explains their theory that the stimulation of large class A alpha fibers is important in closing the gate (substantia gelatinosa) [63].

A more recently described ascending system that may have importance in pain is the spinocervicothalamic system (SCT) [94]. Information about this system is sketchy. It is described by Morin [67] as being prominent in carnivores and has also been identified in man [34]. It arises from Clark's nucleus (Rexed's laminae IV and V) and ascends ipsilaterally to synapse with third-order neurons in the lateral cervical nuclei. This nucleus, only recently described, is located in the reticular formation of the upper cervical segments (C_1C_2) in man, but is represented throughout all segments in the rat [33]. The fibers arising from this nucleus ascend contralaterally with the medial lemniscus to the thalamus while sending collaterals to the cerebellum. Little is actually known about the function of the nucleus. Mechanoreceptors of large peripheral fields and, to some extent, pain and temperature activate this system. Its fibers are fast acting and travel with the medial lemniscus, but its origin from lamina IV and V (subject to descending modulation) relates it to the spinothalamic system. The spinocervicothalamic tract (SCT) may serve as an important alternate proprioceptive route by bypassing of the lemniscal system. Its existence accounts for the persistence of kinesthetic sense, pallanesthesia, and touch after total interruption of the posterior funiculus [46]. Brown in 1974 [14], studying control of class C fibers, focused on the spinocervicothalamic system. He found, as did others [32, 65], that it could be excited by both A and C fibers. They also found that C fiber input on the discharge of the SCT cells produced by A fibers had no conditioning effect. They examined this very carefully, but failed to observe facilitation as demanded by the gate theory of Melzack and Wall [63]. They concluded that for transmission through the SCT, cutaneous C fibers either excite a neuron or have no effect. However, Brown [14] did note that SCT neurons stimulated by C fibers were inhibited by descending axons in the spinal cord (i.e., dorsal column, dorsolateral, and ventromedial funiculi stimulation) (Fig. 2-5). This study of C-fiber inhibition suggested that discharges produced in the SCT are very effectively inhibited by both descending and segmental systems. Its precise role in pain, if any, awaits description.

Central Pain

Cassinari and Pagni [16], after a systematic study of surgical procedures used to relieve pain, concluded that central pain ("central sensory syndrome") was experienced after partial or total damage to the neospinothalamic (paucisynaptic) system. Their research indicated that when the neospinothalamic system is interrupted, impulses tend to be switched via collaterals from the posterior root to the paleospinothalamic (polysynaptic) system which results in central pain if this latter system is still intact. Nashold et al [70], studying central pain, concluded that a "variety of painful and unpleasant sensations occurs in man and animals when the dorsolateral region of the midbrain tegmentum is electrically stimulated." The lateral portion of this midbrain area contains both the neospinothalamic and paleospinothalamic pathways. Further, in 1974, these same authors associated midbrain integration of pain pathways with the emotional aspects of pain perception [71]. Pathophysiological changes within the midbrain were identified as being responsible for the pain and suffering that occurs after protracted periods of painful experience. Clinical data, however, do not support this hypothesis.

Watkins [101], however, supports changes in the central thalamus with prolonged pain relief without peripheral sensory loss. Bowsher [13] and Mehler [59] have presented data to support this. Collins [19], Albe-Fessard and Kruger [6], and Whitlock and Perl [105] have shown that responses in the thalamus are evoked by peripheral (natural, noxious, and electrical) stimuli which also supports thalamic origin of central pain. Andrew and Watkins [9], using stereotactic thalamotomy as therapy for relief of pain in 42 patients, later on autopsy confirmed that lesions created in the central thalamus were the most successful in relieving pain.

It is commonly held that cellular and tissue injury activates specific "pain receptors," nociceptors. This may be by direct damage or by release of chemicals that stimulate the endings. Once the impulse is created via receptor it is then transmitted via A delta and C fibers over a chain of specific neurons to reach a higher pain center in the brain. The impulse created, however, is varied—as are the specific ascending pathways to the brain.

It is obvious that the concept of central pain is becoming more important in the study of pain as man experiences it. Clinically, however, pain is usually still considered in terms of peripheral receptors, nerves, and their spinal pathways even though central control and the multisynaptic afferent system (MAS) are recognized as very important and the concept is gaining momentum in clinical evaluation of pain.

It would seem that if pain is to be controlled, transmission of the pain impulse must be controlled. Therefore, it is not surprising to see clinicians attempting to control pain by controlling the substantia gelatinosa, performing thalamotomy, or creating descending inhibition.

The implication of fine, slow-conducting A delta and C fibers in pain has gained strong support with refinement of research methodologies. When large, fast-conducting A alpha fibers fail to function with a consequent loss of their inhibitory effect, C fibers take over and pain ensues.

Various mechanisms operate to create a discrepancy in the proportion of A and C fibers. There may be an actual decrease in the number of large A fibers. The reduction can be created by surgery, e.g., rhizotomies, cordotomies, or amputations.

Inhibition of the small A delta and C fibers may not occur if large numbers of A alpha fibers are damaged, inactivated, or removed. Recognition that destruction of the large, fast-conducting A alpha fibers allows slow-conducting A delta and C fibers to function without inhibition thus raises questions about the therapies used for relief of pain, especially those that interfere with the anterolateral spinothalamic fibers. Reducing these fibers allows the slow fibers of the paleospinothalamic tract to take over without restraint. While not reducing the number of fibers, inflammation affects the functioning of large fibers rather than the smaller A delta and C fibers. Myelin, which is characteristic of A fibers, has been shown to be susceptible to damage by both neurolytic drugs and inflammatory exudates. This phenomenon became evident in ethyl alcohol injection studies. Fourth-degree injury of nerves was demonstrated by "coagulation necrosis characterized by a diffuse eosinophilic staining with complete loss of details in axons, myelin sheath, nodes of Ranvier, and Schwann cells" with no regeneration [21]. Phenol injection produced similar degeneration, but regeneration did occur after two months. Mehta [60] indicates that dilute solutions of local analgesics have a greater effect on thinner, nonmyelinated fibers than on the larger, myelinated nerves. Postmortem studies of the effects of neurolytic blocking agents on nerve tissues were reviewed by Swerdlow [92]. Following subarachnoid injection of alcohol, axis cylinders in the dorsal roots showed signs of degeneration; in dorsal root ganglia, swelling and chromatolysis had taken place; and dorsal roots were demyelinated. When the neurolytic agent was phenol, more damage was found in the dorsal root than in the ventral root. Damage sustained was demonstrated by patchy degeneration of nerve roots and myelin sheaths, and this degeneration initiated changes in the nerves in the dorsal columns.

Another mechanism that operates in pain is fiber regeneration. Although A delta and C fibers are cut, destroyed, or removed concomitantly with A fibers, regeneration is faster with the former types of fibers in that they are smaller and have little or no myelin. In the regenerative process the growth of a large number of axons, with an increase in the number of sprouts, takes place. Until these attain their full size and are fully myelinated, they act as slow conductors. Hence, an alteration of impulse conduction occurs. Noordenbos [73] indicated that when a nerve was sutured, a full year was required before it fully recovered function and until then these nerves were thin and were slow conductors.

Demonstration of these phenomena is seen clinically. Loesser [57] identified pain that returns after rhizotomies as being due, among other things, to a decrease in afferent impulses and to an alteration in conduction due to the regenerative process. Further illustration of this is offered by Pagni and Mapes.

Pagni and Mapes [77] and Pagni [75, 76] in discussing phantom limb pain suggest that reduction in afferent input by performing a rhizotomy creates an imbalance in the dorsal horn. In addition, Noordenbos [73] considers altered receptor sites as basic to the problem of phantom limb since neuromas act as receptor organs. However, in addition to input from the altered receptors, input from the denervated skin flap, pressure of the stump, and altered proprioceptive impulses because of muscle amputation all contribute to altered input. Pain associated with the phantom limb is attributed to activity of small fibers, finely myelinated or nonmyelinated, because amputation of a part eliminates large-fiber input from that part. In addition a shortening of the nerves caused by the amputation creates a time lag so that those large fibers that are left cannot inhibit the activity of the small fibers.

Causalgia, another clinical manifestation of pain, is related theoretically by Noordenbos [73] to large-fiber damage. This phenomenon, he states, is found more frequently during war since damage is usually associated with a high-velocity phenomenon. The space created by an object rapidly propelled through an area will exert pressure on the surrounding tissue including nerves. This compression and expansion will cause damage to the nerve and speculation is that myelinated fibers may be more susceptible than others to this type of trauma.

Later studies by Meyer and Fields of injuries sustained in the war in Vietnam reported observations of causalgia. Causalgia rarely occurred after complete nerve resection. It did occur with partial nerve injuries. The pain was attributed to small-diameter afferents. The definition of causalgia for their study was "a severe burning, intractable pain which is referred to (or perceived in) the distribution of partially damaged peripheral nerve and is intensified by emotional and certain sensory stimuli" [66]. Their findings, they believe, supported the gate control theory of pain in that the gate was more open and severe pain occurred because large fibers were affected by the injury, and thus inhibition of pain was not possible.

Destruction of nerve fibers by inflammation is seen clinically in postherpetic neuralgia. An earlier study by Noordenbos [73], with the help of Waddell, was done comparing healthy intercostal nerves with those damaged by herpes. In the latter, an increase in nonmyelinated fibers was found; afferent input from skin to intercostal nerves was decreased, and the fibers in the affected skin were finer than those in skin not affected by herpes. They concluded that there was an increase in the small fibers of slow conduction. Similar findings were reported by Dam and vive Larsen [21] who suggest that postherpetic neuralgia resulted from inflammation which affected the large fibers, primarily, with more rapid regeneration of the fine fibers. Regeneration of the large fibers was slow, but they also became slow-conducting. They concluded that with the scarcity of fast-acting fibers, the inhibitory capacity was lost and the multisynaptic system was overactivated, and spontaneous pain resulted.

Summary

What then is pain? A sensation, a feeling, a warning? After intensive study it is still not definable. We know it consists of complex circuits of cellular communication and integration in response to a noxious stimulus created at the periphery. The message is transferred to the central system via first-level afferent neurons in the dorsal root or cranial nerve ganglia.

In the spinal cord this nociceptive pain message ascends via at least three systems. One is a very direct neospinothalamic system that ascends to synapse in central thalamus and projects to neocortex for conscious awareness of the message as pain and as to localization of the peripheral origin of the stimulus. Simultaneously, the message is ascending via the indirect paleo-spinothalamic system, which involves many neurons, much delay, integration, and relay in the reticular core that ultimately reaches the neocortex. Since the neocortex is known to modify the reticular core via descending systems such as the limbic system, this is then responsible for the personal affect of the pain experience as modified by memory of past experience of pain. A message also ascends via the dorsal columns' lemniscal system, which activates an as yet unknown descending system, which feeds back to modulate the cells of the dorsal horn of the spinal cord where the other systems just described originate. All three systems function simultaneously in a concerted way to help man receive, identify, and react to a potentially harmful stimulus in a personal, unique way (Fig. 2-7).

In certain settings the providers of health care spend a great deal of time in the presence of patients who are experiencing pain. Reliance is placed on these individuals to obtain data related to the status of the patient, to provide care, and to make judgments about both. From the preceding discussions, however, several conclusions can be drawn that need to be recognized if the providers of health care are to be effective practitioners of, consumers of, and contributors to, research. There is a need for a far stronger knowledge base than these professionals usually possess. This base may be somewhat difficult to acquire because of the following variables: A time lag exists between acquisition of knowledge by basic scientists and communication of knowledge to the clinician. Communication is hindered by semantics, ambiguous definitions, inadequate follow-up or evaluation, and inadequate reporting. Theories of pain have been derived at times from minimal data and may have little neurophysiological or neuroanatomical support.

True, the clinician makes observations, but of what value are they if these observations are isolated facts unrelated to any other behaviors the patient is presenting? Which of the relationships between empirical referents will give meaning to the pattern of behavior? What relationship is there between

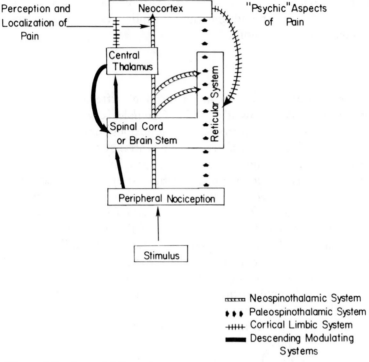

Figure 2-7 A model for pain.

what is seen, what the patient says, what the laboratory findings reveal, and what is written in the literature?

With the vast amount of literature extant, the problem lies in locating that which is most pertinent and in being able to discard the extraneous. Perhaps the most useful way for one to make use of the findings theoretically and empirically is to have a knowledge of anatomy and physiology, of cell structure and function, and of the nervous system.

The health professionals must gain this necessary knowledge in order to care for their patients; they need to read the pain literature and communicate findings to others through self-teaching and continued learning. Knowledge of the concepts of cellular structure and function, communication, perception, and response provides a matrix for inferences about patients' behavior. Cellular structure and function have to change in order to adapt when injury occurs to any part of the body, as previously discussed. This injury may be the result of trauma, disease, or therapy. The greater the knowledge base, the more astute the observations can be because then seemingly unrelated behaviors actually become important clues to what is occurring in the patient. If empirical data are collected systematically, patterns of behavior emerge. Generalizations from these patterns of behavior can be drawn, conceptualization takes place, and appropriate interventions may be hypothesized.

With this base the various theories of pain can be understandable. Utilizing the relationships of these concepts within a theory of pain can make empirical data more meaningful. Or, observations of the patient can then be related to the concepts that are significant in various theories of pain, and interventions can then be supported with theoretical knowledge. Theories provide a framework for communication so that knowledge of the concepts subsumed under the various theories enables the practitioner to read more discriminately and to intervene more appropriately.

Melzack and Chapman [62] identify two therapeutic implications for the gate control theory of pain. Both of these (but particularly the first) have implications for use by providers of health care. By massage or tactile stimulation, large fibers, i.e., A fibers, can be stimulated and pain thus decreased. Control of central mechanisms can be achieved by suggestion and distraction techniques which many nurses as well as others have used, not on a theoretical basis, but on an empirical basis, knowing that these activities usually worked.

Theories of pain are formulated, explored, maybe discarded, only to be resurrected again. Parts of them are perhaps found to be significant again, and serve as a basis for reenergizing further study, if only in an attempt to disprove them.

Such is the case of Melzack and Wall [63] who in 1965 proposed the gate control theory of pain. Briefly stated, the gate (substantia gelatinosa) is closed by large fibers, opened by small fibers, and modulated by descending fibers. Because it attempts to integrate the psychological and physiological aspects of pain, it has become a popular pain hypothesis. The physiological hard facts to support this theory are lacking and it has become suspect because of the results of some pain studies [14, 17, 27, 109]. Despite the neurologists' reluctance to support the gate theory [43, 44, 85], it has given new impetus to the research of pain and, lacking hard physiological facts or not, the theoretical base of the gate theory is being applied clinically and with a great deal of success. Perhaps this quest will lead to a solution to the problem of pain, even if a theoretical base does not emerge.

References

1. Abraham, V. C. An induction of prolonged change in the functional state of the spinal cord. In Bonica, J. J., ed., *Advances in Neurology* (Vol. 4). New York: Raven Press, 1974. P. 243.
2. Adrian, E. D. Impulses produced by sensory nerve endings. Part 1. *J. Physiol.* 61:49, 1926.
3. Adrian, E. D. The impulses produced by sensory nerve endings. Part 4. Impulses from pain receptors. *J. Physiol.* 62:13, 1926–27.
4. Adrian, E. D., and Zotterman, Y. The impulses produced by sensory nerve endings. Part 2. Impulses set up by touch and pressure. *J. Physiol.* 61:151, 1926a.

5. Adrian, E. D., and Zotterman, Y. The impulses produced by sensory nerve endings. Part 3. Impulses set up by touch and pressure. *J. Physiol.* 61:465, 1926b.

6. Albe-Fessard, D., and Kruger, L. Duality of unit discharges from cat centrum medianum in response to natural and electrical stimulation. *J. Neurophysiol.* 25:3, 1962.

7. Albe-Fessard, D., Levante, A., and Lamour, Y. Origin of spinothalamic and spinoreticular pathways in cats and monkeys. In Bonica, J. J., eds., *Advances in Neurology* (Vol. 4). New York: Raven Press, 1974. Pp. 157–168.

8. Anderson, P., Eccles, J. C., Schmidt, R. F., and Yokota, T. Slow potential waves produced in the cuneat nucleus by cutaneous volleys by cortical stimulation. *J. Neurophysiol.* 27:78, 1964.

9. Andrew, J., and Watkins, E. S. *A Stereotaxic Atlas of the Human Thalamus and Adjacent Structures. A Variability Study.* Baltimore: The Williams & Wilkins Company, 1969.

10. Angevine, J. B. The nervous tissue. In Bloom, W., and Fawcett, D. W., eds., *A Textbook of Histology.* Philadelphia: W. B. Saunders Company, 1975.

11. Besson, J. M., Guilband, G., and Le Bars, D. Descending inhibitory influences exerted by the brainstem upon the activities of dorsal horn lamina V cells induced by intra-arterial injection of bradykinin into the limbs. *J. Physiol.* 248:725, 1975.

12. Bishop, G. H. Fiber size and myelinization in afferent systems. In Knighton, R. S., and Dumke, P. R., eds., *Pain.* Boston: Little, Brown and Company, 1964. Pp. 83–89.

13. Bowsher, D. Termination of central pain pathway in man: The conscious appreciation of pain. *Brain* 80:606, 1957.

14. Brown, A. G., Haman, W. C., and Martin, H. G., III. Descending and segmental control of C fiber input to the spinal cord. In Bonica, J. J., ed., *Advances in Neurology* (Vol. 4). New York: Raven Press, 1974.

15. Burgess, P. R. Patterns of discharges evoked in cutaneous nerves and their significance for sensation. In Bonica, J. J., ed., *Advances in Neurology* (Vol. 4). New York: Raven Press, 1974.

16. Cassinari, V., and Pagni, C. A. *Central Pain.* Cambridge: Harvard University Press, 1969.

17. Christensen, B. N., and Perl, E. R. Spinal neurones specifically excited by noxious or thermal stimuli: Marginal zone of the dorsal horn. *J. Neurophysiol.* 33:293, 1970.

18. Collins, W. F., Jr., Nulsen, F. E., and Randt, C. T. Relation of peripheral fiber size and sensation in man. *Arch. Neurol.* 3:381, 1960.

19. Collins, F., Jr., Nulsen, F., and Shealy, N. C. Electrophysiological studies of peripheral and central pathways conducting pain. In Knighton, R. S., and Dumke, P. R., eds., *Pain.* Boston: Little, Brown and Company, 1966.

20. Dale, H. H., Feldberg, W. W., and Vogt, M. Release of acetycholine at voluntary motor nerve endings. *J. Physiol.* (Lond.) 86:353, 1936.

21. Dam, W., and vive Larsen, J. J. Peripheral nerve blocks in relief of intractable pain. In Swerdlow, M., ed., *Relief of Intractable Pain.* New York: Excerpta Medica, 1974.

22. Del Bianco, D. L., Del Bene, E., and Sicuteri, F. Heart pain. In Bonica, J. J., ed., *Advances in Neurology* (Vol. 4). New York: Raven Press, 1974.

23. Erlanger, J., and Gasser, H. S. The action potential in fibers of slow conduction in spinal roots and somatic nerves. *Am. J. Physiol.* 92:43, 1930.

24. Evans, J. H. Neurophysiology and neurophysiological aspects of pain. In Swerdlow, M., ed., *Relief of Intractable Pain.* New York: Excerpta Medica, 1974. Pp. 1–20.

25. Feltz, P., Krauthammer, E., and Albe-Fessard, D.   Neurons of the diencephalon. I: Somatosensory responses and caudate inhibition. *J. Physiol.* 30: 55, 1967.
26. Fidler, S. M. R.   Unpublished data, Iowa City, 1975.
27. Franz, D. N., and Iggo, A.   Dorsal root potentials and ventral root reflexes evoked by non-myelinated fibers. *Science* 162:1140, 1968.
28. Friedman, A. P., Rowan, A. J., and Wood, E. H.   Recent observations in migraine with particular reference to thermography and encephalography. In Bonica, J. J., ed., *Advances in Neurology* (Vol. 4). New York: Raven Press, 1974.
29. Gardner, E.   *Fundamentals of Neurology*, 6th ed. Philadelphia: W. B. Saunders Company, 1975.
30. Goodman, L. S., and Gilman, A., eds.   *Neurohumoral Transmission and the Autonomic System. The Pharmaceutical Basis of Therapeutics*, 3rd ed. New York: Macmillan Inc., 1970. P. 406.
31. Gray, E. G.   The granule cells, mossy synapses, and purkinje spine synapses of the cerebellum: Light and electron microscope observations. *J. Anat.* 95:345, 1961.
32. Gregor, M., and Zimmerman, M.   Characteristics of spinal neurones responding to cutaneous myelinated and unmyelinated fibres. *J. Physiol.* 221: 555, 1972.
33. Gwyn, D. G., and Waldron, H. A.   A nucleus in the dorsolateral funiculus of the spinal cord of the rat. *Brain Res.* 10:342, 1968.
34. Ha, H., and Liu, C. N.   Organization of the spino-cervico-thalamic system. *J. Comp. Neurol.* 127:445, 1966.
35. Hallin, R. G., and Torebjork, H. E.   Activity in unmyelinated nerve fibers in man. In Bonica, J. J., ed., *Advances in Neurology* (Vol. 4). New York: Raven Press, 1974.
36. Harbarth, K. E., and Kerr, D. I. B.   Central influences on spinal afferent conditions. *J. Neurophysiol.* 17:295, 1954.
37. Hassler, R.   Die zentrale systeme des schmerzes. *Acta Neurochir.* (Wien) 8:353, 1960.
38. Hassler, R.   Afferent systems. In Janzen, R., Keidel, W. D., Herz, A., and Steichele, C., eds., *Pain: Basic Principles—Pharmacology—Therapy*. Baltimore: The Williams & Wilkins Company, 1972.
39. Head, H., Rivers, W. H. R., and Sherren, J.   The afferent nervous system from a new aspect. *Brain* 28:99, 1905.
40. Heavner, J. E.   The spinal cord dorsal horn. *Anesthesiology* 38:1, 1973.
41. Herrick, C. J., and Bishop, G. H.   In Proctor, L. D., et al, eds., *Reticular Formation of the Brain*. Boston: Little, Brown and Company, 1958.
42. Iggo, A.   The case for "pain" receptors. In Janzen, R., Keidel, W. D., Herz, A., Steichele, C., Payne, J. P., and Burt, R. A. D., eds., *Pain*. Baltimore: The Williams & Wilkins Company, 1972. Pp. 60–61.
43. Iggo, A.   Critical remarks on the gate control theory. In Janzen, R., Keidel, W. D., Herz, A., Steichele, C., Payne, J. P., and Burt, R. A. D., eds., *Pain*. Baltimore: The Williams & Wilkins Company, 1972. P. 127.
44. Iggo, A.   Activation of cutaneous nociceptors and their actions on dorsal horn neurons. In Bonica, J. J., ed., *Advances in Neurology* (Vol. 4). New York: Raven Press, 1974.
45. Ingram, W. R.   *A Student's Introduction to Neurology*. Iowa City: State University of Iowa, 1964.
46. Ingram, W. R.   *A Review of Anatomical Neurology*. Iowa City: University of Iowa, 1974.

47. Jacobson, M., and Hunt, R. K. The origins of nerve-cell specificity. *Sci. Am.* 228:26, 1973.
48. Kapeller, K., and Mayor, D. The accumulation of NOR adrenaline in constricted sympathetic nerves as studied by fluorescence and electron microscopy. *Proc. R. Soc.* (Biol.) 167:282, 1967.
49. Keele, K. D. *Anatomies of Pain.* Springfield: Charles C Thomas, Publisher, 1957.
50. Keele, K. D., and Armstrong, D. *Substances Producing Pain and Itch.* London: Arnold, 1964.
51. Kruger, L. The thalamic projection of pain. In Knighton, R. S., and Dumke, P. R., eds., *Pain.* Boston: Little, Brown and Company, 1965.
52. Leavitt, F. *Drugs and Behavior.* Philadelphia: W. B. Saunders Company, 1974.
53. Lele, P. P., and Weddell, G. Sensory nerves of the cornea and cutaneous sensibility. *Exp. Neurol.* 1:334, 1959.
54. Lim, R. K. S. Pain mechanisms. *Anesthesiology* 28:106, 1967.
55. Lim, R. K. S. Pain. *Ann. Rev. Physiol.* 32:269, 1970.
56. Lindahl, O. Pain, a general chemical explanation. In Bonica, J. J., ed., *Advances in Neurology* (Vol. 4). New York: Raven Press, 1974. Pp. 46–47.
57. Loesser, J. Dorsal rhizotomy: Indications and results. In Bonica, J. J., ed., *Advances in Neurology* (Vol. 4). New York: Raven Press, 1974.
58. Longo, V. C. *Neuropharmocology and Behavior.* San Francisco: W. H. Freeman and Company, Publishers, 1972.
59. Mehler, W. R. The mammalian "pain tract" in phylogeny. *Anat. Rec.* 127:332, 1957.
60. Mehta, M. *Intractable Pain.* London: W. B. Saunders Co., Ltd., 1973.
61. Melzack, R. *The Puzzle of Pain.* New York: Basic Books, Inc., Publishers, 1973.
62. Melzack, R., and Chapman, C. R. Psychological aspects of pain. *Postgrad. Med.* 53(6):69, 1973.
63. Melzack, R., and Wall, P. D. Pain mechanisms: A new theory. *Science* 150:971, 1965.
64. Melzack, R., and Wall, P. D. Psychophysiology of pain. *Anesth. Clin.* 8:3, 1970.
65. Mendell, L. M. Physiological properties of unmyelinated fiber projection to the spinal cord. *Exp. Neurol.* 16:316, 1966.
66. Meyer, G. A., and Fields, H. L. Causalgia treated by selective large fibre stimulation of the peripheral nerve. *Brain.* 95:163, 1972.
67. Morin, F. A new spinal pathway for cutaneous impulses. *Am. J. Physiol.* 183:245, 1955.
68. Müller, J. *Elements of Physiology* (Vol. 2). London: Taylor and Walton, 1843.
69. Nashold, B. S., and Friedman, H. Dorsal column stimulation for pain: A preliminary report on 30 patients. *J. Neurosurg.* 36:590, 1972.
70. Nashold, B. S., Jr., Wilson, W. P., and Slaughter, D. G. Sensations evoked by stimulation of the midbrain of man. *J. Neurosurg.* 30:19, 1969.
71. Nashold, B. S., Jr., Wilson, W. P., and Slaughter, D. G. The midbrain and pain. In Bonica, J. J., ed., *Advances in Neurology* (Vol. 4). New York: Raven Press, 1974.
72. Noback, C., and Demarest, R. J. *The Human Nervous System,* 2d ed. New York: McGraw-Hill Book Company, Inc., 1975.
73. Noordenbos, W. *Pain.* New York: Elsevier Publishing Co., 1959.
74. Noordenbos, W. Physiological correlates of clinical pain syndromes. In

Soulairic, A., Cahn, J., and Charpentier, J., eds., *Pain.* New York: Academic Press, Inc., 1968.

75. Pagni, C. A.   Pain due to central nervous system lesions: Physiopathological considerations and therapeutical considerations. In Bonica, J. J., ed., *Advances in Neurology* (Vol. 4). New York: Raven Press, 1974.

76. Pagni, C. A.   Place of stereotactic technique in surgery for pain. In Bonica, J. J., ed., *Advances in Neurology* (Vol. 4). New York: Raven Press, 1974.

77. Pagni, C. A., and Mapes, P. E.   A new approach to the surgical treatment of phantom limb pain. In Janzen, R., Keidel, R. W. E., Herz, A., Steichele, C., Payne, J. P., and Burt, R. A. P., eds., *Pain.* Baltimore: The Williams & Wilkins Company, 1972.

78. Pearson, A. A.   Role of gelatinous substance of spinal cord in conduction of pain. *Arch. Neurol. Psychiatr.* 68:515, 1952.

79. Pfenninger, K., Sandri, C., Akert, K., and Augster, C. H.   Contribution to the problem of structural organization of the presynaptic area. *Brain Res.* 12:10, 1969.

80. Pomeranz, B., Wall, P. D., and Weber, W. V.   Cord cells responding to fine myelinated afferents from viscera, muscle and skin. *J. Physiol.* 199:511, 1968.

81. Ranson, S. W., and Billingsley, P. R.   Conduction of painful afferent impulses in the spinal nerves. *Am. J. Physiol.* 40:571, 1916.

82. Rexed, B.   The cytoarchitectonic organization of the spinal cord of the cat. *J. Comp. Neurol.* 96:415, 1952.

83. Robbins, S. L., and Angell, M.   *Basic Pathology.* Philadelphia: W. B. Saunders Company, 1973.

84. Schildkraut, J. J.   Neuropharmocology of the affective disorders. *Annu. Rev. Pharmacol.* 13:427, 1973.

85. Schmidt, R. F.   The gate control theory of pain: An unlikely hypothesis. In Janzen, R., Keidel, W. D., Herz, A., Steichele, C., Payne, J. P., and Burt, R. A. P., eds., *Pain.* Baltimore: The Williams & Wilkins Company, 1972. P. 124.

86. Shealy, C. N., Mortimer, J. J., and Hagfors, N. R.   Dorsal column electroanalgesia. *J. Neurosurg.* 32:560, 1970.

87. Shepherd, G. M.   The neuron doctrine: A revision of functional concepts. *Yale J. Biol. Med.* 45:584, 1972.

88. Sherrington, C.   *The Integrative Action of the Nervous System.* New York: Charles Scribner's Sons, 1906.

89. Sicuteri, F.   Floor discussion: Peripheral nerve disorders. In Bonica, J. J., ed., *Advances in Neurology* (Vol. 4). New York: Raven Press, 1974.

90. Stent, G. S.   Cellular communication. *Sci. Am.* 227:42, 1972.

91. Swanson, A. G., Buchan, F. C., and Alvord, E. C., Jr.   Anatomic changes in congenital insensitivity to pain. *Arch. Neurol.* 12:121, 1965.

92. Swerdlow, M.   Intrathecal and extradural block in pain relief. In Swerdlow, M., ed., *Relief of Intractable Pain.* New York: Excerpta Medica, 1974.

93. Taub, A.   Floor discussion: Peripheral nerve disorders. In Bonica, J. J., ed., *Advances in Neurology* (Vol. 4). New York: Raven Press, 1974. P. 318.

94. Taub, A., and Bishop, P. O.   The spinocervical tract; dorsal column linkage, conduction velocity, primary afferent spectrum. *Exp. Neurol.* 13:1, 1965.

95. Trevino, Daniel L., Coulter, J. D., Maunz, R. A., and Willis, W. D.   Location and functional properties of spinothalamic cells in the monkey. In Bonica, J. J., ed., *Advances in Neurology* (Vol. 4). New York: Raven Press, 1974.

96. Uchizono, K.   Characteristics of excitatory and inhibitory synapses in the central nervous system of the cat. *Nature* 207:642, 1965.

97. Wagman, I. H., and McMillan, J. A. Relationships between activity in spinal sensory pathways and "pain mechanisms" in spinal cord and brain stem. In Bonica, J. J., ed., *Advances in Neurology* (Vol. 4). New York: Raven Press, 1974.

98. Wall, P. D. The laminar organization of dorsal horn and effects of descending impulses. *J. Physiol.* 188:403, 1967.

99. Wall, P. D. The sensory and motor role of impulses traveling in the dorsal column toward the cerebral cortex. *Brain* 93:505, 1970.

100. Wall, P. D. Floor discussion: Ascending pathways in spinal cord. In Bonica, J. J., ed., *Advances in Neurology* (Vol. 4). New York: Raven Press, 1974.

101. Watkins, E. S. The place of neurosurgery in the relief of intractable pain. In Swerdlow, M., ed., *Relief of Intractable Pain*. New York: Excerpta Medica, 1974.

102. Weddell, G., Palmer, E., and Pallie, W. Nerve endings in mammalian skin. *Biol. Rev.* 30:159, 1955.

103. Weiss, P. A. Neuronal dynamics and neuroplasmic flow. In Schmitt, F. O., Quarton, G. C., Melnechuk, T., and Adelman, G., eds., *The Neurosciences Second Study Program*. New York: Rockefeller University Press, 1970.

104. Werle, E. On endogenous pain producing substances with particular references to plasmakinins. In Janzen, R., Keidel, W. D., Herz, A., Steichele, C., Payne, J. P., and Burt, R. A. P., eds., *Pain*. Baltimore: The Williams & Wilkins Company, 1972.

105. Whitlock, D. G., and Perl, E. R. Thalamic projections of spinothalamic pathways in monkey. *Exp. Neurol.* 3:24, 1961.

106. Whittaker, V. P. The synaptosome. In Lajtha, A., ed., *Handbook of Neurochemistry* (Vol. 2). New York: Plenum Publishing Corporation, 1969.

107. Williams, P., and Warwick, R. *Functional Neuroanatomy of Man*. Philadelphia: W. B. Saunders Company, 1975.

108. Wilson, M. E. The neurological mechanisms of pain. *Anesthesia* 29:407, 1974.

109. Zimmerman, M. Dorsal root potential after C-fiber stimulation. *Science* 160:896, 1968.

110. Zotterman, Y. Studies in the peripheral nervous system mechanism of pain. *Acta Med. Scand.* 80:185, 1933.

111. Zotterman, Y. Touch, pain, and tickling—an electrophysiological investigation on cutaneous nerves. *J. Physiol.* 95:1, 1939.

3

Sociocultural and Psychological Aspects of Pain

Ada K. Jacox

Recognition that the psyche and the soma are interrelated in complex ways is the basis for much health- and illness-related research and practice. The assumption that psychological and sociocultural factors influence how a person experiences pain is well accepted by most contemporary clinicians and researchers. In contrast to agreement on the broad assumption regarding the importance of psychological and sociocultural factors in pain, there is little consensus about the specific ways in which these factors operate. This lack of agreement is because of the complexity of the pain experience and because systematic efforts to examine psychological and sociocultural aspects of pain are relatively recent. The study of pain, however, is increasingly the focus of behavioral scientists, and health professionals are rapidly expanding their treatment approaches to include psychological and sociocultural facets.

Pain has been defined in many ways. Richard Sternbach, who defines pain broadly, says that pain is "an abstract concept which refers to (1) a personal, private sensation of hurt; (2) a harmful stimulus which signals current or impending tissue damage; (3) a pattern of responses which operate to protect the organism from harm" [108].

Ronald Melzack and Patrick Wall [71], in proposing their gate control theory (see Chapter 1), also view pain as a complex phenomenon, and try to synthesize previous theoretical approaches to pain definition. While most of Melzack and Wall's research has been on the physiological basis of pain, they suggest how the cognitive evaluation of pain sensations takes place in the terms of past experience, psychological state, and attitudes toward pain. Their theory provides the necessary link between the physiological and psychosocial factors that operate in the pain experience.

Definitions of pain reflect its complexity and subjectivity and offer a way to organize a discussion of the research conducted on psychological and sociocultural factors that influence a person's experience with pain. Such factors operate at every point in the pain experience, contributing to the illness or condition with which the pain is associated, the interpretation of the pain sensation, the response to the sensation, the tendency to report the pain to another person, the assessment process, the methods chosen to alleviate the pain, and the person's response to the treatment.

While no clear-cut distinctions between psychological and sociocultural factors are made in the discussion, it is useful to know generally how these terms are being used in this chapter. *Psychological* factors are those that relate to the mental processes of the individual and include personality characteristics, emotional states, and cognitive processes. The term *social* refers to interrelationships between individuals or groups and includes such factors as family and occupational roles and social class. *Cultural factors* pertain to beliefs, values, and customs that are transmitted from one generation to another. It is apparent that overlap and interrelationships exist among the terms psychological, social, and cultural. What is important to emphasize here is that how a person experiences pain is a function not only of physiological condition but also of sociocultural and psychological factors and their interrelationships with the person's physiological condition.

Influences on Production of Illness and Associated Pain

The study of sociocultural factors as they contribute to illness and pain involves the identification of these factors and how they act through the intervening processes of personality characteristics to contribute to conditions such as coronary heart disease, rheumatoid arthritis, and other painful illnesses [89]. Sociocultural factors often function to produce illness and associated pain in a nonspecific way. That is, persons from lower socioeconomic classes who live in poor housing and whose diets and medical care are inadequate are much more likely to develop a wide variety of illnesses than those in higher socioeconomic classes.

The practices of particular ethnic groups in a society have been identified as important in the production of pain and illness. The health of black Americans, for example, has been considerably poorer than that of whites. Blacks generally have less access to high quality health care than whites. In addition, Hines [49] suggests that the concept of preventive medical care is largely a development of middle-class culture in America and that an orientation to prevention has not been shared by black Americans, which contributes to their higher incidence of illness.

At another level, social factors may influence the emotional and cognitive states of individuals, which in turn may make them more vulnerable to illness and pain. For example, an occupational role that has a great deal of stress associated with it can produce a high level of anxiety in an individual—anxiety, which, in turn, may be associated with illness or pain.

As noted earlier, social conditions generally have been related to illness in a nonspecific way, with few reports of sociocultural factors related to specific illnesses. In contrast, psychological factors frequently are associated with specific illnesses and conditions, although they also may be related to illness in general. One study reported that employees in a biological laboratory who were psychologically vulnerable tended to be more hypochondriacal, more depressed, and reported a poor state of health and history of illness more frequently [20]. It is common, however, for psychological characteristics to be linked with specific conditions, and, in this respect, cancer has perhaps received the greatest attention.

Numerous studies [18, 61] report relationships between neoplastic disease and certain types of psychological situations. According to one reviewer [61], the most consistently reported, relevant psychological factor has been the loss of a major emotional relationship prior to the first noted symptoms of a neoplasm. There also may be some relationship between personality characteristics and the type or location of a cancer. Depression and a sense of guilt have been identified as prominent in patients with cancer, and observers have noted the development of cancer secondary to emotional upsets [82]. Not only the development and location of a cancer, but also the rate of growth, has been related to personality characteristics or states [61, 82].

Blumberg and others [12] suggest that it may be useful to look at resistance in the cancer patient in terms of ability to reduce or adapt effectively to stresses induced by environmental and emotional conflicts.

Grinker clearly expresses the uncertainty about the role of psychological factors in the production of cancer. He suggests that

the conscious and unconscious awareness of the presence of the illness and the defenses that are mobilized might have something to do with the activity of the organism to combat or to facilitate the development of cancer. I don't think it is all a question of the embryonic nature of the cells nor of the location of the tumor, but there may be certain psychosomatic patterns which are facilitative for the growth of an already existing cancer and might even adequately circumscribe it. We know that there is a number of cancers which are accidentally found in autopsy which seem to have had nothing to do with the death of the patient. What then would stir these up into activity? What role does a psychological process have in relation to other factors in facilitating or stirring up new growths after they have been quiescent for some time? This whole area is of extensive importance, and about it so far little is known [40].

As Shawver notes in Chapter 17 of this volume, pain may or may not accompany the progression of a neoplasm. The studies of cancer illustrate the general relationship between personality characteristics and the incidence and progression of a disease.

Other studies relate personality characteristics to particularly painful illnesses or conditions. One of the most common areas for such study is headaches, particularly migraine headaches. A variety of psychological factors have been reported to be either predisposing or precipitating causes of migraine headache. Among the predisposing factors have been various personality attributes, neurosis, and other psychiatric disorders. Some of the precipitating factors identified are emotional reactions, changes in life situations, various psychosocial stresses, periods of overactivity, and let-down periods [90]. Persons who experience migraine are commonly identified as those who react to many life situations with aggression but are unable to express anger directly [8]. Some investigators differentiate between the personality characteristics associated with migraine headache and those associated with tension headache. One group, for example, found that migraine patients exhibited an inhibited personality but that they were not as angry as patients with tension headaches, who were more openly hostile and disorganized [5].

Another condition commonly associated with pain is low back dysfunction. Some studies have shown that low back pain is clearly related to the type of work done in particular occupations, with weight lifting and bending as commonly ascribed causes. Early onset of low back pain occurs in bank clerks, heavy industry workers, farmers, and nurses, suggesting that the physical activity required in such occupations may be significant in the causation or triggering of low back pain [63]. Not only do persons experiencing low back pain often perform work of a heavy physical nature, but they also tend to be in subordinate positions and dissatisfied with their jobs, according to one study [116]. Sternbach and others [109] noted that patients seen in a low back pain clinic show some traditional characteristics associated with psychophysiological disorders. They were depressed, had a life-style of invalidism, and played what Sternbach terms "pain games" with doctors. The contribution of social, psychological, and physiological factors to the development of low back pain is another area in which there are many unanswered questions (see Chapter 21).

Other painful conditions that have been related to personality characteristics are chronic pelvic pain [21], facial pain [105], and rheumatoid arthritis [91].

It is commonly recognized that pain may be a symptom of psychiatric illness, since some persons attempt to express psychological conflict through bodily symptoms. Elsewhere in this volume, Merskey discusses in detail the three principal mechanisms in the psychological etiology of pain: the occurrence of pain as a hallucination, associated either with schizophrenia or endogenous depression; the presence of psychological factors, such as anxiety, which produce muscle tension and other conditions that, when they persist, cause pain; and conversion hysteria (see Chapter 4).

Anxiety, depression, and other psychological states not only can produce pain themselves, but also can influence the intensity of pain present from other causes. Personality characteristics associated with the intensity of pain are discussed later in this chapter.

The discussion thus far has focused on how sociocultural and psychological factors influence the production and progression of various painful conditions and illnesses. An additional consideration appropriate in the relation between psychological factors and pain is the probability that the existence of chronic illness and pain itself may influence the psychological state of a person. Increasingly, investigators are recognizing that having pain over a long period of time may influence the person's personality. Resentment and depression not only may be forerunners to the development of illnesses but they may also be the results of experiencing pain and illness for a very long time.

The findings of a study of patients treated for chronic pain by stereotaxic percutaneous cordotomy lends support to the notion that chronic pain can produce personality changes [13]. In this study, neuroticism and extraversion were measured before and after surgery. While there was divergence from the normal pattern of personality scores before surgery, there were changes toward the normal when the severe pain was relieved.

Robinson et al [91] studied patients with rheumatoid arthritis, other forms of arthritis, and other forms of chronic pain including ruptured lumbar disks or neck problems following automobile accidents. They found that patients in all of these pain groups were significantly more introverted than were normal controls. They suggest that the presence of a painful disease of any kind may lead to greater introversion because of the increased self-concern and withdrawal from social contact. It might be expected that a person with a chronic painful disease would respond with anxiety and depression. The personality traits of such persons may reflect attempts to cope with stresses related to the illness, rather than factors that in themselves produce the illness.

Reporting of Illness and Pain
An issue closely related to the presence of illness is the identification of those who report pain and illness. Many symptoms of illness, including pain, are viewed by persons in lower socioeconomic classes not as something to seek medical attention for but simply as nuisances to be tolerated [57]. They are viewed as a part of one's normal everyday existence.

Irving Zola [122] observed that a socially conditioned, selective process may be operating in the kinds of illnesses and conditions for which persons seek medical treatment. That is, many persons may have conditions that are undiagnosed simply because either they do not view the condition as abnormal or they deny its existence unconsciously and do not seek medical attention. Zola raises the question of whether it is the "differential response to deviation rather than the prevalence of the deviation which accounts for many reported group and sub-group differences" [122]. He reports on a study in which cultural beliefs are related to the symptoms or complaints that a patient presents to his physician. Zola found "compared to the Irish, Italians presented significantly more symptoms, had symptoms in significantly more bodily locations, and noted significantly more types of bodily dysfunction" [122]. He commented that the Irish generally handle their troubles by denial, while Italians handle theirs by dramatization, and that these coping strategies are reflected in the way they communicate about illness. Zola argues that the labeling and definition of a symptom as a problem is part of a social process. A specific focus of the study was on how these patients perceived and tolerated pain with the Irish tending more often to deny that pain was a feature of their illness than did Italians. This tendency was true even for patients who had the same disorder. These findings support the notion that ways of communicating about illness reflect major values and preferred ways of handling problems within the culture itself. Certain cultural practices may produce personality characteristics or emotional states in a cultural group's members which in turn influence whether or not pain is reported.

A similar study was done with 30 patients hospitalized with cancer [75]. Patients' conscious knowledge of their illness and how this knowledge related to when they first noted their symptoms and when they first visited a physician about the symptoms were studied. There was a relationship between level of awareness and education with those who had more education being more aware of the implications of the symptoms. Patients who had only minimal awareness of their symptoms delayed seeking medical care, while those with a higher level of awareness sought help more quickly. Lack of awareness of symptoms, of course, could result either from ignorance about the symptoms or from a denial that they existed. In any case, level of awareness of illness clearly was related to level of education. The self-selection of symptoms to take to a physician was influenced in this case by education factors, which in turn were related to awareness of the illness.

In women with advanced cancer of the uterus, a relationship was noted between personality characteristics of neuroticism and extraversion and reporting or complaint behavior of women [15]. Patients in the study were requested to keep a record of their pain, and the researchers also obtained a record of analgesic drugs received. The women were subdivided into three groups. The first group, who had no pain, were women who had low neuroticism and high extraversion scores and did not receive analgesics. The authors suggest that these women may be representative of those persons in whom awareness of physical symptoms, including pain, is diminished but who react in an outgoing manner to whatever stimuli they do experience. They speculate that these may be persons who seek medical advice late in the course of the illness or disease. They also are recognized as individuals who do not complain by medical and nursing staff. A second group was comprised of patients low in extraversion and high in neuroticism. They experienced pain but did not communicate this to the staff and did not receive drugs. Neuroticism is closely related to anxiety, and a number of studies have shown that as anxiety or neuroticism increases, so does the intensity of pain experienced. Thus, patients in this second group had been experiencing pain but were introverted and did not communicate about their pain. These patients also were regarded as persons who do not complain by hospital and medical personnel. The third group of patients had both high neuroticism and high extraversion scores, suggesting that the pain intensity was increased and that they also were freer to communicate about their pain. This group, in contrast to groups one and two, did receive analgesic drugs. Bond and Pearson's work [15] illustrates clearly the relationship between personality characteristics and patients' experience with and communication about pain.

The emphasis in this section is on how personality characteristics influence communication of pain. Related and important questions are how such characteristics are associated with the perception of the pain sensation and how much pain a person will tolerate before seeking relief.

Influences on Pain Threshold and Tolerance

Numerous studies have been conducted on pain threshold and tolerance. Findings often are contradictory, and the reason for the contradictions resides in part in the definition of terms used by various researchers.

Following Beecher's early work, pain researchers usually have distinguished between *sensation* and *reaction*. Sensation means the output from the sensory receptors that derives from stimulation and is translated as afferent nerve impulses, which emerge in the central nervous system to become a recognized sensation or perception [6]. Beecher calls these events including the eruption of the sensation into consciousness "the original sensation" and calls the succeeding events a secondary response or "reaction," that is, the processing of the sensation. He notes that processing of the sensation probably begins even before the sensation erupts into consciousness, further confusing the relationship between the sensation and the response to it. By reaction, Beecher means the mental process set up by the original stimulation. Many investigators subsequent to Beecher separated the pain experience into the pain sensation and the pain reaction.

The terms *pain threshold* and *pain tolerance* also are commonly found in the literature. Pain threshold is sometimes equated with pain sensation, with the intent of the investigator being to measure the intensity of the noxious stimulus necessary for the subject to perceive it as pain. The reaction, then, is considered in terms of the patient's tolerance for pain.

Sternbach defines pain threshold as the intensity of the noxious stimulus necessary for the person to perceive pain. Tolerance is the "duration of time or the intensity at which a subject accepts a stimulus above the pain threshold before making a verbal or overt pain response" [108].

Some researchers refer to the pain threshold as the point at which pain is just perceived; pain tolerance is the point at which pain is no longer tolerated voluntarily. The difference between the pain threshold and the pain tolerance is referred to as the *pain sensitivity range* [117]. Merskey and Spear [73] noted that pain threshold is more dependent on physiological factors, while pain tolerance is more dependent on psychological factors.

More recently, some investigators have begun to distinguish between two thresholds. One is a *sensation threshold*, the lowest noxious stimulus intensity at which a sensation such as warmth or pressure is first reported. This threshold seems to be relatively constant across people, assuming that the neurological system is intact [68]. The second threshold is the *pain perception threshold,* "the lowest stimulus level at which a person reports feeling pain" [68]. This threshold is influenced by psychological and sociocultural factors. Thus, the distinctions between when a sensation is first perceived as a sensation, when that sensation is perceived as pain, and when that pain can no longer be voluntarily accepted by the patient (pain tolerance) are useful. A recent study [24] of men and women of different ages reported differences between men and women in sensory threshold, as well as in pain threshold, which may explain some of the contradictory findings presented in the literature by investigators who do not commonly distinguish between these two thresholds. In much of the work reported, these two thresholds— sensory and pain perception—have been treated as one.

The fact that the terms sensation, reaction, threshold, tolerance, pain sensitivity range, and others are used in various ways by different authors has made the comparison of research findings in this area difficult. Trying to generalize from studies of experimentally induced pain carried out in laboratories to pathological pain experienced as part of an illness or injury is another problem related to pain threshold and tolerance. Such generalizations must be done with caution and with realization of the potential error involved. Not only is generalizing from experimental to clinical pain problematical, but also, generalizing from one type of experimentally induced pain to another poses difficulties. One investigator [117] used several methods of inducing pain: three were cutaneous methods, and included cold pressor method, radiant heat method, and electrical stimulation method. Two methods caused deep somatic pain: the injection of hypertonic saline and the insertion of needle electrodes into the muscle. The analysis of these methods of inducing pain showed that the effects of the cutaneous and deep somatic pain were clearly distinguishable in patients' threshold and tolerance of pain.

In reviewing the many studies of influences of pain threshold and tolerance, then, one cannot assume that pain is pain. Neither can it be assumed that factors that influence pain in the experimental situation will necessarily influence it in the same way in the clinical situation. Studies of pain tolerance probably have more clinical significance than do studies of pain threshold, which usually are done in the laboratory setting. The determination of threshold in a clinical setting would be difficult, since the application of the amount of noxious stimulus is not under the control of the researcher or the clinician as it is in a laboratory situation.

Several of the factors considered in this section—age, sex, and race—are biological rather than psychological or sociocultural. Although these factors are biological, there often are social norms associated with being young or old, white or black, female or male, which can influence a person's threshold or tolerance for pain. To what extent differences in pain threshold and tolerance are a function of biological or psychosocial factors is difficult to determine. A great number of the studies of pain threshold and tolerance do consider age, sex, and race, however, and will be considered here.

AGE   There is great disagreement in the literature in regard to how age is related to pain threshold and tolerance. Several studies [22, 23, 42, 101, 104] of cutaneous pain threshold using radiant heat as the stimulus reported that the pain threshold increases with age. Wolff and Jarvik [118], producing deep somatic pain by saline injections, found that pain thresholds increased with age in men, but not in women. In a study of female and male children aged 5 to 18 years, Haslam [46], using a pressure algometer to induce pain, reported a positive correlation between age and pain threshold.

Researchers who studied pain sensitivity in five body areas—the forehead, the upper arm, the forearm, the thigh, and the leg—found that overall pain sensitivity was fairly constant until the 50s, when it showed a sharp decline [101]. The decline in pain sensitivity was not the same for all body areas; it began at different ages for different body areas.

Contrary to the above studies, Collins and Stone [27] found that pain threshold was negatively related to age in a group of soldiers. That is, the older the man, the lower his pain threshold. Still other laboratory studies [43, 103, 113] suggest that there is no relationship between age and pain threshold.

Clark and Mehl [24], in a study using radiant heat, distinguished between the ability to first feel the sensation (warmth) and the point at which subjects felt "faint pain." Using a sample of normal male and female volunteers, they found that older subjects were less able to distinguish among the sensations of warmth, heat, and faint pain. Discriminability was lower for older females, suggesting that their sensory input had undergone attenuation and that they actually experienced less pain than did the males and younger females. The researchers speculated that although an equal amount of moderate pain was experienced by males and young females, they reacted verbally to the same sensory experience in different ways. The young men and women were much more apt to label the experience as painful than were the older men. It seems likely that many of the contradictory reports of age and sex differences in pain threshold are caused by variations in how much of the sensation a person will accept before labeling it pain rather than in the ability to perceive the sensation originally.

According to Clark and Mehl [24], older men and, to a lesser extent, older women endured greater pain before reporting it. The authors note that older women tend to lose their sensitivity and, in addition, tolerate higher levels of pain than do younger men and women. Older men apparently do not lose sensitivity but do tolerate more pain than do younger men or women.

Other studies [12, 27] of tolerance report that older persons have decreased tolerance for pain. In a group of psychiatric patients, complaints of persistent pain were more common in older persons than in younger ones, who tended to deny pain [72]. Whether complaints were related to pain threshold, tolerance, complaint behavior, or all three is not clear.

A study [88] of factors related to the management of pain in patients with cancer reported that older patients tended not to receive powerful analgesics and not to be given pain medication on the initiative of nursing staff. Also of interest was the fact that the location of lesions tended to be related to age, which may contribute to an explanation of the findings that older patients receive less powerful analgesics.

Studies relating age to pain threshold are inconclusive, although there seems to be more evidence that pain threshold increases with age. There are fewer systematic studies of pain tolerance and of complaint behavior in relation to age, and these studies present contradictory evidence.

SEX In the studies reported in the previous section, there were few differences in pain threshold noted between females and males. The one exception was the Clark and Mehl study that reported that while there was no difference in the pain threshold, older women tended not to be able to discriminate mild sensations as well as older male subjects.

The literature is contradictory and inconclusive in regard to the impact of sex differences on the pain experience. Petrie [84], in a study of perception, identified two perceptual styles: a tendency to enlarge upon the intensity of incoming stimuli (called *augmenters*) and a tendency to reduce an estimate of size or intensity of stimuli (called *reducers*). She has shown that reducers have greater pain tolerance and that women tend to reduce less than men. Thus, women are reported to have lower pain tolerance than men. Petrie suggests that "a woman's perception of pain is inextricably interwoven with the survival of the race, and a tendency of adult females not to reduce sensation much could have survival value" [84]. Petrie suggests that both cultural factors and differences in basic perceptual styles may account for the sex differences that she asserts exist in pain tolerance.

Petrovich [85], using pictures of men anticipating or undergoing various painful experiences, found that estimated pain intensity and duration of pain were evaluated as greater by women than by men. Sex differences were negligible for clerical workers, while women health professionals judged the portrayed events as more painful than did men health professionals. Occupational socialization apparently is in part responsible for sex differences, a point that has some interesting implications for health professionals.

Woodrow et al [120], using pain induced by pressure to the Achilles tendon, found that men tolerated more pain than women did. This difference held across age, with the oldest men having a higher average pain tolerance than even the youngest women. In addition, pain tolerance varied less among women than among men.

In psychiatric patients and college students, there were no sex differences in pain threshold, but men tolerated higher levels of pain than did women [80]. Jacox and Stewart [51] reported in a study of patients with rheumatoid arthritis that women evaluated the intensity of pain as being greater than did men. Other studies reported no sex differences in medical personnel, using radiant heat [113], and no difference in threshold or tolerance using electrical stimulation in undergraduate students [37].

Interesting sex differences were found in how patients with cancer communicated their pain [16]. The researchers placed patients into two categories: those who recorded pain but did not communicate it to the nursing staff, and those who recorded pain and received pain medication either by requesting it or through initiation of the nursing staff. The pain intensity scores of women in the first group were significantly lower than those of women in the second group. For men, there were no differences in pain intensity between the two groups. Some men who felt pain did not request pain medication, while some who recorded no pain asked for analgesics. Nurses tended to respond more favorably to requests from women, and they also gave medications on their own initiative only to women. The authors offer two alternative explanations for these findings. One is that men have a greater need to communicate their distress, and the second is that female nurses identify more closely with their own sex and have a more therapeutic relationship with women than with men. There are sex differences in how anxiety, hostility, and depression are related to pain ratings, an issue that is discussed later in this chapter.

While the findings related to sex are contradictory, there seems to be some consensus that pain threshold does not vary between men and women and that pain is tolerated better by men than by women.

ETHNIC GROUPS   Anthropological reports often refer to aspects of the pain experience in relation to various cultural groups.

Perhaps the best known study is one by Zborowski [121] in which he describes the pain response patterns of four cultural groups in America. Wolff and Langley [119], in a review of cultural factors in response to pain, summarize the research that has been done in this area. While a number of studies appear in the literature, they are of varying degrees of quality.

Many investigators study attitudes toward pain and give anecdotal accounts of how persons from various cultural groups react to pain. These are summarized by Wolff and Langley in the following way:

Although there is a wealth of anthropological material in which pain is discussed, there is nevertheless a dearth of studies in which both the pain response and cultural factors are directly and experimentally controlled. The few experimental pain studies that do exist suffer from anthropological naiveté, while the anthropological reports lack experimental control of pain. . . . There is thus a need for cultural anthropologists to combine forces with medical scientists in order to add to our knowledge about the human pain response [119].

A number of studies have investigated the relationship between race and pain threshold or tolerance. Chapman and Jones [23] reported that southern Negroes had a lower pain threshold and were able to tolerate less pain than

Americans of European ancestry. Racial differences were found among whites, blacks, and Orientals when pain was induced through pressure on the Achilles tendon [120]. Whites showed the highest average pain tolerance, blacks were next, and Orientals had the lowest average pain tolerance.

In contrast, a study by Merskey and Spear [74] reported no significant differences between Afro-Asians and white students in their reports of pain threshold. Similarly, in a study of lower-class Negro and white obstetric patients, no differences were found in patients' evaluations of the intensity of their pain experience nor in the amount of pain experienced by the two groups as assessed by physicians and nurses rating the patients [115].

In general, few studies have been done in which race is related to pain threshold and tolerance, and those that have been done are contradictory.

PERSONALITY CHARACTERISTICS   The influence of various personality factors on pain threshold and tolerance has been widely studied. Two characteristics frequently considered are extraversion and neuroticism. The instrument most frequently used to measure neuroticism and extraversion is the Eysenck Personality Inventory (EPI). According to Eysenck's theory, a person high in *extraversion* (E) is outgoing, impulsive, has many social contacts, is carefree, easygoing, optimistic, and does not keep his feelings under tight control. Introverts reportedly have lower sensory thresholds and greater reactions to sensory stimulation; thus, extroverts can tolerate pain better.

Studies relating extraversion to pain threshold and tolerance have produced conflicting findings. Schalling [97] suggests that some of the contradictions may be due to the different kinds of painful stimuli used by investigators. Studies [47, 62, 83] using radiant heat stimulation have found that persons high on extraversion tolerated pain better. Schalling and Levander [100], using continuously increasing electrical stimulation, studied male employees at an air base. They reported only a low correlation between extraversion and pain tolerance and suggested that extraversion may be related more to threshold than to tolerance. Davidson and McDougall [30], using both cold pressor and radiant heat tests, found no significant correlation between extraversion and pain tolerance.

Using electrical shock, Leon [60] found no significant differences in pain perception level related to extraversion for either male or female American college students. Pain perception level was defined by Leon as the difference in voltage between the first shock felt and the voltage of the first shock perceived as painful.

In a study of primipara patients on maternity wards, the intensity of labor pains, as recalled by the women, was greater in women with higher extraversion scores [34]. The research suggested that, even though they have a higher tolerance for pain, extroverts tend to exaggerate the painfulness of an event.

Studies relating extraversion to the pain experience have generally shown that patients with chronic painful conditions tend to be more introverted than do normal controls [91]. Further, extraversion *is* related to pain threshold and tolerance, although the findings are inclusive.

Neuroticism (N) is the second dimension of the Eysenck Personality Inventory. *Neuroticism* is defined as emotional lability, overresponsiveness, and a tendency to develop neurotic disorders under stress. The neuroticism dimension of the EPI is highly related to anxiety as measured by other inventories. There is evidence that increased anxiety or neuroticism is associated with increased pain, perhaps because anxiety decreases the pain threshold, decreases pain tolerance, or both. In women with advanced carcinoma of the cervix, those who reported experiencing no pain had significantly lower neuroticism scores than those who experienced pain [14]. In a study using a radiant heat stimulation test, as neuroticism increased, subjects were less able to tolerate the experimentally produced pain [62]. Another study [100] showed that anxiety-prone delinquents were more sensitive to pain induced by electric shock than were less anxious subjects.

Some studies of neuroticism and pain have not supported the above findings. Several investigators have reported nonsignificant correlations between pain tolerance and neuroticism [30, 100]. Petrie [83] found no relationship between neuroticism and pain tolerance either with clinical pain or experimentally induced pain, and Eysenck [34] reported low, nonsignificant correlations between neuroticism and ratings of pain intensity in her study of primipara patients.

The relationship between neuroticism and pain threshold and tolerance is not clear, but increased neuroticism generally seems to be associated with increased pain.

In addition to extraversion and neuroticism, other personality characteristics have been studied in relation to pain. In a study quoted earlier, Petrie suggested that persons who tend to be reducers or to reduce incoming stimuli tolerate pain better [3]. A study by Blitz et al [10] of the relationship between pain tolerance and kinesthetic size judgment supported Petrie's proposition that subjects with lower pain tolerance tend to make larger errors in estimating the size of an object than subjects with higher pain tolerance.

Another psychological mechanism that has been considered by several investigators is the use of denial and repression. A study [55] that used chemically induced pain demonstrated that subjects who were less tolerant of pain showed greater use of denial, repression, and symptomatic complaints than did more tolerant subjects. Using painful electric shocks to study the effect of repression of responses to pain and admissions to feeling anxiety, Scarpetti [94] found that those persons who tended to repress admitted to less anxiety but reached physiologically more strongly to the shock than did those who did not repress. He suggests that the use of repression may cause someone to deny anxiety when, in fact, that person is very sensitive to anxiety-arousing stimuli.

The relationship of anxiety, hostility, and depression to pain in patients in a rehabilitation center was studied by Rosillo and Fogel [92]. Findings indicated that these variables were differentially related to sex. In men, the lower the depression, the higher the pain ratings while in women, the greater the depression, the greater the pain ratings. Similarly, in men, greater hostility is associated with lower pain ratings while greater hostility in women is associated with higher pain ratings. Females with higher pain reported more anxiety, depression, and hostility than did females with less pain. For males, lower ratings on the personality variables were associated with higher pain levels. The authors suggest that different conditioning experiences and cultural expectations for males and females were responsible for these differences.

Males may receive secondary gratification from pain in a wider variety of ways than is available for females. The secondary gratification effects a masking of perception of pain as a negative experience. Consequently females would be likely to interpret pain in a purely negative manner. The mechanism of suppression may also contribute to sex differences in the reaction of pain. Due to cultural influences similar to those . . . males may more vigorously suppress negative affects the more pain increases . . . females may have more motivation to directly suppress the noxious features of pain [92].

Dependence is another psychological variable studied in relation to pain threshold and tolerance. Dependence is a term which has many dimensions and is used by investigators to express various phenomena. Sweeney and Fine [111] used the concept of field dependence to describe a perceptual style. They demonstrated in soldiers that those more independent of their surroundings tend to have lower thresholds of pain. Field-dependent perceivers have a higher threshold of pain.

Adler and Lomazzi [1], using a modified ischemic muscle pain test with male physicians and medical students, demonstrated that more field-dependent persons have greater pain tolerance than more independent persons only as long as certain psychological factors do not interfere. These psychological factors were identified as anxiety, the use of coping behaviors, relating negatively to the experimenter, or showing a negative attitude toward the experiment. In another study, Schalling et al [98] used the term dependence as an indication of the degree to which a person responds to social influences. They found consistent negative relationships between pain threshold and tolerance and dependence as measured by the Marlow-Crowne Social Desirability Scale.

These findings again emphasize the complexity of the relationship between personality variables and reactions to pain. These studies seem to indicate that under certain conditions, persons who are more dependent, whether the term is used to mean a perceptual style or response to social influence, also tend to have higher pain thresholds.

In a review of the relationship between various personality characteristics and tolerance for experimentally induced pain, Schalling [97] noted wide variation in how specific personality characteristics were related to pain tolerance, depending on the method used to induce the pain. Schalling advises that "in discussing relations between pain measures and personality, it appears that it is advisable to specify the type of stimulation used in each case" [97]. Her own work [99] indicates that the method of stimulation is an important factor. When constant stimulation increase was used, pain measures were related to certain variables; when discrete stimulation (shocks) was administered, pain measures were related to other variables.

MISCELLANEOUS Several studies have related level of education to pain threshold and tolerance. In a study using radiant heat, subjects from higher socioeconomic groups of college students had higher pain threshold than did a group of unemployed skilled and unskilled workers [101]. The findings of others [24, 120], however, showed that educational level was not related to pain tolerance in any significant or consistent way.

Another variable investigated in recent years has been the relationship of birth order to pain, based on Adler's suggestion that ordinal position in the family can influence personality characteristics. Schachter [96] reported that firstborn and only children tend to be more sensitive to pain than later-born children. A study [31] of dental pain supported this assertion, finding that firstborn children were rated by dentists as more sensitive to pain and more fearful than later-born children. In another study [114], early-born children were significantly more upset by the threat of injections than were later-born children.

It has been noted frequently in the literature that a person's interpretation and response to pain are influenced by his past experience with it. Melzack and Casey [69], for example, state that past experience is one of the factors that has a profound effect on pain response. McCaffery [65] also cites this as one of the psychological determinants of a person's pain behavior. There are, however, few systematic studies that indicate how past experience influences later pain interpretation and response. One of the major studies usually referred to in support of the assertion was done on dogs [70].

Using soldiers as subjects, pain threshold and tolerance were positively related to the degree of childhood protection experienced by each subject and negatively related to the amount of independence the subject recalled having as a child [25]. In another study, Petrovich [86] divided a group of white male patients in a veterans hospital into three groups, according to their own estimate of whether they had experienced above-average, average, or below-average amounts of pain during their lifetimes. He found a tendency for those who assessed their previous pain experience as greater to estimate that pain associated with a series of painful events would be greater.

Other researchers, studying patients waiting to be seen in a dental clinic, found no relationship between recollections of pain suffered in previous dental procedures and present anxiety about the procedures [87].

Although it does seem reasonable to assume that past experience with pain and illness influences current painful experiences, assertions about how past experience operates seem to be based primarily on informal clinical observations and case studies rather than on carefully designed investigations.

This section has been concerned with the relationship of various psychological and sociocultural factors on pain threshold and tolerance. A great number of studies have been done, often with conflicting findings, to explore this relationship. Contradictory findings have been explained by a combination of factors, including small sample sizes, varying methods of experimentally stimulating pain, and differing uses of the term "threshold."

Increasing Pain Tolerance Through Cognitively Based Interventions

Knowledge that psychological and sociocultural factors influence pain threshold and tolerance has led to attempts to try to manipulate such factors to increase pain threshold and tolerance. These attempts have taken many forms, most of them using experimentally induced pain but some conducted in the clinical area with pathologically derived pain. The methods to increase threshold and tolerance, or either of these factors, can be grouped into two broad and overlapping categories, one in which the effort is centered primarily within the person experiencing the pain, and the other in which someone other than the person experiencing the pain tries to increase the threshold or tolerance. Examples of the first category include giving the person information that will reduce anxiety associated with pain and thus reduce the pain, reinterpreting sensations to encourage the person to view the experience more positively, giving the person control over when and how much pain will be experienced, and using biofeedback to help the person regulate his own responses. Examples of the second category are distraction, hypnosis, social modeling, and operant conditioning. In the following sections each of these approaches to increase pain threshold or tolerance will be discussed separately, although it is acknowledged that there is a great deal of overlap among them and that they are based on the common assumption that a person's threshold or tolerance of pain, or both of these, can be increased through the intentional use of psychological and socially based interventions.

Giving Information

That threat or anticipation of an unpleasant experience causes anxiety has been well documented in the literature. In one study [50], for example, one group of subjects was exposed to a threat of strong electric shock, and another group was not. The anxiety level as measured by heart rate was significantly higher in the experimental group than in the control group. In addition, subjects who had reported moderate-to-high fear of shock two months before the experiment showed greater heart-rate acceleration than subjects who reported little or no fear. This finding suggests that how a person defines a situation prior to experiencing it influences his response during the situation.

Helping a person to define a situation in a particular way has been the basis for much preoperative teaching and other attempts to prepare persons for potentially threatening events. The basic notion underlying this approach to decrease pain by decreasing anxiety is this: If the uncertainty surrounding a situation can be reduced and the person can better understand what to expect, this understanding will reduce his anxiety which, in turn, will reduce pain. Some researchers have given different kinds of information to persons anticipating a painful or otherwise distressing experience. Staub and Kellett [106], using male college students as subjects, gave students varying kinds of information regarding the sensations themselves and the apparatus and procedure used to produce the sensations. Those who received both kinds of information accepted more intensive shocks than subjects receiving only one type of information or no information at all. Johnson [52], in a similar set of studies conducted in both laboratory and clinical settings, showed that a message concerning a description of procedure and one focused on a description of the sensations to be experienced were both effective in reducing anticipatory distress. In addition, those receiving the sensation-description message demonstrated fewer indications of tension during the procedure than those receiving the procedure-description message.

Interpretation of Sensations

Closely related to giving persons information regarding details of a procedure and the sensation they will feel is the situation in which people are encouraged to interpret a given sensation in one way rather than another. Some investigators have suggested that, when a person is unsure what is causing a particular bodily state, his understanding of that state can be manipulated. Schachter [95] demonstrated that a state of arousal produced by epinephrine could be interpreted by subjects as pleasant or unpleasant, depending on the information the subject was given about what was producing the sensations. Nisbett and Schachter [79], in a test of this phenomenon, gave placebos to several groups of subjects. One group was told that the placebo would cause sensations that are known to be associated with electric shock. Another group was told that the placebo would produce other common irrelevant symptoms. The first group, who thought the shock-produced sensations were the effects of the placebo, found the shock less painful and were willing to tolerate more of it.

Other investigators [9] instructed subjects to define low-intensity shocks as discomfort and to define them as pain only "when the experience begins to be clearly painful and not just strong discomfort." Here, the notion was that a relabeling of a bodily state as something less unpleasant (discomfort) would enable the subjects to tolerate higher levels of shock. The researchers showed that instructing the subjects to distinguish between pain and discomfort elevated the pain threshold. They noted the potential clinical significance of their study in using electric shock because it produces sensations of vibration, aching, and burning, all of which make it difficult for a person to distinguish between discomfort and pain. Use of ambiguous noxious stimuli produces experiences similar to clinical pain in which the somatesthetic experience tends to be poorly defined.

Neufeld [77], using radiant heat applied to the forearm, instructed three groups of subjects (1) to deny the pain, thinking of it as being pleasurable, (2) to intellectualize the pain, thinking of it as a protective reaction, and (3) to ignore the pain, thinking of it as a blank wall. The use of denial or thinking of the pain as being pleasurable (reinterpreting it) was the most effective approach.

A study [78] to test several aspects of anticipating pain showed no difference in tolerance to radiant-heat pain when subjects rehearsed pain vicariously or cognitively. Vicarious rehearsal meant watching another subject undergo the experience; cognitive rehearsal was hearing a detailed description of the experience. There was no difference in pain tolerance whether the person was watching someone else experience the pain or whether he was given an explanation of what would happen. For some of the subjects, rehearsal of the experience was very similar to what would be expected. For other subjects, the rehearsal was irrelevant, meaning that what they rehearsed was not related to what they would experience. Subjects who experienced relevant rehearsal had higher pain tolerance than those whose rehearsal was irrelevant, after the first exposure to pain.

Subject Control Over Events

An extension of the idea that having information about an anticipated experience can reduce anxiety is that having some control over the unpleasant sensation will increase the person's tolerance for it. A person who expects to have some control or actually has control over the initiation and termination of potentially stressful stimuli will experience less anxiety [64].

A series of studies has shown, using electric shock as the threat, that persons who have some control over the onset and duration of the shock can tolerate higher shock levels than persons who have no such control. Ball and Vogler [3] found that most persons preferred shocking themselves to passively waiting to receive a random shock. In another study [107] subjects who had control over the intensity of shock and could predict when the shocks would occur judged the shocks as less uncomfortable and tolerated more shock than did persons who did not have such control and predictability.

Bowers [17] proposed that perceived lack of control over shock should increase the pain that the shock produced. He found that persons who viewed themselves as usually characterized by the ability to control events influencing them were more anxious under the no-control condition than were persons who see themselves as more externally controlled. Persons who viewed control as external to themselves perceived shock as less painful but tended to be more anxious. The perception of control in this situation increased the anxiety of subjects who typically view significant reinforcers as being outside their personal control.

In another study [38], pain was experimentally produced through electric shock in two groups of subjects. Both groups received a series of three-second shocks during the study. The first group was told that by decreasing their reaction time to the shock they would decrease the duration of the shock. The second group was simply told that they would receive the shocks. Those who believed that their reaction time was influencing the duration of the shocks had less response to the shock than subjects who did not feel they had control. The authors concluded that the *perception* of effective control, even if it is not actual control, can affect autonomic responses.

All of the above experiments used shock as the stimulus. Kanfer and Siedner [54] used immersion of the hand in ice water as a stimulus. A previous study [53] had shown that viewing travel slides was effective in increasing tolerance in a cold pressor test. In the later study, they examined the effects of having the subjects themselves advance the slides versus the experimenter advancing the slides versus no slides at all. Those subjects who had control over advancing the slides tolerated the most pain; next in order were those for whom the experimenter advanced the slides; and the least pain tolerated was by those who did not observe any slides at all.

Finally, two investigators [76] instructed a group of subjects in the use of breathing exercises and distraction. Prior to teaching them the techniques, the researchers obtained baseline measures of pain threshold of the subjects. They found that both males and females who used the exercises and distractions during pain induced by inflating a blood pressure cuff had higher pain thresholds than those who did not use the techniques.

Biofeedback

A recent development in pain-control techniques is biofeedback training. In this technique, a person is given nearly immediate information or feedback about his body's bioelectric responses. As he receives the information, he becomes aware of what actions to take to change his body's responses. Biofeedback's major usefulness in dealing with pain has been with subjects in whom the pain is associated with muscle tension such as muscular tension headaches. By observing the levels of muscular tension through use of a monitoring device, the person becomes aware of how to relax the tenseness and decrease the pain. See Chapter 12 of this text for a detailed discussion of the use of biofeedback techniques for pain relief.

Distraction

Another approach to increasing pain tolerance in experimentally determined pain is the use of distraction. Sadler et al [93] showed that for subjects who were given a task involving memorizing words, the autonomic responses to pain produced by cold were reduced.

In a study of self-distraction, Blitz and Dinnerstein [11] used a reinter-pretation of sensations as a method of distraction. One group of subjects was told to imagine it was a very hot day, the subjects were in a hot desert, and the water was refreshing and pleasantly cool. They were instructed to try to interpret it as pleasant. Another group was instructed to try to focus their attention and concentrate on the cold and to ignore or focus away from the part of the sensation that was discomfort or pain. The most effective method for raising the pain threshold was directing the attention away from one aspect of the noxious stimulus, that is, the pain or discomfort aspect. This redirection was different from the usual distraction techniques in that the attention was focused on one aspect of the experience, and another aspect was ignored.

It represents a type of dissociation of stimulus qualities, separating one quality heavily loaded with emotional characteristics from others. Such restructuring of pain perception might be a useful technique in some types of clinical pain, where complete distraction cannot be achieved [11].

The researchers found that neither type of instruction raised the pain toler-ance, and noted that greater ability is required to direct focus of attention away from pain at higher levels of intensity than at lower levels.

In another study [4] of distraction, subjects were exposed to pain caused by pressure and simultaneously exposed to distractions, including listening to a story, adding aloud, or counting aloud. The intensity of pain perceived was reduced during the first minute of pain but not during the second.

In a related study [36], the influence of an external cue on heart rate was tested as persons were awaiting electric shock. Persons who observed a clock in the six minutes prior to receiving the shock exhibited increased heart rate in the last minute prior to the shock in comparison to persons who could not see the clock. However, those who watched the clock recovered more quickly following the application of the shock, as measured by decreased heart rate. The researchers suggested that the external cue facilitated coping with the impending event. This study again emphasizes the importance of persons having knowledge of when a stressful or painful event will occur. In this case, it helped the person to recover from the event more quickly.

Hypnosis

The use of hypnosis to increase pain threshold is probably one of the most well-known uses of psychological methods [44, 45, 48, 59, 66, 67]. Hypnosis has been widely used in attempts to reduce both experimentally induced and pathologically determined pain. Chapter 10 in this book reviews the theory and research in the use of hypnosis in the relief of pain.

In a variation of the usual method of hypnosis, Green and Rayher [39] combined hypnosis with use of visual imagery. Subjects were first hypno-tized to produce analgesia. For a second method, they were instructed to imagine a "pleasant enjoyable situation." Finally, hypnotic analgesia and visual imagery were combined for the subjects. The method most effective in increasing tolerance of electric shock was hypnotic analgesia. Use of hypnosis plus pleasant imagery was next highest, and pleasant imagery alone, lowest. An interesting finding was that the content of the pleasant imagery had differential effects on pain tolerance. Imagined situations that were directly body-oriented, such as lying on the beach feeling the warmth of the sun, were less effective in raising tolerance than were images that were not body-oriented, including attending a sister's marriage. The researchers suggest that these findings tend to support Szasz's [112] assertion that a primary requisite for reduction in pain is an ego orientation away from the body.

Social Influences

The vicarious experience of watching another person undergo pain has been reported to influence a subject's own response to pain. That is, if the person observed seems to be tolerating high levels of pain, the subject will do likewise. Craig and Weiss [29] administered pain through electric shock to subjects observing models who were responding to amounts of pain supposedly similar to those received by the subject. Pain thresholds of those observing a model tolerating pain well were three times greater than the thresholds of subjects observing a less tolerant model.

Social modeling also was implicit in the Neufeld and Davidson [78] study mentioned earlier. Here, it was demonstrated that observing another person experiencing an anticipated pain did not produce any significantly greater pain tolerance than did hearing a detailed set of instructions regarding what was going to happen. This comparison of vicarious versus cognitive rehearsal of pain showed that both approaches were effective in increasing pain tolerance.

In a study building on earlier results, Craig and Weiss [28] found that subjects paired with models who demonstrated progressively less tolerance to pain became progressively less tolerant themselves. That is, two groups of subjects were given similar levels of pain intensity. One group watched a confederate model react as if the shocks were increasing. The subjects observing the model rated the shocks as greater than subjects not observing the model.

A number of studies explore the relationship between pain reaction and social conditions under which pain is experienced. Testing the hypothesis that strong identification with a group will result in greater pain tolerance, Buss and Portnoy [19] administered electric shock to groups of men. American college students who were told that, on the average, Russians have a greater tolerance for pain than Americans significantly increased their pain tolerance over two periods of administration of shock. The researchers concluded that strong group identification increases pain tolerance as an indication of the individual's desire to defend the reputation of that group, even at the cost of personal discomfort.

Operant Conditioning

The use of operant conditioning as a treatment in chronic pain has been developed within the past several years. Use of this technique is based on the assumption that patients learn to exhibit certain behaviors as they experience chronic pain. People may develop behaviors designed to avoid pain that persist when the pain no longer remains. In addition, the behavior of others toward an individual experiencing pain can serve to reinforce pain behaviors. The aim of operant conditioning is to reinforce behavior that is healthy or does not reflect pain. This technique has been used in pain clinics in recent years, and an example of its use in such a clinic is given in the Greenhoot and Sternbach article that is Chapter 13 of this book. A more elaborate account is given in Fordyce's article, which appears as Chapter 11 in this volume.

Patients' Responses to Treatment

Earlier in the chapter, the influence of psychological and sociocultural factors on pain threshold and tolerance was discussed. Such factors also influence the patient's response to methods designed to treat the pain.

A subject that has received a great deal of study is the personality characteristics of persons susceptible to hypnosis. It may be that the dynamics involved in positive reactions to placebos and to hypnosis are similar, with reactions to both treatments depending on the degree of susceptibility of subjects to suggestion. Placebo responders are reported to be more sensitive to social influences and less dominant and self-confident [56]. In addition, suggestibility appears to operate when that which is suggested is consistent with what the subject expects about an anticipated event. That is, if the person's perceptions, memory, and judgments are consistent with what is suggested, he will be more susceptible to the hypnotic suggestion.

In review of factors related to positive response to placebos, Shapiro [102] identified anxiety as the most frequently supported characteristic of placebo reactors. He reported consensus among many investigators that suggestibility increases with increased stress. Equally important in the placebo response is that the therapist's interest in the patient, treatment, and results is related to success in treatment and placebo effects.

The evidence of the importance of the therapist's interests includes many clinical studies of many patients with varying diagnoses and backgrounds, and treated with different methods by many therapists with diverse orientations and experience. The generality of the evidence is supported by similar findings and clinical and experimental psychology, and by the observations and conclusions of many physicians, psychotherapists, psychologists, and other investigators. It includes the placebo effect, brief and long psychotherapy, psychoanalysis, hypnosis, psychochemotherapy, insulin coma treatment, projective tests, general medical treatment, and experiment and laboratory data. The evidence is no longer isolated, fragmentary or quantitative, and has reached a qualitative stage which has established a generality of the phenomena [102].

Earlier discussions related neuroticism to the intensity of pain experienced. Neuroticism also influences how patients respond to surgery. A study by Parbrook et al [81] of male patients undergoing peptic ulcer surgery and female patients having elective cholecystectomies demonstrated that neuroticism is related to postoperative vital capacity impairment and to postoperative incidence of complications. In the male patients, but not as strongly in female patients, neuroticism was related to the severity of postoperative pain.

Age was reported earlier as being related to pain threshold with older persons generally having higher thresholds. Age is also related to reports of effectiveness of drugs. In an extensive study of use of drugs for relief of acute postoperative pain, Bellville et al [7] reported that age was highly correlated with pain relief reports, in that the older person reports more pain relief.

These data are consistent with results of earlier studies of experimental pain, as well as with the results of studies of the response of patients with placebos. We believe it is more important to adjust dosage of a narcotic analgesic in relation to height or other patient characteristics [7].

The literature on factors affecting a person's responses to pain relief attempts is sparse, except for studies of placebo reactions.

Psychological and Sociocultural Influences in the Interaction Between Assessors/Observers of Pain and the Subject Experiencing the Pain

Most studies of pain have focused on the person experiencing the pain. A number, however, consider the influence of attitudes and behavior of the persons assessing or treating pain, both on the assessment made and on the patient's response to treatment. This is potentially a rich area for identification of factors that influence how pain is experienced and responded to by a person. The previous section included the observation of how important the therapist's attitude is in the patients' acceptance of a suggestion that a treatment will be effective.

Melzack, for example, reports on the phenomenon of "audioanalgesia," in which use of music and noise were used to control dental pain, with contradictory results. He summarizes the original report and the research designed to resolve the contradictions in the following way:

These data, gained by laboratory experiment, provided an insight into the mechanism underlying "audioanalgesia." They suggested that the device could be effective in the hands of dentists with strong personalities, who could suggest convincingly to their patients that they would feel no pain, but not in the hands of those who use the machines with trepidation or simply place earphones over the patients' ears and began their operations. Moreover, there was indication from dentists that the patient's personality was an important variable; some people are more suggestible than others, and this variable, of course, would interact with the dentist's personality. It is not surprising, therefore, that the enthusiasm for "audioanalgesia" first exhibited by the dental profession fell rapidly, and the machines were soon relegated to the attic of dental history [68].

The findings as summarized by Melzack are familiar to experienced clinicians who realize that a strong suggestion accompanying a treatment often makes the treatment more effective. Similarly, patients respond more enthusiastically and positively to health professionals who appear to have a great deal of confidence in themselves and in the treatments they are prescribing and carrying out. Thus, research as well as practical experience supports the notion that the care-giver's attitude and behavior toward the pain and treatments for reducing it influence the effectiveness of the treatments.

A series of studies have reported on biases of health professionals toward patients experiencing pain. A study by Baer et al [2] found that of three groups of health professionals, social workers tended to infer that patients have the greatest degree of pain, while physicians and nurses inferred less pain. The authors speculated that persons who have constant contact with patients in pain may feel so overwhelmed by the person's pain that they protect themselves by denying it, or that health professionals become so familiar with pain that they tune it out.

Thomas Hackett [41] identifies a series of prejudices exhibited by physicians and other health-care workers. He asserts that health professionals are reluctant to believe that patients have pain unless they have a demonstrated organic basis. Second, health professionals use a model of acute pain to evaluate all pain, including chronic pain, for which such a model is inappropriate. Third, health professionals tend to undermedicate patients and to overemphasize the seriousness of iatrogenic drug addiction with patients who have chronic pain problems. Fourth, physicians use placebos in erroneous ways, and fifth, they call in psychiatrists usually when all else has failed, rather than early in the case of long-standing pain of uncertain etiology. Hackett discusses the implications of such attitudes by health professionals in terms of the unnecessary suffering experienced by patients.

Some studies indicate that health professionals attribute more pain to certain groups of patients than others. Zola [122] reported a tendency among physicians to consider Irish patients as being in more urgent need of treatment than Italian patients, even though there were no differences in the seriousness of the patients' disorders, according to physicians' ratings. Enelow and McKie [33] reported a study in which patients with persistent painful somatic symptoms not explained by organic findings were found to have angry relationships with their doctors. The doctors referred to the patients as "angry crocks." The patients were all found to have a "demanding attitude."

Attributions of prejudices are directed toward some health-care workers who have a tendency to view many complaints, including complaints of pain, in women as indicative of neurosis rather than as organically based [58]. With the women's movement has come an increased interest in the study of how symptoms reported by women are treated by health professionals.

A study by Drew and Shapiro [32] is one of the few studies of pain that adopt a sociological perspective. They found that the use of drugs on medical services varied by sex and socioeconomic status, with females on ward service using the fewest drugs. Obstetrical ward patients on the average used fewer postpartum analgesics and narcotics than did private patients. Within the ward group, Negro patients received more postoperative analgesics for a longer time than did white patients. The author suggests that the public female patient either tolerates her illness with less expression of anxiety and pain than male public patients or female private patients or she expresses her symptoms in a less visible fashion to nurses. Clearly the administration of analgesics in hospital wards is related to sex and socioeconomic status.

Winsberg and Greenlick [115] partially refute others' findings of differences in staff attitudes toward patients from different racial groups. Obstetric interns, residents, nurses, and attendants all reported that there is no difference in Negro and white patients of similar social class in their cooperation, pain response, and estimated degree of pain. They did believe that older and higher-parity patients were more cooperative and stoical. In this study, patients tended to see their pain as more intense than did the medical and nursing staff.

Finally, a study by Neufeld [77] indicated that the status of a person suggesting that a treatment will be effective influences the extent to which subjects believe the suggestion. Hypothetical treatment endorsements given by ninth-grade students and by nurses' aides were found to be much less effective in increasing pain tolerance than endorsements supposedly given by physicians.

Recently, some studies have been done that consider the influence of patterns of interaction in hospital wards on the management of pain in patients Fagerhaugh [35], focusing on pain expression and control on a burn unit, identifies the barriers to effective pain management with such patients. Because many pain-inflicting treatments are necessary in such units, it is often not possible to eliminate pain completely. The suggestion was made that patients be used more in support of other patients' tolerance of their pain. In a related study Strauss et al [110] asserted that staff in hospitals are not accountable for much of their behavior toward patients and pain. They suggest that until staff do become accountable for what they do in regard to patients' pain, there will be little improvement in patient care.

Viewing the staff as a whole, we predict that there will be little improvement in pain work until it becomes a matter of collective concern and organizational accountability. When that day comes, the staff will talk about pain care and pain work rather than "pain management," and about patients "reporting" their perceived pain rather than "complaining" about it [110].

SUMMARY   This chapter summarized and discussed some of the research on sociocultural and psychological factors that contribute to a person's experience with pain. These factors are influential in many aspects of the pain experience, starting with the condition or illness with which the pain is associated, including pain threshold and tolerance, how people report pain, how health professionals assess pain, methods chosen for pain relief, and patients' response to such methods.

Although a great deal of research has been done, much of it is inconclusive, with findings of one study contradicting the conclusions of another. There are several reasons for the inability to achieve scientific consensus thus far. Terms such as threshold and tolerance have been defined differently by investigators; the subjective nature of the pain experience makes measurement difficult; different methods of experimentally inducing pain produce different responses to pain; a significant amount of investigation has been done in laboratory settings and findings are not generalizable to the clinical areas; and much of the clinical research is of an anecdotal, case study nature.

In spite of such problems, interest in the study of psychosocial aspects of pain is increasing and many promising new methods of pain relief are being developed and tried in clinical settings. These include giving various kinds of information concerning anticipated procedures or pain, distraction, social modeling, hypnosis, operant conditioning, and biofeedback.

References

1. Adler, R., and Lomazzi, F. Psychological factors and the realtionship between perceptual style and pain tolerance. *Psychother. Psychosom.* 22:347, 1973.
2. Baer, E., Davitz, L. J., and Lieb, R. Inferences of physical pain and psychological distress: 1. In relation to verbal and nonverbal patient communication. *Nurs. Res.* 19:388, 1970.
3. Ball, T. S., and Vogler, R. E. Uncertain pain and the pain of uncertainty. *Percept. Mot. Skills* 33:1195, 1971.
4. Barber, T. X., and Cooper, B. J. Effects of pain of experimentally induced and spontaneous distraction. *Psychol. Rep.* 31:647, 1972.
5. Baroline, G. S. Psychology and neuropsychology in migraine. *Res. Clin. Stud. Headache* 3:126, 1972.
6. Beecher, H. K. *Measurement of Subjective Responses.* New York: Oxford University Press, 1959. P. 158.
7. Bellville, J. W., Forrest, W. H., Jr., Miller, E., and Brown, B. W., Jr. Influence of age in pain relief from analgesics. *JAMA* 217:1835, 1971.
8. Bihldorff, J. P., King, S. H., and Parnes, L. R. Psychological factors in headache. *Headache.* October 1971. P. 117.
9. Blitz, B., and Dinnerstein, A. J. Effects of different types of instruction on pain parameters. *J. Abnorm. Psychol.* 73:276, 1968.
10. Blitz, B., Dinnerstein, A. J., and Lowenthal, M. Relationship between pain tolerance and kinesthetic size judgment. *Percept. Mot. Skills* 22:463, 1966.
11. Blitz, B., and Dinnerstein, A. J. Role of attentional focus in pain perception: Manipulation of response to noxious stimulation by instructions. *J. Abnorm. Psychol.* 77:42, 1971.
12. Blumberg, E. M., West, P. M., and Ellis, F. W. A possible relationship between psychological factors and human cancer. *Psychosom. Med.* 16:277, 1954.
13. Bond, M. R. Personality studies in patients with pain secondary to organic disease. *J. Psychosom. Res.* 17:257, 1973.

14. Bond, M. R.   The relation of pain to the Eysenck Personality Inventory, Cornell Medical Index and Whiteley Index of Hypochondriasis. *Br. J. Psychiatry* 119:671, 1971.
15. Bond, M. R., and Pearson, I. B.   Psychological aspects in women with advanced cancer of the cervix. *J. Psychosom. Res.* 13:13, 1969.
16. Bond, M. R., and Pilowsky, I.   Subjective assessment of pain and its relationship to the administration of analgesics in patients with advanced cancer. *J. Psychosom. Res.* 10:203, 1966.
17. Bowers, K. S.   Pain, anxiety and perceived control. *J. Consult. Clin. Psychol.* 32:596, 1968.
18. Brown, F., Katz, H., and Kaufman, M. R.   The patient under study for cancer: A personality evaluation. *Psychosom. Med.* 23:166, 1961.
19. Buss, A. H., and Portnoy, N. W.   Pain tolerance and group identification. *J. Pers. Soc. Psychol.* 6:106, 1967.
20. Canter, A., Imboden, J. B., and Cluff, E.   The frequency of physical illness as a function of prior psychological vulnerability and contemporary stress. *Psychosom. Med.* 28:344, 1966.
21. Castelnuovo-Tedesco, P., and Krout, B. M.   Psychosomatic aspects of chronic pelvic pain. *Psychiatr. Med.* 1:109, 1970.
22. Chapman, W. P.   Measurements of pain sensitivity in normal control subjects and in psychoneurotic subjects. *Psychosom. Med.* 6:252, 1944.
23. Chapman, W. P., and Jones, C. M.   Varieties in cutaneous visceral pain sensitivity in normal subjects. *J. Clin. Invest.* 23:81, 1944.
24. Clark, W. C., and Mehl, L.   Thermal pain: A sensory decision theory analysis of the effect of age and sex on d′, various response criteria, and 50% pain threshold. *J. Abnorm. Psychol.* 78:202, 1971.
25. Collins, L. G.   Pain sensitivity and ratings of childhood experience. *Percept. Mot. Skills* 21:349, 1965.
26. Collins, L. G., and Stone, L. A.   Family structure and pain reactivity. *J. Clin. Psychol.* 22:33, 1966.
27. Collins, L. G., and Stone, L. A.   Pain sensitivity, age, and activity level in chronic schizophrenics and in normals. *Br. J. Psychiatry* 112:33, 1966.
28. Craig, K. D., and Weiss, S. M.   Verbal reports of pain without noxious stimulation. *Percept. Mot. Skills* 34:943, 1972.
29. Craig, K. D., and Weiss, S. M.   Vicarious influences on pain-threshold determinations. *J. Pers. Soc. Psychol.* 19:53, 1971.
30. Davidson, P. O., and McDougall, C. E. A.   Personality and pain tolerance measures. *Percept. Mot. Skills* 28:787, 1969.
31. DeFee, J. F., Jr., and Himelstein, P.   Children's fear in a dental situation as a function of birth order. *J. Genet. Psychol.* 115:253, 1969.
32. Drew, F. L., and Shapiro, A. P.   Sociological determinants of drug utilization in a university hospital. *J. Chronic Dis.* 17:983, 1964.
33. Enelow, A. J., and McKie, R. R.   A psychiatrist's view of pain. *Occup. Health Nurs.* 15:18, 1969.
34. Eysenck, S. B. G.   Personality and pain assessment in childbirth of married and unmarried mothers. *J. Ment. Sci.* 107:417, 1961.
35. Fagerhaugh, S. Y.   Pain expression and control in a burn care unit. *Nurs. Outlook* 22:645, 1974.
36. Gaebelein, J., Taylor, S. P., and Borden, R.   Effects of an external cue on psychophysiological reactions to a noxious event. *Psychophysiology* 11:315, 1974.
37. Gatchel, R. J.   Sensation threshold, pain tolerance level, and magnitude-estimation sensitivity: Reliability of prediction. *Percept. Mot. Skills* 27:529, 1968.

38. Geer, J. H., and Davison, G. C. Reduction of stress in humans through nonveridical perceived control of aversive stimulation. *J. Pers. Soc. Psychol.* 16:731, 1970.

39. Greene, R. J., and Reyher, J. Pain tolerance in hypnotic analgesic and imagination states. *J. Abnorm. Psychol.* 79:29, 1972.

40. Grinker, R. R., Sr. Psychosomatic aspects of the cancer problem. *Ann. N.Y. Acad. Sci.* 125:876, 1966.

41. Hackett, T. P. Pain and prejudice: Why do we doubt that the patient is in pain? *Med. Times* 99:130, 1971.

42. Hall, K. R. C., and Stride, E. The varying response to pain in psychiatric disorders: A study in abnormal psychology. *Br. J. Med. Psychol.* 27:48, 1954.

43. Hardy, J. D., Wolff, H. G., and Goodall, H. *Pain Sensations and Reactions.* Baltimore: The Williams & Wilkins Company, 1952.

44. Hartland, J. Clinical applications of hypnosis in general practice. *Postgrad. Med.* 50:76, 1970.

45. Hartley, R. B. Hypnosis for alleviation of pain in treatment of burns: A case report. *Arch. Phys. Med. Rehabil.* 49:39, 1968.

46. Haslam, D. R. Age and the perception of pains. *Psychonomic Sci.* 15:86, 1969.

47. Haslam, D. R. Individual differences in pain threshold and level of arousal. *Br. J. Psychol.* 38:139, 1967.

48. Hilgard, E. R., MacDonald, H., Marchall, G., and Morgan, A. H. Anticipation of pain and of pain control under hypnosis: Heart rate and blood pressure response in the cold pressor test. *J. Abnorm. Psychol.* 38:561, 1974.

49. Hines, R. H. The Health Status of Black Americans: Changing Perspectives. In Jaco, E. G., ed., *Patients, Physicians and Illness: A Sourcebook in Behavioral Science and Health*, 2d ed. New York: The Free Press, 1972.

50. Hodges, W. F., and Spielberger, C. D. The effects of threat of shock on heart rate for subjects who differ in manifest anxiety and fear of shock. *Psychophysiology* 2:287, 1966.

51. Jacox, A., and Stewart, M. *Psychosocial Contingencies of the Pain Experience.* Iowa City, Iowa: University of Iowa College of Nursing, 1973.

52. Johnson, J. E. Effects of structuring patients' expectations on their reactions to threatening events. *Nurs. Res.* 21:489, 1972.

53. Kanfer, F. H., and Goldfoot, D. A. Self-control and tolerance of noxious stimulation. *Psychol. Rep.* 18:79, 1966.

54. Kanfer, F. H., and Seidner, M. C. Self-control: Factors enhancing tolerance of noxious stimulation. *J. Pers. Soc. Psychol.* 25:381, 1973.

55. Klapper, J. A., McColloch, M. A., and Merkey, R. P. The relationship of personality to tolerance of an irritant compound. *J. Pers. Soc. Psychol.* 26:110, 1973.

56. Knowles, J. B., and Lucas, C. J. Experimental studies of the placebo response. *J. Ment. Sci. (Br. J. Psychiatry)* 106:231, 1960.

57. Koos, E. *The Health of Regionsville: What the People Thought and Did About It.* New York: Columbia University Press, 1954.

58. Lennane, J. K., and Lennane, R. J. Alleged psychogenic disorders in women—a possible manifestation of sexual prejudice. *N. Engl. J. Med.* 288:288, 1973.

59. Lenox, J. R. Effect of hypnotic analgesic on verbal report and cardiovascular responses to ischemic pain. *J. Abnorm. Psychol.* 75:199, 1970.

60. Leon, B. N. Pain perception and extraversion. *Percept. Mot. Skills* 38:510, 1974.

61. Leshan, L. Psychological states as factors in the development of malignant disease: A critical review. *J. Natl. Cancer Inst.* 22:1, 1959.

62. Lynn, R., and Eysenck, H. J.   Tolerance for pain, extroversion and neuroticism. *Percept. Mot. Skills* 12:161, 1961.
63. Magora, A.   Investigation of the relation between low back pain and occupation. *Scand. J. Rehabil. Med.* 6:81, 1974.
64. Mandler, G., and Watson, D. C.   Anxiety and the Interruption of Behavior. In Spielberger, C. D., ed., *Anxiety and Behavior*. New York: Academic Press, 1966.
65. McCaffery, M.   *Nursing Management of the Patient with Pain*. Philadelphia: J. B. Lippincott Company, 1972.
66. McGlashan, T. H., Evans, F. J., and Orne, M. T.   The nature of hypnotic analgesic and placebo response to experimental pain. *Psychosom. Med.* 31:227, 1969.
67. Meares, A.   Teaching the patient control of organically determined pain. *Med. J. Aust.* 11:12, 1967.
68. Melzack, R.   *The Puzzle of Pain*. New York: Basic Books, Inc., 1973.
69. Melzack, R., and Casey, K. C.   Sensory, Motivational, and Central Control Determinants of Pain: A New Conceptual Model. In Kenshado, D., ed., *The Skin Senses*. Springfield, Illinois: Charles C Thomas, Publisher, 1968.
70. Melzack, R., and Scott, T. H.   The effects of early experience and the response to pain. *J. Compr. Physiol. Psychol.* 50:155, 1957.
71. Melzack, R., and Wall, P. D.   Psychophysiology of pain. *Int. Anesthesiol. Clin.* 8:3, 1970.
72. Merskey, H.   Psychiatric patients with persistent pain. *J. Psychosom. Res.* 9:299, 1965.
73. Merskey, H., and Spear, F.   *Pain: Psychological and Psychiatric Aspects*. London: Baillière, Tindol and Cassell, 1967.
74. Merskey, H., and Spear, F.   The reliability of the pressure algometer. *Br. J. Soc. Clin. Psychol.* 3:130, 1964.
75. Moses, R., and Cividoli, N.   Differential levels of awareness of illness: Their relation to some salient features in cancer patients. *Ann. N.Y. Acad. Sci.* 125:884, 1966.
76. Mulcahy, R. A., and Janz, N.   Effectiveness of raising pain perception threshold in males and females using a psychoprophylactic childbirth technique during induced pain. *Nurs. Res.* 22:423, 1973.
77. Neufeld, R. W. J.   The effect of experimentally altered cognitive appraisals on pain tolerance. *Psychonomic Sci.* 20:106, 1970.
78. Neufeld, R. W. J., and Davidson, P. O.   The effects of vicarious and cognitive rehearsal on pain tolerance. *J. Psychosom. Res.* 15:329, 1971.
79. Nisbett, R. C., and Schachter, S.   Cognitive manipulation of pain. *J. Exp. Soc. Psychol.* 2:227, 1966.
80. Notermans, S. C. H., and Tophoff, M. M. W. A.   Sex differences in pain tolerance and pain apperception. *Psychiatr. Neurol. Neurochir.* 70:23, 1967.
81. Parbrook, G. D., Dalrymple, D. G., and Steel, D. F.   Personality assessment and postoperative pain and complications. *J. Psychosom. Res.* 17:277, 1973.
82. Perrin, G. M., and Pierce, J. R.   Psychosomatic aspects of cancer: A review. *Psychosom. Med.* 21(5):397, 1959.
83. Petrie, A.   *Individuality in Pain and Suffering*. Chicago: University of Chicago Press, 1967.
84. Petrie, A.   Some psychological aspects of pain and the relief of suffering. *Ann. N.Y. Acad. Sci.* 86:13, 1960.
85. Petrovich, D. V.   The pain apperception test: An application to sex differences. *J. Clin. Psychol.* 15:412, 1959.
86. Petrovich, D. V.   The pain apperception test: Psychological correlates of pain perception. *J. Clin. Psychol.* 14:367, 1958.

87. Pillard, R. C., and Fisher, S. Aspects of anxiety in dental clinic patients. *JADA* 80:1331, 1970.
88. Pilowsky, I., and Bond, M. R. Pain and its management in malignant disease. *Psychosom. Med.* 31:400, 1969.
89. Reader, L. G. Social Epidemiology: An Appraisal. In Jaco, E., ed., *Patients, Physicians and Illness: A Sourcebook in Behavioral Science and Health*, 2d ed. New York: The Free Press, 1972. P. 98.
90. Rees, W. L. Personality and psychodynamic mechanisms in migraine. *Psychother. Psychosom.* 23:11, 1974.
91. Robinson, H., Kirk, R. F., Jr., Frye, R. F., and Robertson, J. T. A psychological study of patients with rheumatoid arthritis and other painful disease. *J. Psychosom. Res.* 16:53, 1972.
92. Rosillo, R. H., and Fogel, M. L. Pain, affects and progress in physical rehabilitation. *J. Psychosom. Res.* 17:21, 1973.
93. Sadler, T. G., Wieland, B. A., Mefferd, R. B., Benton, R. G., and McDaniel, C. S. Modification in autonomically mediated physiological responses to cold pressor by cognitive activity: An extension. *Psychophysiology* 4:229, 1967.
94. Scarpetti, W. C. The repression-sensitization dimension in relation to impending painful stimulation. *J. Consult. Clin. Psychol.* 40:377, 1973.
95. Schachter, S. The interaction of cognitive and physiological determinants of emotional state. In Leidermann, P. H., and Shapiro, D., eds., *Psychobiological Approaches to Social Behavior*. Stanford, California: Stanford University Press, 1964.
96. Schachter, S., and Heineman, F. Cognition, Anxiety and Time Perception. Unpublished manuscript cited in Schachter's *The Psychology of Affiliation*. Stanford, California: Stanford University Press, 1959.
97. Schalling, D. Personality and Tolerance for Experimentally Induced Pain. Report #305 from the Psychological Laboratories. The University of Stockholm, August 1970. P. 6.
98. Schalling, D., Rissler, A., and Edman, G. Pain Tolerance, Personality and Autonomic Measures. Report #304 from the Psychological Laboratories. The University of Stockholm, August 1970.
99. Schalling, D. Tolerance for experimentally induced pain as related to personality. *Scand. J. Psychol.* 12:271, 1971.
100. Schalling, D., and Levander, S. Ratings of anxiety-proneness and responses to electrical pain stimulation. *Scand. J. Psychol.* 5:1, 1964.
101. Schludermann, E., and Zubeck, J. P. Effect of age on pain sensitivity. *Percept. Mot. Skills* 14:295, 1962.
102. Shapiro, A. K. The Placebo Response. In Howell, J. G., ed., *Modern Perspectives in Psychiatry*. New York: Brunner/Mazel Inc., 1971. P. 607.
103. Sherman, E. D. Sensitivity to pain. *Can. Med. Assoc. J.* 48:437, 1943.
104. Sherman, E. D., and Robillard, E. Sensitivity to pain in the aged. *Can. Med. Assoc. J.* 83:944, 1960.
105. Smith, D. P., Pilling, L. F., Pearson, J. S., Rushton, J. G., Goldstein, N. P., and Gibilisco, J. A. A psychiatric study of atypical facial pain. *Can. Med. Assoc. J.* 100:286, 1969.
106. Staub, E., and Kellett, D. S. Increasing pain tolerance by information about aversive stimuli. *J. Pers. Soc. Psychol.* 21:198, 1972.
107. Staub, E., Tursky, B., and Schwartz, G. E. Self-control and predictability: Their effects on reactions to aversive stimulation. *J. Pers. Soc. Psychol.* 18:157, 1971.
108. Sternbach, R. A. *Pain: A Psychophysiological Analysis*. New York: Academic Press, Inc., 1968. Pp. 12, 63.

109. Sternbach, R. A., Wolf, S. R., Murphy, R. W., and Akeson, W. H.   Aspects of chronic low back pain. *Psychosomatics* 14:52, 1973.
110. Strauss, A., Fagerhaugh, S. Y., and Glaser, B.   Pain: An organizational-work-interactional perspective. *Nurs. Outlook* 22:560, 1974.
111. Sweeney, D. R., and Fine, B. J.   Pain reactivity and field dependence. *Percept. Mot. Skills* 21:757, 1965.
112. Szasz, T.   *Pain and Pleasure: A Study of Bodily Feelings.* New York: Basic Books, Inc., 1957.
113. Verghese, A.   Some observations on cutaneous pain threshold. *Med. J. Aust.* 2:263, 1968.
114. Vernon, D. T. A.   Modeling and birth order in response to painful stimuli. *J. Pers. Soc. Psychol.* 29:794, 1973.
115. Winsberg, B., and Greenlick, M.   Pain response in Negro and white obstetrical patients. *J. Health Soc. Behav.* 8:222, 1967.
116. Westrin, C., Hirsch, C., and Lindegard, B.   The personality of the back patient. *Clin. Orthop.* 87:209, 1972.
117. Wolff, B. B.   Factor analysis of human pain responses: Pain endurance as a specific pain factor. *J. Abnorm. Psychol.* 78:292, 1971.
118. Wolff, B. B., and Jarvik, M. E.   Relationship between superficial and deep somatic thresholds of pain with a note on handedness. *Am. J. Psychol.* 77:589, 1964.
119. Wolff, B. B., and Langley, S.   Cultural factors and the response to pain: A review. *Am. Anthropologist* 70:150, 1968.
120. Woodrow, K. M., Friedman, G. D., Siegelaub, A. B., and Collen, M. F.   Pain tolerance: Differences according to age, sex and race. *Psychosom. Med.* 34:548, 1972.
121. Zborowski, M.   *People in Pain.* San Francisco: Jossey-Bass Inc., Publishers, 1969.
122. Zola, I. K.   Culture and symptoms—an analysis of patients' presenting complaints. *Am. Sociol. Rev.* 66:615, 1966.

4

Psychological Aspects of Pain

H. Merskey

Interest in pain never ceases. The present survey is intended to indicate some of the main current psychiatric approaches to the elucidation and treatment of pain syndromes.

Significance of Pain

'Unprofessional persons are always accustomed to associate together the ideas of pain and danger; yet the physician well knows that the most fatal maladies are often the least painful' [104]. The author of this remark was an astute physician who distinguished between the pains of angina pectoris and neuralgia, by which he meant what would now be called effort syndrome or psychogenic pains. Despite such views, pain is normally held to be prima facie evidence of physical disease [93]. To anyone trained in biology and especially in neuroanatomy and physiology it is natural to think of pain as evidence of some physical disturbance. Yet, as Williams and Stengel have pointed out, there is much to suggest that pain is often a sign of psychological disturbance. This is particularly true if headache is included in the discussion. As a symptom, it is very common, particularly in psychiatric patients; thus 6.6% of all the patients in a general practice had headache [20] and 8.7% of a population of army recruits undergoing selection [102] while its frequency rose to 48.7% in cases rejected by the U.S. services on psychiatric grounds. For this and other reasons it has been firmly suggested [37] that most headaches are psychological in origin. Further, in considering pain as a symptom affecting any part of the body, Klee *et al.* [54] found that 61% of a series of psychiatric patients had pain and Spear [90] obtained similar figures. In a medical clinic Devine & Merskey [29] found that 38% of the patients with pain and 40% of those without pain were there because of psychological illness. These findings tend to confirm what the experienced clinician has always recognized: that something which is called 'pain' is a result of emotional disturbance in at least a substantial minority of patients.

Reprinted from *Postgraduate Medical Journal* 44:297, 1968, by permission.

A review of the literature [75] suggests that this is probably true in many different branches of medicine and surgery.

It has also long been recognized that emotional factors could abate the severity of pain or abolish it altogether, despite the presence of extensive wounds. Montaigne [78] wrote 'We feel one cut from the surgeon's scalpel more than ten blows of the sword in the heat of battle'. Baron Larrey [21] observed a similar indifference to wounds by soldiers during the Napoleonic wars and comparable observations have been made by many others, either about battle [77] or other exciting situations [58, 82]. In particular, Beecher [11] showed in a systematic study that wounded soldiers, for whom the wound represented an honourable release from danger, were far less in need of analgesics than civilians with lesions of comparable size, for whom the lesions represented a largely unwelcome disturbance of their normal lives. Some of the difference between soldiers and civilians may be due to different effects from injuries due to high-speed missiles as compared with surgery. There are indications that high-speed injuries are less painful than others [65] but this cannot account for all the situations reported. Thus far it can be said with certainty that psychological factors quite often cause pain and frequently augment its severity. They may also serve to abate or abolish it even in the presence of extensive physical trauma. These considerations have an important bearing on what we mean by pain.

It is a commonplace experience to hear doctors talking of pain arising at nerve-endings, passing along pain fibres, travelling up the spinothalamic tracts and reaching higher centres. Walters [100] points out, in effect, that no such thing happens. Certainly noxious stimulation affects the activity of these parts—although not perhaps so specifically as we used to think [69, 79, 101]. But pain is always a psychological event. It is something we talk about as part of our experience. As Walters indicates, the impulses in the pain fibres and tracts 'are no more the pain than the visual impulses from the retina are the perceptual fields of color and pattern that present to us when our eyes are open'. Szasz [94], in an important theoretical discussion from the psychoanalytic aspect, takes the same view. It is therefore preferable always to talk of 'noxious stimulation' rather than painful stimulation, despite the convenience of the latter expression.

This argument may seem abstract, but ignoring it leads to trouble. It leads to doctors telling patients, who are convinced they have pain, that they do not have it because no organic disorder has been found. Most clinicians are familiar with the unfortunate and avoidable consequences of making this error. If so, they may well find it helpful to agree that the patient has an experience which to him is pain, even though no causative physical mechanism seems likely. It may be easier to do so in the light of the evidence that psychological factors are so common as causes for pain. It has accordingly been argued [71, 74, 75] that an operational definition of pain should be adopted as follows: 'An unpleasant experience which we primarily associate with tissue damage or describe in terms of such damage, or both'. This emphasizes the relationship of pain with the experience of damage to the body and, without making any assumption as to causes, it provides a framework whereby the statements of patients who describe bodily experiences like burning, aching, stabbing, etc., can be assessed, investigated and compared. It follows that by 'psychogenic pain' one should mean pain whose causes are mainly or wholly psychological and by 'organic pain' one means pain whose principal causes are physical. There is no necessary difference between these cases in the subjective experience which the sufferer attempts to describe. In each case it is felt as being like the experience of damage to the body. As a corollary to these views it is worth mentioning that 'mental pain' is a metaphorical expression and does not connote any experience of bodily damage. It is thus distinct from 'psychogenic pain'.

Mechanisms of Psychogenic Pain

Three principal mechanisms are recognized in the psychological aetiology of pain. The first, which is relatively rare, is the occurrence of pain as a hallucination, in association either with schizophrenia or endogenous depression [15, 76, 85]. Most psychiatrists have seen one or two instances of this. In schizophrenia the pain is usually one of a number of other delusional experiences, e.g. that the body is changing in size or being interfered with or that electricity or radar is being directed at the patient. Similarly, in endogenous depression any such hallucinatory pain, occurring independently of a physical mechanism, is usually part of a well-defined syndrome. Occasionally with these illnesses pain is the sole definite symptom and the diagnosis can only be made after some fresh development has occurred in the illness.

The second mechanism or group of mechanisms in psychogenic pain is represented by pain due to muscle tension where that tension itself is due to psychological causes. Another variant on the same theme is the pain of vascular distension, as in migraine, where the process can be initiated by psychological factors.

Sound evidence has been available for some years to suggest that pain often originates by such psychosomatic processes [109]. This evidence has not been seriously challenged. Indeed, investigators have continued to present data [66, 67] that anxiety gives rise to local muscle contraction which, if persistent, causes pain. The possible chemical mediator of these processes is still in doubt [32, 106]. Perhaps some of these mechanisms have been used too widely in explanation since demonstrable myographic differences only account for part of the variance in the experimental studies quoted, but it is easy to see how tempting this type of explanation must be, particularly when many headaches and other pains are undoubtedly relieved by reassurance, relaxation and sedatives.

The third main possible psychological mechanism is that of conversion hysteria. The concepts of hysteria and of the unconscious owe much to Freud [17] but did not originate with him. Brodie [18], of Brodie's abscess fame, said that 'In upper-class women' four-fifths of joint-pains were hysterical, and claimed that 'fear, suggestion and unconscious stimulation were the primary factors'. This is quite representative of other comments scattered through the literature of the last two centuries [97].

It is of particular interest that, in the four women whom Freud described fully in his first essays on hysteria, pain was a prominent symptom. However, the actual frequency of hysteria as a cause of pain is very difficult to assess. Although the validity of the diagnosis of hysteria has been disputed [87] and it certainly carries hazards, there is some evidence that hysterical mechanisms are important in the development at least of persistent pain in psychiatric patients. What is of considerable importance is the idea that a pain may arise not as a result of any physiological process but by an intelligible chain of psychological events. There is also good evidence that there is a group of hypochondriacal patients whom most psychiatrists would recognize as having hysteria and in whom pain is a prominent symptom [41]. It has to be noted that in these cases with intractable hypochondriasis the current sources of emotional conflict are sometimes few and the theory that a conflict exists has to be based upon assumptions about the patients' earlier experiences, particularly in childhood, which are not always demonstrable. But the pattern of the symptoms and the patient's personality can indicate a resemblance with those hysterical symptoms whose causes are more accessible.

Perhaps the most striking illustration of pain as a symptom solving unconscious conflicts and serving to symbolize unconscious attitudes is the couvade syndrome. This word, derived from the Basque, *couver*, meaning to sit on eggs, describes the behaviour of fathers who may act as if suffering from labour pains or lie in bed after their wives' childbirth while the women continue with their normal occupations. Such behaviour occurs in many cultures, is well known to anthropologists and was discussed in some detail by Reik [81]. It is not so attractive to the father as it may sound since many rules of abstinence may have to be observed by him. The term has also been used to cover pains and other physical complaints without organic basis which are found in expectant fathers. As such, the couvade syndrome is still known to occur in Indians of many different social levels [9, 10], in mining communities [28; P. Crann, personal communication, 1965] and in modern urban society [26, 95]. The latter authors gave a useful description of some cases and showed a significant incidence of such symptoms in a survey. The point about this syndrome, relevant to our present discussion, is again to emphasize the psychogenesis of pain as a symptom felt to occur in the body and yet not owing its existence to any physiologic mechanism. Having reiterated this possibility we can now consider the particular psychiatric diagnoses with which pain is most associated.

Pain Due to Psychiatric Illness

It has been indicated that schizophrenia may be accompanied by hallucinations of pain but this is rare. In several other common psychiatric illnesses pain abounds. Thus it is a frequent symptom in neurotic depression, in anxiety states and in hysteria. It does not have such a marked association with obsessional neurosis, the organic confusional states, subnormality, psychopathic personality nor, as a spontaneous symptom, with the sexual perversions.

In many instances of course the pain considered is usually transient and responds to suitable reassurance with or without sedation. Or, once it has been established that the problem is psychiatric, attention is directed away from the symptom of pain while appropriate treatment is instituted and the pain then usually resolves with the illness.

The largest series of psychiatric patients with pain has been described by Walters [99] who reported on 430 cases seen for intractable pain. As in other series, the head and neck were the commonest site. Walters distinguished three separate ways in which psychological factors can evoke pain, as follows:

1. Psychogenic magnification of physical pain.
2. Psychogenic muscular pain (as a result of tension).
3. Psychogenic regional pain.

He recommends this last term in place of the older one of hysterical pain because these patients do not conform to the traditional picture of calm and contented hysteria. They are often depressed and anxious even though they may have some form of conversion symptom.

The writer considers this classification only partly satisfactory. The first category is acceptable but lends itself too readily to the concepts of a small, real 'organic' pain which is 'exaggerated' for psychological reasons. It must be acknowledged, however, that no more satisfactory term has been offered for this common situation which the category describes. The second category is acceptable but the third is the least satisfactory. Pain which fulfills the third set of criteria may be capable of inclusion under the other two. Walters' article is well worth attention, however, for the clinical data it contains, e.g., the finding that the descriptions of pain are often not dramatic (a point made also by Wilson [105], Gittleson [38], and Devine & Merskey [29]). In addition, it gives a realistic and helpful picture of the way in which a combination of both general medical and psychiatric techniques of assessment is necessary and the ways in which psychiatric treatment is beneficial.

At the other end of the scale there has been a very large number of papers describing the psychodynamics and treatment of individual patients with chronic pain of psychological origin. Hart [47] and Merskey & Spear [75] list most of these and discuss their implications. The authors considered generally see the condition as some form of hysteria but do not offer systematic or comparative evidence in favour of their views. They also emphasize the association of pain with resentment and guilt.

Menninger [70] gave more evidence of the masochistic attitudes of these patients and stressed the frequency with which they underwent unnecessary operations. Greenacre [40] made the same points in a very telling description of a single case.

A further contribution has been made by Engel [33, 36] who described twenty patients (nineteen of them women) with facial pain. He regarded his subjects as suffering from an hysterical conversion symptom but he emphasized that they possessed a 'masochistic' character structure, showing many varieties of self-punitive behaviour, i.e., behaviour which repeatedly placed them in unhappy situations. Like Menninger and Greenacre he stressed the frequency with which his patients underwent unnecessary operations. He also noted the gusto with which they would tolerate pain due to physical causes. This approach requires some change in the commonly held idea that psychiatric patients are more 'sensitive' to pain, even though that idea is undoubtedly partly justified. In his later paper, Engel [36] named this type of patient the pain-prone patient. Although there is no direct comparison with other patients the volume of evidence which Engel describes supports his argument well.

In order to try and clarify which psychiatric patients were liable to pain, to obtain more data on them and to obtain some check on the foregoing theories, the writer [71, 72, 73] examined a series of 100 psychiatric patients who denied having pain in association with their illness. It was found that the commonest association of persistent pain in psychiatric illness was with hysteria, anxiety neurosis and neurotic depression. Although there were patients with endogenous depression and with schizophrenia who had persistent pain it was relatively less common with those diagnoses. Whilst the material was not confined like Engel's to patients with facial pain this provides systematic support for his general views. A study by Spear [90] both confirms and complements these findings. Spear had studied psychiatric patients with and without pain but had included patients whose pain was not persistent. He, too, found pain to be associated relatively more often with diagnoses of hysteria and anxiety than with the psychoses.

Personality Characteristics and Pain

It has been indicated that certain attitudes, frequently unconscious, have been attributed to patients with pain of psychological origin. These attitudes include hostility, resentment and guilt. Knopf [57] was one of the first to suggest that these traits occurred in those migrainous subjects who were liable to have their headache precipitated by psychological factors. Wolff [109] supported these views. Largely similar attitudes have, however, been attributed not only to patients with pain in any part of the body but also to patients with asthma, eczema, dysmenorrhoea, ulcerative colitis and the other supposedly psychosomatic illnesses as well as to a number of frank psychiatric illnesses. It therefore seems desirable to know whether these particular factors are more pronounced in patients with psychogenic pain than in others. There is no doubt that they are prominent in some instances and that this is sometimes due to mutual antagonism developing between patients and doctors, as a vivid paper by Bender [13] bears witness. Spear [90] looked for the expression of overt or covert hostility and found no difference between psychiatric patients with pain and those without. Similarly, the writer [73] found no difference in actual acts of aggression in such groups. Merskey did find, however, that spoken expressions of resentment were more common in his patients with pain. In four out of thirty instances this resentment was directed exclusively at doctors, in nine at doctors and others impartially and in seventeen at others to the exclusion of doctors. Another study with positive results was made by Eisenbud [31]. During treatment of a man suffering from amnesia and headaches he concluded that this particular patient was unconsciously hostile to his father. Since this hostility was unacceptable to the patient's conscious mind he was liable to be made anxious and hence to develop conversion symptoms under any circumstance that might bring it to light. One such event was his father's admission to hospital and the headache this caused was relieved by abreaction under hypnosis which permitted a subsequent conscious adjustment to the problem. Eisenbud then conducted a careful series of experiments to test the hypothesis that unconscious hostility would cause headache, but not other unconscious conflict. He did this by inducing 'artificial complexes' under hypnosis. It turned out that hostile or aggressive complexes did have this effect in his patient but not erotic ones. The limited systematic evidence that is available does thus suggest that resentment and, to a lesser extent, hostility are specially relevant to the hysterical type of pain. But it is not clear whether hostility and guilt are markedly more relevant to pain than to other psychiatric and psychosomatic complaints.

Other characteristics to which pain has been related include low social class, low ordinal position in the family, frigidity, dysmenorrhoea and other psychogenic bodily complaints. In many studies, not just those concerned with pain, it has been shown that the chronic clinic attender or patient with persistent pain is of low social status—most characteristically from an economic level equivalent to social classes 3 and 4 of the Registrar-General's classification [39, 50, 83, 92]. This applies even when correction is made for selection factors as in the American epidemiological studies by Hollingshead & Redlich and by Srole *et al.*, and has been interpreted as meaning that the less sophisticated patients will tend to visit the doctor and express depression or emotional conflict in 'body language' rather than in psychological terms. Even this view has its limitations, however, for Baker & Merskey [3] taking all forms of pain—acute and chronic—found no social class-difference in the distribution of pain in patients in a semi-rural general practice. As to birth order, the claim that this is relevant [39] has not been confirmed [90]. Birth-order investigation in fact, while one of the most superficially attractive topics in psychiatric research, has produced sadly conflicting results. Frigidity, however, is traditionally associated with hysteria and seems likely to be relevant [59, 73]. In regard to dysmenorrhoea neither Spear nor the writer found a significant excess of this symptom in patients with psychogenic pain but other work [53] leaves little doubt that some association does exist between dysmenorrhoea and psychiatric illness and may be shown by different survey methods.

In summarizing this section it may be helpful to say that while there are numerous variations on the basic theme the most typical psychiatric patient with pain is a married woman of the working or lower-middle class, possibly once pretty and appealing, but never keen on sexual intercourse, now faded and complaining, with a history of repeated negative physical examinations and investigations, frank conversion symptoms in up to 50% of cases in addition to the pain, and a sad tale of a hard life; together with depression which does not respond to anti-depressant drugs. But anyone who relies too literally on this pen-picture for the purpose of diagnosis does so at his own risk. It represents a statistical mode amongst the clinical patterns, from which actual patients will frequently diverge.

Appendicectomy and Neurosis

Appendicectomy and neurosis is a problem of particular interest to the surgeon. Experienced surgeons [48] and gynaecologists [2] are prone to emphasize the importance of psychological causes of acute abdominal pain. Hinton indeed gives the following list of its causes:

1. Anxiety neuroses with conversion symptoms or other psychogenic factors.
2. Physiologic conditions such as painful ovulation.
3. True organic diseases which require surgical care.

Nevertheless, a history of appendicectomy has been reported as occurring frequently in patients with abdominal pain in association with neurotic illness [25]. Lee [64], in a statistical study, concluded that there was an excess of such operations, especially in young women, and that some 7000–8000 unnecessary appendicectomies were performed annually in England and Wales. Harding [44] concluded that 39.6% of a series of 1300 appendices examined histologically were completely normal, and the proportion of normal appendices removed approached two-thirds in females aged between 11 and 20 years. Wallace, Loane & Quinn [98] obtained similar data and Ingram, Evans & Oppenheim [51] considered that unsatisfactory results were obtained in those patients who had had normal appendices removed.

Most of this could easily have been predicted in the light of a paper by Blanton & Kirk [14] where sixty-one patients were studied for the presence of psychological disturbance and organic pathology. Of forty-four patients with an organic pathology thirteen were emotionally disturbed. The remaining seventeen with normal appendices all had psychiatric conditions. A chi-square computation of these figures shows a significant association of neurosis and normal appendices at the level $P<0.001$. But the thirteen neurotics with diseased appendices highlight the clinician's problem. A similar but less urgent problem has been demonstrated by Apley [1] in respect of children with recurrent abdominal pain. Here the experience of pain can clearly be seen to be a learnt response—often patterned on parental attitudes.

Psychological Theories of Pain

Spear [91] points out that psychiatric work to date has led to the development of three main theories of pain. In the first it is suggested that pain is a consequence of hostility [31, 33, 34, 103], in the second that pain arises in patients of a certain personality-type who use the complaint as a means of communication [35, 36]. Mention has already been made of these theories. The third approach comes from Szasz [94] who argues that pain arises as a consequence of a threat to the integrity of the body. Here the body is regarded as an object of concern to the self. The threat may not be apparent to an outside observer and the pain will then be classed as 'psychogenic'. These theories are not mutually exclusive and are all wholly psychological, i.e., they attempt to deal with pain as a psychological event in relation to those other psychological events which cause it. The theory of Szasz, in particular, utilizes the Freudian concepts of ego, id and super-ego, the ego being the part of the mind which relates both to the forces of the other two systems and to external reality. Szasz suggests that the ego perceives the body as an object and postulates that pain arises when a threat to the body is perceived, either for objective reasons or for emotional ones. The question of whether the symptom is considered organic or functional depends on the observer's assessment of the reality of the threat to the body.

Once this assessment has been made the meaning of the symptom can be considered and it is postulated that this meaning may be interpreted at three levels of symbolization. At the first level the communications are facts having to do with the sufferer's experience of the bodily symptom. At the next level pain is used as a communication which requests help. This function is always involved in any complaint of pain, the two levels being inextricably bound. Communication at the third level of symbolization is more complex and here pain can persist as a symbol of rejection, the repetition of the complaint may become a form of aggression and the continued experience of pain may serve to expiate guilt.

If these hypotheses are looked at together it would seem that Engel's views fit well as a subtheory within the system of Szasz. It has been seen that some of Engel's arguments have had factual confirmation. The same is true for Szasz's concepts. In particular it has been shown [91] that psychiatric patients with pain show more concern with their physical health and bodily state than others who do not experience pain as part of their illness; and this concern is wider than the single symptom of pain.

Perhaps the most important aspect of the theory of Szasz is that it emphasizes the communicative significance of pain. This is something long recognized and liable to be forgotten and re-discovered by successive generations of doctors. Further, while the reader who is unaccustomed to psychoanalytic models may have found the theory difficult to follow, it does have the merit of clarifying the logical status and semantics of pain. Anyone who has thoroughly absorbed Szasz's argument is thus less liable to make the sort of errors which Walters [100] has criticized. As a practical corollary the theory of Szasz leads to an examination of the modes of description of pain and the function which these modes serve. Before doing so it should be mentioned that important current physiological theories of pain have been offered by Noordenbos [79] and Melzack & Wall [69] and that these theories can be reconciled with the psychological ones [75].

Descriptions of Pain

Brain [16] observed 'Our vocabulary for the description of pain is relatively poor and we tend to fall back on terms which describe a pain by describing the way in which it might have been produced, even though in the particular instance it has not been so produced. Thus we speak of pricking pain, stabbing pain, shooting pain, burning pain, bursting pain and so on'. The implication of damage to the body is obvious. Klein & Brown [55] found that 58% of patients in a medical clinic used metaphors of violence to describe their pain. Descriptions of this sort are bound to be somewhat dramatic. It is often said that psychiatric patients use bizarre terms when they complain of pain. Dana [27] gave a long list of such unusual descriptions, e.g., 'a pain in the ovary when excited, helmet sensation, sensations of the body being filled and stuffed with pricking burrs and a pricking as of pine-needles sticking out of the scalp'. As indicated in the discussion of Walters' work this view is not entirely confirmed. Thus Devine & Merskey [29] found that only thirteen of 100 psychiatric patients with persistent pain (usually severe) gave notably bizarre descriptions of their pain and fifty-one gave very simple descriptions. The same authors noted in patients who attended a medical clinic that those with 'psychogenic' pain gave similar descriptions to those with 'organic' pain and some of the most odd descriptions were somatically strictly accurate, e.g., a patient with a rectal carcinoma spoke of a 'strong pain a few inches inside my seat—drawing the seat down as if I was going with it'. The worse a patient felt his pain to be, the more words and the more peculiar similes he used to describe it so that there was a statistically significant trend for patients who said their pain was severe to give more elaborate and complex descriptions of it than those who said their pain was mild. This after all is common sense. Severe pains will provoke far more attention than mild ones. The qualitative description of pain is thus likely to reflect the importance of the pain to the patient and how much it matters to him. It is an earnest of the degree of his concern—and not particularly likely to be a sign of its causation.

Differentiation of Causes of Pain

The qualitative description of pain is clearly an unreliable guide in differential diagnosis. The characteristics of pain of psychological origin which are most typical are as follows [75]: Pain of psychological illness has never apparently been shown actually to rouse a patient from sleep. It is usually continuous from day to day (except at night) or else lasts upwards of 1 hr. It often involves more than one area of the body and it is commonest in the form of headache and often bilateral and symmetrical. Apart from the tendency not to disturb sleep, none of these characteristics is exclusive.

The differentiation of causes thus still depends upon clinical skill in establishing the presence of a valid physical or psychiatric diagnosis. Clearly the presence of positive physical signs (e.g., tenderness, spasm) or other evidence of physical disease is helpful. Similarly, positive evidence of psychiatric illness, the presence of the characteristics just outlined, evidence of the relevant personality traits discussed earlier and an appropriate response to psychiatric treatment may also be helpful. There are times, however, when neither physician, surgeon nor psychiatrist can find reliable evidence of a particular illness to account for a patient's pain. In these circumstances the best course is to suspend judgement, continue observation and treat the patient empirically with non-addictive analgesics.

Treatment

Progress both in diagnosis and treatment of chronic pain has been fostered in several centres by 'Pain Clinics' [68, 86]. These rely for their operation on regular consultation between several specialists, usually anaesthetists, neurosurgeons, radiotherapists and psychiatrists. Their work is evidently fruitful, as might be expected, since each of these disciplines has contributed much that is useful to the treatment of chronic pain. Anaesthetists have made a special contribution by extensive studies of the placebo response and the comparative effects of different drugs, again showing how much the abatement of fear may reduce pain. The same point is well recognized by those concerned with the care of the dying [49] and of women in childbirth [21, 80].

It has long been thought that hypnosis would modify or abolish pain at operation. There is reason to believe [4, 5] that hypnosis is not a special trance state but rather a situation in which the subject accepts the possibility of various unusual changes in his behaviour and then produces them on the suggestion of the hypnotist. Thus Barber [7] suggests that the records of operations under hypnosis sometimes point not to an absence of pain but to an unwillingness to state that pain was experienced. Pain as an experience is not absent but is denied; and there are no greater changes in the physiological responses to noxious stimulation than can be produced by direct suggestion without hypnosis [8]. As a manoeuvre directed towards allaying anxiety, however, hypnosis is successful, like other methods of suggestion, in allaying even chronic pain [6, 19, 30].

Apart from these general factors the specific psychiatric treatment of pain is frequently successful. Normally this occurs where there is a well-defined condition responsive to standard psychiatric treatments, e.g., anti-depressant drugs or ECT for endogenous depression, sedation and some form of psychotherapy in neurotic illnesses. Unfortunately, where there is a well-marked persistent hypochondriacal or hysterical attitude, without marked evidence of anxiety or depression, treatment is less helpful. Despite favourable reports of the use of ECT [42] and anti-depressant drugs [61, 62] for chronic pain there is no really satisfactory evidence that these measures are helpful in the absence of a significant degree of anxiety or depression. Similarly, chlorpromazine which can be useful in central pain [63] or in terminal carcinoma [84] is rarely useful in pain of neurotic origin. Perhaps when it is effective this is because of its action upon the reticular activating system. Occasionally, the above treatments work to the surprise of the psychiatrist, but too rarely for him who hopes to treat all psychogenic pain with drugs, so that there remains a group of patients in which the psychiatric contribution is limited to helping the patient to bear with his infirmity and the physician to bear with his patient. These usually are the hypochondriacal patients for whom the diagnosis of hysteria seems appropriate.

With regard to leucotomy for pain, similar considerations obtain as with anti-depressant drugs or ECT. It has been generally accepted for some years that leucotomy is useful if there is much anxiety, tension or depression evident. The combined use of ECT and drugs has, however, greatly reduced the frequency with which it is considered. To relieve pain (including that of carcinoma), in the absence of anxiety or depression, leucotomy must be extensive and will then cause undesirable personality changes. This may be acceptable in terminal illness.

Treatment by stereotaxic surgery may also be appropriate and from this Cooper [24] has made a particularly illuminating contribution to the understanding of cerebral mechanisms of pain.

Experimental Psychology

A substantial literature has accumulated on this topic showing the influence of emotions on the occurrence of pain. Numerous investigations both by this method and others followed the introduction of the Hardy-Wolff-Goodell dolorimeter for heat-pain [12, 22, 23, 43, 45, 46, 60, 75, 88, 89, 96, 107, 108]. This is a field in which positive achievements have been made but in which opinion and emphasis have varied considerably. Dispute has particular centred on the validity and interpretation of so-called Pain Perception Thresholds and Pain Reaction Thresholds. The interested reader is referred to the references cited.

Acknowledgments

I wish to thank Dr. R. Gwyn Evans and Dr. E. G. Oram for helpful comments.

References

1. Apley, J. *The Child with Abdominal Pains.* Oxford: Blackwell Scientific Publications, 1959.
2. Atlee, H. B. *Acute and Chronic Iliac Pain in Women.* Springfield, Ill.: Charles C Thomas, Publisher, 1966.
3. Baker, J., and Merskey, H. Pain in general practice. *J. Psychosom. Res.* 10: 383, 1967.
4. Barber, T. X. Hypnosis as perceptual cognitive restructuring: II. Post-hypnotic behaviour. *Int. J. Clin. Exp. Hypn.* 6:10, 1958.
5. Barber, T. X. The concept of hypnosis. *J. Psychol.* 45:115, 1958.
6. Barber, T. X. Toward a theory of pain: Relief of chronic pain by prefrontal leucotomy, opiates, placebos and hypnosis. *Psychol. Bull.* 56:430, 1959.
7. Barber, T. X. The effects of 'hypnosis' on pain. *Psychosom. Med.* 25:303, 1963.
8. Barber, T. X., and Hahan, K. W. Physiological and subjective responses to pain-producing stimulation under hypnotically-suggested and waking-imagined 'analgesia'. *J. Abnorm. Psychol.* 65:411, 1962.
9. Bardhan, P. N. The fathering syndrome. *U.S. Armed Forces Med. J.* 20: 200, 1965a.
10. Bardhan, P. N. The couvade syndrome. *Br. J. Psychiatry* 111:908, 1965b.
11. Beecher, H. K. Relationship of significance of wound to the pain experienced. *JAMA* 161:1609, 1956.
12. Beecher, H. K. Measurement of subjective responses. In *Quantitative Effects of Drugs.* New York: Oxford University Press, 1959.
13. Bender, B. Seven angry crocks. *Psychiatrics* 5:225, 1964.
14. Blanton, S., and Kirk, V. A psychiatric study of 61 appendicectomy cases. *Ann. Surg.* 126:305, 1947.
15. Bleuler, E. *Lehrbuch der Psychiatrie,* 10th ed. Berlin: Springer, 1960.
16. Brain, Lord. Presidential address in Keele, C. A., and Smith, R., *The Assessment of Pain in Man and Animals.* Edinburgh: Livingstone, 1962.
17. Breuer, J., and Freud, S. *Studies on Hysteria. Complete Psychological Works of Freud.* Standard Edition, Vol. 2. London: Hogarth Press, 1955.
18. Brodie, B. *Lectures Illustrative of Certain Nervous Affections,* No. 2. London, Cit. Zilboorg, G., and Henry, G. W., *A History of Medical Psychology.* London: Allen & Unwin, 1941.
19. Butler, B. The use of hypnosis in the care of the cancer patient. *Cancer* 7:1, 1954.
20. Carne, S. J. Headache. *Br. Med. J.* ii:233, 1967.

21. Chertok, L. *Psychosomatic Method in Painless Childbirth* (Trans. by D. Leigh). London: Pergamon Press, Inc., 1959.
22. Cheymol, J., Gay, Y., and Duteuil, J. Des différents tests proposés pour l'étude d'un analgésique. *Thérapie* 14:210, 1959a.
23. Cheymol, J., Montagne, R., Dallon, S., Paeile, C., and Duteuil, J. Contribution au test de la stimulation électrique de la dent du lapin pour l'étude expérimentale des analgésiques. *Thérapie* 14:350, 1959b.
24. Cooper, I. S. Clinical and physiologic implications of thalamic surgery for disorders of sensory communication. I. Thalamic surgery for intractable pain. *J. Neurol. Sci.* (Amst.) 2:495, 1965.
25. Crohn, B. B. The psychoneuroses affecting the gastrointestinal tract. *Bull. N.Y. Acad. Med.* 6:155, 1930.
26. Curtis, J. I. A psychiatric study of 55 expectant fathers. *U.S. Armed Forces Med. J.* 6:937, 1955.
27. Dana, C. L. The interpretation of pain and the dysaesthesias. *JAMA* 56:787, 1911.
28. Dennis, N., Henriques, F., and Slaughter, C. *Coal Is Our Life.* London: Eyre & Spottiswoode, 1956.
29. Devine, R., and Merskey, H. The description of pain in psychiatric and general medical patients. *J. Psychosom. Res.* 9:311, 1965.
30. Dorcus, R. M., and Kirkner, F. J. The use of hypnosis in the suppression of intractable pain. *J. Abnorm. Soc. Psychol.* 43:237, 1948.
31. Eisenbud, J. The psychology of headache. *Psychiatry Q.* 11:592, 1937.
32. Elkind, A. H., and Friedman, A. P. A review of headache: 1955 to 1961. I–III. *N.Y. State J. Med.* 62:1220, 1962. Pp. 1444, 1649.
33. Engel, G. L. Primary atypical facial neuralgia. An hysterical conversion symptom. *Psychosom. Med.* 13:375, 1951.
34. Engel, G. L. Studies of ulcerative colitis: IV. The significance of headaches. *Psychosom. Med.* 18:334, 1956.
35. Engel, G. L. 'Psychogenic' pain. *Med. Clin. North Am.* 42:1481, 1958.
36. Engel, G. L. 'Psychogenic' pain and the pain prone patient. *Am. J. Med.* 26:899, 1959.
37. Friedman, A. P., Finley, K. H., Graham, J. R., Kunkle, C. E., Ostfeld, M. O., and Wolff, H. G. Classification of headache. Special report of the Ad Hoc Committee. *Arch. Neurol.* 6:173, 1962.
38. Gittleson, N. L. Psychiatric headache: A clinical study. *Br. J. Psychiatry* 107:403, 1961.
39. Gonda, T. A. The relation between complaints of persistent pain and family size. *J. Neurol. Neurosurg. Psychiatry* 25:277, 1962.
40. Greenacre, P. Surgical addiction—a case illustration. *Psychosom. Med.* 1:325, 1939.
41. Guze, S. B., and Perley, M. J. Observations on the natural history of hysteria. *Am. J. Psychiatry* 119:960, 1963.
42. Hagen, K. O. von Chronic intolerable pain. *JAMA* 165:773, 1957.
43. Hall, K. R. L. Studies of cutaneous pain: A survey of research since 1940. *Br. J. Psychol.* 44:281, 1953.
44. Harding, H. E. A notable source of error in the diagnosis of appendicitis. *Br. Med. J.* 2:1028, 1962.
45. Hardy, J. D., Wolff, H. G., and Goodell, H. Studies on pain. A new method for measuring pain threshold: Observations on spatial summation of pain. *J. Clin. Invest.* 19:649, 1940.
46. Hardy, J. D., Wolff, H. G., and Goodell, H. *Pain Sensations and Reactions.* Baltimore: The Williams & Wilkins Company, 1952.
47. Hart, H. Displacement, guilt and pain. *Psychoanal. Rev.* 34:259, 1947.

48. Hinton, J. W.   The surgical significance of acute abdominal pain. *Calif. Med.* 69:418, 1948.
49. Hinton, J.   *Dying.* Harmondsworth: Penguin Books, 1967.
50. Hollingshead, A. B., and Redlich, F. C.   *Social Class and Mental Illness: A Community Study.* New York: John Wiley & Sons, Inc., 1958.
51. Ingram, P. W., Evans, G., and Oppenheim, A. N.   Right iliac fossa pain in young women; with appendix on the Cornell Medical Index Health Questionnaire. *Br. Med. J.* 2:149, 1965.
52. Keele, C. A., and Smith, R.   *The Assessment of Pain in Man and Animals.* Edinburgh: Livingstone, 1962.
53. Kessel, N., and Coppen, A.   The prevalence of common menstrual symptoms. *Lancet* 2:61, 1963.
54. Klee, G. D., Ozelis, S., Greenberg, I., and Gallant, L. J.   Pain and other somatic complaints in a psychiatric clinic. *Md. State Med. J.* 8:188, 1959.
55. Klein, R. F., and Brown, W. A.   Pain as a form of communication in the medical setting. Unpublished abstract, 1965.
56. Knighton, R. S., and Dumke, P. R.   *Pain: Henry Ford Hospital International Symposium.* London: Churchill, 1966.
57. Knopf, O.   Preliminary report on personality studies in thirty migraine patients. *J. Nerv. Ment. Dis.* 82:270, 400, 1935.
58. Kraepelin, E.   *Allgemeine Psychiatrie,* 7th ed. Leipzig: Barth, 1903.
59. Kreitman, N., Sainsbury, P., Pearce, K., and Costain, W. P.   Hypochondriasis and depression in out-patients at a general hospital. *Br. J. Psychiatry* 111:607, 1965.
60. Kutscher, A. H., and Kutscher, N. W.   Evaluation of the Hardy-Wolff-Goodell pain threshold apparatus and technique. *Int. Rec. Med.* 170:202, 1957.
61. Lance, J. W., and Curran, D. A.   Treatment of chronic tension headache. *Lancet* 1:1236, 1964.
62. Lascelles, R. G.   Atypical facial pain and depression. *Br. J. Psychiatry* 112:651, 1966.
63. Lassman, P. L., Moody, J. F., and Gryspeerdt, G. L.   Central pain due to cerebral ischaemia. *Folia Psychiat. Néerl.* 62:34, 1959.
64. Lee, J. A. H.   Appendicitis in young women. *Lancet* ii:815, 1961.
65. Livingston, W. K.   Silas Weir Mitchell and his work on causalgia. In R. S. Knighton and P. R. Dumke, eds., *Pain: Henry Ford Hospital International Symposium.* London: Churchill, 1966. P. 561.
66. Malmo, R. B., and Shagass, C.   Psychologic study of symptom mechanisms in psychiatric patients under stress. *Psychosom. Med.* 11:25, 1949.
67. Malmo, R. B., Shagass, C., and Davis, J. F.   Electromyographic studies of muscular tension in psychiatric patients under stress. *J. Clin. Exp. Psychopathol.* 12:45, 1951.
68. McEwen, B. W., de Wilde, F. W., Dwyer, B., Woodforde, J. M., Bleasel, K., and Connelley, T. J.   The pain clinic. *Med. J. Aust.* 52:676, 1965.
69. Melzack, R., and Wall, P. D.   Pain mechanisms: A new theory. *Science* 150:971, 1965.
70. Menninger, K. A.   *Man Against Himself.* New York: Harcourt Brace Jovanovich, Inc., 1938.
71. Merskey, H.   *An Investigation of Pain in Psychological Illness.* D.M. thesis, Oxford University, 1964.
72. Merskey, H.   The characteristics of persistent pain in psychological illness. *J. Psychosom. Res.* 9:291, 1965a.
73. Merskey, H.   Psychiatric patients with persistent pain. *J. Psychosom. Res.* 9:299, 1965b.

74. Merskey, H., and Spear, F. G.   The concept of pain. *J. Psychosom. Res.* 11: 59, 1967a.
75. Merskey, H., and Spear, F. G.   *Pain: Psychological and Psychiatric Aspects.* London: Bailliére, Tindall & Cassell, 1967.
76. Michaux, L.   Les aspects psychiatriques de la douleur somatique. In T. Alajouanine, ed., *La Douleur et les Douleurs.* Paris: Masson, 1957.
77. Mitchell, S. W., Morehouse, G. R., and Keen, W. W.   *Gunshot Wounds and Other Injuries of Nerves.* Philadelphia: J. B. Lippincott Company, 1964.
78. Montaigne, Me. E. de.   J. V. le Clerc, ed., *Essais.* Book 1, Chap. 40. Paris: Garnier Frères, 1965. P. 374.
79. Noordenbos, W.   *Pain: Problems Pertaining to the Transmission of Nerve Impulses Which Give Rise to Pain.* Amsterdam: Elsevier, 1959.
80. Read, G. D.   *Childbirth Without Fear.* London: Heinemann, 1943.
81. Reik, T.   Couvade and the psychogenesis of the fear of retaliation. In *Ritual: Psychoanalytic Studies.* London: Hogarth, 1931.
82. Rivers, W. H. R.   *Instinct and the Unconscious.* Cambridge, Eng.: Cambridge University Press, 1920.
83. Ruesch, J.   Chronic disease and psychological invalidism: A psychosomatic study. *Psychosom. Med. Monographs No. 9.* New York: Am. Soc. Res. Psychosom. Problems, 1946.
84. Saunders, C.   The treatment of intractable pain in terminal cancer. *Proc. R. Soc. Med.* 56:195, 1963.
85. Schneider, K.   *Clinical Psychopathology* (Trans. by M. W. Hamilton). London: Grune & Stratton, Inc., 1959.
86. Simpson, D. A., Saunders, J. M., Rischbieth, R. H. S., Rees, V. E., Burnell, A. W., and Cramond, W. A.   Experiences in a pain clinic. *Med. J. Aust.* 52: 671, 1965.
87. Slater, E.   Diagnosis of 'hysteria'. *Br. Med. J.* i:1395, 1965.
88. Smith, R.   The Dynamics of Pain. In L. Halpern, ed., *Problems of Dynamic Neurology.* Jerusalem: Grune & Stratton, Inc. 1963.
89. Smith, R.   The use of pressure and chemical stimulation to investigate pain. *Proc. R. Soc. Med.* 59:73, 1966.
90. Spear, F. G.   *A Study of Pain as a Symptom of Psychiatric Illness.* M.D. thesis, Bristol University, 1964.
91. Spear, F. G.   An examination of some psychological theories of pain. *Br. J. Med. Psychol.* 39:349, 1966.
92. Srole, L., Langner, T. S., Michael, S. T., Opler, M. K., and Rennie, T. A. C. *Mental Health in the Metropolis: The Midtown Manhattan Study,* Vol. 1. New York: McGraw Hill Book Company, Inc., 1962.
93. Stengel, E.   Pain and the psychiatrist. *Med. Press* 243:23, 1960.
94. Szasz, T. S.   *Pain and Pleasure. A Study of Bodily Feelings.* London: Tavistock, 1957.
95. Trethowan, W. H., and Conlon, M. F.   The couvade syndrome. *Br. J. Psychiatry* 111:57, 1965.
96. Truchaud, M.   *Étude des Variations du Seuil de la Douleur sous l'Influence de l'Altitude Simulée.* Paris: Romand & Beurel, 1965.
97. Veith, I.   *Hysteria: The History of a Disease.* Chicago: University of Chicago Press, 1965.
98. Wallace, W. F. M., Loane, R. A., and Quinn, J. T.   A study of appendicectomies in Belfast in 1958. *Ulster Med. J.* 32:199, 1963.
99. Walters, A.   Psychogenic regional pain alias hysterical pain. *Brain* 84:1, 1961.
100. Walters, A.   The psychological aspects of bodily pain. *Appl. Ther.* 5:853, 1963.

101. Weddell, A. G. M.   Observations on the anatomy of pain sensibility. In Keele, C. A., and Smith, R., eds., *The Assessment of Pain in Man and Animals*. Edinburgh: Livingstone, 1962.
102. Weider, A., Mittelmann, B., Wechsler, D., and Wolff, H. G.   The Cornell Selectee Index: A method for quick testing of selectees for the armed forces. *JAMA* 124:224, 1944.
103. Weiss, E.   Psychogenic rheumatism. *Ann. Intern. Med.* 26:890, 1947.
104. Williams, J. C.   *Practical Observations on Nervous and Sympathetic Palpitation of the Heart, as well as on Palpitation, the Result of Organic Disease*, 2d ed. London: Churchill, 1852.
105. Wilson, H.   Psychogenic headache. *Lancet* i:367, 1938.
106. Wolff, B. B.   Drug studies in experimental and clinical pain. Symposium on assessment of drug effects in the normal human. 74th Annual Convention of Am. Psychol. Assoc., New York, 1966.
107. Wolff, B. B., Kantor, T. G., Jarvik, M. E., and Laska, E.   Response of experimental pain to analgesic drugs. I. Morphine, aspirin and placebo. *Clin. Pharmacol. Ther.* 7:224, 1966a.
108. Wolff, B. B., Kantor, T. G., Jarvik, M. E., and Laska, E.   Response of experimental pain to analgesic drugs. II. Codeine and placebo. *Clin. Pharmacol. Ther.* 7:323, 1966b.
109. Wolff, H. G.   *Headache and Other Head Pain*. London: Oxford University Press, 1948.

5

Measurement of Clinical Pain

Mary L. Stewart

The relief of pain in patients under their care is a prime concern of clinicians, while the multiple contingencies of the pain experience are the concern of researchers studying pain. Clinicians cannot say that pain has been relieved unless pain relief has somehow been assessed. Researchers cannot study pain until they understand what pain is; such an understanding is basic to a knowledge of pain analysis and measurement. This chapter has been written for those who want to measure clinical or pathological pain for research purposes. Chapter 6 in this volume is written for the clinician interested in pain assessment.

Before the researcher can measure pain, he must be fully cognizant of the subjectivity of the pain experience. The interpretation of certain stimuli as being "painful" is overlaid with past history as well as present circumstance. The quality as well as the intensity of a pain experience is personal and can never be fully assessed by an observer. This is especially true of clinical pain where there is no control of stimulus intensity and where the experience is not the same from person to person even though it may involve undergoing identical pain-producing procedures. Pain researchers are dealing with a psychophysiological phenomenon that can be fully measured only when taking into account the emotional as well as the sensory aspects.

In focusing on *clinical* pain, the intent is to distinguish this from *experimental* pain, in which an experimenter administers a noxious stimulus to a subject, carefully controlling the intensity and quality of the stimulus, and terminating it when so instructed by the subject.

The manipulation and measurements of pain threshold and tolerance levels have been carried out largely in the laboratory rather than in the clinical setting. Experimental pain measurement has for the most part been concerned with the determination of pain threshold and pain endurance in healthy subjects. While some of the methods discussed in this chapter, particularly the section on psychophysical measurements, are relevant to the measurement of experimental pain, the major emphasis is on the measurement of clinical pain for research purposes.

Generally there have been three basic approaches to the measurement of clinical pain. These are (1) eliciting the person's subjective report of pain, either through verbal or written accounts; (2) observing a person's behavior—for example, restlessness, agitation, grimacing, or crying; and (3) using instruments to measure autonomic signs of pain, such as increase in blood pressure and pulse or excessive perspiration. This chapter focuses on the first approach, eliciting the person's subjective report of pain. The second approach, behavioral indicators that are helpful in clinical pain assessment, are discussed in Chapter 6. For an example of a research study that incorporates observable behaviors (restlessness, respiration, perspiration) into a pain rating scale, the reader is referred to a report from Ohio State University School of Nursing [28]. The third approach, using instruments to measure autonomic signs of pain, is not satisfactory in the measurement of clinical pain because such indicators also reflect other emotions or stresses, and other physiological conditions, which makes it very difficult to detect a pattern of responses that is unique or specific to pain.

A person's own subjective report is probably the best single indicator of pain, and is an essential complement to any of the other methods. Generally if someone says he is in pain, then very probably he *is* in pain; if he says he is having a lot of pain, then usually it is best to assume that he is indeed having a lot of pain. A report of pain is a subjective interpretation that does not necessarily reflect the amount of tissue damage present. The frequent disparity between extent of cellular pathology and the subjective report of associated pain is central to research on pain, and is frequently misunderstood by the clinician. The disparity does not mean that the person is actually experiencing less or more pain; it means only that how a noxious stimulus is perceived, interpreted, and reported varies greatly from person to person. The investigation of the "how" and "why" of the differences in interpretation is the target for the pain researcher.

Since the pain experience is a product of interpretation by the mind, the intensity felt can be increased or decreased by conscious and unconscious thoughts or emotions. Similarly, the content or timing of the pain report itself is subject to cognitive processes involving events both inside and outside the body. A person may make a decision (consciously or unconsciously) to report more or less pain than what is actually being felt—a situation resulting in inadequate medical and nursing care and misguided research on many occasions. Usually the error is in the direction of reporting less pain. This is especially true under conditions in which pain is being induced or manipulated experimentally. Often when investigators think they have successfully manipulated a person's actual pain threshold or endurance they have manipulated only his criteria for endurance or tolerance of pain. A person's personal criteria for pain reporting has considerable ramifications in the assessment of clinical pain where, for example, a patient may have learned that being "good" means not to report or complain of pain. When the patient does not complain of pain, the assumption is too frequently made that he is not experiencing pain.

To reiterate, how pain is experienced is determined not only by the extent of pathology but also by psychological contingencies such as depression or anxiety. In addition, the report itself is dependent upon conscious or unconscious decision making and therefore may not reflect the actual intensity of pain as experienced by the person. In the former case, one is dealing with the actual *experience* of pain while in the latter the experience of pain is not affected—only the criteria for reporting the experience. The "error" of the pain experience itself frequently is in the direction of pain enhancement, while the "error" in the reporting criteria usually is to de-emphasize pain. Chapter 3 in this volume elaborates on the psychosocial factors that influence how a person interprets and reports pain.

Psychophysical Measurements

The psychophysical measurement of pain generally refers to the experimental induction of pain in the laboratory setting. In the literature, four variables can be identified: (1) pain threshold—a point at which pain is just perceived; (2) pain tolerance—that point at which pain can no longer be tolerated; (3) the pain sensitivity range (PSR)—the difference between pain threshold and pain tolerance; and (4) just noticeable difference (JND)—the smallest unit of discriminability between successive pain intensities. It is not the purpose of this section to review or analyze the various measurement techniques used in the laboratory or to report on the multiplicity of findings. Those interested in this aspect of measurement may refer to some of the classic studies by Hardy, Wolff, and Goodell [12, 13], or to studies by Gelfand [10], Merskey and Spear [26], and Wolff [40], or to a more recent study by Wolff [41] in which three of the psychophysical variables have been factor-analyzed in an attempt to extract pain factors.

The difficulties in arriving at scientific consensus about these variables have been twofold. First, there is little agreement among experimenters about levels of pain tolerance and sensitivity, which in large part is due to the variability both within and between individuals. Even the concept of pain threshold, once thought to be a physical constant or relatively stable measure for a given individual, is now suspect as a useful entity. Researchers are finding that any of the above variables can be manipulated under certain experimental conditions. Whether the thresholds themselves are being changed or whether the change is simply in the *reporting* of them is another question that is gaining attention.

A direct approach to this problem has been reported by Clark [8], who uses "signal detection theory," renaming the method "sensory decision theory," to demonstrate how a person's report of pain can be distinguished from other sensory experiences induced by noxious stimuli. Essentially

"Sensory decision theory" identifies two determinants of threshold performance. The first, d', measures discriminability and provides an index of sensory functioning which remains unaltered when variables such as attitude and expectation are varied. The other determinant, L_x, indexes the observer's criterion for emitting a particular response, and is a function of psychological (attitudinal) variables [8, p. 272].

Clark reports in his comparison of conventional analysis with sensory decision theory analysis that in utilizing the former, the pain threshold would have been reported as raised; whereas, under sensory decision theory, the experimenter effect of suggestion was seen to raise only the withdrawal criterion for pain tolerance. In other words, the pain sensitivity was not changed, but only the criteria for reporting pain. For some, this issue can be important, especially for those who have maintained that the pain sensory mechanism and especially the pain threshold has biological stability.

A second related difficulty with determination of the psychophysical variables has been the apparent equivocal relationship with clinical pain. All four variables have been measured and manipulated primarily in the laboratory setting using experimentally induced pain. Beecher [1, 2, 3] has been one of the strongest proponents of the position that experimental pain cannot be equated with clinical pain. He asserts that because there are important differences in the meaning of the pain attributed to the two situations, the reaction component will not be the same. Experimental pain, artificially produced and controlled by the experimenter, represents no real threat to the person, while pathological pain with its many uncertainties produces anxiety. Beecher contends that this difference in meaning for the subject is the reason why morphine is not dependable in the relief of experimental pain but is highly effective in the relief of pathological pain. Similarly, this difference in the meaning of pain accounts for the fact that placebos are not as effective in experimental laboratory research as they are in the clinical setting. Sternbach [37], on the other hand, feels that it is possible to produce a response to severe pain in the laboratory that is comparable to pathological pain. This type of pain is the slowly developing sustained pain, such as that produced by a tourniquet method.

The difficulty in trying to apply techniques and conclusions from the laboratory setting to the clinical setting becomes apparent for the prospective pain researcher. As long as one stays within the experimental laboratory [11, 22, 27, 32, 41], there are good techniques available to measure pain thresholds. The relevant application of given psychophysical measurements or findings to the clinical area has still not been determined. Pain threshold, for example, has not been found to have a demonstrable relationship to pain tolerance, so that determining a patient's pain threshold prior to surgery may not be helpful in predicting how well he might tolerate pain postoperatively.

Wolff [41] has reported on a study in which three pain variables (pain threshold, pain tolerance, and pain sensitivity range) were measured on presurgical arthritic patients and then subjected to a factor analysis. One of the factors ("pain endurance") was found to be correlated .42 with a psychological prediction rating of painful rehabilitation outcome following surgery. The same factor had a significant but low correlation of .23 with a six-month postoperative surgical outcome rating. While a correlation coefficient of .23 (thought to be due in part to poor inter-rater reliability) enables a very low level of predictability, this study represents one of the more sophisticated approaches to statistical manipulation and modeling of pain variables and does support the possibility of a relationship between experimental and clinical pain as Wolff suggests.

Types of Pain Scales

One of the most common ways to measure pain has been to ask a person to indicate the intensity of the pain he is experiencing. Figure 5-1 shows four such scales. Each scale represents a different approach to the quantification of pain intensity, and each has particular advantages and disadvantages.

Simple Descriptive Scale

The simple descriptive scale (Fig. 5-1A) reflects the most basic approach to pain assessment and generally serves the researcher well because of its ease

A.   SIMPLE DESCRIPTIVE SCALE

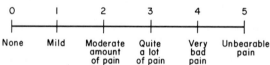

B.   MELZACK'S SCALE

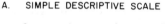

C.   0-100 NUMERIC SCALE

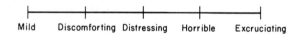

D.   VISUAL ANALOGUE SCALE OR GRAPHIC RATING METHOD

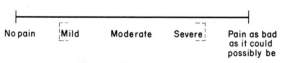

Figure 5-1   Examples of pain scales.

in administration. The average subject has no difficulty in using the scale to indicate a level of pain. Yet, like all scales of its type, there is a problem with words having different meanings for different people. Mild, moderate, quite a lot, very bad, and unbearable are relative descriptors that have no universal anchorage. They are concepts that vary from person to person as well as from time to time for the same person. The difficulty with such a scale can be decreased somewhat by presenting the subject fewer categories to choose from—for example, no pain, mild pain, moderate pain, and severe pain. The reduction in the number of choices gives a more reliable, albeit less sensitive, estimate of the pain.

The investigator should understand that while the anchor words are assigned numerical values on the scale, one cannot assume equal intervals between points. In other words, quite a lot of pain does not necessarily mean twice as much pain as mild pain. The numbers help to convey relative pain levels, but the investigator needs to be aware of this limitation for interpretation and statistical analysis.

Melzack's Scale

The Melzack scale was developed by Melzack and Torgerson [25] in their investigation of a new approach to pain measurement. In testing numerous pain descriptors, Melzack and Torgerson found these words to have the linear relationship shown in Fig. 5-1B. It is important to note that these words describe an emotional or qualitative aspect of the pain experience, and for this reason they should not be considered simply as substitutes for the measurement of pain *intensity*. When used jointly, there is a high correlation between ratings on the simple scale and on the Melzack scale, but not total agreement. This lack of total agreement is not necessarily undesirable, for the Melzack tool was developed to measure a dimension of the pain experience qualitatively different from intensity. Depending upon the needs of the investigator, measurement of the affective quality of the pain experience rather than its intensity may be what is desired.

There are several potentially limiting factors to the Melzack scale that can be easily remedied. The scale as developed does not allow for a "no pain" category, a category that may be necessary depending upon pain status of the projected population. If a "no pain" point is needed, it does not violate any basic assumptions to extend the continuum and have "0" represent the lack of pain. Another potential difficulty lies in the word "excruciating" which is not always understood by persons with little education. The researcher needs to be aware of this possibility in case interpretation is needed. Also, as in the Simple Descriptive Scale, equal intervals between word-points cannot be assumed.

0 to 100 Numeric Scale

The next scale (0 to 100) features an extended continuum that permits more definable choices, which increases the sensitivity of the instrument. The anchor words shown in Fig. 5-1C are arbitrary and may be replaced by others, or only the endpoints of the scale may be given anchorage—e.g., "no pain" and "pain as bad as it possibly can be." While the subject rating pain on this scale is encouraged to utilize the numerical values to indicate level of intensity, some anchor words and clear instructions are necessary if the subject is expected to conceptualize pain sensation in terms of numbers. For statistical analysis, equal interval can be assumed.

Visual Analogue or Graphic Rating Scale

Another example of a pain scale is a line that represents a continuum with the ends marked for the two extremes of the pain. Such a scale is called a visual analogue scale when only the endpoint descriptors are used, such as "no pain" and "pain as bad as it could possibly be." It is a graphic rating scale if "levels" are referenced with the words mild, moderate, and severe, as indicated with the broken line in Fig. 5-1D.

This type of scale has been used to measure such concepts as anxiety, depression, and sleep. Clarke and Spear [7] used the visual analogue scale for the measurement of well-being and concluded that the method is both reliable and sensitive. The method was adopted and modified by Pilowsky and Kaufman [31] and Pilowsky and Bond [30]. For their pain studies, the analogue scale was set to 10 cm in length. The subject was asked to place a mark at some point on the line to indicate his pain intensity; the pain score was the distance of the mark from the left end measured in millimeters.

The main advantage of the visual analogue scale is the avoidance of numbers or word descriptors. The subject is not required to relate specific words or numbers to his or her pain experience, but is free to indicate on a continuum the intensity of the pain sensation relative to the two extremes. Also, the assumption of equal intervals can be met, which simplifies quantification and analysis.

While the visual analogue and graphic rating scales are potentially more sensitive than the simple scale, the subject will not always take advantage of the sensitivity but instead may use only points corresponding to the descriptive terms. A study by Berry and Huskisson [5] comparing the graphic rating scale with the simple descriptive method illustrates this phenomenon. The authors found that 73 percent of the patients used only the levels indicated by the descriptive terms. The problem did not occur with the analogue scale where the descriptive words are used only for the ends of the scale. This pitfall can also be partially avoided by using the descriptive terms to designate areas rather than actual points on the scale (as shown in Fig. 5-1).

Another potential limitation of this type of scale is that some patients may not easily understand how the scale is to be used. In fact, some persons will not be able to use or will refuse to use the scale. The general concept is probably too abstract for many, especially if mental acuity is at low ebb. Because of this potential problem, researchers who use this type of scale may find it necessary to use more thorough explanations or to omit certain subjects from the study.

Johnson's Two-Component Scales

Johnson [18, 19], who developed another type of pain measurement scale, separated two components of the pain experience—the sensory-discrimination component and the reactive component. The two dimensions are measured separately by asking subjects to conceptualize pain as a physical sensation with levels of intensity and make an independent judgment as to how much distress is caused by the sensation. Sensation is defined for the subject as "the physical feel of the pain," and distress as "how much those sensations bother you." While these two components are highly correlated, they do act differentially and can be separately analyzed, especially where different pain reduction methods are being investigated.

Note that while the pain sensation scale (Fig. 5-2) is marked for intervals ranging from zero to ten, it is comparable to the 0 to 100 scale. Johnson's scale, like the 0 to 100 scale and the visual analogue scale, has the advantage that a rank ordering of words symbolizing pain intensity can be avoided.

A Johnson-type scale has this potential disadvantage: the quality of abstractness and ambiguity of a word such as "maximum" may make it difficult to perceive this word as an endpoint of a continuum. This ambiguity can present a problem for some people who are able to project feelings and attitudes only in a very concrete sense.

Summary

The simple descriptive scale offers ease in administration and scoring. However, it is limited in that the descriptive words and their associated points cannot be considered to be at equal intervals, even though they are assigned equally distanced numerical values. More patient-subjects will prefer to use

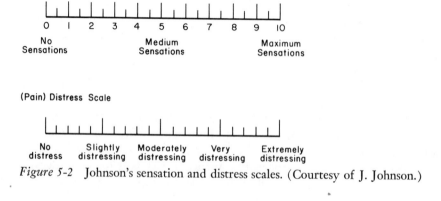

Figure 5-2 Johnson's sensation and distress scales. (Courtesy of J. Johnson.)

this scale rather than the other types of scales. The 0 to 100 scale is probably the most functional, especially where research data requires repeated testing. The scoring can assume interval level of measurement; the scale has an increased sensitivity; and while it is difficult for some subjects to use this type of scale, clear instructions can help to overcome any confusion.

The visual analogue scale moves closer to a "pure" continuum, but its quality of abstractness is its most limiting characteristic. Many people simply will not be able to conceptualize their pain intensities in reference to a line with no guideposts. However, if mental acuity is not impaired and if the researcher is willing to give thorough instructions, this type of scale can be a useful instrument.

If one is concerned with quality of pain experience in addition to its intensity then the Melzack Scale and Johnson's dual measurement of sensation plus reaction are options. Melzack's scale is simpler to administer. It is probably best employed within the total context of the McGill-Melzack Questionnaire, an instrument geared toward quantification of qualities of the pain experience other than intensity. The total instrument is presented in a later section of this chapter.

Sensory Matching Method

A method that departs from the use of paper-and-pencil measures of pain is sensory matching. Sensory matching employs a method of simultaneously comparing experimentally induced pain (or other sensation) with the clinical pain. When the two pain sensations are subjectively judged to be equal, the degree of stimulus producing the experimental pain is considered to be an analogue of the pathological pain. For example, Hardy et al [13] suggested that pathological pain could be measured by matching pain induced by heat. The pathological pain is given an intensity value in dols according to the matched intensity of the heat-produced pain.

Another method developed by Kast [20] uses an apparatus operated by the patient which applied pressure to the fingertip. The amount of air pressure required to establish intensity of experimental pain equal to the pathological pain serves as a measurement of the pathological pain. In the same study, Kast simultaneously compared other methods of pain assessment (patient report on pain relief, behavioral signs, experimenter's own estimate of the pathological pain) with the pressure method and found all four methods to correlate highly with each other.

In the above studies, pain intensity is being compared with pain intensity. Another approach is cross-modality sensory matching such as one reported by Peck [29]. Peck used a simple audiometer to produce a signal whose intensity (measured in decibels) became the auditory analogue of the clinical pain. Patients were asked to manipulate the intensity of sound until the loudness of the noise signal matched the intensity of the pain. The process was repeated several times and an average sound intensity obtained to indicate the relative intensity of their clinical pain.

The theoretical basis for sensory matching is depicted in Figure 5-3. The advantages of this method of measurement are: (1) there is a quantified measurement of pain that can be considered to be interval-level. (2) Two *sensations* are being compared rather than the symbolic representation (a point on a scale) of pain to the sensory experience of pain. The method is more straightforward because communicative difficulties or styles are avoided. It is also possible to check the reliability of the patient-subject's responses by repeating the test several times for any given period. Variance can be checked and averages used for a final value.

The major difficulties in the sensory matching method are: (1) The patient must be in pain at the time of the comparison estimate. (2) The severity of the clinical pain may be so extreme that an inducement of either experimental pain or noise tone for comparison is ethically or physiologically impossible. In other words, the technique is limited to individuals with relatively mild pain. (3) The mental concentration and cooperation required are difficult to obtain from sick or medicated people.

A Note on the Comparison and Validation of Different Approaches

Woodforde and Merskey [43] concluded that Peck's "thymometric" (audiometer) method, the ten-centimeter analogue scale, and a simple verbal description of pain were all significantly correlated, especially the analogue scale with the simple description. Their study was based on two groups of patients—those who had an organic disease associated with their pain and those with no apparent organic evidence for their pain. This finding has been supported in the author's work where high correlations between the simple descriptive and the ten-centimeter analogue scales have been found with both clinical and experimental pain.

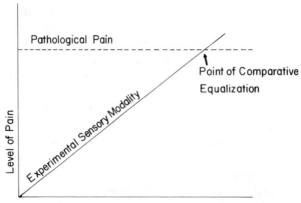

Figure 5-3   Theoretical basis for sensory matching.

Applied Sensory Matching—A Clinical Example

Sternbach et al [38] have combined a verbal estimate of pain with a comparative method estimate that capitalizes on the advantages while seemingly avoiding the disadvantages of both techniques. Their subjects are inpatient referrals to a pain unit in a veterans administration hospital in La Jolla, California. The typical patient is one with a chronic pain syndrome of either known or unknown origin. Low-back-pain problems are by far the most frequent, as is the case in many pain clinics. These patients are not terminally ill or too sick to be able to cooperate with the procedure. In fact, Sternbach's patients are under a contractual agreement to cooperate with the regime presented at the clinic.

Sternbach and his colleagues use a method that avoids pain assessment based entirely on the patient's description of pain, a procedure that invites contamination and confounding of both psychological and sociocultural factors. Two pain measurements are obtained from patients at the clinic. One measure is the patient's own "pain estimate," which is a numerical pain-intensity rating based on a scale from 0 to 100. The instructions given the patient are:

We need to get a more accurate idea of how severe your pain is. On a scale of 0 to 100, in which 0 is no pain at all, and 100 is pain so severe you'd commit suicide if you had to endure it more than a minute or two, what number would you give your *average* pain? What is your average pain *these days?* [38, p. 281].

The second pain measurement, obtained with the sensory matching technique, employs ischemic pain as the physical stimulus against which the patient is to match his clinical pain. Ischemic pain is believed to produce a deep and slowly increasing intensity of pain that is similar to many types of pathological pain. The method employed is the submaximum effort tourniquet technique developed by Smith et al [35, 36].

The technique yields two direct measures: the time at which the induced ischemic pain and average clinic pain are matched in severity, and the time required to reach an unbearable level of pain (maximum pain tolerance). The technique requires the use of a blood pressure cuff, stretch bandage, and a hand exerciser. The procedure as used by Sternbach et al is presented below:

Sternbach's Tourniquet Pain Test Procedure (as adapted from Smith et al) [from a private printing—courtesy of R. Sternbach].
  1. Have patient lie down.
  2. Identify which is nondominant arm (opposite from one used for writing). Ask patient if there is anything wrong with that arm. If the nondominant arm is o.k., it will be used for the test on each occasion. Otherwise, the dominant arm should be used.
  3. Have patient remove any jewelry (watch, rings, etc.) from arm to be used.
  4. Explain the basic procedure to the patient in a brief fashion and mention that he may ask questions if he wishes.
  5. Raise the arm to be used, and then begin wrapping arm with rubber Esmarch

bandage. Wrap the arm very tightly, starting with the top of the finger tips to just slightly beyond the elbow. Tuck any extra bandage roll into the wrappings.

6. Inflate blood pressure cuff to 250, with the cuff placed in the normal position, and just at the end of the Esmarch bandage.
7. Remove Esmarch bandage.
8. Lower arm and begin stopwatch for a 60-second pause. During this period, make sure the cuff stays at 250.
9. Give patient hand exerciser and tell him to squeeze-release, every 2 seconds for 20 squeezes. When the second hand passes 1 minute 20 seconds, he will have completed 20 squeezes.
10. *Restart* stopwatch by pressing side button. Timing begins when last squeeze completed.
11. Ask patient to tell when what he feels in his arm feels similar to: (1) the average pain he has had for the past week; and (2) the "unbearable" level (the most he can take).
12. When patient says the pain in his arm is unbearable, stop the watch by pressing the large center knob and release the cuff. That is the end of the test.
    Note: Be sure patient compares arm feeling to pain he has had. Question him if he says it is "unbearable" and hasn't mentioned clinical pain.

If patient does not reach "clinical" level in 15 minutes, stop the test and remove cuff.

Note that the basic unit of measure is "the amount of time (in seconds) from the cessation of exercise until the pain reaches a given level" [38, p. 284].

The Sternbach group uses several pain measures—clinical pain level, maximum pain tolerance, the difference between the two or the "pain ratio" which is the proportion of clinic to maximum pain multiplied by 100

$$\frac{\text{clinical pain in seconds}}{\text{maximum pain in seconds}} \times 100$$

and the difference between the pain estimate (discussed earlier) and the pain ratio. By multiplying the proportion by 100, the ratio assumes comparable status to the pain estimate with its range of 0 to 100. Sternbach sees the difference between the patient's pain estimate and the pain ratio having a useful diagnostic function. "When the former is much higher—and it is often very much higher—we assume the patient is exaggerating the severity of his pain, and we discuss the difference with him. If the Pain Estimate is much lower, as occasionally happens, we assume the patient is unusually stoical for some reason, and we discuss that with him" [38, p. 287].

The *general* validity of the ischemic pain–clinical pain comparison method is apparent. Smith et al [35, 36] reported supporting evidence of validity by testing ischemic pain measures associated with relief from various analgesics. Validity is also supported in the Sternbach et al [38] study in that the measures reflected expected pain levels before and after surgery (pain levels are reduced following surgical intervention). However, there is some question of validity when one looks at the maximum tolerance pain estimate of the tourniquet pain test. Theoretically, these levels should stay approximately the same over weeks of testing even though the *clinical* pain varies. However, when one looks at the data presented, the maximum pain varies with the clinical pain. When clinical pain is reduced, so is the maximum tolerance. The association between clinical pain and maximum tolerance tends to dampen the differential values of the pain ratio. An interesting note is that the apparent psychological factor of pain relativity—one's perception of maximum pain tolerance—is always higher than current perceived clinical pain (using this technique), but apparently one does not endure the same high level of maximum tolerance when clinical pain is low. The judgment of maximum pain tolerance is relative to the current clinical pain.

Retesting of the tourniquet (ischemic) pain measures over time by Sternbach et al showed them to be reliable with correlations in the .70s to .90s for the low-back-pain group but lower (high .40s to .70s) in the chronic-pain group (patients on the pain unit)—a phenomenon attributed by the authors to nonspecific treatment effects. The matched clinical pain correlations were generally lower than repeated measurements in which patients were asked to indicate when the tourniquet pain was slight, moderate, severe, or unbearable. The lower correlations for clinical pain measurement are assumed to be a reflection of the inherent variability in clinical pain. However, the repeated measures of "unbearable" (with tourniquet pain) had correlations only in the .60s to low .70s for the *inpatient group* (chronic pain)—a probable function of the questioned validity in "maximum tolerance" discussed above—while the figure for repeated tests on "normals" for indicating unbearable pain was .89. One would question whether chronic pain patients are somehow less able to authenticate their pain experience, or are their lower correlations again a function of relative adjustment to a fluctuating clinical pain?

Stewart Pain-Color Scale and Pain Circles

The author has developed another approach to sensory matching in an attempt to avoid the limitations of high sound intensities for comparison measurement of clinical pain. Sensory stimuli, either in the form of light intensity or color intensity, can also be provided via sight. Color intensity was selected for development of pain measures when it became apparent that nearly all people will pick red to represent pain when given the chance to choose from an array of primary colors. Further, if asked to associate degree of pain intensity with color hue, subjects show high agreement in the choice of color. Oranges or orange-reds were chosen for milder pain with stronger or redder hues selected to indicate increasing pain intensity. Some subjects chose purples and blacks to represent projected severe pain. In other words, there is an almost natural ranking of red shades that can be associated with degree of pain intensity.

Figure 5-4 presents the Stewart Pain-Color Scale, an assessment instrument that presents the subject with a chromatic array of yellow-orange-red-black. A sliding pointer can be set by the subject to indicate the redness that best represents his pain. The anchor words for each end of the color continuum were added after pilot work confirmed that subjects with little or no pain would freely use the left side of the scale (yellow, orange), those with severe pain would choose colors to the far right, and those having moderate pain intensities would use the middle range of the scale. The color scale has been easily used by patients with a variety of characteristics and painful conditions—medical, surgical, burns, cancer, little pain, extreme pain, young and old.

There are two dimensions to the color continuum: pain quality or intensity that increases to a brilliant red, and pain quality or intensity that increases to a shade of black. The first dimension seems to be associated with the intensity of the pain and the second, with the affective component. The correlation coefficient of 0.60 between the color scale and the simple descriptive scale, based on 163 patients, was found to be significant at the 0.001 level.

Because both red and black can represent pain, a projective technique was developed in an attempt to capture the emotional feeling tone accompanying the pain. The instrument consists of six circle-figures, with the colors red and black having interchangeable positions as inner or outer circles (see Fig. 5-5). In the instructions, subjects are asked to choose a figure (1 to 6) that represents their pain *now* and a figure (1 to 6) that represents their pain at its *worst*. They also are asked which color-circle (red or black) represents "self" and which represents "pain." At the same time, pain intensity measurements were obtained on the pain-color scale described above and on the simple descriptive scale described in a previous section.

Both the color scale and the circle-figures were tested on a sample of hospitalized patients at a large university hospital in Iowa. The patients belonged to one of three pain groups according to pathology—rheumatoid arthritis, cancer, and cholecystitis or hernia patients undergoing surgery. These groups were termed Short-term pain (surgery), Long-term pain (arthritis), and Progressive pain (cancer) to denote a different meaning that the pain holds for different group members. Table 5-1 shows the distribution of circle-figures chosen for "pain now" and "pain worst."

Table 5-1 presents strong evidence of the differentiating power of the six circle-figures. Because patients generally are interviewed when their pain intensity is relatively low, it is expected that the intensity of their worst pain would be higher than their current pain. This expectation is reflected in the shift of figures chosen to represent each state. The figures containing less red or black (figures 1, 3, 5) are chosen 68 percent of the time with "pain now" and only 15 percent of the time for "worst pain," while figures 2, 4, 6 shift from 32 percent for "pain now" to 85 percent for "worst pain." Circle-figure 4, with the larger black outer circle, is the most frequently chosen circle for "worst pain," followed closely by circle-figure 6 with a large red inner circle and circle-figure 2, which has the large red outer

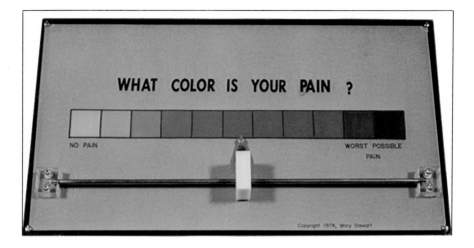

Figure 5-4 Stewart Pain-Color Scale.

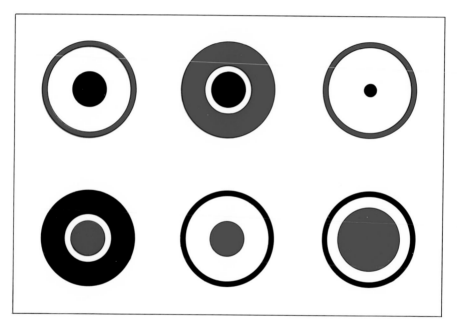

Figure 5-5 Stewart's pain circles.

Table 5-1 Percentage distribution of circle-figures under two pain conditions

Circle-figure	Pain now (%)	Pain worst (%)
1	14	5
2	18	22
3	37	3
4	8	33
5	17	7
6	6	30
N = 157		

circle. Pain intensity measurements on the color and simple scales associated with circle-figure 4 are also the highest (see Table 5-2), especially with measurements on current pain. Higher intensity measures for circle-figures 2 and 6 are close seconds. One-way analysis of variance tests for differences across the circle-figures on pain measurement yielded differences significant for both the color and simple scales in both pain conditions.

Table 5-3 shows the distribution of circle-figures chosen, according to pathological classification.

In the "worst pain" column, two points are designated with a box showing where there are marked differences between arthritic and cancer patients on the one hand and postsurgical patients on the other. Only 18 percent of the surgical patients chose circle-figure 4 (black outer circle) as compared with 41 and 42 percent of the arthritic and cancer patients. The surgical group preferred circle-figures 2 and 6 for their worst pain—figures with more red relative to smaller black circles.

Patients also were asked to decide which circle, red or black, represented *pain* and which represented *self*. Table 5-4 depicts the data for the color chosen to represent *pain*—the other color-circle would then represent *self*. All figures, with the exception of circle-figure 1 for "pain now," show a clear color preference for indicating pain.

Not only does the choice of color need to be considered, but also the re-

Table 5-2 Pain intensity means for circle-figures under two pain conditions

| Circle-figure | Pain Now | | Pain Worst | |
	Color scale (range 1–11)	Simple scale (range 0–5)	Color scale (range 1–11)	Simple scale (range 0-5)
1	2.7	1.0	6.7	1.8
2	5.8	2.3	8.1	2.9
3	2.7	1.0	5.8	2.1
4	7.6	2.7	8.9	3.1
5	4.3	1.9	6.5	2.7
6	5.9	2.3	8.4	3.1
N = 157				

Table 5-3 Circle-figures rated under two pain conditions according to pathology

Circle-figure	Pain now			Pain worst		
	Surgical %	RA %	Ca %	Surgical %	RA %	Ca %
1	17	8	18	9	2	3
2	23	19	10	23	24	19
3	32	38	44	7	2	0
4	9	9	3	18	41	42
5	14	19	21	7	4	10
6	4	7	5	36	26	26
N =	65	53	39	65	53	39

lationship of *self* to *pain*. For circle-figure 2, the majority of patients chose the red *outside* circle for *pain* and the *inner* black circle as *self*. For circle-figure 6, most patients chose the large red inner circle to represent *pain*. With circle-figure 4, where 97 percent chose black to represent their worst pain, the *pain* component of the figure again surrounds the *self*.

The choice of color seems especially significant in view of the preponderance of arthritic and cancer patients who chose circle-figure 4 to represent their "worst pain." For circle-figures 1 and 3, a higher percentage of the patients preferred black to represent their pain, with the exception of circle-figure 1 for "pain now," where there was a 50–50 percent choice. For these two circle-figures, the black circle is contained within the outer red circle; also, there is less pain associated with these two than with the others (Table 5-2). Circle-figure 5 has black as the outside circle; and the red circle, preferred by the majority of patients to represent their pain, is the inside circle (surrounded by self). The choice of figure and color is assumed to be determined in large by the level of pain they were experiencing. Circle-figure 5 represents less pain (Table 5-2) than circle-figures 2, 4, or 6, but more

Table 5-4 Color chosen to represent pain in circle-figures under two pain conditions

Circle-figure	Pain Now		Pain Worst	
	Red %	Black %	Red %	Black %
1	50	50	17	83
2	69	31	89	11
3	29	71	25	75
4	33	67	3	97
5	93	7	87	13
6	67	33	97	3
N =	83	74	83	74

pain than circle-figures 1 and 3. There is less red in circle-figure 5 than in circle-figures 2 and 6.

Why many of the patients chose black to represent their pain for circle-figures 1 and 3 is not completely understood at this time. The sample size is too small for relevant comparisons or conclusions. Further testing is being done to determine whether such factors as despondency, locus of control, and denial have some part in the decision process. Also, neuroticism will be further analyzed since there is an indication that those subjects who chose black to represent pain are higher on this personality dimension than those who chose red.

The possible reasons for the choice of color and rating of the pain-self relationship are highly speculative at this time, but there are certain aspects of color theory that lend themselves to an explanation. The choice of the color red to represent pain was empirical, as was the choice of black. According to the literature [6, 21, 33, 34], red is said to be exciting, stimulating, and when chosen in large quantities, to represent impulsive affect or impulsive extroverted emotionality. Black, on the other hand, is said to be indicative of inhibition and blocking of feelings of inadequacy; it is also a signal of depression, sadness, and to some, a sign of evil, darkness, and fear. Patients with rheumatoid arthritis or cancer were much more likely to choose circle-figure 4 with black for their worst pain color than were surgical patients. This choice of black would be associated theoretically with the "darker" depressive component of their pain, as compared with the relatively short-term pain of the surgical patient. Most of the arthritic patients have had to cope with pain, the crippling effects of their disease, and the knowledge that it is incurable, while the pain of cancer is associated with an extremely fearful and depressing condition that may ultimately end in death. The choice of circle-figure 6 for some patients points to an all-encompassing focus on pain. The fact that many of these patient-subjects do seem by observation to have characteristics of impulsive affect or extroverted emotionality points to the need for further investigation.

The Stewart circle-figures represent a new approach to pain measurement. The instrument is still in its early developmental stages but shows promise as a means of assessing qualitative aspects of the pain experience that serves to differentiate individuals as well as groups.

The McGill-Melzack Pain Questionnaire

The McGill-Melzack Pain Questionnaire, which is a relatively new instrument in the quest for quantification of clinical pain, attempts to measure something more than just the intensity component of the pain experience. The questionnaire is based on classes of word descriptors specifying different aspects of the pain experience. The classes of words were developed from an earlier study by Melzack and Torgerson [25]. Words are categorized into 16 subclasses comprising the three major classes.

The classes are: (1) words that describe the *sensory qualities* of the experience in terms of temporal, spatial, pressure, thermal and other properties; (2) words that describe *affective qualities*, in terms of tension, fear, and autonomic properties that are part of the pain experience; and (3) *evaluative* words that describe the subjective overall intensity of the total pain experience. Each subclass . . . consists of a group of words that are considered . . . to be qualitatively similar. Some of these words are undoubtedly synonyms, others seem to be synonymous but vary in intensity, while many provide subtle differences or nuances (despite their similarities) that may be of importance to a patient who is trying desperately to communicate to a physician [24, p. 278].

The words within each subgroup were determined by Melzack and Torgerson to be ranked according to pain intensity. For example, pounding pain is considered worse than pulsing pain and stabbing implies more pain than boring which, in turn, represents more pain than pricking. The words can be assigned a ranking number (the word in each subclass implying the least pain is given a value of 1, the next word a value of 2, and so forth). A pain intensity score can thereby be obtained for each subclass (sensory, affect, evaluative, and miscellaneous) or obtained from the total scores of all the chosen words.

Melzack also uses a pain-rating index that is based on scale values derived from the original Melzack-Torgerson study. Their values were determined by asking a group of doctors and a group of patients to assign each word in a given category a position on a five-point word-number scale where the words mild, discomforting, distressing, horrible, and excruciating served as anchor words. The values 1 and 5 represented the lowest and highest pain values respectively. The actual scale values are not included in this chapter but can be obtained from the Melzack-Torgerson reference [25, pp. 54–55]. Two pain-rating indexes can be obtained: (1) the total of the scale values chosen in a given category (sensory, affective, or evaluative) or for all categories and (2) the total of the rank values of words chosen by a patient for each category, or a total score. Another accounting of overall pain evaluation is simply the total number of words chosen. The McGill-Melzack Pain Assessment Questionnaire [24] is shown in its entirety on pages 126 and 127.

Part 1 (Where Is Your Pain?) of the questionnaire is useful in the delineation of pain location, especially as progress is being assessed. More important, the body drawing offers an easy mode for the patient or client who has difficulty in communicating. The drawing of the body should be of a neutral figure such as the drawing included in this chapter that has been relatively successful in its portrayal of a sexless figure.

Part 2 contains the words and categories discussed earlier. Group numbers 1 to 10 constitute the *sensory* subclass; numbers 11 to 15 make up the *affective* subclass; category 16 is the only group in the *evaluative* class, and groups 17 to 20 (added at a later date) are classified under miscellaneous. The latter group (17 to 20) may present difficulty if used for pain intensity purposes since it is not clear whether words in each subgroup can be assumed to be in rank order except perhaps for subgroup 19. For example, "piercing" seems to have a different connotation than "spreading," but does it imply higher intensity?

Part 3 includes words for describing the pattern of pain and information-seeking questions regarding relief and aggravation of pain. The answers to these questions, while not easily quantified, may provide meaningful research information. Part 4, which elicits information on the subject's perception of pain intensity, utilizes anchor words derived from the Melzack and Torgerson [25] study. These words carrying a more affective quality of the pain experience were discussed in the earlier section on scales. While Part 4 reportedly provides information on the patient's tendency to rate pain at the low or high end of the pain scale, its usefulness has not yet been demonstrated. Part of the weakness seems to lie in the difficulty in interpretation of the obtained values. However, the entire tool is still in the pioneering state and will undoubtedly undergo further refinement.

Melzack [24], reporting on the properties and scoring methods of the questionnaire, discusses the method of administration and analysis. This article should be referred to if the reader intends to use the questionnaire. Melzack maintains that four types of quantitative data can be obtained from the questionnaire (in addition to the information from other sections): the two pain-rating indexes based on scale values and on the ranking of the words in each subcategory; the total number of words chosen; and the present pain intensity, which is the number-word combination (Part 4), used as an indicator of the overall pain intensity. Whether a total score in Part 4 across all items, a subtotal based on the clinical pain items, or only a value for "pain now" should be used would depend in part on the objectives and interests of the researcher.

Since the words in each group purportedly assume different pain intensities, the values of the chosen words should have some correlation with the intensity of pain indicated in Part 4. Melzack [24] reports that correlations between the "overall present pain intensity" (Part 4) and the pain-rating indexes (scale or rank values of words in each word group) are between .30 and .40, which suggest there is little relationship; he contends that the variance in the pain intensity score of Part 4 is associated with factors other than those indicated by the word descriptors. Similar correlations between the two independent pain measurement parts of the questionnaire were found in this author's work based on samples of hospitalized patients with multiple diagnoses [39]. Melzack states that the verbal descriptors represent specification of the properties of pain (involving multiple choices) and are therefore not as subject to the psychological impendencies of the moment as is the word-number estimate of pain which, by contrast, involves a single choice. In other words, the relative rank of the descriptor word(s) chosen may be a more stable and reliable, albeit rough, indicator of pain intensity than is a chosen value on the word-number scale. In fact, Melzack does find the word-number estimate of pain less satisfactory for reflecting

A

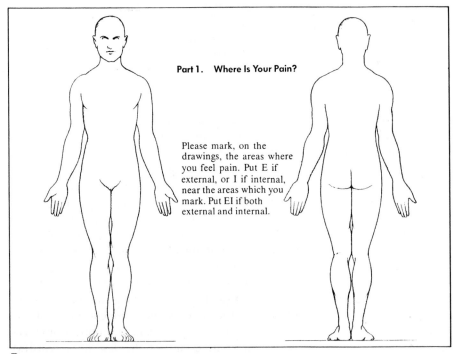

B

Figure 5-6 McGill-Melzack Pain Assessment Questionnaire. (Courtesy of R.
Melzack.) A. Cover Sheet. B. Part One. C. Part Two. D. Parts Three and Four.

Part 2. What Does Your Pain Feel Like?

Some of the words below describe your present pain. Circle ONLY those words that best describe it. Leave out any category that is not suitable. Use only a single word in each appropriate category--the one that applies best.

1	2	3	4	5
Flickering	Jumping	Pricking	Sharp	Pinching
Quivering	Flashing	Boring	Cutting	Pressing
Pulsing	Shooting	Drilling	Lacerating	Gnawing
Throbbing		Stabbing		Cramping
Beating		Lancinating		Crushing

6	7	8	9	10
Tugging	Hot	Tingling	Dull	Tender
Pulling	Burning	Itchy	Sore	Taut
Wrenching	Scalding	Smarting	Hurting	Rasping
	Searing	Stinging	Aching	Splitting
			Heavy	

11	12	13	14	15
Tiring	Sickening	Fearful	Punishing	Wretched
Exhausting	Suffocating	Frightful	Gruelling	Blinding
		Terrifying	Cruel	
			Vicious	
			Killing	

16	17	18	19	20
Annoying	Spreading	Tight	Cool	Nagging
Troublesome	Radiating	Numb	Cold	Nauseating
Miserable	Penetrating	Drawing	Freezing	Agonizing
Intense	Piercing	Squeezing		Dreadful
Unbearable		Tearing		Torturing

C

Part 3. How Does Your Pain Change With Time?

1. Which word or words would you use to describe the pattern of your pain?

1	2	3
Continuous	Rhythmic	Brief
Steady	Periodic	Momentary
Constant	Intermittent	Transient

2. What kind of things relieve your pain?

_____
_____
_____
_____

3. What kind of things increase your pain?

_____
_____
_____
_____

Part 4. How Strong Is Your Pain?

People agree that the following 5 words represent pain of increasing intensity. They are:

1	2	3	4	5
Mild	Discomforting	Distressing	Horrible	Excruciating

To answer each question below, write the number of the most appropriate word in the space beside the question.

1. Which word describes your pain right now? _____
2. Which word describes it at its worst? _____
3. Which word describes it when it is the least? _____
4. Which word describes the worst toothache you ever had? _____
5. Which word describes the worst headache you ever had? _____
6. Which word describes the worst stomach-ache you ever had? _____

D

changes in clinical pain than the pain index based on the rank value of the descriptor words. He writes,

Thus, some patients reported that their pain was still at the same PPI level [pain intensity based on number-word scale], but had changed in a way that was difficult to describe—it was somehow less sharp, less gnawing, not as exhausting and miserable as before. These changes were clearly reflected in the PRI (R) [pain index based on rank value of word] which showed a substantial percentage change even though the PPI remained unchanged [24, p. 291].

The total number of words chosen seems to be indicative of the pain as a major problem in the patient's life. Patients who have selected a higher number of words (not necessarily of higher intensity rating although the two are correlated) are seemingly those whose whole life is centered or focused on their present pain. Their reaction to the pain has consumed their whole being. Melzack [24], reporting on the analysis of several pain syndromes, found that of the following categories—menstrual, arthritis, cancer, dental, back, phantom-limb, and postherpetic pain—those with back pain utilized more descriptor words (with postherpetic a close second) than the others; the menstrual group had the fewest number. Why those with dental pain used the same number of words as those with arthritic and phantom-limb pain is not clearly understood. It may have to do with the fact that many of the descriptor words are so "descriptive" of dental pain, or it may be that dental pain is more readily described. Jacox and Stewart found in their study [17] that patients with rheumatoid arthritis (long-term pain) will choose a significantly higher number of words to describe their pain than will patients whose pain stems from surgical procedures such as herniorrhaphy and cholecystectomy. Patients with cancer also selected a greater number of words than did the surgical patients (not statistically significant) but less than the arthritis patients.

Overall, the McGill-Melzack Pain Assessment Questionnaire does appear to show promise in its ability to provide useful information. Melzack [24] substantiates its usefulness in the determination of relative effectiveness for different procedures in the treatment of clinical pain and to provide information about the relative effects of a given treatment not only on the intensity quality of pain, but also on the affective or more reactionary components of pain. For example, Melzack [23] reports " . . . we are now convinced that morphine acts primarily on the affective rather than the sensory components of the pain experience" [p. 13]. The potential user, however, should keep in mind that while this tool has considerable potential, it has been used primarily at pain clinics, is still in a developmental form, and will no doubt have further revisions made.

Other Forms of Pain Indexes

A Pain Symptom Scale

Other indexes for pain measurement can be adopted from a method used by Ingham [14, 15]. The procedure was developed out of a need to reduce if not eliminate response bias, response sets, or any other factors that other-wise influence a person's ability or readiness to report symptoms of illness. Since symptoms are not all-or-none events, Ingham feels that it is better to think of them along a continuum. Five scales for assessing backache, fatigue, anxiety, headache, and depression devised by Ingham are reportedly satis-factory in consistency of response patterns and discriminatory power. The headache and backache scales are shown below.

Backache:
1. My back never bothers me at all.
2. My back hardly ever bothers me.
3. I sometimes have a twinge of pain in my back.
4. I often have a twinge of pain in my back.
5. Often my back hurts quite a lot.
6. I often have really bad backache.
7. I have really bad backache all of the time.

Headache:
1. I never have headaches.
2. I very occasionally have a slight headache.
3. I have a headache quite often.
4. I quite often have a rather bad headache.
5. I often have a really bad headache.
6. I get a lot of very severe headaches.
7. I have constant very bad headaches that are almost unbearable.

Adopting the format of Ingham's scales, this author developed a scale for more general pain. Preliminary results using this scale on hospitalized pa-tients indicate that there is a high rate of consistency; where there is not gen-eral agreement at least the source of error is known. In this case, either the questionnaire can be repeated, or the data not used where valid measurement is required for research purposes. The "general pain index" is shown below:

1. I never have any pain or discomfort.
2. I occasionally have some pain.
3. I have some pain quite often.
4. I quite often have rather bad pain.
5. I often have really bad pain.
6. I am in very bad pain a lot of the time.
7. I have constant very bad pain that is almost unbearable.

While any number of statements regarding symptoms can be used, the basic number of seven used by Ingham was selected to provide more sensi-tivity; more than seven items tends to become unwieldy with too much burden on the patient.

The statements are presented to the subject in pairs and he or she is re-quired to choose the statement that is "closer to the truth." Not all possible pairs need to be presented to the subject. For seven statements, a maximum of eleven pairs is required to establish both a position on the scale and pat-terns of consistency. By this method the same number of scoring categories is obtained as when all possible pairs are presented, thus retaining discriminat-

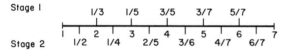

Figure 5-7 Midpoints of scale values (From Ingham).

ing information. The statements can be typed on 3- x 5-inch index cards with a random ordering of severity of statements—half with the more severe degree at the top, and half with it on the bottom. Midpoints of the scale values are shown in Figure 5-7.

The method devised by Ingham for the presentation of pairs is done in two stages. For the first stage, pairs (1, 3), (1, 5), (3, 5), (3, 7), and (5, 7) are presented to the subject one at a time in random order. From this information, a determination can be made of an approximate position on the scale, as well as information gained concerning the consistency of response.

For the second stage, two further pairs are presented according to the scoring position obtained in the first stage. One pair determines the scale position and the other consistency information. A scoring guide can be set up in the fashion of Figure 5-8.

If pluses are scored for choice of the higher intensity statement of the pairs, and a minus whenever the statement of lesser severity is chosen, a position on the scale as well as a consistency pattern can be seen. For example, a subject selects statement 3 of card one and statement 5 of card two, but 3 instead of 5 and 7 on cards three and four, and 5 instead of 7 on card five. This indicates a consistent pattern and places the subject between 1/5 and 3/5 on the scale (he is higher than 3, closer to 5 than 1, but closer to 3 than 5) at the midpoint area between 2 and 5. At this level, pairs 1 and 2, and 2 and 5 are presented. The choice between 2 and 5 enables a further subdivision for people located on the left (selected 2) of midpoint 2/5 or to the right of midpoint 2/5 (selected 5). Pairs 1, 2 provide the consistency information. Notice that the same two pairs are used for subjects located to the left of midpoint 1/3 (selected 1 rather than 3), but in this case 1, 2 provides the scale position and 2, 5 the consistency information. Notice that on the scoring guide, this would mean that no pluses would be given in stage 1 because the less severe statement was always chosen. This position is indicated by the minus on the scoring guide. Subjects located between 3/7 and 5/7 (pluses given up to and through card four) have indicated they are closer to 7 than 3, but closer to 5 than 7 or are at midpoint 4/7. The two further pairs presented in stage 2 are 1, 4 and 4, 7—the former providing consistency and the latter, a finer scale locus. The same two pairs are presented for subjects located between 1/3 and 1/5 but now pair 1, 4 provides scale location and 4, 7 the consistency information.

The inconsistency patterns can be spotted whenever pluses are not adjacent to each other, or do not start with the less severe statements. Two examples of inconsistency patterns in stage 1 are shown below:

	Pairs	
Card 1	1, 3	+
Card 2	1, 5	+
Card 3	3, 5	−
Card 4	3, 7	+
Card 5	5, 7	−

	Pairs	
Card 1	1, 3	+
Card 2	1, 5	+
Card 3	3, 5	−
Card 4	3, 7	+
Card 5	5, 7	+

Of course, an inconsistency may not show up until stage 2—for example:

	Pairs		*Pair:*	
Card 1	1, 3	+		
Card 2	1, 5	+	1, 2	1 is selected
Card 3	3, 5	−		rather than 2
Card 4	3, 7	−		
Card 5	5, 7	−		

CARD NO.	ITEM NO'S		ITEM NO'S		ITEM NO'S
	(minus)	⟶	(1, 2) _____	/(2, 5) _____	
1.	(1, 3) _____	⟶	(1, 4) _____	/(4, 7) _____	
2.	(1, 5) _____	⟶	(1, 2) _____	/(2, 5) _____	
3.	(3, 5) _____	⟶	(3, 6) _____	/(6, 7) _____	
4.	(3, 7) _____	⟶	(1, 4) _____	/(4, 7) _____	
5.	(5, 7) _____	⟶	(3, 6) _____	/(6, 7) _____	

Figure 5-8 Method of scoring pain symptom scale.

Ingham reports a very low inconsistency percentage based on the five symptom scales he devised (between 1.3 and 1.8 percent, based on 1,550 responses). The author's own preliminary work utilizing the general pain items supports Ingham's findings in that there has been an extremely low inconsistency rate. Although the sample is too small at this time for any definitive evaluation, the measurement tool is showing strong evidence of both reliability and validity.

The general pain index can also be reworded for past tense so that a "pain history" can be obtained. Currently, the pain history is being tested as a possible pain predictor for surgical patients by running a correlation postoperatively with the general pain index. This type of scale can be modified for assessment in many areas. Further, the use of a seven-point continuum for degrees of severity has the advantage that it is generally easier for the subject to express himself with seven choices rather than two yes-no answers. The uniqueness and potential strength of the instrument are in the method by which the subject has to choose between paired statements but is given more than one opportunity to select a level of pain.

An Item Checklist for Pain

Because of the abstractness of many pain intensity measures—e.g., mild, moderate, severe—and the difficulties with semantic anchorage, one may wish to use a more concrete checklist. An example of this approach is shown in Figure 5-9 which lists various physical and mental aspects associated with a painful condition (surgical pain in this case) that may be scored by the patient on a Likert-type rating scale. The checklist may be adapted to other painful conditions such as arthritis, for example, by changing several of the items to read "my joints ache," "I am bothered by stiffness," and so forth.

Note that several of the items are scored in the opposite direction to reduce response set. A total may be obtained (reverse scores on items 3 and 7) or any single item may be looked at separately. The usefulness of this approach to pain measurement is that different areas as well as different aspects of the pain experience are being questioned in a specific or more concrete manner. The advantages are that communication problems or unreliable answers can be identified by the comparison of antagonistic items—for example item numbers 7 and 12. The Likert scale, compared with simple Yes or No statements, provides more sensitivity and avoids the difficulty some people have in making a more limited forced choice. These forms were used in the Jacox pain study [16] and were found to have stability (reliability) over days when the pain was assumed to be fairly constant, as with arthritic patients. The forms also have validity, as reflected in expected changes in pain, such as with postoperative patients who were improving each day. The pain forms also were more highly related and responsive to effects of pain interventions and other factors under investigation than were the simple pain intensity scales. The reason for the enhanced responsiveness over the pain scales is not entirely clear but seems to be associated with a greater specificity

Name_____   Date_____

DIRECTIONS: A number of statements which people have used to
describe themselves are given below. Read each statement and
then circle the appropriate number to the right of the statement
to indicate how you have generally felt today.

There are no right or wrong answers. Do not spend too much time
on any one statement but give the answer which seems to describe
your present feelings best.

	Not at all	Sometimes	Most of the time	All of the time
1. I feel aching.	1	2	3	4
2. My pain is depressing.	1	2	3	4
3. I am free of pain.	1	2	3	4
4. I have annoying sensations	1	2	3	4
5. I feel tired	1	2	3	4
6. I have stabbing sensations.	1	2	3	4
7. My body is comfortable.	1	2	3	4
8. The pain is sickening.	1	2	3	4
9. It hurts to move around	1	2	3	4
10. My abdomen hurts.	1	2	3	4
11. I feel sharp sensations	1	2	3	4
12. My body feels miserable	1	2	3	4
13. I have pulsing sensations	1	2	3	4
14. I am nauseated.	1	2	3	4
15. I feel depressed	1	2	3	4

Total [   ]

Figure 5-9   Pain checklist for postoperative patients.

and sensitivity of the pain form to the patient's overall condition than can be
provided by the simple scales.

The forms discussed above have not been standardized; they are presented
only as examples of a different approach to pain measurement. The items
could be modified to better fit any specific condition, deleted or augmented
according to the needs of the investigator.

Further Considerations of Pain Measurement

Many factors to be considered in pain measurement have been discussed in
previous sections. This final section deals with measurement problems that
relate generally to reliability and validity.

The clinician, researcher, or assistant should use a consistent, standardized approach in the collection of pain data from subjects-patients. Such standardization is especially necessary in the clinical area where a patient is likely to be anxious about his illness or pain as well as about his dependency on a medical-care system. The data collector can be neither indifferent nor over-solicitous so that the patient feels either a lack of concern or an overconcern for his well-being. In the former case, the patient may not take the collection of data seriously and so may give invalid responses; and in the latter case, he may become more sensitized to his own feelings of anxiety or to the needs and biases of the data collector, or to both. An unhurried, neutral approach must be maintained consistently in order for the patient to report his pain as objectively as possible.

Generally, it is considered best to have several pain measurements over any given time period and then use averages. This approach will better accommodate pain level fluctuations and also allow for improved reliability. With some patients, however, it may not be appropriate or perhaps even ethical to solicit repeated pain measurements. Some patients may need to be directed away from their pain rather than required to think about it, such as a patient with cancer who may be denying his pain and the accompanying fear and anxiety. Only the researcher in the situation can best decide about any given patient.

If there is a need to get repeated measures over time, it may be necessary in some cases to sacrifice the more subjective and easily quantifiable data and turn to other means of assessment, such as observing behavioral expressions. Observations of limitation in range of motion or other physical activity or impairment in the ability of the patient to focus attention on things outside himself—reading, TV, conversation—can be used as indicators of pain. One of the problems with behavioral data is that it is not generally sensitive to pain of milder intensity. That is, a person may easily be able to control behavioral expressions of mild pain and may use TV, for example, for distraction from pain of mild or moderate degree, but he may not find such distraction helpful or possible when the pain becomes more severe, longer in duration, or accompanied by great fear. What one may be assessing in many instances is a person's coping or reactive mechanisms. Degree of pain and coping are confounded in these kinds of measures; this confounding is not necessarily undesirable as long as the clinician or researcher is aware of its existence and knows what kind of information is desired and how to use it. Another independent measurement is a record of daily analgesic consumption. Such consumption can be quantified in roughly equal units across drugs by using morphine as a comparative standard. A gross evaluation of the level of pain can be estimated from the frequency and dosage level.

Any pain measurement instrument should be checked for reliability and validity. For validity, a reasonable evaluation can be made on any group of subjects in whom the pain is known to change; for example, postoperative patients with no complications will have decreasing levels of surgical pain each day, a process that should be reflected in the pain data. Depending on the sensitivity of the instrument, these changes can even be perceived over a matter of hours rather than days. Whether or not the type of data collected provides the information needed can be ascertained by the clinician/researcher only with some preliminary testing. The value of pilot testing for any research efforts cannot be stressed enough.

The reliability of any pain estimator instrument is very difficult to establish because one is dealing with a subjective response that can vary markedly, sometimes from minute to minute. In controlled laboratory settings where the intensity of the pain stimulus is known, reliability can be established more readily. In the clinical setting, one has to accept a wider margin of error because of so many chance factors that may influence the pain response. Generally, however, one can find certain groups of patients in whom pain is assumed to be fairly stable over several days, and testing can be done with relative satisfaction. Knowledge and control of extraneous influences during these periods of testing are important. Reliability and validity can also be determined by using a multiple measurement approach, comparing the results of the several indicators.

In summary, there is no single instrument or method of pain measurement that can be judged to be the best under all circumstances. The measurement of pain is replete with difficult problems because of the inherent nature of the pain experience. Yet, significant strides are being made, especially in the areas of sensory matching and sensory decision. For the clinical researcher, pain measurement can probably be achieved to a satisfactory level if the researcher is sensitive to the potential problems with the various instruments and procedures and is willing to cope with the possible means of error reduction that require time and patience. For those who will experiment with new approaches to pain measurement, there remains a real challenge.

References

1. Beecher, H. K. Generalizations from pain of various types and diverse origins. *Science* 130:267, 1959.
2. Beecher, H. K. *Measurement of Subjective Responses. Quantitative Effects of Drugs*. New York: Oxford University Press, 1959.
3. Beecher, H. K. Increased stress and effectiveness of placebos and "active" drugs. *Science* 132:91, 1960.
4. Beecher, H. K. Pain: One mystery solved. *Science* 151:840, 1966.
5. Berry, H., and Huskisson, E. C. A report on pain measurement. *Clin. Trials* 9:13, 1972.
6. Canter, C. An Investigation of the Psychological Significance of Reactions to Color on the Rorschach and Other Tests. Ph.D. dissertation, State University of Iowa, 1950.
7. Clark, P. R. F., and Spear, F. G. Reliability and sensitivity in the self-assessment of well-being. *Bull. Br. Psychol. Soc.* 17, 1964.
8. Clark, W. W. Pain sensitivity and the report of pain: An introduction to sensory decision theory. *Anesthesiology* 40:272, 1974.

9. Davidson, P. O., and Neufeld, R. W. J. Response to pain and stress: A multivariate analysis. *J. Psychosom. Res.* 18:25, 1974.
10. Gelfand, S. The relationship of experimental pain tolerance to pain threshold. *Can. J. Psychol.* 18:36, 1964.
11. Hardy, J. D. Pharmacodynamics of human disease. II. The pain threshold and the nature of sensation. *Postgrad. Med.* 34:579, 1963.
12. Hardy, J. D., Wolff, H. G., and Goodell, H. S. Studies on pain. A new method for reviewing pain threshold: Observations on spatial summation of pain. *J. Clin. Invest.* 19:649, 1940.
13. Hardy, J. D., Wolff, H. G., and Goodell, H. S. *Pain Sensations and Reactions.* Baltimore: The Williams & Wilkins Company, 1952.
14. Ingham, J. G. A method for observing symptoms and attitudes. *Br. J. Soc. Clin. Psychol.* 4:131, 1965.
15. Ingham, J. G. Quantitative evaluation of subjective symptoms. Proceedings of the Royal Society of Medicine. *Proc. R. Soc. Med.* 62:492, 1969.
16. Jacox, A., and Stewart, M. L. Psychosocial Contingencies of the Pain Experience. College of Nursing, University of Iowa, 1973.
17. Jacox, A. Psychosocial Contingencies of the Pain Experience. U.S.P.H.S. Research Grant NU00387–02.
18. Johnson, J. Effects of structuring patient's expectations on their reactions to threatening events. *Nurs. Res.* 21:499, 1972.
19. Johnson, J. The effect of accurate expectations about sensations on the sensory and distress components of pain. *J. Pers. Soc. Psychol.* 27(2):261, 1973.
20. Kast, E. C. An understanding of pain and its measurement. *Med. Times* 94:1501, 1966.
21. Kouwer, B. J. *Colors and Their Character.* The Hague: Martinus Nijhoff, 1949.
22. McCarty, D. J., Gatter, R. A., and Phelps, P. A dolorimeter for quantification of articular tenderness. *Arthritis Rheum.* 8:551, 1965.
23. Melzack, R. Using the language of pain. *Pain: Curr. Concepts Pain Analg.* 2:1, 1974.
24. Melzack, R. The McGill Pain Questionnaire: Major properties and scoring methods. *Pain* 1:277, 1975.
25. Melzack, R., and Torgerson, W. S. On the language of pain. *Anesthesiology* 34:50, 1971.
26. Merskey, H., and Spear, R. G. The concept of pain. *J. Psychosom. Res.* 11:59, 1967.
27. Mills, R. J., and Renfrew, S. Measurement of pain threshold by thermal contact. *Lancet* 738, 1971.
28. Newton, M. E., Hunt, W. E., McDowell, W. E., and Hanken, A. F. *A Study of Nurse Action in Relief of Pain.* Unpublished report, The Ohio State University School of Nursing, 1964.
29. Peck, R. E. A precise technique for the measurement of pain. *Headache* 189, 1967.
30. Pilowsky, I., and Bond, M. R. Pain and its management in malignant disease. *Psychosom. Med.* 31:400, 1969.
31. Pilowsky, I., and Kaufman. A. An experimental study of atypical phantom pain. *Br. J. Psychiatry* 111:1185, 1965.
32. Ryan, E. D., and Kovacic, C. R. Pain tolerance and athletic participation. *Percept. Mot. Skills* 22:383, 1966.
33. Schaie, K. W., and Heiss, R. *Color and Personality.* Bern, Switzerland: Hans Huber, 1964.
34. Scott, I., ed. *The Luscher Color Test.* New York: Random House, Inc., 1969.

35. Smith, G. M., and Beecher, H. K. Experimental production of pain in man: Sensitivity of a new method to 600 mg. of aspirin. *J. Pharmacol. Exp. Ther.* 10:213, 1969.
36. Smith, G. M., Egbert, L. D., Markowitz, R. A., Mosteller, F., and Beecher, H. K. An experimental pain method sensitive to morphine in man: The submaximum effort tourniquet technique. *J. Pharmacol. Exp. Ther.* 154:324, 1966.
37. Sternbach, R. A. *Pain: A Psychophysiological Analysis.* New York: Academic Press, Inc., 1968.
38. Sternbach, R. A., Murphy, R. W., Timmermans, G., Greenhoot, J. H., and Akeson, W. H. Measuring the severity of clinical pain. *Adv. Neurol.* 4:281, 1974.
39. Stewart, M. L. *Studies in Pain Measurement.* Unpublished report, 1974.
40. Wolff, B. B. The relationship of experimental pain tolerance to pain threshold: A critique of Gelfand's paper. *Can. J. Psychol.* 18:249, 1964.
41. Wolff, B. B. Factor analysis of human pain responses: Pain endurance as a specific pain factor. *J. Abnorm. Psychol.* 78:292, 1971.
42. Wolff, B. B., and Jarvik, M. E. Quantitative measures of deep somatic pain: Further studies with hypertonic saline. *Clin. Sci. Mol. Med.* 28:43, 1965.
43. Woodforde, J. M., and Merskey, H. Some relationships between subjective measures of pain. *J. Psychosom. Res.* 16:173, 1972.

6

Assessment of Clinical Pain

Marion Johnson

This chapter will focus on the evaluation of pain in the clinical setting, particularly upon pain evaluation as it pertains to nursing practice. Clinical pain generally signifies either a symptom of a disease condition or a temporary aspect of treatment; in either case the expectation ordinarily exists within both the patient and the clinician that pain will be alleviated. Pain is frequently the symptom for which the patient seeks medical help. According to Szasz [30] the client seeks help, usually from the physician, because pain is being perceived as an indication that something is wrong with the structural or functional integrity of the body. A primary responsibility that the physician assumes in relation to clinical pain is the evaluation of pain for the purpose of diagnosing and treating the disease process or pathology causing the symptom; however, other aspects of the pain experience must also be considered in the clinical setting.

Clinical pain is a reaction of the whole personality to a much greater extent than is experimentally produced pain [29]. Therefore, the clinician is dealing not only with the pathophysiology of pain but also with the patient's perception of the pain experience.

Although the client initially may seek assistance only from the physician, all other health professionals will eventually have contact with the person experiencing pain and each health worker may assist the patient in diverse but complementary ways. The professional nurse assumes responsibility for pain assessment for the purpose of providing information that will assist the physician in diagnosis and therapy, and that will assist the nurse in (1) making a nursing diagnosis, (2) evaluating and instituting nursing care measures or prescribed therapy for pain relief, (3) helping the individual with chronic pain achieve positive adaptive mechanisms, and (4) evaluating the effectiveness of interventions by determining the degree of relief obtained. In order to assess pain effectively, the nurse must understand the pain experience.

Pain is one of life's paradoxes—it is one of the most common and universal experiences of man but it is also a phenomenon so complex and with so many ramifications that most attempts at definition have been less than satisfactory. No definition has met the test of being universally acceptable or usable, because most definitions reflect inadequacies in comprehensiveness or clarity.

However, these attempts have not been without value and a brief review of some of the theories that have been proposed can provide a better understanding of the problems inherent in pain assessment in the clinical setting.

Aspects of Pain

Prior to the 19th century most authorities followed Aristotle's lead and placed pain in the realm of the emotions; its opposite was pleasure. As knowledge about sensory physiology was expanded, the concept of pain as an emotion was replaced by the concept of pain as a sensation. This gave rise to the specificity theory, which described pain in terms of a sensory reaction to a noxious stimulus. This reaction was dependent upon impulses traversing a specific pain pathway. The consideration of pain as a sensation implied a direct, invariable relationship between stimulus and response and this view could not be supported by observation of clinical pain.

A number of investigators began to study pain more systematically in the 1950s and to stress the difference between sensory and reactive aspects of pain. Work done by others supported this view and Beecher identified two components of pain—the "original sensation" and the "reaction component."

The description of pain as an experience having sensory and reactive or response components is reflected in much of the present literature. Each component of the pain experience has unique characteristics that can often be evaluated independently. The sensory component is dependent upon neurophysiological function and is similar in organization and response to other sensory systems. It allows one to estimate the descriptive characteristics of the pain experienced, such as location and quality. The reaction component, which varies markedly among persons, is dependent upon personality, social, and cultural factors. It can be thought of as the emotional response and is evaluated in terms of the distress that occurs with the pain. The reaction component can be observed through the autonomic, motor, and verbal responses and statements that occur with pain.

A definition that takes into account these various components of the pain experience has been provided by Richard Sternbach, a psychologist [28]. Sternbach has defined pain as an "abstract concept which refers to (1) a personal, private sensation of hurt; (2) a harmful stimulus which signals current or impending tissue damage; (3) a pattern of responses which operate to protect the organism from harm." This definition encompasses the subjectivity of the pain experience and allows one to consider pain as both a sensory stimulus and a response. It also points out that although we can separate these components for the purpose of study or discussion, they overlap or occur simultaneously when an individual experiences pain.

Although this definition of pain presents the various components of pain it does not sufficiently reflect the different types of pain based upon pathology and duration. There appear to be two distinct types of pain in relation to duration—acute pain and chronic pain. Acute pain with visible symptoms of discomfort is the pain model typically used by health workers despite the fact that it does not sufficiently describe symptoms associated with chronic pain.

Acute transient pain functions to inform the individual of noxious stimulation or to warn that something is wrong. It is usually produced by external agencies or by internal disease and results in typical patterns of response that contribute to homeostasis [6]. Examples of such response patterns are the reflex muscle spasm and automatic splinting that occur as a protective reaction with a fracture, and the avoidance of foods that increase the pain and chemical irritation of peptic ulcer. Acute pain is frequently of sudden onset and leads to action undertaken to relieve the source of the pain. There is every likelihood of complete relief because the cause can be identified and is self-limiting or readily corrected [22].

Chronic pain may begin as an acute pain episode or may be more insidious making it difficult to identify when pain began. At some point one characteristic becomes predominant; the pain exists without a known time limit. The pain may be continuous or intermittent; it may vary in intensity or remain the same while it becomes a constant companion, to be controlled if possible but always to be lived with. The source of the pain may be recognized but an effective treatment not be available or the source may be uncertain so that a diagnosis cannot be made. If treatment is provided without the person obtaining relief or if the pain exists without demonstrable disease, it is referred to as intractable.

Le Shan has identified some of the qualitative aspects of chronic pain [19]. He compares chronic pain to a nightmare in that terrible things are occurring with worse threatened, outside forces are in control, and there is no time limit known. Chronic pain becomes not an event but a state of existence in which the need to react is threatened and the suffering individual is limited to bearing the pain. Lishman also points out that chronic pain provides nothing external about which to feel angry and there is no immediate action readily available that the individual can pursue to protect himself [21].

Another question being raised in relation to chronic pain is the extent to which it is learned behavior. Fordyce [11] states that when pain responses occur over a long period this leads to learned pain behavior. He suggests that reinforcement of pain behaviors will lead to optimal learning of such behaviors. This may occur when individuals receive attention only when they experience pain and the attention is withdrawn if they are comfortable. As knowledge about pain increases it may become possible to identify the role that learning plays in the development of chronic pain; this role may vary in pain conditions due to progressive disease, such as terminal cancer, and in pain conditions in which the etiology is less readily apparent.

There is agreement that chronic pain in and of itself imposes stress on the individual; emotional, physical, and financial stress all may be incurred. Bonica identifies chronic pain as the most common disabling condition, imposing a cost of over ten billion dollars annually on Americans [5]. He points out that individuals do not become accustomed to chronic pain but seem to suffer more with the passing of time as it produces physical and mental depletion [6]. Lishman [21] also notes that the mental and physical resources of the patient become exhausted and lead to changes in behavior. Mehta [22] has observed that "unrelieved pain is a disease in itself and saps the moral and physical strength of even a phlegmatic individual." Under these conditions the world of the patient can become centered on the pain and all of his energies consumed by the pain. The smallest amount of additional discomfort may become intolerable. Hackett states that chronic pain either exhausts and destroys the individual or results in the individual's somehow adapting to the pain, which then becomes more bearable and less visible [13].

Although clinicians and investigators are only beginning to study chronic pain systematically there is enough evidence to support the fact that acute and chronic pain differ in many important respects and may lead to different types of pain behavior.

Pain, whether acute or chronic, often has been viewed as psychogenic pain or organic pain depending upon whether the source of the pathology is psychological or physiological. There has been a tendency to think of these as a dichotomy—organic or "real" pain versus psychogenic or "imaginary" pain—and to assume a lack of suffering when pathology cannot be demonstrated. If we consider the various components of pain, there is probably no "pure" organic pain nor "pure" psychogenic pain. Pain might better be thought of as a continuum in which physiological or psychological factors play greater or lesser roles. Determination of the degree to which psychological factors are important is useful in determining the method of treatment that will be most successful in providing pain relief. (For further discussion of pain which is primarily psychogenic, see Chapter 4. For discussion of specific psychosocial factors that influence pain perception and reaction, see Chapter 3.)

The Pain Evaluation Process

Evaluation of pain in the clinical setting by nurses is done for a number of reasons cited earlier in this chapter. The process of pain evaluation may be broken down into a number of steps: (1) the determination that pain exists, (2) evaluation of the descriptive characteristics of the pain, (3) evaluation of the physiological and behavioral responses that occur with pain, (4) evaluation of the individual's perception of pain and the meaning that pain has for him, and (5) evaluation of the adaptive mechanisms being used to cope with the pain. Although the evaluation that pain is present is the first step in the process, this step will be discussed last because it is dependent upon knowledge that will be discussed in the other steps of pain evaluation. The first aspect of assessment to be considered is evaluation of the characteristics of the pain experience.

Characteristics of Pain

Determination of the descriptive characteristics of pain is the portion of pain assessment with which nurses probably are most familiar and comfortable. It is the component of clinical assessment about which most is known and the literature on the neuroanatomical aspects of pain provides a reliable source of information for this aspect of pain assessment.

Factors to be assessed primarily focus on the sensory component of the pain experience and include: (1) location, (2) intensity, (3) quality, and (4) chronology of the pain experience. These factors should be evaluated once the determination is made that pain exists. Questions initially should be phrased to elicit the information required but not to lead the patient; for example, "describe (or point out) the location of the pain" is preferable to "is the pain in the lower back?" More specific questions reflecting or enlarging upon the individual's response may be needed later in the pain evaluation process. Pain is difficult to describe and it may be easier for the patient to agree with a partially correct statement than to attempt to clarify points of discrepancy between the statement and his pain experience.

Pain characteristics may be more easily described by the individual suffering acute pain than by one suffering chronic pain, since a subjective change may appear in the interpretation of the original sensation or in the way it is perceived when pain persists over weeks or months. Expected differences between acute and chronic pain will be considered as each aspect is discussed.

The source of pain determines many aspects of the sensory characteristics of pain. Three general pain sources which will be considered are: (1) cutaneous, which includes superficial somatic structures located in skin and subcutaneous tissue; (2) deep somatic, which includes bone, nerve, muscle, and other tissues supporting these structures; (3) viscera, which includes all body organs located in the trunk.

LOCATION   Pain is always assigned a body location. It can be experienced only in reference to a particular body part or preexisting part, such as a phantom limb.

Pain location should be described as specifically as possible and should include extent or spread of pain as well as areas in which pain is absent in the case of diffuse pain. Cutaneous pain and some visceral or deep pain may be delineated by having the patient point to the painful areas. Terms that are used to describe location include:

localized—confined to site of origin
projected—transmitted along the course of a nerve distribution
radiates—extends from the site of origin
referred—occurs in a part of the body other than the source

Several factors are known to affect the ability to localize pain. Acute pain usually can be described in terms of location; even when the pain is diffuse, painful and nonpainful areas generally can be identified. Chronic pain may or may not be as easily localized. If the chronic pain projects along a nerve distribution the location may remain constant, as with the neuralgias. If the chronic pain occurs with progressive pathology, it may vary in terms of extent and radiation, making it difficult for the patient to identify consistently painful or nonpainful areas. Anatomically those body structures that are most highly innervated allow pain to be localized most precisely. The skin, for example, has many nerve endings and thus pain is easier to localize than in the bowel, where the nerve endings are sparse. Severity of the pain also may affect the ease with which it can be localized: mild pain is closest to pure sensation and is generally well localized [4]; intense pain may be more diffuse and in fact may envelop the entire body with pain or tenderness.

Cutaneous or superficial pain can be well localized since skin and mucous membranes are innervated with receptor endings widely distributed over the body surface. It may be delineated by having the patient point to the painful areas. Cutaneous pain may occur along dermal segments, each segment representing a portion of the body surface innervated by one dorsal root as illustrated in the dermatome chart (Fig. 6-1). Although the dermatome boundaries are shown as distinct on a dermatome chart, there is in actuality an overlap of nerve distribution and irritation of one posterior root, for example T_6 will give rise to pain experienced in the adjacent dermatomes, T_5 and T_7, as well as T_6.

Deep somatic structures are not innervated as well as cutaneous surface areas and the distribution of a single nerve supplies a larger area. The scleratome, or area supplied by one posterior nerve root, is less well defined than a dermatone and does not correspond with a dermal segment; therefore somatic pain will generally be more diffuse than cutaneous pain. Deep structures vary in degree of pain sensitivity. Deep fascia, tendons, ligaments, joints, periosteum of bone, blood vessels, and nerves are all highly sensitive. Skeletal muscle is sensitive to stretching and ischemia [4], while bone and cartilage respond only to extremes of pressure [22]. In general, deep somatic pain is diffuse although pain arising from the highly sensitive structures may be better localized. Pain from deep structures frequently radiates from the primary site; pain due to muscle spasm, for example, may gradually spread from the original site. Pain from a nerve root or trunk usually will project along the afferent fiber, as with pain that travels along the sciatic nerve from a lumbar disk. As the duration of deep pain lengthens, the pain tends to become more diffuse and may be referred to other deep structures, usually located in the same scleratome [22]. In contrast to superficial pain which is located along a line, deep pain may be felt as three-dimensional.

Viscera are also sparsely innervated compared to the cutaneous area; therefore visceral pain tends to be diffuse but may become better localized as the pain continues. Nerve fibers innervating these organs follow the sympathetic nerves to the spinal cord, which may account for the fact that autonomic symptoms frequently accompany visceral pain. Visceral pain may also be

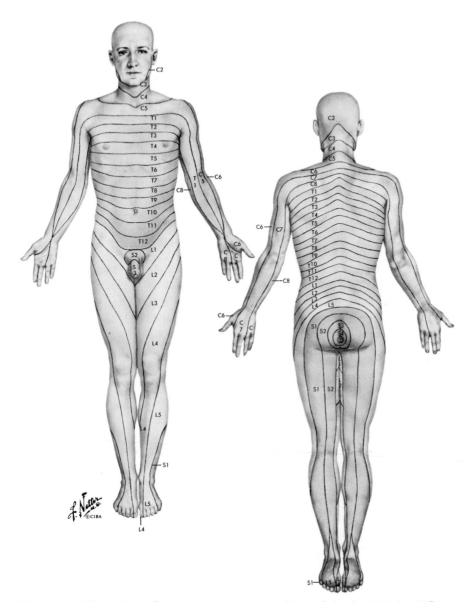

Figure 6-1 Illustration of dermatome segments. (Copyright © 1974, by CIBA-Geigy and F. H. Netter. Used by permission.)

accompanied by the referral of pain or tenderness to the body surface in cutaneous locations either adjacent to or remote from the painful organ.

Much referred pain occurs in consistent patterns that can be used to diagnose the source of the pain. Referred pain due to visceral disease follows dermatome patterns whereas somatic referred pain does not [6]. Examples of common patterns of referred pain include the pain of coronary heart disease felt in the left axilla or radiating down the inside of the left arm, pleural pain of the diaphragm felt in the shoulder, and pain of cholecystitis felt in the back and in the angle of the scapula. Common sites of referred pain are demonstrated in Figure 6-2. Phantom pain is a complex type of referred pain in which the pain is experienced as occurring in an absent or phantom limb. Referred pain frequently is associated with cutaneous hyperalgesia (increased sensitivity to pain) or cutaneous tenderness. There are often trigger zones that when stimulated cause pain in the referred site and in the diseased organ [26].

INTENSITY   Pain intensity may be the most difficult characteristic to assess accurately, perhaps because it is readily influenced by the subjectivity of the person experiencing it. Pain intensity reflects a combination of both the sensation experienced and the distress caused by the sensory component. Unlike the other sensations the intensity of the pain does not need to parallel the intensity of the stimulus and pain may in fact occur without demonstrable noxious stimulation. Studies have demonstrated that the pain threshold level—the point at which pain is perceived—is relatively uniform, while the toler-

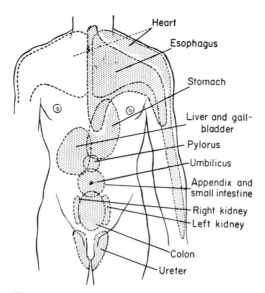

Figure 6-2 Surface areas of referred pain from different visceral organs. (From Guyton, A. C. *Basic Human Physiology.* Philadelphia: Saunders, 1971. Used by permission.)

ance or reaction level varies both among individuals and within the same individual at different times. A previous chapter has discussed those factors known to affect pain tolerance levels (see Chapter 3).

As mentioned earlier the sensation of pain is not dependent upon the presence of noxious stimulation; the severe pain of tic douloureux, for instance, can be triggered by a slight touch. When a noxious stimulus and intact nervous system are present, however, the sensation of pain will be experienced as tissue damage begins to occur. Noxious stimulation intense enough to produce severe pain eventually will destroy the pain fiber and surrounding tissue [16]. Consequently, high-intensity pain resulting from intense stimulation and tissue damage must be of short duration or alternate with pain-free periods, whereas low-intensity pain resulting from mild stimulation can be supported by the tissues indefinitely [16]. The perceived pain intensity can be altered by the amount of psychological distress present as well as by the intensity of the stimulus and the degree of tissue damage. The average person can tolerate the most severe pain of short duration much better than less severe pain if prolonged. If the pain becomes chronic and persists over months or years, a change may appear in the way the sensation is perceived and make it difficult to evaluate the degree of intensity.

While interviewing patients with terminal cancer, we found that they frequently would describe sensations caused by ascites, shortness of breath, lymphedema, pressure in the abdomen, and so forth as being uncomfortable but not painful; however they would often add that the sensation was painful when they first experienced it.* Patients who have suffered a cervical fracture and are being treated with Crutchfield or Vinke tongs to immobilize the neck may initially experience an ache in the shoulders that for some becomes increasingly painful over the period of weeks required for treatment. Melzack's comment [26] that pain might "refer to a category of experiences, not to a specific sensation that varies along a single intensity dimension" suggests a reason for the difficulty in trying to assess the intensity of pain accurately.

Clinically, pain intensity is most often evaluated by ranking the degree of pain along a scale such as none, mild, moderate, severe, intolerable, or overwhelming. The individual can be asked to compare the intensity of the present pain with previous pain experiences; for example, "is it more or less intense than a toothache?" (or a headache, surgical incision, and so forth). It is also possible to ask the individual to equate the current pain with the most severe pain he has ever experienced. This type of comparison will provide some indication of how the individual reports pain intensity. Perhaps one person reports all pain as mild to moderate, while another views all pain as severe or intolerable.

Source of the pain may also influence the degree of pain experienced. The intensity of cutaneous pain may correlate quite closely with the intensity of

* Grant No. NU 00467-03 from the Division of Nursing, Bureau of Health Manpower Education, Public Health Service.

the stimulus; that is, a mild stimulus may cause sensations, such as itch or tingling, that become perceived as pain as the intensity of the stimulus increases. Deep somatic pain of more than short duration frequently is accompanied by segmental muscle contraction which increases the discomfort and may increase the perceived pain intensity. This is true in conditions such as ruptured vertebral disk or pulled or torn tendons or ligaments. Visceral pain due to muscle contraction of an obstructed passage, such as renal or biliary colic, is one of the most severe pains experienced. Visceral pain of moderate intensity often will become more severe if allowed to continue without relief, as in the case of pain caused by a peptic ulcer. As was noted previously cutaneous tenderness may occur with both referred or deep somatic pain, for example, the body surface areas to which pain is referred or the area over a fractured bone may give rise to pain.

Pain intensity can be modified by body activities and physiological processes. Cutaneous pain usually will increase with stimulation of the involved area and may decrease with gentle stimulation, massage, or warmth of adjacent noninvolved areas. This is noted when a patient rubs the area around an infiltrated IV site or benefits from moist heat. Muscle activity will increase the pain of skeletal muscle and moveable skeletal parts whereas resting the involved body part generally will decrease the amount of pain experienced. Visceral pain can be increased with peristaltic activity, pressure, and movement and decreased by eliminating these stimuli. This is one reason why antispasmodic medications, nasogastric tubes, and nothing by mouth can decrease pain of gastrointestinal origin. Pain arising from vessels will be increased with systole or with increased pressure in the cardiovascular system; the throbbing migraine headache is a typical example.

The individual's own description of the degree of pain being experienced is almost the sole guide in this area of assessment. Assisting the person to compare the present sensation with previous pain may enable him to be more objective in his evaluation of the sensation but it should be borne in mind that intensity will reflect other components of the pain experience and cannot be viewed only as an indication of the severity of the stimulus causing the sensation. (The psychosocial factors that influence pain intensity have been considered in Chapter 3.)

CHARACTER AND QUALITY The English language does not contain a specific vocabulary that describes the quality of pain, but a variety of words and similes are used to describe pain qualities. Specific types of pain seem to produce relatively consistent sensations that are described in similar terms. Clinicians have long relied upon this consistency in pain description to assist in identification of the source of pain.

Cutaneous pain often is described as a bimodal sensation; an initial bright, prickling, sharp sensation is followed by a dull, burning sensation of longer duration. This bimodal response may be labeled as "first" and "second" pain or "fast" and "slow" pain and is believed to be related to the type of periph-

eral fiber being stimulated. Abnormal sensations that may occur with cutaneous pain include:

1. hyperalgesia—excessive sensibility to pain [32]
2. cutaneous tenderness—pain or discomfort, or both, elicited by a stimulus
   that is normally insufficient to cause pain
3. paresthesia—abnormal sensation without objective cause, such as numbness, prickling, and tingling [32]

Deep pain commonly is described as dull, aching, or boring. It is often
accompanied by cutaneous tenderness, muscle rigidity, and a sensation of
deep tenderness, such as occurs with the pain of inflamed or arthritic joints.
Visceral pain also may be described as a dull, aching pain and be accompanied by muscle rigidity or spasm over the involved viscus, as in the pain of
an inflamed kidney. If visceral pain continues without relief it may assume a
sharper, stabbing quality, often noted with pancreatitis when pain becomes
intense. Obstruction of the intestine or biliary tree produces a cramping
pain, as noted in renal colic, which may be characterized as twisting, grip-
ing, or cramping. Pain caused by such obstruction ordinarily occurs in
waves, with episodes of intense pain alternating with pain-free periods. Ul-
ceration of the upper gastrointestinal tract often produces a pain described
as sharp and burning. Pleuritis produces a stabbing, knifelike pain that occurs
with inhalation and decreases with exhalation.

A number of factors may affect the descriptions of pain given by the patient. The person may be limited by vocabulary or by an "indescribable
pain." The severity of the pain or the importance that the pain has for the
individual also may affect pain descriptions. Merskey found that more attention is focused on severe pain or pain of particular concern to the patient
with the result that a more elaborate description of pain may be related by
the patient (see Chapter 4). A number of attempts have been made to determine if differences exist in the description of "psychogenic" pain and "organic" pain without any conclusive results.

Acute pain most often can be described rather precisely. The character of
chronic pain also may be described quite precisely as in the burning sensations common with causalgia, or it may be impossible for the person to describe the pain except as a constant ache or soreness. Both acute and chronic
pain may be mixed with other body sensations, such as pressure, pulling,
and so on, making it more difficult to describe the pain sensation.

Melzack and Torgerson have reported results of research done to cate-
gorize and scale words used in describing pain [24]. Words were categorized
into three main classes: (1) words that describe *sensory* qualities of pain,
(2) words that describe *affective* qualities, and (3) *evaluative* words that describe the subjective intensity of the pain experience. Table 6-1 presents an
ordering of words in the various classes for which there was strong agreement on the classification into which the word fell. Since there was quite

Table 6-1 Classes and subclasses of pain descriptors as rated by patients

Category	Descriptors	Category	Descriptors
SENSORY			Hurting
Temporal	Flickering		Aching
	Quivering		Drawing
	Pulsing		Blurred
	Thumping		Steady
	Throbbing		Heavy
	Beating	AFFECTIVE	
	Pounding	Autonomic	Nauseating
Spatial	Jumping		Sickening
	Flashing		Suffocating
	Spreading		Choking
	Radiating	Sensory misc.	Tender
	Shooting		Taut
Punctate pressure	Pricking		Rasping
	Boring		Splitting
	Drilling		Tearing
	Stabbing	Tension	Nagging
	Lancinating		Fatiguing
	Penetrating		Tiring
	Piercing		Exhausting
Incisive pressure	Sharp		Dragging
	Cutting	Punishment	Racking
	Lacerating		Punishing
Constrictive	Pinching		Grueling
pressure	Nipping		Cruel
	Tight		Vicious
	Squeezing		Killing
	Pressing		Torturing
	Binding		
	Gnawing	EVALUATIVE	Annoying
	Biting		Bearable
	Cramping		Troublesome
	Gripping		Miserable
	Crushing		Distracting
Traction pressure	Tugging		Agonizing
	Pulling		Ugly
	Wrenching		Intense
Thermal	Hot		Intolerable
	Burning		Unbearable
	Scalding		Savage
	Searing		Violent
Brightness	Tickling	Fear	Fearful
	Tingling		Frightful
	Itchy		Terrifying
	Smarting		Dreadful
	Sticking	Affective-	Grinding
Dullness	Dull	evaluative-	Wretched
	Sore	sensory misc.	Awful
	Numbing		Blinding
			Wicked

Source: Adapted from Melzack, R., and Torgerson, W. W. "On the Language of Pain." *Anesthesiology* 34:1, January 1971, pp. 54–55.

consistent agreement on the qualities of pain described by these words, they might be useful to the clinician in assisting with interpreting the descriptions given by the patient. The list of words also can be given to a patient with instructions to check those qualities that best describe the sensation he is experiencing; this may be helpful in situations where the individual has been unable to verbalize the quality of the pain sensation.

CHRONOLOGY   Chronology is used to refer to the sequence of events that occur in relation to the pain experience. Factors to be assessed, if not self-evident, when considering the chronology of pain include: (1) the mode of onset, (2) precipitating factors, (3) variations in time of occurrence, (4) variations in character, and (5) duration of the pain experience.

The mode of onset and precipitating factors may be obvious when pain is due to traumatic injuries, incisions, or other external causes. Other types of pain may be insidious in onset or may be perceived as another type of sensation—pressure, pulling, tingling—which gradually becomes perceived as painful if the sensation continues. These types of pain experiences may be more difficult to identify in terms of onset or precipitating factors.

The occurrence of pain may vary in relation to time over a twenty-four hour period or over longer periods or with seasonal changes. This may be related to the pathology involved, such as in arthritic pain that occurs with changes in the weather or in migraine headache that may occur at specific points in the menstrual cycle. It also may be associated with the availability of distracting factors: pain that has been successfully ignored when a person is busy becomes noticeable when he tries to rest.

Changes in character of the pain can be related to the involved organ or the pathology. Pain due to an inflamed pleura will increase as stretching occurs with each breath. Pain caused by obstruction of a hollow organ or tube attempting to expel its contents will occur in rhythmic waves. The pain will mount in intensity over 10 to 20 seconds, be maintained for about a minute, and then subside, and the entire cycle will be repeated with each peristaltic wave. Inflamed tissue can give rise to a throbbing pain as blood vessels fill during systole or to a steady pain and tenderness due to the continued release of noxious chemicals. Changes in character of the pain should be elicited and may include the following patterns: constant, steady pain; intermittent variable pain; throbbing pain; pain that peaks and falls off in a cycle; mounting pain that becomes progressively more severe. All of these factors may be more readily identified in acute pain than in chronic pain or when the pain becomes more intense, thereby increasing the degree of attention given to the sensation.

The duration of pain can extend from a few minutes to a lifetime and can be a factor that causes considerable modification in the pain sensation. Intense but brief pain does not produce the same pain experience as possibly less severe but permanent pain. "Pain will create its own conditioning, its physical and psychological repercussions which will transform the patient. Time introduces a considerable transformation factor into pain" [7]. When dealing with acute pain episodes one can expect that deep pain and visceral pain will persist longer after the stimulus is removed than cutaneous pain that is more transient. The point at which pain begins to recede may reflect alterations in the underlying pathology, alterations in psychological factors affecting pain perception, or damage to pain pathways.

A profile of the characteristics of pain that have been discussed in this section in relation to the source of the pain is given in Table 6-2. This provides a guide for commonly occurring aspects of pain as related to source but it should be borne in mind that subjective factors within the individual may influence the way in which pain is perceived and described. For example, cutaneous pain may be described by the patient as a vague, poorly localized pain rather than a sharp, well-demarcated area of pain. The assessment of these factors may be important in providing the physician with information helpful in making a medical diagnosis and should be accurately recorded.

Pain Response

The responses that occur as a part of the pain experience include a complex sequence of events that may be described in physiological, behavioral, or

Table 6-2 Characteristics of pain as commonly related to source of pain

Source	Location	Intensity	Quality	Chronology
Cutaneous	Well localized	Correlates with intensity of stimulus.	Bimodal sensation may occur. Sharp, tingling, stinging. Abnormal surface sensations may occur.	Correlates with stimulus changes, tissue damage. May be steady or throbbing in inflamed tissues.
Deep somatic	Poorly localized. May localize with tendon, periosteum, ligament pain. May be referred to body surface.	Correlates with intensity of stimulus and with movement of involved area.	Vague, aching, boring, dull. Cutaneous tenderness may accompany.	May be steady or change in character with stimulus change or movement. Correlates with stimulus changes.
Visceral	Poorly localized. May localize as duration extends. May be referred to body surface.	May be severe with colic. May increase if not relieved. Correlates with intensity of stimulus.	Vague, dull, aching, burning. If continues may become sharper. If due to obstruction may be gripping, cramping, twisting.	Obstructive pain generally occurs in cycles. Untreated pain may mount. Correlates with stimulus changes.

affective terms. One pattern identified by Melzack and Wall [23] illustrates the complexity of these responses.

Sudden, unexpected damage to the skin is followed by (1) a startle response; (2) a flexion reflex; (3) postural readjustment; (4) vocalization; (5) orientation of the head and eyes to examine the damaged area; (6) autonomic responses; (7) evocation of past experience in similar situations and prediction of the consequences of the stimulation; (8) many other patterns of behavior aimed at diminishing the sensory and affective components of the whole experience, such as rubbing the damaged area, avoidance behavior, and so forth.

This aptly illustrates the variety of behaviors that may occur with even a minor pain experience. The typical pain response seems designed to protect the individual from harm and may be similar to behavior patterns typical of fight, flight, or withdrawal responses. Some of the behaviors are automatic or reflexive while other behaviors have been learned as methods for coping with pain.

A number of factors that will affect the pain response are: (1) integrity of the central nervous system, (2) level of consciousness, (3) training and previous experience in pain control, (4) attention and distraction, (5) fatigue, and (6) anxiety.

PHYSIOLOGICAL RESPONSES   The physiological responses which occur as a part of the pain experience are largely a result of activation of the autonomic nervous system. Typical responses that occur with stimulation of the sympathetic and parasympathetic portions of the autonomic nervous system are listed in Table 6-3. These responses are a great deal more complex than they are made to appear here. Only responses which can be useful for pain assessment have been listed in the table; other responses occur with stimulation of the autonomic nervous system but have been omitted. The typical response occurring with pain is characteristic of activation of the sympathetic branch. Although this response may predominate, it does not occur consistently and

Table 6-3   Physiological responses which occur with stimulation of the autonomic nervous system and may be useful in pain evaluation

Response	Sympathetic stimulation	Parasympathetic stimulation
Pupil size	Dilated	Constricted
Perspiration	Increased	No effect
Rate and force of heartbeat	Increased	Decreased
Blood pressure	Increased	Decreased
Depth and rate of respiration	Increased	No effect
Urinary output	Decreased	No effect
Peristalsis of GI tract	Decreased	Increased
Basal metabolic rate	Increased	No effect

in fact the physiological effects of pain may represent a mix of sympathetic and parasympathetic responses. Emotions, particularly anxiety and fear, also may initiate the same or similar response patterns thereby augmenting or altering physiological changes that occur with pain. Despite these limitations physiological measures can be a useful index in pain assessment.

Changes indicative of sympathetic stimulation are seen most consistently with superficial or cutaneous pain. An increase in pulse rate, elevation of systolic and diastolic blood pressure, and pallor due to cutaneous vasoconstriction may be present. Both respiratory rate and depth of respirations may be increased unless pain involves the chest or abdominal wall, in which case splinting of the painful area may limit the usual respiratory changes. Perspiration, gooseflesh, and dilated pupils are other physiological changes that may occur and should be noted. Nausea and vomiting may occur with cutaneous pain, but this is not usual. Alterations indicative of parasympathetic or mixed stimulation are not common in superficial pain but may occur with any prolonged, severe pain or with visceral or deep pain. These symptoms may precede collapse and are indicative of the body's inability to maintain homeostasis. Under these circumstances pulse rate and blood pressure will decrease and may be accompanied by nausea, vomiting, pallor, and increased perspiration. This state of incipient collapse is not common with pain and therefore pain may be overlooked as a contributing factor with these symptoms, particularly if the patient is not alert and able to verbalize the degree of pain he is experiencing.

As mentioned earlier, autonomic responses will be modified in cases of prolonged or chronic pain. The body cannot sustain such prolonged sympathoadrenal activity without either collapse or adaptation intervening. As adaptation occurs the autonomic symptoms previously discussed will be altered or reduced and therefore appear less evident to the observer.

The startle response and flexion or withdrawal reflex are automatic motor reactions that are initiated by pain of cutaneous origin. These reflexes are primitive spinal cord responses designed to remove the body from a noxious stimulus. They are not usually present with visceral or deep somatic pain although motor behaviors indicative of total body withdrawal may occur with this type of pain.

BEHAVIORAL RESPONSES   Gross motor activity and verbal expressions are common pain responses. A person may react with increased motor activity and agitation or with inhibition of activity and withdrawal depending upon the type of pain and the personality and coping style of the individual. Acute pain with intense local stimulation, such as in renal or biliary colic, does not allow for the development of individual response patterns and pain behavior tends to be relatively uniform. With pain of longer duration, cardiac pain, headache, or backache, the personality structure of the individual is of greater importance in the development and expression of pain behaviors and responses will be more diverse [9]. Behavioral responses, both motor and verbal, represent important sources of information in pain assessment, since pain usually is inferred from these responses.

Motor behaviors may fall into typical patterns frequently encountered with pain experiences. The flexion and withdrawal reflexes have already been discussed. Spasms of smooth or skeletal muscle frequently accompany visceral or deep somatic pain. They occur as a protective, often involuntary response early in the pain experience but may be maintained for long periods and actually exacerbate the pain.

Many of the voluntary behaviors elicited by pain represent protective actions taken in an attempt to decrease the pain. Behaviors may represent an increase in body activity—rubbing or supporting a painful area, frequent change in body position, walking or pacing; or they may represent reduction of activity—resting an extremity, protecting an area from any stimulation, and decreasing body movement by lying quietly. The behaviors chosen will reflect those behaviors that previously have been effective in reducing pain and that are suited to the type of pain experienced and to the personality of the individual. Generally as pain builds up in intensity activity decreases or ceases; one noticeable exception is visceral pain due to muscle spasms. With colic or cramping abdominal pain the individual frequently assumes a rolled-up or kneeling position while rocking the entire body. Although decreasing activity may be the usual behavior with increasing pain some individuals have been known to respond with increasing activity as pain increases; sometimes this behavior may be detrimental and represent a loss of ability to reason rationally as pain becomes unbearable.

Facial expressions are almost intuitively observed when assessing pain. Pinched features, a knotted brow, dilated pupils, facial grimaces, and perspiration present a portrait of pain to the observer. Any of these may occur with acute pain or exacerbations of chronic pain but may be absent in chronic pain or in stoic individuals who control such expressions of pain. The patient with chronic pain may have a tired, drawn look, or the eyes alone may reflect the suffering that is being endured.

A wide range of verbal behaviors can appear as a result of pain. Responses can include sighing, moaning, screaming, crying, repetition of words or phrases, as well as statements about the pain. Statements about pain can relate to any aspect of the pain experience from describing the pain to questioning why the pain is present. Verbal communication is the only available means of determining the subjective aspects of the pain experience. Pain may be recognized without specific statements and the degree of suffering may be inferred from other behaviors, but pain discussion is the only method available to the clinician to attempt to grasp the full implication of the pain experience for the patient.

AFFECTIVE RESPONSES   Almost any affective state can accompany pain, especially pain that becomes chronic; however, some responses seem to occur with greater frequency. Depression is often present with chronic pain

[14, 21], although it is sometimes difficult to determine whether the depression is caused by or preceded the pain. When depression is present and is treated the pain problem may improve. (See Chapter 4 for further discussion of the point.)

Regression, either as an egocentric response in which demands for attention are increased or a passive response in which weeping and dependent behavior predominate, may occur [28]. Pain frequently evokes an increase in anxiety which may in turn decrease the amount of pain that can be tolerated, thereby causing the individual to be caught in a vicious cycle of increasing anxiety and pain. Decreasing anxiety levels may alter this cycle and enable the individual to tolerate the pain better.

Behaviors may occur that indicate the development of aggressive, hostile, or manipulative states. "It is the *usual* situation that pain responses consist of reflexive protective behavior *and* regressed expression of anxiety and interpersonal manipulating maneuvers" [28].

Pain may disrupt normal behaviors; for example, learning time and reaction time may be adversely altered. Changes reflecting deviations from the individual's normal behavior patterns may also occur; for example, irritability or withdrawal.

Any changes in behavior should be assessed, especially with chronic pain, to determine the need for treatment of underlying behavior states.

Perception and Meaning of Pain

Perception is the process that defines the way one experiences the world of objects, people, and events [25]. Except for automatic or reflexive responses, the behaviors and reactions observed with a pain experience will be a result of the processing of the original stimulus by the central nervous system. It is this process that is modified and influenced by the cultural, psychological, and social background of the individual and it is this process that will determine the significance of the pain and the presence or absence of suffering.

The individual's perception of pain can be inferred from statements about the intensity and quality of the pain and from behaviors that accompany the pain experience. The evaluative terms used by the patient to describe the intensity of the pain will provide clues as to the degree of suffering being experienced. It is important to be aware that suffering may be present in the absence of the pain sensation. Copp, in a nursing study of pain and suffering [8], found that some hospitalized patients reported that suffering seemed to begin even before the pain and was focused on the anticipatory fears about the forthcoming pain.

Determining the significance and meaning that pain has for the individual becomes increasingly important as the duration of the pain is extended. If the pain is caused by a condition that can be cured, thereby eliminating the pain, the experience may hold no other meaning than that of a temporary distressing event; furthermore, painful treatments or surgery may be readily endured if they "cure" the pathology. The surgical pain of a cholecystectomy or removal of a stone in the ureter may be perceived as minimal when it means the elimination of painful renal or biliary colic. This type of acute or intermediate pain is usually "expected pain" and is handled quite well by both the patient and the clinician since both relief and curative measures can be provided.

There are, however, some types of pain that although expected and of known duration may nevertheless become highly significant if they lead to loss of a body part or function. The surgical amputation of a limb may fall into this category whereby a "cure" can be attained but at considerable expense. In this type of pain the anxiety level may indicate the significance attached to the lesion, the treatment, or the pain.

As pain continues and it becomes apparent that the source of the pain cannot be diagnosed or cannot be cured, assessing the meaning that pain has may become progressively important if the patient is to receive the utmost help in coping with the experience. Le Shan [19] has identified the fact that individuals with chronic pain attempt to give some meaning to the pain but receive little assistance from our culture in which no positive meaning is assigned to pain. Some of the meanings that patients in Copp's study attached to pain were the following [8]:

39 patients (26%) reported value in the pain experience.
Strong religious connotations were frequent.
33 patients (22%) described pain as a struggle, a fight.
19 patients (13%) reported pain as punishment with some redeeming aspects.
16 patients (11%) described pain as a challenge and assumed emotional and/or spiritual benefits would result.

It is interesting to note that the majority of these patients were for the most part able to ascribe some positive meaning to the pain—even the group that viewed pain as punishment identified some redeeming aspects.

This assignment of a meaning to pain is philosophical and must be consistent with the needs and values of the individual. It is important that the ideas of patients be respected whether or not the clinician agrees with them. This aspect can be assessed only by listening to and helping to clarify the individual's thoughts about the pain experience as it relates to his personal life.

The personal meaning that is placed on pain may be influenced by the way in which pain alters the life-style of the individual. These changes can be assessed with pertinent questions. Has the pain hampered physical activities? Does this affect self-care, occupation, leisure activities? How much time is spent up and how much down? Is this change seen as negative or does it have some positive value for the person? Does the pain interfere with personal relationships—in the family, with friends, with co-workers? Does the person associate pain with an uncertain prognosis? Does it mean a disease is becoming progressively more severe, impending death, or eventual loss of function or a body part? Has it changed his self-concept? Does he see himself as less productive, less useful, a drain on others? Or as an individual who can still contribute to life although the method of contribution may be different? Are pain and suffering to be endured—either quietly or not so quietly? Or are they seen as a challenge to be overcome?

Assessment of these factors may take days or weeks; it will require a relationship of trust and an ability to listen to what the patient tells the clinician both verbally and nonverbally. The information becomes meaningful in terms of helping the patient only to the degree that this process has helped the patient to clarify his thoughts about pain and has helped patient and staff to develop attainable goals for the patient's care.

Coping Mechanisms

A complete evaluation of chronic pain states will include an assessment of the methods being used to cope with the pain. This will allow the nurse to provide those methods that have been most helpful to the patient and can be used in the hospital setting. It will also allow staff to assist the patient in developing positive methods of coping if he has not already done so. Although this part of assessment is essential with chronic pain, it need not be limited to long-term pain; knowing how an individual normally handles or "copes" with pain may provide clues to providing relief with acute or transient pain. To help with this aspect of pain evaluation some of the coping mechanisms that may be used will be discussed.

The process of coping with a physical illness can be defined as "all cognitive and motor activities which a sick person employs to preserve his bodily and psychic integrity, to recover reversibly impaired function and compensate to the limit for any irreversible impairment" [20]. The process will be a combination of the individual's normal style of coping and techniques used to deal specifically with illness. The process may be considered adaptive or maladaptive depending upon how appropriate it is for the patient in a particular situation and how well it achieves maximum recovery [20].

Observation of patient behavior and response to illness can provide clues about the coping method that is being used. The patient may attempt to deal with pain by minimizing its existence. Behaviors that could be indicative of this style of coping include: denial of the pain, concealing the pain, and retaining "well" behaviors. When using these methods to minimize pain, the patient may not be able to verbalize their use without altering their effectiveness for him. The clinician will need to rely on observation to assess these techniques. In some settings treatment modalities used with chronic pain may actually focus on changing responses so that the patient minimizes pain behaviors thereby allowing him to conceal pain and retain normal activity.

Behavior may indicate the patient's efforts to control the pain being experienced. The individual may seek information about the pain or the pathology causing pain in an attempt to learn how to control the pain. Various methods of focusing, such as counting, repeating phrases, or of distraction may be used. Judicious timing of medication may be a control measure learned by the patient. Purposeful diversionary activities may be developed and prove helpful in pain control. Almost any type of physical or cognitive activity may prove beneficial depending upon the person and the situation. To determine the strategies used by the patient it is important to *ask* how he normally controls pain.

The individual may cope with pain by using techniques which actually increase the suffering experienced. They may focus all attention on the sensations experienced. Fear and anxiety about the illness may contribute to increased awareness of and attention to all symptoms, including pain. The individual may cling to the pain if the sick role provides a way of gaining attention and support. Szasz [31] has noted that severe, chronic illness does not necessarily lead to pain but "unless the patient can find something more interesting and worthwhile to attend to, the career of pain is apt to last till death" [31]. Techniques that increase suffering can be inferred from the observed responses and need to be recognized before a decision can be made about assisting the patient to develop more adaptive methods of coping.

While assessing coping strategies, fatigue, anxiety, and fear of impending pain should be evaluated. These factors can decrease pain tolerance and interfere with the individual's ability to use pain control techniques.

An assessment guide containing a number of factors that have been discussed and should be considered when evaluating pain follows. This is only a guide, not a pain history. It should be altered to meet the needs of specific groups of patients; some items may not be relevant for all patients and other items may need to be expanded greatly for pain related to specific conditions.

Assessment Guide for Evaluation of Pain—Factors To Be Considered

A. Characteristics of pain
   1. Location
      a. Areas of pain
      b. Areas without pain
   2. Intensity
      a. Mild
      b. Moderate
      c. Severe
      d. Overwhelming
   3. Quality of pain—words patient uses to describe pain
   4. Chronology
      a. Mode of onset
      b. Precipitating factors
      c. Variations in intensity and quality

B. Pain responses
   1. Physiological responses
      a. Note changes in pulse, blood pressure, respirations
      b. Note presence of dilated pupils, perspiration, nausea, vomiting, pallor

2. Behavioral responses
   a. Body activity increased or decreased
   b. Protection of painful areas
   c. Body position
   d. Facial expression
3. Affective responses

C. Pain communication
   1. How does the patient describe the pain and the degree of suffering?
   2. Is the patient groping for a meaning for the pain or does he ascribe some meaning to the pain?
   3. Does the pain interfere with physical activity? Personal relationships?
   4. How does the patient relate pain to the pathology?

D. Coping techniques
   1. Does the patient use any method to control the pain?
   2. If not, what does he do when the pain occurs or increases in severity?

E. Factors that can affect pain
   1. Is fatigue consistently present?
   2. Does the patient appear to be anxious, depressed, frightened?
   3. Is the patient worried about the illness? Does he have questions about it that have not been answered?
   4. What are the patient's expectations in relation to the pain? Does he want complete relief or just enough control to be able to pursue certain activities? What activities have a high priority for him?

F. Sources that should be used in assessing pain include
   1. The patient
   2. Close family members
   3. The medical record
   4. Information about expected pain patterns that occur with the diagnosed pathology

The Presence of Pain

The first step in the process of pain assessment is the determination that pain exists. Evaluation of pain as previously discussed presupposes that the clinical judgment—this individual is experiencing pain—has been made. The determination that pain exists may seem an elementary step but knowledge about information used by nurses in arriving at this initial phase of clinical decision is limited. Although the index most frequently recommended for pain assessment is the patient's verbal report of pain, there is indication that this recommendation is not widely accepted or practiced by nurses. In 1966 Hammond and associates [15] reported the results of a study that analyzed the inference process and resultant nursing action taken in the care of patients with postoperative pain. They found a very large number of cues were being used and reported by nurses with no single cue or grouping of cues transmitting a significant amount of information in determining the state of the patient.

In an exploratory study concluded in 1973 by Jacox and Stewart, nurse subjects were asked to describe one patient situation in which it was diffi-

Table 6-4 Categories of cues used by nurses in pain assessment

Behavior	Percent of responses identified under "difficult"	Percent of responses identified under "easy"
1. Characteristics of affect or disposition	46	54
2. Oral expression, excluding verbal complaints	35	65
3. Verbal communication	44	56
4. Facial expressions	21	79
5. Body movements	22	78
6. Vital sign changes	22	78
7. Other physiological signs	20	80

cult to assess pain and one in which it was easy to assess pain.* Four hundred and forty-three nurses responded to the questionnaire and a total of 46 patient behaviors were identified from the descriptions given. By classifying all of the behaviors into the categories shown in Table 6-4, it became evident that this group of nurses reported physiological signs and behaviors as easier indexes to use in pain assessment than verbal communication. Two factors must be considered when relying on physiological symptoms, particularly changes in vital signs. These changes are due to activation of the autonomic nervous system and may occur with emotional states other than pain and secondly, although they occur with acute pain, they are absent or sharply modified with chronic pain. These indexes can be useful adjuncts in determining that pain exists if one keeps their limitations in mind. For example, an elevated blood pressure in the immediate postoperative period may be an indication of pain, although the patient may be too drowsy to state that he has pain.

Since verbal communication would seem to be the most accurate method of assessing a symptom as subjective as pain, it would be helpful to know why this measure was difficult to use. The problem most frequently identified in the Jacox and Stewart study was the fact that patients' verbal expressions of pain were not consistent with other patient behaviors considered indicative of pain; that is, a patient said he was in pain but did not appear to be so or the patient appeared to be in pain but did not complain of pain or denied it when questioned. In an attempt to clarify this discrepancy an assessment guide was prepared, based upon the behaviors as previously identified. Research staff used these as a tool for pain assessment and collected data on a small group of surgical patients and patients with metastatic cancer (Table 6-5). Three cues appeared quite consistently in the cancer patient—

* The study cited here and in subsequent pages was part of a research program conducted at the University of Iowa College of Nursing from 1971–1976. Grant No. NU-00387-02 and No. NU-00467-03 from Division of Nursing, Bureau of Health, Manpower, Education.

Table 6-5 Cues used in assessing pain in surgical patients and cancer patients

Behavior	Surgical patient N = 30	Cancer patient N = 30
1. Characteristics of affect or disposition		
Unable to concentrate on anything except pain	2	12
Anxious, tense	3	10
2. Oral expressions, excluding verbal complaints	3	2
3. Verbal communications	18	26
4. Facial expressions		
Grimacing, clenched jaw	14	6
Distressed appearance	16	25
Painful look in eyes	7	22
5. Body movements		
Lying rigid	17	20
Splinting, etc.	19	15
6. Other physiological changes		
Diaphoresis	4	0
Flushed skin	4	1
Pallor	0	14

verbal communication, a distressed appearance, and a painful look in the eyes. A cue that was not written into the guide but was frequently added by the assessor was exhaustion or fatigue. No cues were used as consistently with the surgical patient, although splinting an area, lying rigidly, and verbal communication were the three that ranked highest. One can speculate that cancer patients might rely upon verbal communication because the other frequently occurring signs of pain are quite subtle and may not be observed and acted upon by the nurse, thereby forcing the patient to use verbal pain communication. With the surgical patient, however, a number of more obvious cues that are present might be observed and acted upon by the nurse without the patient having to initiate statements about pain. This would support Hackett's assertion that clinicians use acute pain with visible signs of discomfort as a model for all pain despite the fact that it is not sufficient to describe chronic pain [13]. Lack of understanding concerning the physiological changes that occur with chronic pain may be one of the reasons for nurses' statements that verbal expressions of pain were not consistent with other behaviors.

The other side of the problem is the patient who appears to be in pain but does not complain about pain or denies having pain. Relying upon the patient to initiate communication about his pain may present an unrecognized problem in pain assessment. Three groups of patients were studied intensively in relation to their pain experience in the study conducted by Jacox and Stewart. The patient population included 102 patients with (1) short-term pain associated with elective surgical procedures, (2) long-term pain associated with rheumatoid arthritis, and (3) progressive pain associated with metastatic cancer. Nearly three-fourths of these patients stated that they did not like to discuss their pain or were ambivalent about doing so [17]. The most common reason given for not discussing pain by both short-term and long-term groups was that "others are not interested in my problems." For the progressive group, the reason given most frequently was the social stigma attached to complaining. Patients in this study also were asked how they generally respond to pain and nearly two-thirds indicated that they attempt to remain outwardly calm [17].

Based upon these findings and the fact that research staff frequently found it necessary to use terms other than "pain" when eliciting responses from patients, the decision was made to explore the use of the terms pain and discomfort. Interviews were conducted with 200 hospitalized patients. Characteristics of the population sample include:

1. Sex: 108 males and 92 females.
2. Age range: 16 to 20, 9 patients; 21 to 40, 64 patients; 41 to 60, 65 patients; 60 to 82, 62 patients.
3. Educational background ranged from not completing grade school to completion of graduate education with the majority of patients having completed between grade 10 and two years of college.
4. Reason for hospitalization: 92 had surgical procedures, most of which would be classified as major procedures; 108 were admitted for medical problems or diagnostic tests.

Patients were asked to rate pain and discomfort being experienced at the time of the interview on a ten-point scale. Ratings showed that 149 patients (approximately 75 percent) were experiencing no pain at the time of the interview. A few of these patients (N = 28) were not experiencing pain at any time but the majority who responded this way had recently received pain medication. In contrast only 84, or 42 percent, were experiencing no discomfort at the time of the interview and only nine had been free of discomfort during this hospitalization. It would appear that the use of terms relating to comfort might elicit more response from the patient than the use of the term pain. The reason given as the cause of pain or discomfort was frequently the same; however, there are some differences as noted in Table 6-6, which lists the most frequently identified cause of pain or discomfort. This group of patients also completed a questionnaire in which they were asked to rate various conditions or procedures. The condition was rated as causing pain, discomfort, neither, or never experienced. Even with this small sample there are some trends; nausea and vomiting, being in one position, and muscle aches were rated as causing discomfort rather than pain. Pain was caused by muscle spasms, throbbing headaches, and incisions according to the ratings given by this sample. During the immediate postoperative period it was most painful to turn, cough, and ambulate, in that order; lying quietly

Table 6-6 Most frequently occurring cause or source of pain and discomfort as identified by 200 hospitalized patients

Cause/Source	D Now	D Hosp.	P Now	P Hosp.
1. Incision	38	56	24	67
2. Lower back and legs	15	21	12	20
3. Head and neck	16	19	7	24
4. Cramps/spasms	5	12	2	13
5. Chest pain or difficulty breathing	5	11	1	13
6. Being in hospital	4	19	0	0
7. Immobility	6	16	0	0

D = Discomfort
P = Pain
Now = during interview
Hosp. = during this hospitalization

was noted as painful in only about 11 percent of the sample. The acute experiences appeared to be the ones causing the patient to label the experience pain—as illustrated by the differences in ratings of muscle spasm and muscle aches.

Statements patients used to characterize pain versus discomfort included: pain is worse, it's shorter, it's all-consuming, it's "pure hurt," while discomfort was characterized as long-lasting, bearable, keeps one from being relaxed. One woman who had undergone a percutaneous cordotomy for pain relief very graphically described comfort as "getting away from pain."

Based on the information that has been obtained from interviewing patients and nurses, the following suggestions should be helpful in determining the presence of pain.

1. Listen to the patient; if he states he is having pain follow this statement up with an evaluation of the pain. Do not assume pain is not present because "the patient doesn't appear to be suffering."
2. Rely on physiological indicators of pain as clues of possible pain in the patient who is less alert than normal either because of drugs or the disease condition or in the patient who does not volunteer information about his state of comfort or discomfort. Follow up these clues by asking about pain or discomfort.
3. Use terms other than pain when trying to determine the patient's state of comfort. Ask if he hurts, if he is sore, if there is any change in the way he feels.
4. Expect that the individual with chronic pain may react differently than the patient with acute pain. The physiological symptoms of pain may be reduced or absent; he may talk about pain or he may deny pain but talk about being uncomfortable. The recognition of pain may be dependent upon the ability of the nurse to listen and observe; patients can relay a

great deal of information about their state of comfort but may do so only if the nurse indicates that she is ready to listen.

Summary

This chapter has attempted to provide some general guidelines that can be useful to the nurse in assessing and evaluating pain. Information pertinent to assessment of the existence of pain, evaluation of pain characteristics and responses, and consideration of the need to evaluate the significance of the pain and the coping mechanisms being used have been discussed. Information pertinent to the evaluation of specific types of pain will be considered as various disease conditions are discussed in the second section of this book.

References

1. Beecher, H. K.   *Measurement of Subjective Responses: Quantitative Effects of Drugs.* New York: Oxford University Press, 1959. P. 188.
2. Beecher, H. K.   An inspection of our working hypotheses in the study of pain and other subjective responses in man. In Keele, C. A., and Smith, R., eds., *The Assessment of Pain in Man and Animals.* London: E. & S. Livingstone Ltd., 1962. P. 163.
3. Beecher, H. K.   The placebo effect as a non-specific force surrounding disease and the treatment of disease. In Janzen, R., Keidel, W., Herz, A., and Steichele, C., eds., *Pain: Basic Principles—Pharmacology—Therapy.* Baltimore: The Williams & Wilkins Company, 1972. Pp. 175–180.
4. Bonica, J. J.   *The Management of Pain.* Philadelphia: Lea & Febiger, 1954. Pp. 48, 166.
5. Bonica, J. J.   Introduction: Management of pain. *Postgrad. Med.* 53:56, 1973.
6. Bonica, J. J.   Fundamental considerations of chronic pain therapy. *Postgrad. Med.* 53:81, 1973.
7. Charpentier, J.   Parameters of pain in man. In Janzen, R., Keidel, W., Herz, A., and Steichele, C., eds., *Pain: Basic Principles—Pharmacology—Therapy.* Baltimore: The Williams & Wilkins Company, 1972. Pp. 28–33.
8. Copp, L. A.   The spectrum of suffering. *Am. J. Nurs.* 74:491, 1974.
9. Delius, L.   Psychosomatic aspects of treatment. In Janzen, R., Keidel, W., Herz, A., and Steichele, C., eds., *Pain: Basic Principles—Pharmacology—Therapy.* Baltimore: The Williams & Wilkins Company, 1972. Pp. 175–180.
10. Engel, G.   Pain. In MacBryde, C. M., and Blacklow, R. S., eds., *Signs and Symptoms,* 5th ed. Philadelphia: J. B. Lippincott Company, 1970.
11. Fordyce, W. E.   An operant conditioning method for managing chronic pain. *Postgrad. Med.* 53:123, 1973.
12. Gatz, A. J.   *Manter's Essentials of Clinical Neuroanatomy and Neurophysiology,* 4th ed. Philadelphia: F. A. Davis Company, 1970. Pp. 20–24.
13. Hackett, T. P.   Pain and prejudice: Why do we doubt that the patient is in pain? *Med. Times* 99:130, 1971.
14. Hackett, T. P.   The surgeon and the difficult pain problem. *Int. Psychiatry Clin.* 4:179, 1967.
15. Hammond, K. R., et al.   Clinical inference in nursing. *Nurs. Res.* 15:134, 1966.
16. Hardy, J. D.   The nature of pain. *J. Chronic Dis.* 4:22, 1956.
17. Jacox, A., and Stewart, M.   *Psychosocial Contingencies of the Pain Experience.* Iowa City: The University of Iowa Press, 1973. Pp. 68–69.

18. Le Masters, R. E. A clinical approach to pain. *South. Med. J.* 67:173, 1974.
19. Le Shan, L. The world of the patient in severe pain of long duration. *J. Chronic Dis.* 17:119, 1964.
20. Lipowski, Z. J. Physical illness, the individual and the coping processes. *Psychiatry Med.* 1:91, 1970.
21. Lishman, W. A. The psychology of pain. In Autton, N., ed., *From Fear to Faith.* London: SPCK, 1971. Pp. 8–22.
22. Mehta, M. *Intractable Pain.* Philadelphia: W. B. Saunders Company, 1973. Pp. 3–17.
23. Melzack, R., and Wall, P. D. Pain mechanisms: A new theory. *Science* 150: 971, 1965.
24. Melzack, R., and Torgerson, W. S. On the language of pain. *Anesthesiology* 34:50, 1971.
25. Melzack, R., and Chapman, R. R. Psychologic aspects of pain. *Postgrad. Med.* 53:69, 1973.
26. Melzack, R. *The Puzzle of Pain.* New York: Basic Books, Inc., Publishers, 1973. Pp. 41, 173–179.
27. Pace, J. B. Management of chronic pain: Concepts, facts, and techniques for family physicians. *Clin. Med.* 82:13, 1975.
28. Sternbach, R. A. *Pain: A Psychophysiological Analysis.* New York: Academic Press, Inc., 1968. Pp. 12, 93.
29. Swerdlow, M. Problems in the clinical evaluation of pain. In Janzen, R., Keidel, W., Herz, A., and Steichele, C., eds., *Pain: Basic Principles—Pharmacology—Therapy.* Baltimore: The Williams & Wilkins Company, 1972. Pp. 49–51.
30. Szasz, T. S. *Pain and Pleasure.* New York: Basic Books, Inc., Publishers, 1957. P. 83.
31. Szasz, T. S. Psychiatric perspective on pain and its control. In Hart, D. F., ed., *The Treatment of Chronic Pain.* Lancaster: Medical and Technical Publishing Co., Ltd., 1974. Pp. 39–61.
32. *Taber's Cyclopedic Medical Dictionary*, 12th ed. C. L. Thomas, ed. Philadelphia: F. A. Davis Company, 1973. Pp. H-69, P-28.

II

Pain Alleviation Generally

7

Surgical and Electrical Stimulation Methods for Relief of Pain

Dennis McDonnell

Introduction

Chronic, intractable pain is not a symptom but a functional disease of the central nervous system. Its effective treatment has been elusive. Surgical approaches to this pain have developed only in the past 80 years. These procedures initially were directed toward the destruction of part of the sensory pathways to the cerebrum [1]. They were performed by open exposure of the cerebrum or spinal cord, usually under general anesthesia. The principle of stereotaxic surgery refined the technical approach and allowed similar lesions to be performed under local anesthesia. This has brought the benefits of relief even to the cachectic, poor-risk terminal cancer patient. The central nervous system inherently tends to protect itself from any ablative procedure, so that eventually suspended function due to the procedure tends to recover and pain tends to recur. The recent concept of extraneous stimulation of the nervous system promises a more physiological approach and hopefully will expand our knowledge and understanding of the mechanisms of chronic pain. This chapter will introduce and explore these techniques and principles. They are presented in a cephalocaudad sequence (Fig. 7-1).

Stereotaxic Encephalotomy

Socrates defined pain as a "passion of the soul" and, as such, intimate with the emotions of the personality leading to anxiety, depression, and introspection. Papez's classic proposal places the emotional center of cerebral function within the limbic system (amygdala, fornix, hypothalamus, anterior thalamus, and cingulate gyrus) [98, 99, 140]. Empirical evidence so far supports this proposal. These structures are phylogenetically old and located on the medial surface of the hemispheres and extend to the central core of the brain stem. The embryological origin and anatomical location support the pri-

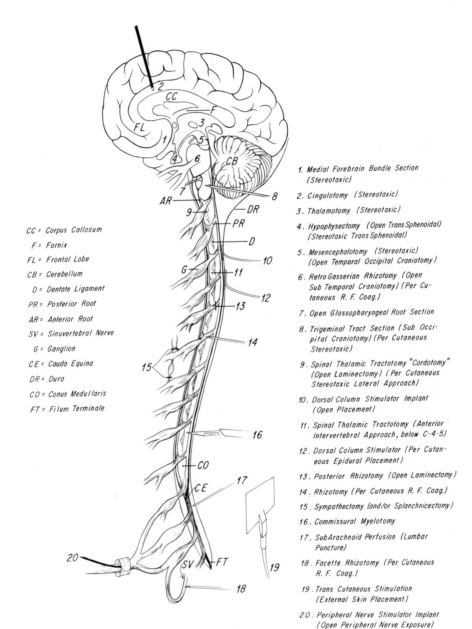

1. Medial Forebrain Bundle Section
   (Stereotaxic)

2. Cingulotomy (Stereotaxic)

3. Thalamotomy (Stereotaxic)

4. Hypophysectomy (Open Trans Sphenoidal)
   (Stereotaxic Trans Sphenoidal)

5. Mesencephalotomy (Stereotaxic)
   (Open Temporal Occipital Craniotomy)

6. Retro Gasserian Rhizotomy (Open
   Sub Temporal Craniotomy) (Per Cutaneous R. F. Coag.)

7. Open Glossopharyngeal Root Section

8. Trigeminal Tract Section (Sub Occipital Craniotomy) (Per Cutaneous
   Stereotaxic)

9. Spinal Thalamic Tractotomy "Cordotomy"
   (Open Laminectomy) (Per Cutaneous
   Stereotaxic Lateral Approach)

10. Dorsal Column Stimulator Implant
    (Open Placement)

11. Spinal Thalamic Tractotomy (Anterior
    Intervertebral Approach, below C-4-5)

12. Dorsal Column Stimulator (Per Cutan-
    eous Epidural Placement)

13. Posterior Rhizotomy (Open Laminectomy)

14. Rhizotomy (Per Cutaneous R. F. Coag.)

15. Sympathectomy (and/or Splanchnicectomy)

16. Commissural Myelotomy

17. SubArachnoid Perfusion (Lumbar
    Puncture)

18. Facette Rhizotomy (Per Cutaneous
    R. F. Coag.)

19. Trans Cutaneous Stimulation
    (External Skin Placement)

20. Peripheral Nerve Stimulator Implant
    (Open Peripheral Nerve Exposure)

CC = Corpus Callosum
F = Fornix
FL = Frontal Lobe
CB = Cerebellum
D = Dentate Ligament
PR = Posterior Root
AR = Anterior Root
SV = Sinuvertebral Nerve
G = Ganglion
CE = Cauda Equina
DR = Dura
CO = Conus Medullaris
FT = Filum Terminale

Figure 7-1 Sagittal view of cerebrum and lateral view of spinal cord and roots—panorama of surgical approaches and procedures.

mary homeostatic function of emotion. This is tempered by the phylogenetically newer neocortex which is most highly developed in man and responsible for intellectual function. The anterior cerebrum and in particular the limbic system receives, transmits, interprets, and is the source of reactive expression of pain. Suffering can therefore be altered by manipulating or interrupting pathways connecting the anterior cerebrum to the limbic system and thalamus.

Freeman and Watts's bifrontal leukotomy for pain (1946) with the attendant devastating personality changes is of historical interest only [43, 79]. This bears no relationship to the precise modern procedures of stereotaxic surgery.

Spiegel and Wycis, 1947, were the first to develop a reliable method of placing a small-bore probe or electrode accurately to a predetermined target within the depths of the brain [198]. Since then many instruments and procedure modifications have further increased the facility and accuracy of this method.

The stereotaxic method involves transferring a particular cerebral target point from an atlas or model brain to the patient's brain by relating the point to intracerebral landmarks in the patient. This requires some contrast procedure, placing either air or an iodinated compound within the ventricular system. The third ventricular boundaries, more specifically the foramen of Monro, anterior and posterior commissures, as well as the width of the ventricles, are visualized radiographically. These are landmarks that can be related to similar landmarks in the atlas or model. The procedure is performed under local anesthesia in the awake, cooperative patient. An instrument is attached to the patient's head that not only secures the head from movement but holds and guides the probe to the target. Thus, any target in the depths of the cerebrum can be approached with no essential damage to the intervening cerebral tissue.

Precisely located, extremely small lesions produced stereotaxically have the best chance of producing the beneficial desired effect, and minimize undesirable side effects such as personality alteration [195]. The lesions are usually produced by radio-frequency coagulation using an electrode or by freezing using a small-bore cooling probe.

Most lesions performed stereotaxically to relieve pain are closely related to the limbic system and thalamus. An early target was the medial forebrain bundle that forms connections between the frontal lobe and thalamus [79]. The cingulum bundle, which lies deep to the cingulate gyrus above the corpus callosum and connects the hippocampus, cingulate cortex, interventricular septal region, and the anterior thalamus, is also an effective target.

Electrical stimulations are always made as the electrode approaches the target. Observation of the responses in the awake patient further increases accuracy of electrode placement.

Cingulotomy

Interruptions of the anterior cingulate bundle are made bilaterally for more permanent pain relief. Lesions in the medial forebrain bundle and cingulum are more effective for "psychogenic" pain disorders since they tend to modify the patient's affective reaction to pain. They are also effective for diffuse visceral pain and pain of head and neck cancer [4, 34, 35, 62, 100, 123, 183].

Thalamic target areas for pain-relieving lesions are primarily in association radiations such as the intralaminar nuclei, the centromedian nucleus, and the pulvinar, but not the primary sensory nuclei (posterior ventral lateral and posterior ventral medial) [106, 108, 109, 157]. These latter nuclei receive the terminal fibers of the lateral spinothalamic tracts. Small lesions here produce marked loss of touch and proprioception with little change in pain. Also, the pain is even more severe and intractable with associated numbness and dystaxia [157]. This pain is worse than the first and is a type of central hyperpathia or anesthesia dolorosa [24]. Such pain can occur following cordotomy and amputation (phantom-limb pain).

Most ascending sensory fibers in the lateral and ventral spinothalamic tracts send collaterals and terminate in the central grey (reticular formation) in the midline of the brainstem, then proceed rostrally with bilateral representation.

Lesions in the dorsal medial and anterior nuclei modify the emotional component to pain similar to medial forebrain bundle section so that there is less preoccupation with pain. Precise target localization is facilitated by observing responses to evoked thalamic activity from distant external cutaneous stimuli as well as to direct stimulation of the thalamic nuclei entered.

Bilateral thalamic lesions are often required even for unilateral pain. Pain relief is usually immediate but pain in 10 to 50 percent will recur [109].

The spinothalamic and trigeminothalamic tracts are small and rather compact in the mesencephalon, and subject to more complete interruption at this site, particularly the more medially placed trigeminal fibers.

Nashold reported 25 patients with 70 percent overall relief from central dysesthesia, phantom-limb pain, and brachial plexus injury pain. He reported eight patients with head and neck carcinoma, all with good relief. There was an incidence of less than 10 percent central dysesthesia overall, and he considers this an excellent procedure for patients with intractable pain from head and neck carcinoma [130, 133].

The precise modern techniques of stereotaxic surgery allow for accurate approach to the desired target. Inherent limitations are the uniqueness of each patient's anatomy that is in variance to the norms used to determine the target, and the variable of individual patient response to stimulation. The procedure requires a contrast study to visualize the ventricular system, and as in most ablative procedures the effect tends to recede with time and pain often recurs [109, 195]. It requires sophisticated instrumentation and carefully aimed radiography, as well as special training. It does offer, however, relief for painful conditions not otherwise treatable, such as the central hyperpathias and thalamic pain, as well as pain about the head, neck, and upper limbs due to neoplasm.

Hypophysectomy

Hypophysectomy (surgical removal of the pituitary gland) is effective in palliative treatment of metastatic carcinoma of the breast and prostate [171, 186]. Diffuse, painful bone metastasis is common with both of these malignancies. Since the painful metastasis is frequently so widely spread, it is difficult to control with a strategically placed single ablative procedure in the spinal cord. These tumors are frequently hormone-dependent, and consequently to some extent under control of the pituitary [23].

Prolactin (a hormone released by the pituitary) and estrogen (a hormone released from the ovary under control of the pituitary) are important in the growth and regression of mammary carcinoma. It is possible that human growth hormone (released from the pituitary) is also a factor in supporting tumor growth. L-Dopa has been shown to reduce prolactin levels in serum and has been reported to relieve pain of osseous metastasis [25, 77].

Removal of the pituitary gland, which reduces or eliminates serum concentration of these hormones, would have a tendency to inhibit growth of these tumors and thus relieve pain of metastatic deposits in bone. This does occur in patients whose tumor cells are dependent on these hormones. About 40 percent of patients with carcinoma of the breast will have a palliative response to endocrine therapy [114].

Recent technical advances in the surgical removal of the pituitary gland, along with availability of oral hormone preparation for replacement (thyroid and cortisone), have brought hypophysectomy to a practical and effective means of palliation in tumor growth and relief of pain for osseous metastasis. The transsphenoidal approach to the sella, either by the stereotaxic method or open microscopic technique, is the presently preferred approach.

The stereotaxic method involves passing a small bored cannula through the nose and sphenoid sinus and then into the sellar region. The pituitary is then ablated by freezing with a cryoprobe [150], heating with radio-frequency electrode [199, 200, 201], or by radiating with implant of radio-isotopes [36, 127]. An inherent drawback to the stereotaxic method is that there may be small parts of the pituitary that survive these measures and continue to be hormonally active, and thus nullify the effect of the procedure.

Hardy has popularized the open transsphenoidal approach to the sella for both pituitary ablation for hormonal control of breast and prostate cancer and removal of pituitary tumors [51, 52].

The procedure is performed under general anesthesia. The incision is underneath the upper lip exposing the nasal cavity. The nasal mucosa is reflected, the nasal septum removed, and the floor of the sphenoid sinus entered. A portable fluoroscope is then positioned so that the sella can be viewed in the lateral projection on an image intensifier. The surgical binocular microscope is positioned so the operative cavity is brightly illuminated and magnified. The floor of the sella is then opened. The pituitary gland can be viewed directly and clearly. It can then be totally removed as a single unit. This method assures total removal of the gland [11, 15, 49, 51].

A recent report showed a 58 percent incidence of tumor remission 12 months following hypophysectomy. Pain relief from osseous metastases has been most gratifying. Surgical morbidity is low and average in-hospital time is less than seven days. Hypophysectomy is a procedure worthy of consideration to relieve pain of metastatic breast and prostatic cancer [186, 196].

Retrogasserian Rhizotomy

Pain involving the trigeminal nerve has been a challenge for centuries. Trigeminal neuralgia, or tic douloureux, consists of sharp, lancinating pain, fleeting but distressingly recurrent in the facial distribution of one or more of the three nerve branches. It can often be triggered by touching a particular place or by eating; chewing or talking may exacerbate it. The successful surgical treatment has generally been directed toward denervating or rendering analgesic the trigger area or distribution area of the pain.

In 1891 Sir Victor Horsley first reported the temporal approach to the Gasserian ganglion intradurally by elevating the temporal lobe. Hartly in the U.S. and Krause in Germany used an extradural approach to the ganglion [54, 76]. Frazier developed the technique of selective root section via the extradural subtemporal approach and it is this technique that is widely used [40, 41, 42, 174].

The procedure is performed with the patient under general anesthesia in the sitting position. The head is secured in a straight-on position with the operated side free. A vertical scalp incision is made in the temporal region 2 cm in front of the ear. A "silver dollar"-sized area from the temporal squama bone is removed. The dura is separated from the floor of the middle fossa and gently lifted. The middle meningeal artery entering through the foramen spinosum is cut, and the mandibular nerve entering its foramen ovale in the middle fossa floor is identified. The dural covering over the nerve is opened and the rootlets proximal to the ganglia are cut or massaged. Care is taken to preserve the motor branch which courses along with the mandibular sensory branch. This is the nerve to muscles of mastication.

If the rootlets are cut, the patient is anesthetic in the area of their distribution. If the rootlets are massaged, then some sensation is preserved, but there is a tendency for pain to recur over a period of years [48, 50, 170, 180].

Dandy, in 1925, proposed sectioning the nerve at the level of the pons [19]. This involves an approach through the suboccipital region with mild retraction of the cerebellum to expose the cerebello-pontine angle [189]. The advantage of this approach is to detect an unsuspected tumor as the cause of the trigeminal neuralgia. This is unusual without other associated symptoms or findings [20, 22].

This route, however is the approach of choice for glossopharyngeal neuralgia [21]. This tic pain involves the glossopharyngeal nerve and was first described by Harris in 1921 [71]. It is an uncommon neuralgia that consists of paroxysms of severe, lancinating pain in the throat and the base of the tongue, occasionally radiating to the ear. The pain may be accompanied by salivation and precipitated by talking or swallowing. Touching the tonsillar pillar may exacerbate the pain [73]. If medical treatment fails to relieve it, then pain can be relieved by sectioning the glossopharyngeal nerve intracranially, using Dandy's method. The nerve is approached through a suboccipital craniectomy. The cerebellum is gently lifted to expose the jugular foramen. The glossopharyngeal nerve is just anterior to the vagus at the foramen. Microscopic magnification and illumination greatly facilitate identifying the nerve for section. The sensory loss in the ipsilateral pharynx is very well tolerated, and the pain is usually cured [21].

Percutaneous Radio-Frequency Retrogasserian Rhizotomy

In 1970 Sweet and Wepsic reported their technique and results in treating trigeminal neuralgia by percutaneously coagulating the trigeminal nerve. Their series was updated in 1974 when, of 214 patients with trigeminal neuralgia, 91 percent had relief of pain [179]. This experience has been confirmed by others, and has led to the great popularization of this procedure in this country [137, 184].

Kirschner in 1931 (Germany) was the first to use electrical current to coagulate the Gasserian ganglion, but difficulty in regulating the heat at the electrode tip led to injury to the carotid artery, extraocular cranial nerves, and unwanted corneal anesthesia [76]. However, with modern radio-frequency electrical generators and accurate electrode-tip thermisters, more precisely regulated lesions can be achieved. The advantages of the procedure in addition to relatively atraumatic ease are selective interruption of the smaller pain fibers and preservation of touch. The lesion can be limited to only the involved roots [179].

The patient is given a neurolept-type anesthetic so as to be alert enough to respond to stimulating current and sensory testing after each lesion is made. A needle is passed under fluoroscopic control into the cheek and through the foramen ovale (exit hole for the mandibular branch) in the floor of the middle fossa. It passes along the mandibular division past the Gasserian ganglion and toward the compact portion of the nerve in Meckles Cave on the petrous ridge (Fig. 7-2). Stimulation responses of the patient determine rootlets in proximity of the electrode. When the electrode is in the desired position, the patient is more deeply anesthetized with a short-acting drug, and the electrode tip is heated from 60° to 80° C. for a measured time (30 to 60 seconds). When the patient is aroused the face is tested for pain

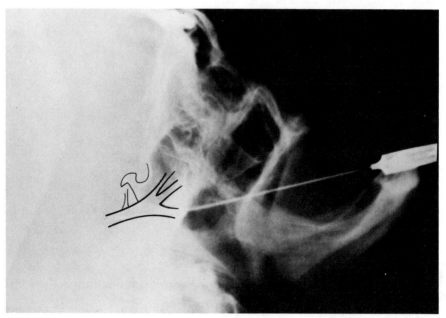

Figure 7-2 Percutaneous retrogasserian radio-frequency rhizotomy. The tri-geminal nerve is heavily outlined, and the dorsum sellae and petroclinoid ligament are lightly outlined. The electrode is placed through the foramen ovale and lies along the mandibular branch of the trigeminal nerve.

and touch. The procedure is repeated until the desired amount of analgesia is obtained. The patient can be discharged the following day free of pain.

The large A beta fibers that carry touch are better insulated from the heating electrode than C fibers and their function is thus preserved. If there is hypoalgesia without analgesia in the pain trigger areas, there is great likeli-hood that neuralgia will recur [179].

Nevertheless, attaining analgesia while preserving touch sensation has been a great advance in the treatment of trigeminal neuralgia.

Vascular Decompression

Dandy initiated the concept that trigeminal neuralgia was due to involve-ment of the posterior root by a tumor or compression by an artery [22]. Jannetta and Rand have determined that the majority of trigeminal neural-gias are due to arteries close to the root pulsating against it, causing irritation [151]. They expose the nerve in the cerebellar pontine angle using light and magnification of the operating microscope [67, 68]. Their approach, how-ever, is subtemporal and transtentorial. Small tortuous branches of the su-perior cerebellar artery pulsating against the trigeminal nerve close to the pons are dissected away from the nerve. It is suggested that sclerotic, elongated vessels encroach and pulsate against the nerve producing focal demyelination or "short circuits" which give rise to the pain. This concept approaches trigeminal neuralgia from its possible etiology and has the advantage of preserving function of the nerve.

Mesencephalic Spinothalamic Tractotomy

Only a relatively small number of fibers from the spinothalamic tract reach the posteroventral sensory nuclei of the thalamus; most fibers turn medially to end in the central core neurons of the reticular formation in the rostral medulla, pons, and mesencephalon [102, 133]. These spinoreticular fibers can then be traced to the internal medullary lamina of the thalamus. The spinothalamic tract in the pons and mesencephalon is rather small and scant. It, however, is located close to the surface of the posterolateral wall of the pons and mesencephalon and can be exposed through an occipital craniotomy by elevation of the occipital lobe [188]. The lesion is placed by marking a small cut on the upper lateral surface of the mesencephalon. Interruption of the tract at this level is directed to relieve pain in the head, neck, and arm [130]. It is at times necessary to make the tractotomy this high because even with high cervical cordotomy there is the tendency for analgesia levels to fall or disappear over a period of several months. Then pain will recur.

Dogliotti in 1938 was the first to report section of the tract at the mesencephalic and pontine levels. In 1942 Walker repeated his section of the tract just ventral to the posterior margin of the superior colliculus. Unfortunately, there is a high incidence of central dysesthesia and loss of analgesia with this procedure because the small C-spinoreticular fibers are more medially placed and are missed by the cut. This, coupled with a high mortality rate, has discouraged the use of this procedure even for head and neck cancer.

Medullary Tractotomy

Medullary tractotomy was introduced by Schwartz and O'Leary in 1941 for pain in the face, neck, and upper limb [160, 161]. Cuts made 2 to 10 mm caudally to the obex avoided the vestibular nuclei and restiform body, so that dystaxia would be less likely to occur. Ipsilateral hypoalgesia in the face occurs with involvement of the descending trigeminal tract. Experience has shown that analgesia is less likely to fade and medullary tractotomy is to be preferred over high cervical cordotomy for relief of pain in the upper limb [9, 16, 38].

Cordotomy

Cordotomy, or interruption of the lateral spinothalamic tract located in the anterior lateral quadrant of the spinal cord, is one of the more widely accepted and used procedures for treating intractable pain. Spiller and Martin

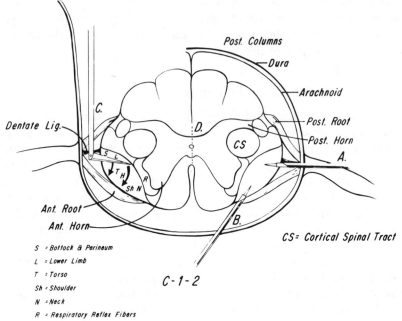

Figure 7-3 Cross section of spinal cord at C1–2. A. Percutaneous lateral approach to lateral spinal thalamic tracts—C1–2 interlaminar space. B. Percutaneous anterior approach—intervertebral disk space below C3–4. C. Open anterolateral cordotomy. D. Commissural myelotomy—usually in the lumbar and sacral segments. Note the somatropic arrangement within the lateral spinothalamic tract and position of respiratory reflex fibers.

[175] in 1912 were the first to report intentional surgical interruption of the anterolateral columns of the cord to relieve pain (Fig. 7-3).

Open Cordotomy

Several series have been reported and procedure modifications have been proposed; indications for open cordotomy have changed as knowledge and experience have expanded [32, 47, 64, 70, 194].

The procedure may be performed under general or local anesthesia, through a small laminectomy when portions of adjacent laminae are removed, exposing the posterolateral dura which is opened longitudinally (Fig. 7-4). The dentate ligament runs the entire length of the cord on either side and inserts on the dura delineating the dorsal half from the ventral half of the cord. This ligament can be exposed and gently lifted to expose the ventrolateral aspect of the cord. A sharp, pointed blade, narrowed and adjusted so as to penetrate the cord for a depth of 4 to 5 mm, is inserted at or just ventral to the insertion site of the dentate ligament; it is then carried forward to transect the ventrolateral cord. Care is taken to avoid rotational dis-

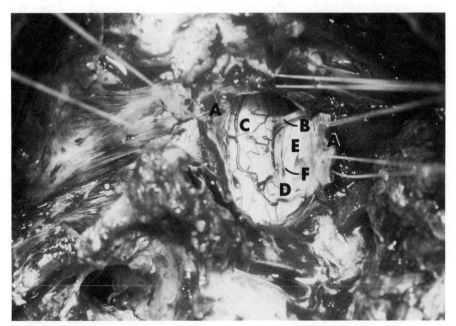

Figure 7-4 Exposed right side of spinal cord at C1–2 for open anterolateral cordotomy. A. Dural flaps being retracted. B. Dorsal root C1. C. Dorsal lateral surface of spinal cord. D. Dorsal root C2. E. Dentate ligament inserting onto inner surface of dura. F. Origin of dentate ligament from lateral surface of cord, marking the dorsal from the ventral half of the cord.

tortion of the pliable cord when manipulated, which would decrease the accuracy of the cut. Also the medial extent of the cut is closely observed to avoid damage to the anterior spinal artery.

Local anesthesia is preferred by some so that effectiveness of analgesic level and pain relief can be documented as the lesion is made. Generally, however, it is performed under general anesthesia, and the cut made strictly anatomically under direct vision without physiological control [194, 195].

If the pain is midline or bilateral, then the spinothalamic tracts must be divided bilaterally to give complete pain relief.

When bilateral lesions are made, one side cut must be separated by three to four segments from the opposite side to avoid transverse section cord changes. This results in lost sensation for pain and temperature two to three segments below the level of the cut on the body side contralateral to the cut. There may be gait unsteadiness for several days due to interruption of the spinocerebellar fibers coursing in the same region.

The high cervical level at C1–2 is preferred for upper limb and shoulder pain. Because of the widened interlaminar space at C1–2, less bone removal is required. The high level affords less chance for analgesic level to fall below the pain level [44]. The larger spinal canal and spinal subarachnoid space allow more room to adjust the cut more safely. The contralateral cut for bilateral lesions is made through a separate "keyhole"-type laminectomy several segments below the C4 level so as to preserve automatic respiratory control and avoid the phrenic-efferent segments of C3 and C4 [195].

Over a period of months to years the level of analgesia may drop several segments, and islands of pain sensation return in the previously analgesic regions. The pain may recur even in an analgesic region. Distressing central burning or dysesthetic pain may begin in an analgesic region. This is of central spinal cord origin and may be more distressing than the original pain.

In general, therefore, this procedure is usually limited to those with pain from metastatic neoplasm where longevity expectation is limited in terms of months rather than years. Tabetic crisis and chronic lumbar arachnoiditis have been indications in the past, but because of recurrent pain and central dysesthesias these indications are less frequent.

Percutaneous Cordotomy

Mullan [125] in 1963 revolutionized spinothalamic tractotomy by his concept of approaching the upper cervical cord percutaneously with a needle under local anesthesia. His lesion was made by a strontium-uranium isotope needle applied against the ventrolateral cord for a measured time in minutes to deliver a tissue-coagulating dose of radiation limited to the ventrolateral quadrant.

Rosomoff modified this by passing the needle from a direct lateral position through the wide interlaminar space at Cl–2 into the subarachnoid space and securing it in a three-coordinate variable vise [158]. Radio-frequency coagulation is used to produce the lesion in gradual increments, and the patient's head is supported gently in a head rest to prevent movement (Fig. 7-5). Emulsified pantopaque is injected to outline the dentate ligament (Fig. 7-6). This is the primary target and is viewed with biplane fluoroscopy (Fig. 7-7).

Additional verification of preferred electrode position is obtained by the patient's response to the stimulation current, using a pulsed square wave current at 25 Hz and 0.01 volts. With this the patient perceives tingling paresthesias in the contralateral side. The electrode can be carefully positioned within the somatotopically arranged tract according to the patient's response. Sacral and lower limb fibers are arranged more laterally, while trunk and upper limb fibers are more medially placed [181].

In this manner the tract may be more selectively interrupted to produce satisfactory pain relief, minimize unnecessary denervation, and avoid motor deficits.

If the cause of pain is midline, i.e., spinal metastasis, or involves bilateral structures, pain will often recur with previous intensity contralaterally to the side of the cordotomy effect, thus requiring a bilateral lesion.

Bilateral cordotomy lesions can be made safely, but only if the second

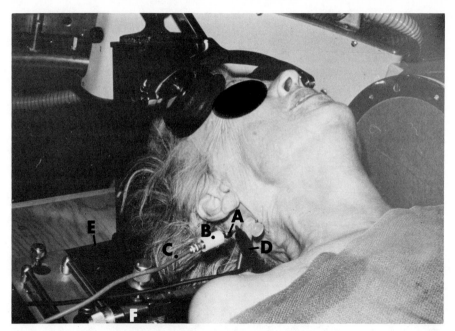

Figure 7-5 Percutaneous cordotomy lateral approach at C1–2. Patient's head is supported on the Rosomoff head rest. A. 18-gauge needle. B. Electrode jack with electrode inserted. C. Active cable to the electrode—one pole. D. Active cable to needle—second pole. E. Head rest.

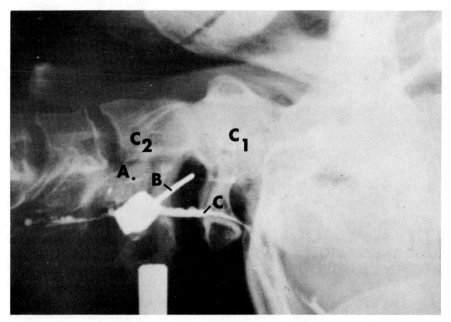

Figure 7-6 C1–2 percutaneous cordotomy radiograph, lateral projection; C1 and C2 vertebral bodies. A. Contrast outlining the dentate ligament. B. 18-gauge needle. C. Contrast outlining the posterior subarachnoid space.

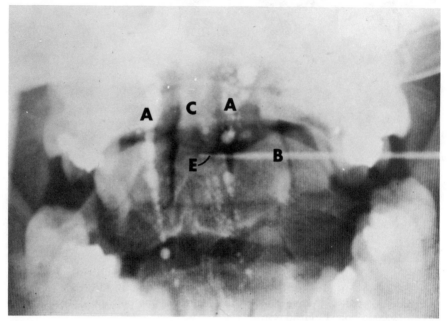

Figure 7-7   C1–2 percutaneous cordotomy radiograph, AP projection. A. Contrast material on the dentate ligament bilaterally. B. 18-gauge thin-walled needle. C. Shadow of spinal cord showing shift of the cord by the needle. E. Tip of electrode.

lesion is delayed by at least two weeks and the patient's respirations carefully monitored with an apnea monitor or in an intensive care facility.

Bilateral high cervical cord lesions interrupt afferent and efferent respiratory reflex pathways coursing deep in the ventrolateral quadrants close to the anterior horns [37, 134]. The respiratory reflexes fail to respond to hypercarbia, causing the patient to become apneic in sleep and expire in respiratory arrest [7, 80]. This phenomenon is known as Ondine's Curse [117]. It is quickly reversed by awakening the patient and encouraging deep, voluntary respirations. This phenomenon is usually self-limited and resolves in several days. It can be minimized by keeping the cordotomy lesion as precise and as small as is effectively possible [126].

Lin and Gildenberg et al in 1966 modified the percutaneous technique by inserting the needle from an anterior to posterior direction through the disk space into the spinal canal and anterolateral quadrant of the cord [45, 46, 87]. This allows interruption of the spinothalamic tract at any cervical interspace below the C1–2 level. Thus, percutaneous lesions can be placed below the diaphragmatic outflow at the C3–4 level preserving respiratory reflexes.

The percutaneous techniques of cordotomy are well tolerated by even the most wasted and debilitated patients who often need the procedure most.

Availability of pain relief to the cancer patient has been greatly increased by advancement of the percutaneous technique.

Dorsal Rhizotomy

One of the axioms in physiology is that sensory impulses enter the spinal cord via the posterior roots and motor impulses exit the spinal cord via the ventral roots. Magendie [101] in 1822 was the first to discover sensory impulses in the posterior roots. Abbe and Bennet [1] in 1889 were the first to surgically cut the posterior root to relieve pain.

The specific skin distribution of sensation from these nerve roots (dermatomes) was determined by Sherrington, Foerster, and Keegan [32, 72]. Considerable overlap has been demonstrated. There are myotomes (muscle) and sclerotomes (bone) that do not correspond in region to dermatomes. Theoretically, then, pain arising from the distribution of a single root could be relieved of all modes of sensation (in contrast to cordotomy). There is less certainty and more controversy regarding the effectiveness of posterior rhizotomy, other than for the trigeminal and glossopharyngeal nerves [90, 91, 138, 139, 193]. The advantage of posterior rhizotomy is that if it is effective initially, there is a tendency for relief to continue, whereas with cordotomy the effect tends to resolve with time. Therefore, rhizotomy is considered more frequently in pain conditions of benign origins [153, 162, 195].

Prior to rhizotomy a temporary paravertebral block of the roots involved is performed under fluoroscopic control [195]. The needle point is directed to the neural foramen, and frequently the patient experiences paresthesias in the distribution of the nerve root. The root is then infiltrated with a local anesthetic. There should be loss of sensation then in the nerve root distribution appropriate to the usual duration of the local anesthetic. Pain should also be relieved for an appropriate time period.

Although paravertebral block is performed and pain relieved, this will not guarantee successful relief of pain if these roots are sectioned. It is possible that paravertebral block itself carries a significant placebo effect, thus limiting the predictability of ultimate rhizotomy effectiveness.

Due to the overlap, several roots are usually sectioned, at least two above and two below the roots involved. Multiple root section is rarely performed for upper or lower limbs because an anesthetic limb is useless even though motor power is normal [193]. Sacral root section will result in sensory neurogenic bladder and impotence [18]. Therefore, rhizotomy is most often applied for thoracic and upper lumbar segments [193].

When rhizotomy is performed the level is marked and x-rays taken to locate the exact root level. The roots are then exposed through a laminectomy procedure. The dura is opened longitudinally. Here the use of the operating microscope allows precise delineation of the posterior roots, which are separated from the ventral roots by the dentate ligament. Small vessels accompanying the roots can then be preserved. The rootlets are then coagulated with bipolar forceps and sectioned. Multiple roots above and below the involved level are similarly identified and cut.

Preferably this is performed under local anesthesia, where each nerve root can be stimulated, and the pain reproduced. Also, the effectiveness of completed rhizotomy can be assessed while the patient is under surgery to assure adequate denervation and to better insure effective relief.

White and Sweet [195] point out that even multiple roots to the upper or lower limbs can be sectioned. So long as sensory innervation of the thumb (C6) is preserved, there will be satisfactory sensation for a usefully functional limb, but they stress that C6 and C7 should be preserved whenever possible. Also either the L5 or S1 root must be preserved in the lower limb. They advocate rhizotomy for benign conditions where there is long life expectancy and advise multiple root sections to compensate the wide overlap in sensory root distribution. The advantages are that areas of anesthesia remain stable through the years and the incidence of central dysesthesia is quite low. The anesthesia is well tolerated even in the upper or lower extremities so long as strategic roots are preserved, C6 in the upper and either L5 or S1 in the lower.

A drawback to the procedure is that many services report poor relief of pain treated by rhizotomy, even when preliminary paravertebral block indicated that good relief should be expected. Therefore, as with any ablative procedure, rhizotomy must be carefully weighed with each individual patient. There is general agreement that pain due to postherpetic neuralgia and adhesive arachnoiditis does not respond to rhizotomy.

Percutaneous Facet Rhizotomy

The causes of chronic back pain are multiple and all too frequently unclear. Obvious causes such as inflammation or marked degenerative arthritis, herniated intervertebral disk, hypertrophic spondylosis, congenital stenotic spinal canal, and neoplasm must be excluded. The pathophysiology may be due to degenerative changes in the articular facet and irritation of its surrounding joint capsule. With degeneration and narrowing of the disk space there are added strains on the facet joint. The patient usually has local tenderness over the involved facet joint [149, 164].

The sinuvertebral (articular) nerves, which are branches of the posterior ramus of the nerve root, supply the facet joint capsule as well as the anulus of the disk [142]. Rees [155] in 1971 proposed interrupting these nerves to relieve chronic back pain and sciatica. Shealy perfected and popularized the procedure of "facet rhizotomy" [163, 164, 165].

Under local anesthesia, and under x-ray and fluoroscopic control, the center of the facet joint is located on both anteroposterior and lateral views. A 12-gauge guide needle is then inserted through the skin to the facet. A thermocouple electrode is then inserted into the needle. The needle is then withdrawn from the skin over the electrode, which is left in place. Using a stimulating current at 25 cps the electrode is manipulated close to the articular nerve; care is taken to avoid the nerve root. Response is usually seen with 1 to 2 volts. The pain produced may be the same as the original pain. When paresthesias, pain, and x-rays indicate the electrode is next to the articular nerve, it is coagulated at 80° C. for 50 seconds. This is usually repeated twice more for a total of 150 seconds.

There have been mixed reports on this procedure [185]. Patient selection will determine results. It has potential as a screening diagnostic as well as a therapeutic procedure. Complications are infrequent when care is used to avoid the main nerve root. No neurological deficit should arise from this procedure.

Percutaneous Radio-Frequency Rhizotomy

Rhizotomy can be performed percutaneously under local anesthesia. Using heat generated in a thermocouple electrode driven by a radio-frequency generator, pain fibers can be selectively coagulated and interrupted while preserving touch, proprioception, and motor function. The principles involved are the same as for radio-frequency coagulation of the trigeminal nerve [141].

Needles are passed under fluoroscopic control into the neural foramen. Stimulation with a biphasic square wave current from 0.5 to 2 volts at 25 to 85 cps produces paresthesias along the nerve root distribution as well as appropriate muscle contraction. When indications confirm proper position of the electrode tip next to the nerve root and away from the subarachnoid space, the root is coagulated at from 50° to 70° C. for 120 seconds. This has been shown to selectively interrupt C fibers while preserving A alpha, beta, and delta fibers. This can be performed at multiple levels from the cervical region to L5–S1 inclusively. The potential advantages of this procedure over the classic open laminectomy and rhizotomy are obvious. Touch and proprioception are preserved. However, the limitations regarding patient selection are the same.

Commissural Myelotomy

Pain in the midline structures, such as low back, perineum, and rectum, has been extremely difficult to control. Spinothalamic tractotomy has been partially effective, but must be done bilaterally with its impendent risks to respiration, bladder function, and motor strength [82]. Sagittal hemisection of the cord over a few segments offers a possible solution [191].

The majority of fibers conveying pain and temperature in the lateral spinothalamic tracts take origin from neurons in the dorsal horns (substantia gelatinosa). These fibers cross to the opposite side ventromedially in the

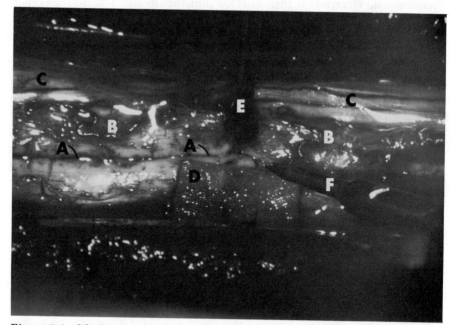

Figure 7-8 Myelotomy—exposed spinal cord through operating microscope. A. Dorsal median sulcus of spinal cord. B. Veins on dorsal surface of cord. C. Nerve rootlets. D. Cottonoid paddy (small sponge). E. Microdissector instrument. F. Knife opening the sulcus; dorsal median sulcus is opened for sagittal hemisection of the spinal cord.

ventral white commissure just beneath the central canal [17]. This anatomical feature allows interruption of pain bilaterally by section of the commissural fibers in the midline [156]. This is performed under general anesthesia through a laminectomy exposing the cord above the root entry of the highest level of pain. The dura is opened over the midline exposing the dorsal columns of the spinal cord. Using the operating microscope for illumination and magnification, the dorsal median sulcus of the cord is separated and the commissure split continuously in a cephalocaudal direction until all segments involved in the pain are sectioned and the cord is halved (Fig. 7-8). Special care is taken to avoid damage to the anterior spinal artery, which might lead to infarction of the bisected cord. Microsurgical techniques minimize the risks of damaging the cord halves. The results of relieving midline perineal pain using this method have been quite encouraging [88, 148, 173].

Sympathectomy

Causalgia and sympathetic dystrophies are severe, debilitating conditions that directly or indirectly involve the sympathetic nervous system [81, 84, 89, 107]. The sympathetic nervous system does not include afferents of pain, but rather is visceral motor in function [123]. Weir Mitchell's description

[122] of the causalgia pain occurring with Civil War wounds remains a classic, and he coined the term causalgia (Greek–*kausos*, heat; *algos*, pain). True causalgia is a specific syndrome consisting of a constant burning pain in the periphery of an extremity following a partial or incomplete peripheral nerve injury [27]. Most commonly the nerve injured is a mixed nerve (motor and sensory, i.e., median nerve in uppers and sciatic nerve in lowers). The pain is exacerbated by even minor stimuli (breeze of cold air, weight of a sheet) and by emotional upset. It may be partially relieved by wrapping in a cool or warm wet compress. The skin in the painful part may become thin, hairless, tight, and pale, with thick, long nails. The pain is usually relieved by block or ablation of sympathetic innervation to the painful part.

Related conditions that usually respond to sympathetic interruption are posttraumatic sympathetic dystrophy and posttraumatic osteoporosis (Sudeck's atrophy). Posttraumatic sympathetic dystrophy is causalgia pain not associated with nerve injury but accompanying fractures or extensive blunt trauma to soft tissues, whereas Sudeck's atrophy is an accelerated osteoporosis in the painful part due to alteration in blood flow to the bone [8, 121].

Initially these conditions are treated by temporary sympathetic block [124]. This is done by injecting a local anesthetic into the cervical sympathetic chain as it courses along the anterolateral border of the C7–T1 vertebrae. A needle is passed under sterile aseptic conditions one inch above and one inch lateral to the suprasternal notch 1 mm back from the anterior aspect of the spinal column. After injection of anesthetic, effective sympathetic blockade is assured when the limb is noted to be warm, dry, and slightly erythematous from increased blood flow in the skin. The superficial veins become more prominent. Also a Horner's syndrome is noted on the ipsilateral side (slight droop of the eyelid and small pupil). The causalgia is completely relieved at least for the duration of the local anesthetic and frequently longer. Satisfactory permanent relief may be obtained by repeated temporary sympathetic blocks. Success with this treatment is more likely if begun very soon after the injury and onset of pain [192]. For pain in the lower limbs a paravertebral block is made at L1–2–3–4 under fluoroscopic control. The needle approach here is from a posteromedial direction.

If repeated sympathetic block is not successful in giving permanent relief but is followed by temporary relief lasting at least for the duration of drug action, then surgical sympathetic ablation is indicated [3]. For upper-limb pain this may be accomplished from an anterior approach exposing the C7–T1 vertebral chain through a cervical incision above the clavicle, or posteriorly through either a paravertebral or intercostal incision [12, 115]. Another alternative approach is through a transaxillary second and third intercostal incision. If the upper half of the stellate ganglion at C7 is preserved, no permanent Horner's syndrome will result [65, 96]. Usually the sympathetic ganglia of T1 to T4 or T5 are removed [55, 85, 86].

For the lower limb an oblique flank incision is made with removal of the 12th rib to visualize the sympathetic chain from L1 through L4 [172, 182].

Splanchnectomy and Thoracic Sympathectomy

Splanchnectomy and thoracic sympathectomy are occasionally used to relieve intractable pain in the biliary ducts or pancreas, particularly chronic pancreatitis. If these are performed they must usually be accomplished bilaterally for effective relief.

Peet [143] in 1935 proposed a posterior approach, resecting the vertebral articulation of the 11th rib and exposing the D10–11–12 chain as well as the greater and lesser splanchnic nerves (the abdominal visceral afferents).

Prior to surgical interruption a coeliac ganglion block is made with local anesthetic using retrograde angiography with selective catheterization of the coeliac artery. It is then injected with iodinated contrast material and viewed fluoroscopically. The artery is then used as a target to guide the needle for coeliac ganglion block. If visceral pain is relieved for a period appropriate to the action duration of the drug, then surgical splanchnectomy is considered.

Preferably the classic thoracotomy and intrapleural approach is used because of better exposure of the sympathetic and splanchnic nerves. The disadvantage of this is that the bilateral interruption must be done in two separate procedures [147].

If the inflammatory process is chronic relapsing pancreatitis involving the surrounding muscles in the retroperitoneal space, then the patient suffers from both visceral and somatic pain [105]. In this instance bilateral dorsal rhizotomy of lower dorsal and upper lumbar roots will be more effective than splanchnectomy. The concern of this denervation is that any warning of a subsequent intra-abdominal catastrophe will be masked, i.e., perforated duodenal ulcer, acute cholecystitis, or appendicitis. These dangers must be carefully assessed prior to this ablative surgery.

Intrathecal Injection

The spinal rootlets and the entry zone of the dorsal roots to the posterior lateral funiculus of the spinal cord are bathed in cerebrospinal fluid within the subarachnoid space. These primary afferent pathways are exposed to and influenced by the cerebrospinal fluid environment. Changes induced in this environment can alter conduction within the spinal rootlets. There is easy access to the spinal subarachnoid space via needle puncture through the interlaminar space of the spinal column. This exposure allows alteration of the cerebrospinal fluid milieu so as to selectively interrupt transmission of the unmyelinated C fibers and small, thinly myelinated A delta fibers. The heavily myelinated A alpha and A beta fibers as well as efferent fibers are relatively resistant to change [74]. A major inherent drawback to this is limiting the alteration to only those segments involving the pain, and the control of a substance once it is injected is haphazard at best.

Alcohol, which is hypobaric (lighter than water), tends to float; it is caustic and destroys nerve fibers [2]. Its position can be controlled by altering the patient's posture on a tilt table. Dogliotti [26] in 1931 reported relief of sciatic pain by introducing alcohol in the lumbar subarachnoid space and maintaining the patient in a head-down position so the alcohol floated up to the cul de sac of the theca and coagulated the sacral rootlets. Sensory loss, bladder dysfunction, and muscle weakness combined to render this procedure undesirable. Also, incomplete sensory fiber destruction allows recurrence of pain [56].

Phenol (carbolic acid) introduced by Maher [103] is a hyperbaric (heavier than water) and tends to sink with gravity; mixing with a viscid substance such as glycerin or radioiodinated lipid tends to hold the phenol in a more localized area. Again, this is caustic to structures other than the pain afferents and thus prone to complication [66, 104, 110].

Usually use of both alcohol and phenol is limited for relief of pain in lower parts of the body, that is, below the umbilicus. Phenol can be injected into the lower thoracic segments using fluoroscopic control to help guide the needle to the desired location. The patient is positioned with the painful segments in a dependent position so the hyperbaric phenol falls to surround the involved nerve roots.

Preciseness of the lesion for pain relief is improved, and untoward complication is minimized by limiting the amount of caustic injected, by aspiration of the agent after the achieved effect, by use of multiple needles, and by careful fluoroscopic control [30].

Subarachnoid irrigation of hypothermic isotonic saline cooled to 4° C. and 0.9% NaCl isotonic saline for treatment of pain was introduced by Hitchcock in 1967 [57]. This produces a more generalized effect on structures bathed in the subarachnoid space and is indicated in the relief of midline pain, visceral pain, and causalgia, where multiple and bilateral segments must be altered to achieve relief. There is controversy regarding the effect of hypothermia on A and C fibers [119].

Savitz and Malis report 11 of 33 patients with carcinoma were relieved by hypothermic isotonic saline injection with no neurological deficits [159]. Hypothermia, however, is only transient and there is some question whether hypothermic perfusion can effectively lower the temperature in the roots enough to affect pain impulse transmission. However, vasospasm has been demonstrated and the effect may be due to relative ischemia of the roots.

Hypertonic saline (5 to 15% NaCl) is probably more effective, but is prone to complication [58, 69, 111]. There have been vascular changes demonstrated in roots on microscopy. There may be depolarization of the roots by the local hyperosmolarity. The injection of hypertonic saline intrathecally is very painful. It induces strong shivering and muscle cramping. There is a profuse sympathetic discharge with elevation of blood pressure and electrocardiographic changes. Therefore, it is usually performed with general or spinal anesthesia or the anesthetic agent is mixed with the hypertonic saline. A general anesthetic can be used, but recent reports indicate spinal anesthesia is more effective in preventing the stress of sympathetic discharge and convulsive muscle twitching [176].

Hitchcock, in 1975, reported a series of 108 patients given 10 to 15% NaCl lumbar intrathecal injections. Fifty percent of patients with pain due to malignancy were relieved of pain three months after injection.

Hitchcock's technique is reported as follows. Under general anesthetic with the patient in a head-up position and the painful segments most dependent (painful side down in lateral decubitus position) a lumbar puncture is made; 20 ml of 12.5 to 15% NaCl is injected rapidly. The patient is moved rapidly to a head-down position for pain in the upper part of the body. Close monitoring of ECG and blood pressure is made during injection and for a 30-minute period following injection because of muscle fibrillation and generalized sympathetic discharge.

At the University of Iowa, 5% NaCl solution with a larger volume (150 cc) and a second lumbar-puncture needle to allow simultaneous drainage of the increased volume of fluid over a 20-minute period is used. This allows more sustained elevation of NaCl concentration, but at low enough NaCl concentration to avoid irreversible damage to the ventral roots.

This procedure has promise in relieving the pain of malignancy, in particular, high midline and visceral pain. However, complications of cardiac arrhythmia, pulmonary edema, paraparesis, cerebral infarction, and urinary bladder dysfunction must be carefully weighed [97].

Stimulation Therapy

Melzack and Wall's gate theory of pain in 1965 [118] is discussed in Chapter 1. Whether the exact details of this theory are correct has yet to be determined. It, however, has had a great impact on the treatment of pain, for it has changed the direction and philosophy of treatment from ablative manipulation to the more physiological, nondestructive electrical inhibition of pain.

As Shealy points out [167], electrical stimulation to relieve pain is not new; Electreat (Electreat, Inc., Minneapolis, Minn.) was patented by a naturopath in 1918. It was a battery-powered skin stimulator sold over the counter for the treatment of pain.

Since A fiber stimulation would tend to close the pain gate, and a great number of these heavily myelinated, fast-conducting fibers is concentrated in the dorsal column, Shealy, Sweet, and Mortimer [168, 178] did preliminary work on stimulating the dorsal column to relieve pain.

Transcutaneous Nerve Stimulation

Transcutaneous electrical nerve stimulation (TENS) arose from the need to screen patients for dorsal column stimulator implants, and it was found that at times this alone was effective in relieving pain (Fig. 7-9) [92, 94, 113, 197].

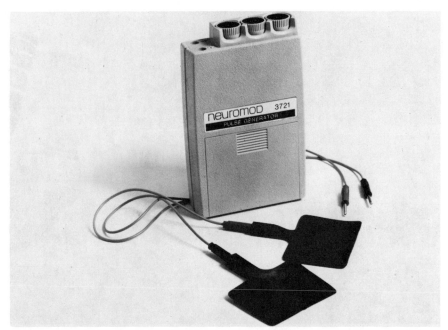

Figure 7-9 Transcutaneous stimulator driven by three AA 1.5 volt batteries. Controls vary voltage, pulse frequency, and pulse width. Carbon silicone rubber electrodes, one positive and one negative, are applied to the skin. (NEUROMOD TNS, Medtronic Corporation, Minneapolis, Minnesota)

The trial program for initial pain evaluation is begun in a manner similar to that described by Long in 1974 [94]. A detailed history and thorough general and neurological examination, followed by psychometric and intelligence testing, are accomplished. The concept of skin stimulation and pain inhibition is carefully explained. The patient is instructed in the use, care, and maintenance of the stimulator. Electrode placement is empirical and depends on the site of the pain.

Usually a superficial nerve close to the pain is chosen for stimulation (i.e., ulnar nerve at elbow for upper-limb pain and common peroneal around the head of the fibula for lower-limb pain). Electrodes of unidirectional stimulation have positive and negative poles and are usually placed within several inches. Power-alternating polarity units allow wide placement of electrodes without diminishing the stimulation effect (Figs. 7-10 and 7-11).

Voltage, pulse width, and pulse rate are all variables that can be controlled by the patient; the optimal settings for these are also empirical and determined by the patient.

Nonsaline aquaphylic electrode jelly is used as a conduction medium between the electrodes and the skin. Ample amounts are used to insure a moist skin-electrode interface and are secured by nonallergenic plastic or paper

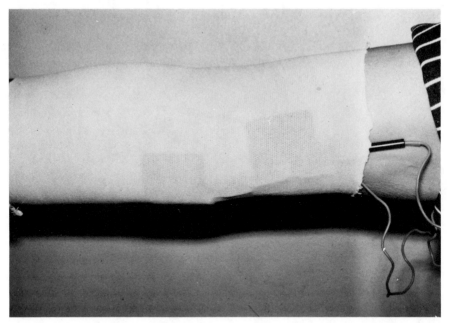

Figure 7-10   Old elastic stocking used to hold electrodes in place over the ulnar nerve.

tape, as well as by various types of elastic wraps. Both skin and electrodes are cleaned and fresh jelly applied every eight hours to insure fresh contact.

Patients are hospitalized three days so that stimulator use and electrode placement can be accurately supervised. If there is even a slight pain relief response to TENS, then an instrument is issued to the patient on loan at no cost for a four-week home trial. If, after this time, the patient continues to get satisfactory pain relief, then a unit is purchased by the patient. Usually TENS is continued 24 hours daily, but this is altered by the patient's need and response.

If stimulation over a nerve is not effective, then electrodes may be placed directly over the painful area or along the course of the involved nerve. For example, with chest wall pain electrodes might be placed side by side along the intercostal nerve or along the paravertebral region. The entire painful area is explored for optimum electrode placement. When local or appropriate peripheral nerve stimulation fails, then areas remote to the pain corresponding to acupuncture meridians may be effective.

Patient understanding, interest, and motivation are considerable factors in the success of TENS. Several reports and our own experience have shown that well over 50 percent of patients gain good to excellent relief with transcutaneous stimulation.

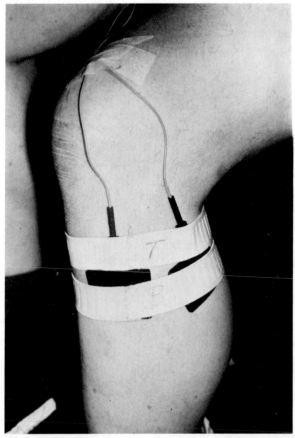

Figure 7-11 Transcutaneous electrodes positioned on lateral left leg over the common peroneal nerve. Secured by homemade garters. "T" for top, "B" for bottom.

Percutaneous Epidural Dorsal Column Stimulation

This procedure involves percutaneous placement of a single (unipolar) or two (bipolar) insulated-wire electrodes into the spinal epidural space. It has been found that the stimulation effect of electrodes placed in the epidural space is similar to the effect obtained if placed in the subdural or subarachnoid space.

This allows temporary, direct dorsal column stimulation as a screening procedure prior to permanent implantation [29, 61]. This is a necessary part of the evaluation of a pain patient to determine candidacy for permanent implantation [60].

The patient is positioned prone on the fluoroscopy table. A C-arm fluoroscope is positioned for lateral projections. Local anesthetic is injected in the soft tissue overlying the interspinous space (usually in the middorsal region). An 18-gauge Touhy needle (curved slightly at the tip) is inserted through the interspinous ligaments in the midline, the depth of puncture being closely observed on the x-ray by lateral-view fluoroscopy.

When the epidural space is entered, the wire electrode is gently passed through the needle into the epidural space. It can then usually be manipulated into the desired position under fluoroscopy. The needle is then withdrawn over the wire electrode, which is left in place and secured. This is repeated either at the same or different interspace for the second electrode. The electrodes are then attached to an external power source, and continuous dorsal column stimulation is controlled by the patient (Fig. 7-12).

Recent equipment improvements allow a receiver to be implanted subcutaneously and attached to the subcutaneous part of these epidural electrodes (the contaminated external parts are discarded), thus converting the percutaneously placed electrodes into a permanent implant stimulation system, and avoiding a laminectomy. This, however, requires optimum initial positioning of the electrodes [154].

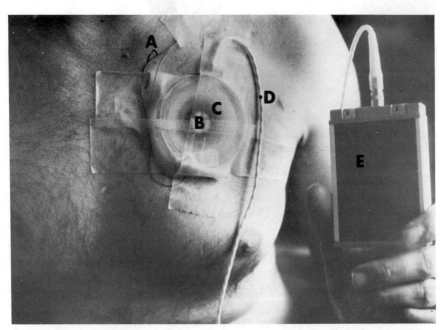

Figure 7-12 Percutaneous electrode epidural stimulation, temporary implant. A. Electrode wires (external portion). B. Receiver (external temporary type). C. Antenna. D. Antenna lead wire. E. Transmitter power unit. External appliances worn in convenient position; wires have been inserted posteriorly between the spinous processes into the epidural space (not shown). (Avery Laboratories, Inc., Farmingdale, New York.)

Dorsal Column Spinal Cord Stimulation

Wall, in 1967, was first to report stimulation of the heavily myelinated afferent fibers to control pain [190]. Electrodes were placed in the cauda equina and stimulation effect varied with change of patients' posture position. When the stimulation effect (paresthesia) was noted in the area of pain, the pain was relieved.

Shealy, in 1957, pioneered the concept of stimulating large myelinated afferent fibers concentrated in the posterior columns of the spinal cord with direct electrode placement [168]. The stimulation effect is then perceived over a wide area of the body below stimulated segments, including the pain area. Long, Nashold, Shealy, and others have reported results in large series [95, 120, 132, 169].

Success with this mode of therapy requires careful patient selection [166]. The pain must be due to a definitely diagnosed organic cause that has been treated by all modes of conventional treatment. Preferably the patient will have had partial relief with transcutaneous nerve stimulation, at least to the degree that the tingling sensation effect is not disturbing or aggravating. A personality and psychology profile should be obtained on all patients. It has been observed that patients having clinically significant profiles in neurosis, hypochondriasis, and depression, as well as those patients with pending litigation, do not respond as well clinically and consequently the results are less than optimal. Preferably initial screening should include percutaneously placed intraspinal epidural insulated-wire electrodes for temporary dorsal column stimulation [29, 60, 61]. If the patient is significantly relieved of pain by these measures, then placement of a dorsal column stimulation implant may be effective in relieving intractable organic pain.

The implant stimulation device is a transisterized receiver imbedded in epoxy resin and smaller than a pocket watch. It is attached to platinum-button or tinsel-wire electrodes which may be monopolar but are more usually bipolar. The electrode is connected to the receiver by an insulated-wire lead.

At operation, a subcutaneous pocket is formed for the receiver. The pocket is usually in the infraclavicular region on the chest wall or in the abdomen close to the belt line, depending on the segment level in which the electrode is implanted. The electrode and lead are passed subcutaneously to a laminectomy incision. The laminectomy is usually performed in the high dorsal region. However, the cervical region is the preferred site of placement if the pain involves the upper limb.

The electrode buttons are imbedded in a rectangular insulation sheet that is inserted between the leaves of the dura. Formerly electrodes were placed in the subdural or subarachnoid space; however, stimulation effect gradually decreased because of arachnoid fibrosis around the electrodes. Also, there was hazard of cerebrospinal fluid leak along the electrode. The interdural placement has eliminated these hazards since the subdural space is not entered.

The receiver is driven by an externally worn power source consisting of a battery-powered radio transmitter and circular antenna. The antenna is centered and worn directly over the receiver, which in turn powers the electrode by induction. The current is a pulsed square wave current which may or may not vary in polarity. The patient can vary the voltage, frequency, and pulse wave duration. The voltage is usually from 1 to 2 volts, and the range between light stimulation effect and intolerable paresthesia is quite narrow. Effective pulse rates are usually between 50 and 150 Hz. The pulse duration is usually from 100 to 300 microseconds. With this the patient perceives a gentle tingling, a buzzing sensation, or a feeling of warmth.

Electrode position over the dorsal column is important, since pain is relieved preferentially in areas of the body to which the stimulation paresthesias are referred. The dorsal columns are somatotopically arranged so that fibers from caudal segments are medial, and those from more cephalad segments are lateral. Bantli et al [5] in 1975 have further emphasized the importance of electrode position. They have shown that there is a wide distribution of evoked electrical activity in many spinal pathways by dorsal column stimulation by both direct and transsynaptic effect; such effect can be varied by electrode position on the cord. Those gaining relief with stimulation are likely to find carry-over relief after stimulation is stopped. This may last from hours to days.

C. H. Sheldon, 1975, reported good results in 8 of 17 patients with metastatic carcinoma. Also, the preoperative psychological attitude correlated more highly with pain relief than any other technical variable.

Results of this treatment are usually judged on the basis of the protocol adopted by the National Study Group for Dorsal Column Stimulation. The criteria used are: degree of pain relief, elimination of analgesics and tranquilizers, etc., and increased activity levels. As Sweet points out, however, the true level of success can be judged only by pain relief that allows the patient to return to productive activity. The credibility of patients who fail to return to work but state that pain is relieved is questioned.

Long and Erickson [29, 95] found that a major serious complication was failure to get stimulation effect into the painful part and thus failure to relieve pain.

In their series of patients with low back pain, multiple surgical procedures, and lumbar arachnoiditis for over a 3½-year period, eight were completely relieved and 40 failed to gain lasting relief compared with an initial 46 gaining at least 50 percent relief; nine failed immediately.

The patient's personality can be a major source of failure. The electrode type and placement, as well as stimulation variables (voltage, waveform, frequency), are equally important.

Shealy reports that of 80 patients only 12 have excellent results, 25 are fair, and 43 are failures after a minimum of seven months' follow-up evaluation [166].

Just as important in the management of these patients is the modification of emotions by using open-end conditioning, autogenic training, and bio-feedback.

Dorsal column stimulation can relieve chronic pain, but the effect diminishes with time; it is Nashold's opinion that dorsal column stimulation is not an established mode of therapy for pain relief and he recommends carefully planned investigation [131]. Most recently Erickson reported total failure in 15 of 16 very carefully selected patients, who initially indicated pain relief with percutaneous dorsal column stimulation, so that true long-term success has yet to be established, but appears less promising than initially expected.

Permanent Implant Peripheral Nerve Stimulation

The stimulation of a peripheral nerve can inhibit pain. In several large series of unselected patients with intractable pain, 50 percent experienced variable but definite relief of pain [92, 94, 113, 197]. This relief is due to a suppression of pain perception. It, however, does not produce a hypoalgesia or interfere with peripheral nerve impulse transmission.

It is logical, therefore, that implant stimulation of a peripheral nerve for pain suppression would be particularly effective in patients having intractable pain referable to a part innervated by a specific nerve or referable to the nerve itself, i.e., trauma to sciatic nerve or herpes zoster of the ophthalmic nerve.

Stimulator implants have been designed for peripheral nerve stimulation. Most are bipolar and are insulated in a silastic flag that is wrapped loosely around the nerve (Fig. 7-13). The electrode is driven by a subcutaneously placed receiver similar to the dorsal column stimulator implant, which in turn is activated by an externally centered concentric antenna by induction from a battery-drive pulse-modulated radio-frequency transmitter (Fig. 7-14).

In stimulating complex peripheral nerves with important efferent as well as afferent components, more precise A alpha fiber afferent stimulation is required to avoid the interference and annoyance of associated muscle contraction. The Avery Corporation has developed a four-plate electrode that can be connected in 28 separate combinations. This is connected under local anesthesia, and each connection combination stimulated and tested to achieve optimum afferent stimulation with minimum efferent muscle stimulation. Presently this electrode is especially designed for sciatic nerve stimulation.

The peripheral nerve stimulation theoretically offers more precise stimulation of the involved painful segments, particularly if pain is limited to an extremity or to a specific nerve. Patients receiving good benefit consistently with transcutaneous nerve stimulation continue to have relief with implant stimulation. Picaza [145, 146] reports 34 of 50 patients with good to excellent relief of previously intractable pain, which is considerably better than results of dorsal column stimulation.

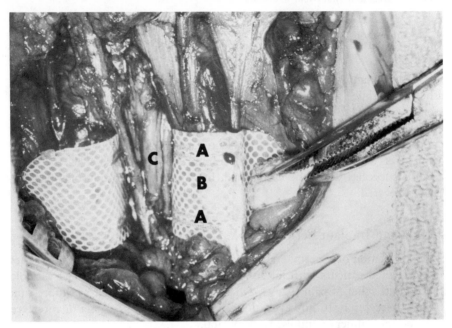

Figure 7-13 Peripheral nerve stimulator electrode implant. Femoral nerve exposed at groin. A. Bipolar electrode wire. B. Dacron mesh–silastic "electrode flag." C. Femoral nerve. (Medtronic, Inc., Minneapolis, Minnesota.)

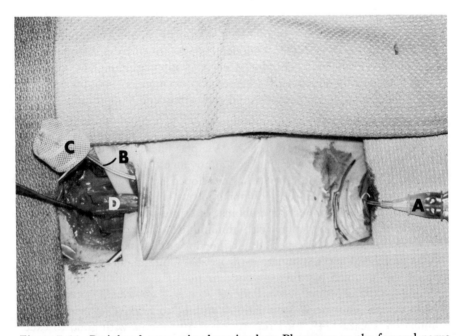

Figure 7-14 Peripheral nerve stimulator implant. Placement on the femoral nerve at the groin. A. Receiver on the abdominal wall. B. Bipolar wire lead. C. Bipolar electrode. D. Femoral nerve. (Medtronic, Inc., Minneapolis, Minnesota.)

198

The complications of peripheral nerve implant stimulation are relatively infrequent and minor. However, Picaza points out the potential hazard of possible nervous system injury from continuous, long-term externally applied electrical stimulation [146]. To date, none has been demonstrated. This, however, emphasizes the fact that stimulation therapy in the treatment of pain is still investigational. Preliminary results indicate considerable promise for relief of pain in conditions previously not effectively treatable—chronic lumbar arachnoiditis, central dysesthesia, herpes zoster neuritis, phantom-limb pain, and the pain of peripheral neuropathy and myelopathy.

References

1. Abbe, R. A contribution to the surgery of the spine. *Med. Rec.* (New York) 35:149, 1889. Reprinted in Wilkins, H., *Neurosurgical Classics*, pp. 512–515. New York: Johnson Reprint Corp., 1965.
2. Adson, A. W. The value of and indications for intraspinal injections of alcohol in the relief of pain. *Minn. Med.* 20:135, 1937.
3. Allen, M. B., Jr., and Moretz, W. H. Sympathectomy. In Youmans, J. R., ed., *Neurological Surgery* (Vol. 3). Philadelphia: W. B. Saunders Company, 1973.
4. Ballantine, H. T., Cassidy, W. L., Flanagan, N. B., and Marino, R. Stereotaxic anterior cingulotomy for neuropsychiatric illness and intractable pain. *J. Neurosurg.* 26:488, 1967.
5. Bantli, H., Bloedel, J. R., Long, D. M., and Thienprasit, P. Distribution of activity in spinal pathways evoked by experimental dorsal column stimulation. *J. Neurosurg.* 42:290, 1975.
6. Bantli, H., Bloedel, J. R., and Thienprasit, P. Supraspinal interactions resulting from experimental dorsal column stimulation. *J. Neurosurg.* 42:296, 1975.
7. Belmusto, L., Brown, E., and Owens, G. Clinical observations on respiratory and vasomotor disturbance as related to cervical cordotomies. *J. Neurosurg.* 20:225, 1963.
8. Bergan, J. J., and Con, J., Jr. Sympathectomy for pain relief. *Med. Clin. North Am.* 52:147, 1968.
9. Birkenfeld, R., and Fisher, R. G. Successful treatment of causalgia of upper extremity with medullary spinothalamic tractotomy. *J. Neurosurg.* 20:303, 1963.
10. Burton, C., and Mauer, D. D. Pain suppression by trancutaneous electronic stimulation. *IEEE Trans. Biomed. Eng.* [*BME*] 21:81, 1974.
11. Ciric, I. S., and Tarkington, J. Transphenoidal microsurgery. *Surg. Neurol.* 3:207, 1974.
12. Cloward, R. B. Upper thoracic sympathectomy: Surgical technique. *Surgery* 66:1120, 1969.
13. Collins, J. R., Juras, E. P., Van Houten, R. J., and Spruell, L. Intrathecal cold saline solution: A new approach to pain (evaluation). *Anesth. Analg.* 48:816, 1969.
14. Collins, W. F. Hypophysectomy: Historical and personal perspective. *Clin. Neurosurg.* 21:68, 1974.
15. Conway, L. W., and Collins, W. F. Results of trans-sphenoidal cryohypophysectomy for carcinoma of the breast. *N. Engl. J. Med.* 281:1, 1969.
16. Crawford, A. S., and Knighton, R. S. Further observations on medullary spinothalamic tractotomy. *J. Neurosurg.* 10:113, 1953.

17. Crosby, E. C., Humphrey, T., and Lauer, E. W. *Correlative Anatomy of the Nervous System.* New York: Macmillan, Inc., 1962. P. 78.
18. Crue, B. L., and Todd, E. M. A simplified technique of sacral rhizotomy for pelvic pain. *J. Neurosurg.* 21:835, 1964.
19. Dandy, W. E. An operation for the cure of tic douloureux. Partial section of the sensory root at the pons. *Arch. Surg.* 18:687, 1929.
20. Dandy, W. E. Section of the sensory root of the trigeminal nerve at the pons. Preliminary report of the operative procedure. *Johns Hopkins Med. J.* 36:105, 1925.
21. Dandy, W. E. Glossopharyngeal neuralgia (tic douloureux): Its diagnosis and treatment. *Arch. Surg.* 15:198, 1927.
22. Dandy, W. E. The treatment of trigeminal neuralgia by the cerebellar route. *Ann. Surg.* 96:787, 1932.
23. Dao, T. L. Ablation therapy for hormone dependent tumors. *Annu. Rev. Med.* 23:1, 1972.
24. Dejerine, J., and Roussey, G. Le syndrome thalamique. *Rev. Neurol.* (Paris) 14:521, 1906.
25. Dickey, R. P., and Minton, J. P. L-Dopa effect on prolactin, follicle stimulating hormone, and luteinizing hormone in women with advanced breast cancer: A preliminary report. *Am. J. Obstet. Gynecol.* 114:267, 1972.
26. Dogliotti, A. M. Traitement des syndromes douloureux de la périphérie par l'alcoolisation sub-arachnoidienne des racines postérieures à leur émergence de la moelle èpiniere. *Presse Méd.* 39:1249, 1931.
27. Doupe, J., Cullen, C. H., and Chance, C. Q. Post-traumatic pain and causalgic syndrome. *J. Neurol. Neurosurg. Psychiatry* 7:33, 1944.
28. Echols, D. H. Sensory rhizotomy following operating for ruptured intervertebral disc: A review of 62 cases. *J. Neurosurg.* 31:335, 1969.
29. Erickson, D. L. Percutaneous trial of stimulation for patient selection for implantable stimulating devices. *J. Neurosurg.* 43:443, 1975.
30. Flanigan, S., and Boop, W. C. Spinal intrathecal injection procedures in the management of pain. *Clin. Neurosurg.* 21:229, 1974.
31. Flanigan, S., and Filbeck, J. Intrathecal alcohol and pain. *J. Arkansas Med. Soc.* 68:184, 1971.
32. Foerster, O. Vorderseitenstrangdurchschneidung in Ruckenmark zur Beseitigung von schmerzen. *Berlin: Klin. Wochenschr.* 50:1499, 1913.
33. Foerster, O. The dermatomes in man. *Brain* 56:1, 1933.
34. Folz, E. L., and White, L. E. Pain "relief" by frontal cingulotomy. *J. Neurosurg.* 19:38, 1962.
35. Folz, E. L., and White, L. E. The role of rostral cingulotomy in "pain" relief. *Int. J. Neurol.* 6:353, 1967.
36. Forrest, A. P. M., Roberts, M. M., and Stewart, J. J. Pituitary ablation by Yttrium-90. *Acta Neurochir.* (Suppl.) 21:137, 1974.
37. Fox, J. L. Localization of the respiratory motor pathway in the upper cervical spinal cord following percutaneous cordotomy. *Neurology* 19:1115, 1969.
38. Fox, J. L. Delineation of the obex by contrast radiography during percutaneous trigeminal tractotomy. Technical note. *J. Neurosurg.* 36:107, 1972.
39. Fox, J. L. Dorsal column stimulation for relief of intractable pain: Problems encountered with neuropacemakers. *Surg. Neurol.* 2:59, 1974.
40. Frazier, C. H. A surgeon's impression of trigeminal neuralgia based on experiences with three hundred and two cases. *JAMA* 70:1234, 1918.
41. Frazier, C. H. Subtotal resection of sensory root for relief of major trigeminal neuralgia. *Arch. Neurol. Psychiatr.* (Chicago) 13:378, 1927.
42. Frazier, C. H., Lewy, F. H., and Rowe, S. N. The origin and mechanism

of paroxysmal neuralgic pain and surgical treatment of central pain. *Brain* 60:44, 1937.

43. Freeman, W., and Watts, J. W.   *Psychosurgery in the Treatment of Mental Disorders and Intractable Pain.* Springfield, Ill.: Charles C Thomas, Publisher, 1950.

44. French, L. A.   Cordotomy in the high cervical region for intractable pain. *Lancet* 73:283, 1953.

45. Gildenberg, P. L.   Percutaneous cervical cordotomy. *Clin. Neurosurg.* 21: 246, 1974.

46. Gildenberg, P. L.   Percutaneous cervical cordotomy for relief of intractable pain. *Cleve. Clin. Q.* 36:183, 1969.

47. Graf, C. J.   On cervical cordotomy—a new technique. *J. Neurosurg.* 15:576, 1958.

48. Graf, C. J.   Trigeminal compression for tic douloureux: An elevation. *J. Neurosurg.* 20:1029, 1963.

49. Guiot, G., and Thibaut, B.   L'extirpation des adenomes hypophysaires par voie trans-sphenoidale. *Neurochirurgie* 1:133, 1959.

50. Hamby, W. B.   Effectiveness of various operations for trigeminal neuralgia. *J. Neurosurg.* 17:1039, 1960.

51. Hardy, J.   Trans-sphenoidal hypophysectomy. *J. Neurosurg.* 34:582, 1971.

52. Hardy, J.   Transnasal-trans-sphenoid approach to the pituitary gland. In Yasargil, M. G., ed., *Microsurgery Applied to Neurosurgery.* New York: Academic Press, Inc., 1969.

53. Harshey, V., Taylor, J., and Coleman, W. S.   Remarks on the various surgical procedures devised for the relief or cure of trigeminal neuralgia (tic douloureux). *Br. Med. J.* 2:1139, 1891.

54. Hartley, F.   Intracranial neurectomy of second and third divisions of the fifth nerve, a new method. *N.Y. State J. Med.* 55:317, 1892.

55. Haxton, H.   Technique and results of upper limb sympathectomy. *J. Can. Vasc. Surg.* (Toronto) 11:27, 1970.

56. Hay, R. C., Yonezawa, T., and Derrick, W. S.   Control of intractable pain in advanced cancer by subarachnoid alcohol block. *JAMA* 169:1315, 1959.

57. Hitchcock, E.   Hypothermic subarachnoid irrigation for intractable pain. *Lancet* 1:1133, 1967.

58. Hitchcock, E., and Prandini, M. N.   Hypertonic saline in management of intractable pain. *Lancet* 1:310, 1973.

59. Hitchcock, E. R., and Tsukamoto, Y.   Physiological correlates in stereotactic spinal surgery. *Acta Neurochir.* (Suppl.) 21:119, 1974.

60. Hoppenstein, R.   Percutaneous implantation of chronic spinal cord electrodes for control of intractable pain: Preliminary report. *Surg. Neurol.* 4:195, 1975.

61. Hosobuchi, Y., Adams, J. E., and Weinstein, P. R.   Preliminary percutaneous dorsal column stimulation prior to permanent implantation. *J. Neurosurg.* 37:242, 1972.

62. Hurt, R. W., and Ballantine, H. T.   Stereotactic anterior cingulate lesions for persistent pain: A report on 68 cases. *Clin Neurosurg.* 21:334, 1974.

63. Hyndman, O. R.   Intractable pain due to cancer: Treatment by neurosurgical methods. *Am. J. Surg.* 75:187, 1948.

64. Hyndman, O. R., and Van Epps, C.   Possibility of differential section of the spinothalamic tract: A clinical and histologic study. *Arch. Surg.* 38:1036, 1939.

65. Hyndman, O. R., and Wolkin, J.   Sympathectomy of the upper extremity. *Arch. Surg.* 45:145, 1942.

66. Iggo, A., and Walsh, E. G. Selective block of small fibers in the spinal roots by phenol. *Brain* 83:701, 1960.

67. Jannetta, P. J. Trigeminal neuralgia. *Curr. Probl. Surg.* February, 1973. P. 49.

68. Jannetta, P. J. Arterial compression of the trigeminal nerve at the pons in patients with trigeminal neuralgia. *J. Neurosurg.* 26:159, 1967.

69. Jewitt, D. L., and King, J. S. Conduction block of monkey dorsal rootlets by water and hypertonic saline solutions. *Exp. Neurol.* 33:225, 1971.

70. Kahn, E. A., and Peet, M. M. The technique of anterolateral cordotomy. *J. Neurosurg.* 5:276, 1948.

71. Karnosh, L. J., Gardner, W. J., and Stowell, A. Glossopharyngeal neuralgia: Physiologic considerations of the role of the ninth and tenth cranial nerves. Report of cases. *Trans. Am. Neurol. Assoc.* 72:205, 1947.

72. Keegan, J. J., and Garrett, F. D. The segmental distribution of the cutaneous nerves in the limbs of man. *Anat. Rec.* 102:409, 1948.

73. Keith, W. S. Glossopharyngeal neuralgia. *Brain* 55:357, 1932.

74. King, J. S., Jewitt, D. L., and Sundberg, H. R. Differential blockade of cat dorsal root C fibers by various chloride solutions. *J. Neurosurg.* 36:569, 1972.

75. Kirklin, J. W., Chenoweth, A. I., and Murphy, F. Causalgia. A review of its characteristics, diagnosis and treatment. *Surgery* 21:321, 1947.

76. Kirschner, M. Die Bchandlung der Trigeminusneuralgie (nach Erfahiurg an 1113 Kranken). *Munch. Med. Wochenschr.* 89:235, 1942.

77. Kleinberg, D. L., Noel, G. L., and Frantz, A. G. Chlorpromazine stimulation and L-dopa suppression of plasma prolactin in man. *J. Clin. Endocrinol. Metab.* 33:873, 1971.

78. Knighton, R. S., and Dumke, P. R., eds. *Pain.* Boston: Little, Brown and Company, 1966. P. 587.

79. Koskoff, Y. D., Dennis, W., Lazovik, D., and Wheeler, E. T. The psychological effects of frontal lobotomy performed for the alleviation of pain. *Res. Publ. Assoc. Res. Nerv. Ment. Dis.* 27:723, 1948.

80. Krieger, A. J., and Rosomoff, H. L. Sleep-induced apnea. Part 1: A respiratory and autonomic dysfunction syndrome following bilateral percutaneous cervical cordotomy. *J. Neurosurg.* 40:168, 1974.

81. Kuntz, A. *The Neuroanatomic Basis of Surgery of the Autonomic Nervous System.* Springfield, Ill.: Charles C Thomas, Publisher, 1949. Pp. 3–76.

82. Laitinen, L., and Singounas, E. Longitudinal myelotomy in the treatment of spasticity of the legs. *J. Neurosurg.* 35:536, 1971.

83. Larson, S. J., Sances, A., Riegel, D. H., Meyer, G. A., Dallman, D. E., and Swiontec, T. Neurophysiological effects of dorsal column stimulation in man and monkey. *J. Neurosurg.* 41:217, 1974.

84. Leriche, R., and Fontaine, R. Chirurgie du sympathique. *Rev. Neurol.* 1:1046, 1929.

85. Leriche, R., and Heitz, J. Des effets physiologiques de la sympathectomie périphérique. *Compt. Rend. Soc. de Biol.* 80:66, 1917.

86. Leriche, R. *The Surgery of Pain.* Baltimore: The Williams & Wilkins Company, 1939.

87. Lin, P. M., Gildenberg, P. L., and Polakoff, P. P. An anterior approach to percutaneous lower cervical cordotomy. *J. Neurosurg.* 25:553, 1966.

88. Lippert, T. G., Hosobuchi, Y., and Nielson, S. L. Spinal commissurotomy. *Surg. Neurol.* 2:373, 1974.

89. Livingston, W. K. *Pain Mechanisms: A Physiological Interpretation of Causalgia and Its Related States.* New York: Macmillan, Inc., 1943. P. 253.

90. Loeser, J. D. Dorsal rhizotomy for relief of chronic pain. *J. Neurosurg.* 36:745, 1972.
91. Loeser, J. D. Dorsal rhizotomy: Indications and results. In Bonica, J. J., ed., *Advances in Neurology* (Vol. 4). New York: Raven Press, 1974. Pp. 615–619.
92. Loeser, J. D., Black, R. G., and Christman, A. Relief of pain by transcutaneous stimulation. *J. Neurosurg.* 42:308, 1975.
93. Long, D. M. Electrical stimulation for relief of pain from chronic nerve injury. *J. Neurosurg.* 39:718, 1973.
94. Long, D. M. External electrical stimulation as a treatment of chronic pain. *Minn. Med.* 57:195, 1974.
95. Long, D. M., and Erickson, D. E. Stimulation of the posterior columns of the spinal cord for relief of intractable pain. *Surg. Neurol.* 4:134, 1975.
96. Lougheed, W. M. A simple method for upper thoracic sympathectomy in patients requiring sympathectomy of the upper limb. *Can. J. Surg.* 8:306, 1965.
97. Lucas, J. T., Ducker, T. B., and Perot, P. L. Adverse reactions to intrathecal saline injection for pain. *J. Neurosurg.* 42:557, 1975.
98. MacLean, P. D. Psychosomatic disease and the "visceral brain." Recent developments bearing on the Papez theory of emotion. *Psychosom. Med.* 11:338, 1949.
99. MacLean, P. D. Contrasting functions of limbic and neocortical systems of the brain and their relevance to psychophysiological aspects of medicine. *Am. J. Med.* 25:611, 1958.
100. Mogani, H., Matsumoto, K., Kakikawa, K., Koshino, K., and Nakatani, S. Treatment of intractable pain by frontal cryocingulotomy. *Brain Nerve* (Tokyo) 17:449, 1965.
101. Magendie, F. Expériences sur les functions des récines des nerfs rachidiens. *J. Physiol. Exp. Pathol.* 2:276, 1822.
102. Magoun, H. W., and McKinley, W. A. The termination of ascending trigeminal and spinal tracts in the thalamus of the cat. *Am. J. Physiol.* 137:409, 1942.
103. Maher, R. M. Relief of pain in incurable cancer. *Lancet* 1:18, 1955.
104. Maher, R. M. Neuron selection in relief of pain. Further experiences with intrathecal injections. *Lancet* 1:16, 1957.
105. Mallet, G. P., and Jaubert de Beaujeu, M. Treatment of chronic pancreatitis by unilateral splanchnectomy. *Arch. Surg.* 60:233, 1950.
106. Mark, V. H., and Ervin, F. R. Role of thalamotomy in treatment of chronic severe pain. *Postgrad. Med.* 37:563, 1965.
107. Mark, V. H., and Ervin, F. R. Stereotactic surgery for the relief of pain. In White, J. C., and Sweet, W. H., eds., *Pain and the Neurosurgeon: A Forty-Year Experience.* Springfield: Charles C Thomas, Publisher, 1969.
108. Mark, V. H., Ervin, F. R., and Yakovlev, P. I. Stereotactic thalamotomy. *Arch. Neurol.* 8:528, 1963.
109. Mark, V. H., Ervin, F. R., and Hackett, T. P. Clinical aspects of stereotaxic thalamotomy in the human: I. Treatment of chronic severe pain. *Arch. Neurol.* 3:351, 1960.
110. Mark, V. H., White, J. C., Zervas, N. T., Ervin, F. R., and Richardson, E. P. Intrathecal use of phenol for the relief of chronic pain. *N. Engl. J. Med.* 267:589, 1962.
111. Mathews, G. J., Ambruso, V. T., and Osterholm, J. L. Hypothermic hyperosmolar saline irrigation of cisterna magna: A new method for the relief of pain. *Surg. Forum* 21:445, 1970.

112. Mayfield, F. H. *Causalgia*. Springfield: Charles C Thomas, Publisher, 1951.
113. McDonnell, D. E. Transcutaneous stimulation in treatment of chronic pain. Presented at Iowa Midwest Neurosurgical Society, November, 1974.
114. McGuire, W. L. A new approach for selecting patients with metastatic breast cancer for hypophysectomy. *Clin. Neurosurg.* 21:39, 1974.
115. McKay, J. J. Improved approach for posterior upper thoracic sympathectomy. *JAMA* 159:1261, 1955.
116. McKenzie, K. G. Trigeminal tractotomy. *Clin. Neurosurg.* 2:50, 1955.
117. Mellins, R. B., Balfour, H. H., Turino, G. M., and Winters, R. W. Failure of autonomic control of ventilation (Ondine's Curse). *Medicine* 49:487, 1970.
118. Melzack, R., and Wall, P. D. Pain mechanisms: A new theory. *Science* 150:971, 1965.
119. Meyer, J. S., and Hunter, J. Effects of hypothermia on local blood flow and metabolism during cerebral ischemia and hypoxia. *J. Neurosurg.* 14:210, 1957.
120. Miles, J., Hayward, M., Mumford, J., Lipton, S., Bowsher, D., and Malony, V. Pain relief by implanted electrical stimulators. *Lancet* 1:777, 1974.
121. Miller, D. S., and DeTakats, G. Post-traumatic dystrophy of the extremities: Sudeck's atrophy. *Surg. Gynecol. Obstet.* 75:558, 1942.
122. Mitchell, S. W. *Injuries of Nerves and Their Consequences*. Philadelphia: J. B. Lippincott Company, 1872. P. 277.
123. Mixter, W. J., and White, J. C. Pain pathways in the sympathetic nervous system: Clinical evidence. *Arch. Neurol. Psychiatr.* 25:986, 1931.
124. Moore, D. C. *Stellate Ganglion Block*. Springfield: Charles C Thomas, Publisher, 1954.
125. Mullan, S., Harper, P. V., Hekmatpanah, J., Torres, H., and Dobbin, G. Percutaneous interruption of spinal pain tracts by means of a strontium 90 needle. *J. Neurosurg.* 20:931, 1963.
126. Mullan, S. Hekmatpanah, J., Dobbin, G., and Beckman, F. Percutaneous intramedullary cordotomy utilizing the unipolar anodal electrolytic lesion. *J. Neurosurg.* 22:548, 1965.
127. Mundinger, F. Stereotaxic Curie-therapy of pituitary adenomas. A long-term followup study. *Acta Neurochir.* (Suppl.) 21:169, 1974.
128. Murphy, G. P., Boctor, Z. N., Gailani, S., and Belmusto, L. Hypophysectomy for disseminated prostatic carcinoma. *J. Surg. Oncol.* 8:81, 1969.
129. Murphy, G. P., Reynoso, G., Schoones, R., Gailani, S., Bourke, R., Kenny, G. M., Mirand, E. A., and Schalch, D. S. Hypophysectomy and adrenalectomy for disseminated prostatic carcinoma. *J. Urol.* 105:817, 1971.
130. Nashold, B. S. Mesencephalotomy. Presented at symposium, The Treatment of Pain. Rush Presbyterian–St. Luke's Medical Center, Chicago, February, 1973.
131. Nashold, B. S. Dorsal column stimulation for control of pain. A three year followup. *Surg. Neurol.* 4:146, 1975.
132. Nashold, B. S., and Friedman, H. Dorsal column stimulation for control of pain. Preliminary report on 30 patients. *J. Neurosurg.* 36:590, 1972.
133. Nashold, B. S., Wilson, W. P., and Slaughter, D. G. Stereotaxic midbrain lesions for central dysesthesia and phantom pain. *J. Neurosurg.* 30:116, 1969.
134. Nathan, P. W. The descending respiratory pathway in man. *J. Neurol. Neurosurg. Psychiatry* 26:487, 1963.
135. Nathan, P. and Wall, P. D. Treatment of postherpetic neuralgia by prolonged electrical stimulation. *Br. Med. J.* 3:645, 1974.
136. Nielson, K. D., Adams, J. E., and Hosobuchi, Y. Experience with dorsal column stimulation for relief of chronic intractable pain: 1968–1973. *Surg. Neurol.* 4:148, 1975.

137. Nugent, G. R., and Berry, B. Trigeminal neuralgia treated by differential percutaneous radiofrequency coagulation at Gasserian ganglion. *J. Neurosurg.* 40:517, 1974.
138. Onofrio, B. M. Rhizotomy: What is its place in the treatment of pain? *Advances in Neurology* (Vol. 4). New York: Raven Press, 1974. Pp. 621–623.
139. Onofrio, B. M., and Campa, H. K. Evaluation of rhizotomy. Review of 12 years' experience. *J. Neurosurg.* 36:751, 1972.
140. Papez, J. W. A proposed mechanism of emotion. *Arch. Neurol. Psychiatr.* (Chicago) 38:725, 1937.
141. Pawl, R. P. Percutaneous radiofrequency electrocoagulation in the control of chronic pain. *Surg. Clin. North Am.* 55:167, 1975.
142. Pederson, H. E., Blunk, C. F. J., and Gardner, E. The anatomy of lumbosacral posterior rami and meningeal branches of the spinal nerves (sinu-vertebral nerves). *J. Bone Joint Surg.* 38(A):377, 1956.
143. Peet, M. M. Splanchnic section for hypertension. A preliminary report. *Univ. Hosp. Bull., Ann Arbor* 1:17, 1935.
144. Peet, M. M., and Schneider, R. C. Trigeminal neuralgia. A review of 689 cases with a followup study of 65% of the group. *J. Neurosurg.* 9:367, 1952.
145. Picaza, J. A., Cannon, B. W., Hunter, S. E., Boyd, A. S., Guma, J., and Maurer, D. Pain suppression by peripheral nerve stimulation. Part I: Observations with transcutaneous stimuli. *Surg. Neurol.* 4:105, 1975.
146. Picaza, J. A., Cannon, B. W., Hunter, S. E., Boyd, A. S., Guma, J., and Maurer, D. Pain suppression by peripheral nerve stimulation. Part II: Observations with implanted devices. *Surg. Neurol.* 4:115, 1975.
147. Polumbo, L. T. Anterior transthoracic approach for upper sympathectomy. *Arch. Surg.* 72:659, 1956.
148. Putnam, T. J. Myelotomy of the commissure. *Arch. Neurol. Psychiatr.* 32:1189, 1934.
149. Putti, V. New concepts in the pathogenesis of sciatic pain. *Lancet* 2:53, 1927.
150. Rand, R. W. Cryosurgery of the pituitary in acromegaly: Reduced growth hormone levels following hypophysectomy in 13 cases. *Ann. Surg.* 164:587, 1966.
151. Rand, R. W. *Microneurosurgery.* St. Louis: The C. V. Mosby Company, 1969. P. 163.
152. Rand, R. W., Dashe, A. M., Paglia, D. E., Conway, L. W., and Solomon, D. H. Stereotaxic cryohypophysectomy. *JAMA* 189:255, 1964.
153. Ray, B. S. The management of intractable pain by posterior rhizotomy. *Res. Publ. Assoc. Res. Nerv. Ment. Dis.* 23:391, 1943.
154. Ray, D. R., and Maurer, D. D. Electrical neurological stimulation systems: A review of contemporary methodology. *Surg. Neurol.* 4:82, 1975.
155. Rees, W. E. S. Multiple bilateral subcutaneous rhizolysis of segmental nerves in the treatment of intervertebral disc syndrome. *Ann. Gen. Pract.* 26:126, 1971.
156. Richards, D. E., Tyner, C. F., and Shealy, C. N. Focused ultrasonic spinal commissurotomy experimental evaluation. *J. Neurosurg.* 24:701, 1966.
157. Richardson, D. E. Thalamotomy for intractable pain. *Confin. Neurol.* 29:139, 1967.
158. Rosomoff, H. L., Carroll, F., Brown, J., and Sheptak, P. Percutaneous radiofrequency cervical cordotomy: Technique. *J. Neurosurg.* 23:639, 1965.
159. Savitz, M. H., and Malis, L. I. Intractable pain treated with intrathecal isotonic iced saline. *J. Neurol. Neurosurg. Psychiatry* 36:417, 1973.
160. Schwartz, H. G., and O'Leary, J. L. Section of spinothalamic tract at the level of the inferior olive. *Arch. Neurol. Psychiatr.* (Chicago) 47:293, 1942.

161. Schwartz, H. G., and O'Leary, J. L. Section of the spinothalamic tract in the medulla with observations on the pathway for pain. *Surgery* 9:183, 1941.

162. Scoville, W. Extradural spinal sensory rhizotomy. *J. Neurosurg.* 25:94, 1966.

163. Shealy, C. N. *Procedure Techniques for Percutaneous Spinal Facet Rhizotomy.* Burlington, Mass.: Radionics, Procedure Technique Series, 1974.

164. Shealy, C. N. Role of the spinal facets in back and sciatic pain. *Headache* 14(2):101, 1974.

165. Shealy, C. N. Percutaneous radiofrequency denervation of spinal facets treatment for chronic back pain and sciatica. *J. Neurosurg.* 43:448, 1975.

166. Shealy, C. N. Dorsal column stimulation optimization of application. *Surg. Neurol.* 4:142, 1975.

167. Shealy, C. N., and Maurer, D. Transcutaneous nerve stimulation for control of pain. *Surg. Neurol.* 2:45, 1974.

168. Shealy, C. N., Mortimer, J. T., and Reswick, J. B. Electrical inhibition of pain by stimulation of the dorsal columns: Preliminary clinical report. *Anesth. Analg.* 46:489, 1967.

169. Shealy, C. N., Mortimer, J. T., and Hagfors, N. R. Dorsal column electroanalgesia. *J. Neurosurg.* 32:560, 1970.

170. Sheldon, C. H. Compression procedure for trigeminal neuralgia. *J. Neurosurg.* 25:374, 1966.

171. Smith, E. J. R., Gurling, K. J., and Baron, N. The effect of hypophysectomy in advanced carcinoma of the prostate. *Br. J. Urol.* 31:181, 1959.

172. Smithwick, R. H. Surgery of sympathetic nervous system. *N. Engl. J. Med.* 220:475, 1939.

173. Sourek, K. Commissural myelotomy. *J. Neurosurg.* 31:524, 1969.

174. Spiller, W. G., and Frazier, C. H. The division of the sensory root of the trigeminals for relief of tic douloureux: An experimental pathological and clinical study with a preliminary report of one surgically successful case. *Philadelphia Med. J.* 8:1039, 1901.

175. Spiller, W. G., and Martin, E. The treatment of persistent pain of organic origin in the lower part of the body by division of the anterolateral column of the spinal cord. *JAMA* 58:1489, 1912.

176. Squire, A. W., Calvillo, O., and Bromage, P. R. Painless intrathecal hypertonic saline. *Can. Anaesth. Soc. J.* 21:308, 1974.

177. Stovner, J., and Endresen, A. Intrathecal phenol for cancer pain. *Acta Anesthesiol. Scand.* 16:17, 1972.

178. Sweet, W. H., and Wepsic, J. G. Treatment of chronic pain by stimulation of fibers of primary afferent neurone. *Trans. Am. Neurol. Assoc.* 93:103, 1968.

179. Sweet, W. H., and Wepsic, J. G. Controlled thermocoagulation of trigeminal ganglion and rootlets for differential destruction of pain fibers. *J. Neurosurg.* 40:143, 1974.

180. Taarnhøj, P. Decompression of trigeminal root. *J. Neurosurg.* 11:299, 1954.

181. Taren, J. A., Davis, R., and Crosby, E. C. Target physiologic corroboration in stereotactic cervical cordotomy. *J. Neurosurg.* 30:569, 1969.

182. Telford, E. D. Sympathetic denervation of the upper extremity. *Lancet* 1:70, 1938.

183. Turnbull, I. M. Bilateral cingulotomy combined with thalamotomy or mesencephalic tractotomy for pain. *Surg. Gynecol. Obstet.* 134:958, 1972.

184. Turnbull, I. M. Percutaneous rhizotomy for trigeminal neuralgia. *Surg. Neurol.* 2:385, 1974.

185. Uematsa, S., Udvarhelyi, G. B., Benson, D. W., and Siebens, A. A. Percutaneous radiofrequency rhizotomy. *Surg. Neurol.* 2:319, 1974.

186. Van Gilder, J. C., and Van Gilder, I. S. Hypophysectomy in metastatic breast cancer. *Arch. Surg.* 110:293, 1975.
187. Von Euler, C. Selective responses to thermal stimulation of mammalian nerves. *Acta Physiol. Scand.* 14 (Suppl. 45):1, 1947.
188. Walker, A. E. The spinothalamic tract in man. *Arch. Neurol. Psychiatr.* (Chicago) 43:284, 1940.
189. Walker, E., Miles, C. F., and Simpson, J. R. Partial trigeminal rhizotomy using suboccipital approach. *Arch. Neurol. Psychiatr.* 75:514, 1956.
190. Wall, P. D., and Sweet, W. H. Temporary abolition of pain in man. *Science* 155:108, 1967.
191. Wertheimer, P. Posterior commissural myelotomy for relief of pain. *Acta Chir. Belg.* 54:28, 1946.
192. White, J. C. Painful injuries of nerves and their surgical treatment. *Am. J. Surg.* 72:468, 1946.
193. White, J. C. Posterior rhizotomy: A possible substitute for cordotomy in otherwise intractable neuralgias of the trunk and extremities of nonmalignant origin. *Clin. Neurosurg.* 13:20, 1966.
194. White, J. C., Sweet, W. H., Hawkins, R., and Nilges, R. Anterolateral cordotomy: Results, complications and causes of failure. *Brain* 73:346, 1950.
195. White, J. C., and Sweet, W. H. *Pain and the Neurosurgeon. A Forty-nine Year Experience.* Springfield, Ill.: Charles C Thomas, Publisher, 1969.
196. Wilson, C. B., and Fewer, D. Role of neurosurgery in management of patients with carcinoma of the breast. *Cancer* 28:1681, 1971.
197. Winter, A., Winter, R. L., and Laing, Y. J. Pain relief—transcutaneous nerve stimulation. *J. Med. Soc. N.J.* 71:365, 1974.
198. Wycis, H. T. Long range results in treatment of intractable pain by stereotaxic midbrain surgery. *J. Neurosurg.* 19:101, 1962.
199. Zervas, N. T. Stereotaxic radiofrequency surgery of the normal and the abnormal pituitary gland. *N. Engl. J. Med.* 280:429, 1969.
200. Zervas, N. T., and Gordy, P. D. Radiofrequency hypophysectomy for metastatic breast and prostate carcinoma. *Surg. Clin. North Am.* 47:1279, 1967.
201. Zervas, N. T., and Hamlin, H. Stereotaxic thermal pituitary ablation. *Acta Neurochir.* (Suppl.) 21:165, 1974.

8

Acupuncture

Margaret E. Armstrong

Acupuncture points are electrically distinguishable from adjacent tissues. And, when a point is stimulated, the meridian which is formed by acupuncture points registers a corresponding change in electrical potential. Maybe there is a scientific basis for this mysterious therapy.

Acupuncture, an unfamiliar term in this country barely a year ago, is becoming a meaningful word to health professionals and laymen alike. It will probably be some time before detailed information is readily available concerning the theoretical basis and practical application of acupuncture. However, enough is now known to begin acquisition of knowledge and assessment of implications of this ancient medical practice. Only if we begin now, will the nursing profession be able to determine its own destiny regarding its role in relation to acupuncture and related techniques.

Puncture Points

The term acupuncture derives its meaning from the Latin *acus*, needle, and *punctura*, a puncture. It is a method of preventing, diagnosing, and treating disease by inserting metal needles into the body at designated locations—acupuncture points—at various depths and angles.

There are now approximately 1,000 known acupuncture points, each nearly 0.1 inch in diameter, which in pathologic conditions become tender when pressure is applied. Any given disease may affect one or several points and the groupings may differ from patient to patient.

Acupuncture points, also known as "hoku points," do not exist in isolation; they form essentially 14 groups. The points in each group are arranged in a line known as a meridian, which is associated with an internal organ. A meridian runs along one of the major parts of the body and terminates at the tips of the fingers or toes. Each meridian is paired with another meridian located on the other side of the body [9].

The pain or sensation indicating disease in that organ is registered along

Reprinted by permission from *American Journal of Nursing* 72:1582, 1972. Copyright © 1972, The American Journal of Nursing Company.

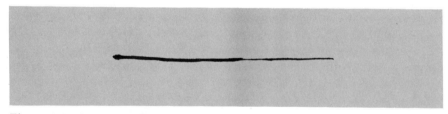

Figure 8-1 Acupuncture needle, shown in actual size, is rotated and inserted downward for treatment.

the path of the meridian for that specific organ [9]. For example, the pain commonly felt in angina pectoris runs along the course of the heart meridian, which runs down the inside of the arm.

Other meridians are associated with the pericardium, lungs, large and small intestines, stomach, spleen, diaphragm, liver, gall bladder, kidneys, bladder, circulation; with sex; and with the function of nervous energy and warmth.

Acupuncture needles are very fine slivers, about 0.01 inch in diameter, and have been made of wood, bamboo, gold, silver, and various other metals. Today, they are usually made of stainless steel, varying in length from one to seven inches with a wire wrapped around the blunt end to aid in handling. They are like fine sewing needles, rather than the hollow needles used for injections.

Most commonly, the needle is inserted by rotating it between the thumb and index finger using slight pressure in a downward direction. The speed and angle of rotation depend upon the intensity of the desired stimulation. The method for insertion is determined in part by the angle and depth of insertion to be used as well as the duration and frequency of the treatments. At this point, one may logically conclude that acupuncture is totally irrational and ought to be discarded in modern medical or nursing practice. But, there is a long history of its use in Western Europe as well as in Asia, indicating, perhaps, that it has proved helpful through the years.

Restoring the Balance

The date of the origin of acupuncture is an approximation at best, but the practice probably began nearly four to five thousand years ago in China. It was introduced in Japan 2,600 years ago [3]. In China its development reached a peak by the mid-1800's and then steadily declined as a result of increasing western influence, initially by Jesuit missionaries and then by medical doctors.

However, the practice continued to develop in Japan and Korea, and returning missionaries and doctors introduced acupuncture to Europe—principally France, Germany, and Holland—and England [9]. With the beginning of the Chinese People's Republic in 1949, interest in acupuncture in China

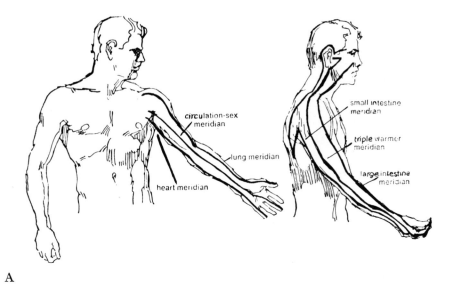

A

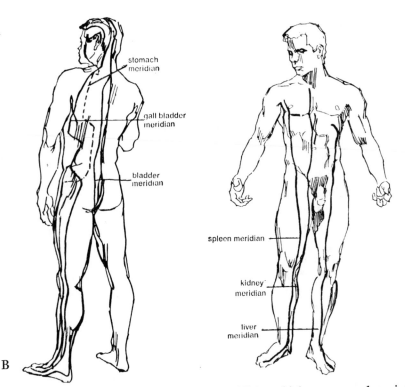

B

Figure 8-2   Acupuncture points form meridians which correspond to internal organs. Cardiac pain, for example, is registered along the heart meridian.

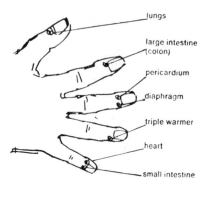

lungs

large intestine (colon)

pericardium

diaphragm

triple warmer

heart

small intestine

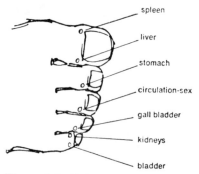

spleen

liver

stomach

circulation-sex

gall bladder

kidneys

bladder

Figure 8-3 Points on fingers and toes can be measured electrically to detect disease.

was rekindled in order to bring health care to the millions of people who were without readily available medical services.

Modern western medicine and traditional oriental methods, including acupuncture, are now used in an increasingly integrated fashion in China and Japan. In 1956, the U.S.S.R. sent several doctors to China to study acupuncture, consequently stimulating extensive research, education, and practice in the U.S.S.R.

Thus, acupuncture is now an integral part of the basic medical education in China, Japan, Southeast Asia, and Russia. There are also acupuncture societies, journals, and practitioners throughout Europe and Scandinavia. Cooperation and exchange of research are carried out through annual meetings of the International Congress of Acupuncture and Moxibustion. There are relatively few doctors in Canada and the United States, however, who have incorporated acupuncture into their medical practice.

The development of acupuncture in China has been deeply embedded in the oriental philosophy concerning the balance in the universe of the antagonistic forces of Yin and Yang. In Old China, the people believed that these two forces had to be in balance for health to exist. Disease and, consequently,

meridians and acupuncture points were classified according to the characteristics of the Yin and Yang philosophy.

The ancient Chinese also believed that Qi, the energy of life, flows through
the meridians in a constant flux which must be maintained for health to exist.
A blockage of Qi, they believed, caused an excess in certain areas of the
body, resulting in a disease corresponding to the sites involved [9].

For believers in Yin and Yang, the universe is thought to be made up of
five basic elements which have a distinct relationship to one another, and
thus maintain a balance for all existence. Organs, emotions, senses, and all
other entities are classified according to the interdependence of these basic
elements.

Viewing health care in terms of balance is difficult for us until we consider
specific examples. For instance, acupuncture is used to restore the balance
between sympathetic and parasympathetic innervation of the stomach in the
treatment of gastric ulcers. It is also used to maintain or restore the balance of
the five to one ratio of sodium and potassium necessary for electrolyte balance. When it is thus illustrated in our own terminology, we are able to
visualize the ancient philosophy of Yin and Yang as used practically in modern medical practice.

Practicing the Art

Preventive medicine has been an important part of oriental life for centuries.
A doctor commonly was paid by the patient when he was healthy; payments
ceased when the patient became ill. The doctor provided medicine and treatment as needed during illness free of charge.

Today, an assessment, recommended yearly although frequency varies
with availability of medical services, is made to determine early signs of disease. The skin's resistance to electric current is measured on acupuncture
points located on the fingers and toes as illustrated in the chart shown above
[9]. A 50 percent or more difference between the readings of the paired
meridians indicates the need for treatment to restore a balance before symptoms of pathology appear. It is believed that increase of pathology can be
prevented during the very early stages of disease when it is difficult to determine a specific diagnosis [14].

Although modern diagnostic techniques are used in conjunction with acupuncture, emphasis is also placed upon interviewing the patient and observing colors, odors, and emotions in great detail. The face, especially the forehead and below the eyes, and the inner aspect of the forearm are carefully
examined for abnormal coloration. It is also believed that any changes in the
sense organs are related to changes in one of the body organs. Vocal expressions, odors, secretions, and emotions are all thought to be related to specific
functions. Table 8-1 provides a summary of these relationships [3].

Auscultation and palpation in oriental medicine are performed to a much
greater extent than in western medicine. In fact, palpating pulses has been

Table 8-1 Observations used in diagnosis

Organs	Color	Sense	Vocal Expressions	Odor
Liver–gall bladder	Blue	Sight	Shouting	Rancid
Heart–small intestine	Red	Taste	Speaking	Scorched
Spleen–stomach	Yellow	Touch	Singing	Fragrant
Lungs–colon	White	Smell	Crying	Rotten
Kidneys–bladder	Black	Hearing	Groaning	Putrid

This information is used with traditional diagnostic methods.

developed to a fine art; various disease entities have been associated with the pulses felt by using varying amounts of pressure and at slightly different locations on the radial artery. There are probably 48 different pulses over the body, but at the location of the wrist over the radial artery there are 2 pulses at six locations for a total of 12 pulses. In diagnosis and in subsequent evaluation of acupuncture treatments, approximately 27 qualities of 12 different pulses in three positions on the radial artery of each hand are assessed.

"If the ball of the finger is lightly placed on the radial artery in these three positions, it will be noticed, except in a perfectly healthy person, that the sensation is different at each place, and if gradually a greater pressure is exerted, suddenly a point is reached where the sensation has a totally different quality. This is a deep position. The superficial position has been compared to the elasticity of the arterial wall, and the deep position to the sensation of the flow of blood within the artery. It has been suggested that the pressure required for the superficial pulse is the diastolic pressure, while that for the deep pulse is the systolic pressure" [9]. Consistent practice is required to make a detailed assessment of these values. Figure 8-5 indicates the relationships that are believed to exist between the deep and superficial pulses and internal organs.

Recently in China, there has been an attempt to treat deafness by acupuncture, especially that caused by childhood disease [15]. Many schools for deaf and mute children have had impressive results with recently developed techniques.

Not all diseases, however, have been effectively treated with acupuncture. Theoretically, it is possible to help or cure any disease that can be affected by a physiologic process. A problem that is purely anatomic or advanced to the stage of being uninfluenced by a physiologic process, such as a kidney stone, advanced osteoarthritis, or a fully formed cataract, cannot be treated successfully by acupuncture.

Considerable publicity has been given to acupuncture as an anesthetic for surgical and dental procedures as well as to its use as an analgesic for postoperative pain. Local and spinal nerve blocks, as well as inhalation anesthesia, are commonly used in China. However, acupuncture for anesthesia, using one or several needles, is an alternative for most surgical procedures with the

Secretions	Emotions
Tears	Anger, irritability, restlessness, instability
Sweat	Joy, excessive laughter
Lymph	Worry, emotional tension, depression
Mucus	Grief, negativism
Saliva	Fear, timidity, easily surprised

possible exception of abdominal surgery when extensive manipulation of abdominal viscera is involved.

Approximately 20 minutes prior to surgery, the needle or needles are inserted into the area for the particular procedure and are rotated manually or connected to a battery operated pulsator [4]. During surgery, the patient is able to converse with the doctors and nurses or read. Fluids and fruit are offered to the patient, and he is frequently allowed to walk from the operating room to his hospital room.

As anesthesia, acupuncture has several advantages over other types of anesthesia. With acupuncture, blood pressure is not lowered and respiratory tract complications do not occur postoperatively. There is no interruption in the patient's hydration and no postoperative nausea or vomiting. The pa-

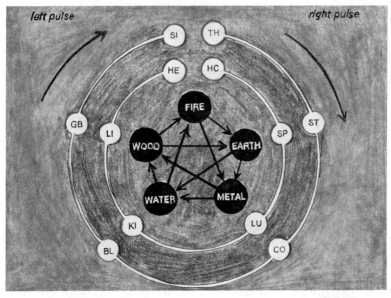

Figure 8-4 Much of acupuncture is based on the theory of the interdependence of five elements; each affects the other by creating (outer arrows) or by destroying (inner arrows) the next. Internal organs relate to the elements and similarly to each other.

Positions of Pulse Diagnosis

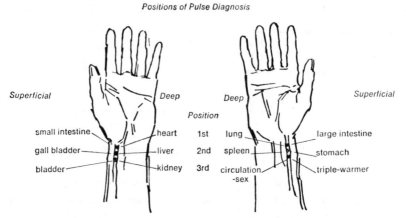

Superficial		Deep	Deep		Superficial
			Position		
small intestine		heart	1st	lung	large intestine
gall bladder		liver	2nd	spleen	stomach
bladder		kidney	3rd	circulation-sex	triple-warmer

Figure 8-5 Diseases can be detected by using varying pressures on the pulses at the radial artery. There are six locations which correspond to internal organs.

tient's pain threshold is increased, making it possible to perform minor procedures associated with the surgery without additional anesthesia [4].

The term moxibustion is frequently used in the literature on acupuncture. Moxibustion, which is stimulation of the acupuncture points by heat, may be used alone or as a supplement to acupuncture and uses acupuncture principles, although it is more generally applied for chronic illnesses [1]. In this technique, sticks or cones made from pulverized artemisia vulgaris (wormwood) are placed over the acupuncture point and are ignited and permitted to burn down to or close to the skin.

Understanding the Art

There is no apparent explanation of why the insertion of needles or the application of heat on the surface of the body should have any, much less definitive and predictable, results in areas and functions far removed from the treatment site.

Commonly, hypnosis, autosuggestion, cultural and political influence, or some aspect of quackery is given as an explanation. Yet, one needs only to survey the results of extensive research in many countries in which the same effects of acupuncture are found in several animal species to realize that these initial answers are not adequate. Indeed, acupuncture is widely used in veterinary medicine for the same purposes as described here for humans.

In looking further for a theoretical basis, it is necessary to sort out aspects of oriental philosophy and superstition from objective data which can be observed, recorded, and analyzed. As theories develop to scientifically plausible levels, one can then look back to ideas of the past and recognize correlations, unhindered by emotional barriers, formed by words and ideas strange to our culture and education.

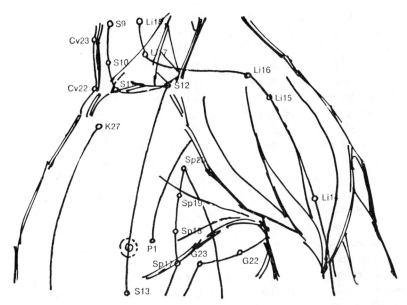

Figure 8-6 Large intestine meridian and acupuncture points Li 15 and Li 14 are located on the meridian of the deltoid muscle. Giving injections in this area may stimulate these points.

Several possible theories have emerged from research activities, mainly in China, Japan, and Russia. In 1893, Sir Henry Head, a British neurologist, published the observation that pain resulting from pathology of various organs was often referred to clearly definable areas on the body surface. These areas, which came to be known as "Head's zones," are similar to the location of the acupuncture meridians associated with the same organs. In 1883, independent of acupuncture research Dr. Weihe claimed he had discovered 195 points in close proximity with the viscera—points quite similar to acupuncture points. Both of these discoveries contributed to the development of therapeutic anesthesia including nerve blocking via injection of a local anesthetic for relief of somatic or visceral pain [10].

There is also a relationship between the arrangement of the meridians and the various layers of cells in the earliest stages of embryonic development. Detailed examination of this relationship reveals inconsistencies, but there is sufficient correlation here to warrant further study.

Another possible relationship may exist between Bonica's theory of trigger points and acupuncture. According to his theory, injury or pathology in muscles causes tenderness not only in the involved muscles themselves, but also in their tissues and associated organs, and the resulting increase in tension causes stiffness and increased tenderness in the muscles [9]. Moreover, Bonica contends that this type of local pain may be projected to other locations as referred or radiating pain.

The gate control theory of pain by Melzack and Wall is another possibility to consider. This theory stems from their discovery that two types of nerves are stimulated when a pain-evoking agent, like a needle, is applied [13]. The fine nerves (delta fibers which are small, myelinated, type A neurons) transmit the pain sensation to the appropriate location in the spinal cord and then to the brain. The other fibers (unmyelinated C fibers) are thicker and have an inhibiting effect on the finer ones. Perhaps because of their larger size, sensory impulses which the thicker fibers conduct arrive at the spinal cord first and close the gate for the sensation of pain carried by the fine nerves. Thus, activity in the larger peripheral sensory nerve fibers carrying nonpainful impulses inhibits pain conduction in the spinal cord from the smaller fibers. According to these authors, pain centers in the brain may then be jammed by the messages of minor pains, such as from acupuncture needle insertions, thereby decreasing awareness or sensation of the more major pain which occurs in surgery.

Dimond reports [2] that researchers in China used electrophysiologic techniques in rabbits and by peripheral pain stimulation produced a standard "induction voltage" in the cerebral cortex of 1 to 2 mm in height. (This measurement is not recorded in the usual manner, but may represent that used in China.) According to Dimond, "Acupuncture when placed appropriately had proved to lower this cerebral induction voltage substantially, even though the painful stimuli application continued. . . . Using humans and a standard stimulation of the tooth as the pain stimulus, they [the Chinese research team] found evidence that the recognized 'tooth' acupuncture anesthesia point on the back of the hand, near the attachment of the thumb, would effectively eliminate this pain stimulus to the patient."

A number of independent investigators have found that acupuncture points have characteristic electrical properties. The electrical resistance of tissue is consistently lower at acupuncture points than that at surrounding tissue; that is, there is a decrease in the skin's resistance to the flow of electrical current. Electrical resistance varies at acupuncture points, but it is fairly consistent over other skin areas. This change in electrical characteristics seems to be influenced by the physiologic processes of the body and by certain emotional states. When an acupuncture point is stimulated, the resistance of other points along the corresponding meridian is also affected. However, these changes along the meridian are transmitted more slowly than are nerve impulses. If the anatomic meridian is cut, the stimulus of an acupuncture point on that meridian is not transmitted to acupuncture points beyond the cut. Similarly, the internal organ with which the meridian is associated is not influenced by the treatment.

These electrical characteristics disappear in patients who have undergone electric or x-ray therapy. But, almost with this sole exception, the acupuncture points can be detected by their electrical resistance measured in microamperes.

Additional confirmation comes from the work of the Kirlians, a Russian couple, who have developed a method of producing photographs from the action of high-energy frequency currents [7]. In this method, nonelectrical properties of the object being photographed are converted into electrical ones through the action of a field with a directed transfer of charges from the object to a photographic plate or screen. This method, now called Kirlian photography, shows emission of energy from the specific areas traditionally called acupuncture points.

A Korean physiologist claims to have found distinct anatomic characteristics which coincide with acupuncture points and meridians. These points are said to ". . . consist of groups of small oval cells surrounded by many blood capillaries" [9]. The structures connecting one acupuncture point to another ". . . consists of clusters of thin tubular cells with round or oval cross-sections, and having a diameter of 20 to 50 microns" [9]. Attempts by a Chinese research team to confirm the results of this study have thus far been unsuccessful.

Much research still needs to be done. But, many possible theories are beginning to emerge and perhaps the anatomic and physiologic basis of this ancient technique will soon be firmly established or rejected on the basis of sound research endeavors.

Acupuncture and Nursing Practice

Several principles of traditional acupuncture are akin to ideas that nursing has been advocating for many years: the importance of preventive health measures, active involvement of the individual patient, detailed observations, and patient teaching are but a few examples. In addition, most references concerning acupuncture stress the importance of the whole man, in whom nothing happens in isolation but in relationship to other events occurring in his internal or external environment. Consequently, there are specific areas within the context of these concepts which have relevance to nursing practice.

Nurses, I believe, are often applying acupuncture principles directly and indirectly and have been doing so for some time. For example, acupuncture points have been used to develop massage techniques by schools of massage throughout the world. Massage used to produce results proximally or distally to precise points of cutaneous stimulation may be called reflexogenous. These fall into two groups: spontaneously painful points and points selected by the therapist. These correspond to acupuncture points and are treated with the hand instead of the needle [5]. Nurses have generally used massage techniques for a local or regional effect or a general feeling of well-being and relaxation.

Since several meridians run longitudinally along the back, neck, and buttocks, studies need to be carried out to determine what effects the massage techniques commonly employed by nurses have upon specific functions far removed from the site of massage. And, what are the distant effects of local heat treatment applied for local results? Compiling such information will aid in planning the procedures needed for desirable and predictable results as well as in avoiding the problems we may have dismissed in the past as being unrelated to a particular procedure.

A natural question arises as to the possibility that we are stimulating known acupuncture points when administering injections, starting intravenous feedings, or withdrawing blood. It now appears that if the common injection sites are correctly chosen, the major acupuncture points in the area can be avoided. For example, look at the illustration of the deltoid muscle in Figure 8-6. The large intestine meridian runs through the midline of the muscle. If injection sites are located in the belly of the muscle just off the midline, the meridian as well as the acupuncture points Li 14 and 15 can easily be avoided.

Common injection sites on the buttocks, anterior thighs, and below the iliac crest present similar situations. The bladder meridian runs longitudinally down the midline of the gluteus maximus muscle leaving the inner aspect of the upper outer quadrant free of major acupuncture points. The midline of the anterior thigh is also void of points. The gall bladder meridian runs down the outer aspect of the thigh but swings anteriorly below the iliac crest leaving the v-shaped area commonly used for injections free of points if the injection site is not in the extreme anterior portion of the v.

Numerous meridians are located in the abdominal area and in the anterior and posterior surfaces of the forearm and hands. Thus, a detailed study of meridians must be done to determine the more important areas to avoid when inserting a needle for whatever purpose in these areas. It is possible that persistent pain or sensation following an injection may be due to stimulation of an acupuncture point with physiologic results in the corresponding organ.

It is also interesting to note that acupuncture points are located on the tips of the fingers. In acupuncture therapy, these points are treated in tonsillitis, fever, sunstroke, meningitis, and intestinal influenza. In patients with high fever, a quick jab with a triangular needle is made with removal of several drops of blood. What effects, then, if any, are brought about by the method commonly used to obtain blood in capillary tubes for hematocrits?

Attempts are now being made to assess the use of acupuncture in this country [3]. In New York City, a ten-man committee of medical specialists to conduct and coordinate acupuncture studies has been formed. Elsewhere, several doctors and medical groups, such as the National Academy of Sciences, have attempted to initiate cooperative research with practitioners in China. And some attempts are being made to seek information from practitioners in this country. In Seattle, for example, approximately 45 doctors and other health related professionals have attended a survey course in acupuncture being taught at the University of Washington's noncredit Experimental College. The 14 week course is taught by Professor Mifoo Hsu, a retired acupuncturist, who has taught and practiced in Hong Kong and Japan.

In preparation for increased practice of acupuncture, the Teamsters Union in San Francisco recently decided to include acupuncture coverage in its health insurance policy [11]. This may be one of the first steps toward popularization of the practice of acupuncture in the United States.

Thus, the process of inquiry has already begun in this country into a medical practice that is thousands of years old and embedded in a culture vastly different from our own. To discard or accept acupuncture as a sound medical and nursing practice would be wrong at this time. Openmindedness with a proper degree of caution would be most helpful while we investigate the practice of acupuncture and related techniques with the hope of making discoveries which will eventually improve nursing care.

Implications for nursing research have been implicit throughout this discussion. As interest in acupuncture increases, nurses and other health professionals can provide accurate information to laymen, and to one another, to avoid inappropriate and overzealous use of acupuncture. As the valid uses of acupuncture are determined, nursing can play a valuable role in judicious integration of these techniques into nursing and medical practice.

References

1. Bechterev, V. M.   Acupuncture research in U.S.S.R. *J. Int. Cong. Acupunct. Moxibustion* 15:272, 1965.
2. Dimond, E. G.   Acupuncture anesthesia: Western medicine, Chinese traditional medicine. *JAMA* 218:1558, 1971.
3. Hashimoto, M.   *Japanese acupuncture.* P. M. Chancellor, ed. New York: Liveright Publishing Corporation, 1968.
4. Hsu, M.   Survey Course of Acupuncture, 1971–1972. Seattle, Washington, University of Washington, Experimental College, 1972.
5. Hsu, M.   Form MH 1001.
6. Huard, P., and Wong, M.   *Chinese Medicine.* New York: McGraw-Hill Book Company, 1968.
7. Kirlian, S. D., and Kirlian, K.   *Photography and Visual Observation by Means of High-Frequency Currents.* Federal Technical Report, FTD-TT-62-1549/1+2+4, Sept. 19, 1959.
8. Kramer, B.   *Wall Street Journal,* March 29, 1972.
9. Mann, F.   *Acupuncture: The Ancient Chinese Art of Healing.* New York: Random House, Inc., 1963.
10. Melzack, R., and Wall, P. D.   Pain mechanisms: A new theory. *Science* 150: 971, 1965.
11. Randel, J.   *Orlando Sentinel,* March 16, 1972, p. 1-C.
12. Schreiber, C.   *Syracuse Herald Journal,* March 21, 1972, p. 1.
13. Schreiber, C.   Mutes regain their speech. *China Reconstructs* 21:2, 1972.
14. Stovickova, D.   About moxibustion. *Far East Reporter* 1:31, 1972.
15. Wallnofer, H., and Von Rottauscher, A.   *Chinese Folk Medicine.* New York: Crown Publishers, 1972.

Addendum: Reflections on Acupuncture

During the five years since 1972, the increase of interest and activity regarding acupuncture in this country has been remarkable. There has been a phenomenal growth in the number of research studies and educational programs addressing the theoretical basis and clinical practice of acupuncture. In addition, there has been a tremendous increase in the number of physicians and nonphysicians adding the modality of acupuncture to their clinical practice. This growth has resulted in rapid changes in the legal status of acupuncture in many states. Lastly and perhaps most importantly, the lay public has received a vast amount of information via television and writings regarding acupuncture, and their interest in the practice has grown accordingly. In turn the public has increasingly exerted pressure for more liberal legislation and more available treatment.

As a result of the increase in research activities, several of the theories used to explain the basis of acupuncture have been developed to a more specific extent or have decreased in popularity. In regard to the basis of acupuncture as an analgesic, the gate control theory of pain remains the best explanation of this action. Although the gate control theory of pain has yet to be fully explained by quantitative data, it remains the clearest and most comprehensive explanation of the central control of pain, as well as the role of acupuncture in decreasing pain, that is available to us. Indeed, several laboratory studies regarding acupuncture have added related data to the dynamics of the gate control theory.

The philosophy and use of meridians has decreased somewhat throughout the world. It has not been possible to gather more specific data on the relevance or existence of actual meridians and thus meridians are used in the main as an international nomenclature for the location of specific acupuncture points.

There continues to be some debate as to the relationship of acupuncture to hypnosis and autosuggestion. However, most studies have shown that although the two modalities are quite similar in what they can accomplish, one cannot be explained solely by the other [5]. Controlled clinical studies, however, have shown that a belief in the modality of acupuncture will enhance the response to the treatment, as is true with other modalities of treatment [6]. However, it should be noted that in instances in which acupuncture is used appropriately in the treatment of a pathology, the percentages of positive responses are generally higher than that which could be expected as a result of either placebo effect, hypnosis, autosuggestion, and/or strong belief on the part of the recipient.

Regarding the use of acupuncture in the treatment of disease, the most common explanation adhered to at the present time is the dynamics of sympathetic nervous system reflexes. The autonomic nervous system and its ability to effect responses in internal viscera to stimuli to the skin have never been fully understood. However, more data are currently being collected as to the role of the autonomic nervous system relative to the accomplishments of acupuncture.

There has also been an increase in studies regarding the biochemical dynamics of acupuncture responses. One of the most notable is a study showing a consistent increase in serotonin in the brainstem following acupuncture treatments, which results in decreased pain [1]. There is also beginning evidence that histamine may be a neurotransmitter in the brainstem. This is particularly relevant since a small red wheal around the hub of the needle during an acupuncture treatment is an indication that the patient will have a positive response.

There has been little additional research regarding the anatomical basis of acupuncture until very recently. A study was recently reported in which a significant amount of collagen tissue was found to exist around the location of acupuncture points compared to nonacupuncture areas [4]. It is expected that more research will be done in this regard.

Although it has commonly been found that humans and various animals respond with a general relaxation response to acupuncture, the specific physiological dynamics taking place during acupuncture treatment is still relatively vague. This writer is currently conducting a study measuring the various physiological responses to a variety of dermal stimuli, including acupuncture, in an attempt to explain this response.

Research funds have primarily been obtained from private and other nonfederal sources. However, a few studies were recently funded by the National Institutes of Health. A directory of research activities and centers working with acupuncture can be obtained [2].

Although there have also been increased attempts to conduct controlled clinical studies of acupuncture, there have been difficulties in adequately controlling the many factors that affect the responses to acupuncture treatments. Fortunately, a greater emphasis is now being placed upon the need for tight control of relevant research variables in clinical acupuncture studies.

The legal status of acupuncture has changed considerably in the recent past. In the past, most states did not have any legislation regarding the practice of acupuncture. During the past two years, most states either have formulated legislation regarding the control of the practice of acupuncture or are currently considering such legislation. Some states have even gone through a revision of their initially formulated laws. Since there is such a variation among the state laws with such rapid change, it is advisable for practicing nurses to check the legal status of acupuncture in their individual states and to keep informed as changes take place. Unfortunately, the majority of legislation does not address itself to the involvement of nurses in the practice of acupuncture as an inherent factor within common nursing activities. Therefore, although there has been money allocated in some states for educational programs for physicians and other providers of medical care, there has been no such funding provided for educational programs for nurses. However, there are now many seminars, workshops, and short courses provided by various groups regarding the research and practice of acupuncture throughout the country. Many of these meetings are open to nonphysicians, including nurses. Unfortunately, the cost of these programs is very often prohibitive. It is to be hoped that this situation will improve.

Several professional and semiprofessional organizations have been formed to encourage research and provide programs regarding acupuncture. Such organizations include the National Acupuncture Research Society, the National Association for Veterinary Medicine, and the National Academy of Acupuncture. There have also been several journals which are now publishing on a regular basis, including *The Journal of New Chinese Medicine, The American Journal of Chinese Medicine, Acupuncture News*, and *The Acupuncture Letter*. A number of companies have begun to produce acupuncture equipment, thereby increasing the accessibility of equipment for researchers and practitioners.

The actual practice of acupuncture has also been refined during the past few years. The traditional methods of utilizing acupuncture points for prevention and diagnosis has been further developed by Dr. Manaka in Japan. He has developed the method termed "Ryodoraku" which means semipermeable points in which key acupuncture points are measured relative to their electrical activity with results of such measurements plotted on charts to indicate existent pathologies. Programs providing information relative to this method are now being offered in this country.

The use of acupuncture as an anesthesia is still very limited in this country, although a reasonable number of attempts have been made to explore this use more fully. The use of acupuncture as an analgesic is currently receiving more attention in both research and practice. Although more research is needed for definite conclusions, the majority of studies indicate that the response to acupuncture for some types of pain is greater than one would normally expect from the placebo effect alone. It is too early to know if this conclusion will stand as further evidence is forthcoming.

The use of acupuncture as a treatment modality has found the greatest amount of popularity as practiced in numerous acupuncture clinics and physician and nonphysician practices. New methods for the administration of acupuncture have also been developed. It has been known for some time that many methods can be used to stimulate acupuncture points including heat, vibration, and finger pressure. References are now readily available regarding application of finger pressure to treat common problems [3]. One of the most popular new methods of applying stimulation to acupuncture points is the use of ultra-sound. Other new forms which have been increasingly used include electrical current and injection of slowly absorbable substances.

Several acupuncture specialties have begun to develop. For instance, some practitioners have begun to specialize in the use of acupuncture points in and around the ear. Others have restricted their practice to hand acupuncture or locally sensitive points around the location of the clinical problem. A very recent development is the use of scalp points for various motor and sensory problems.

Information is constantly being gathered as to newly identified problems which have been successfully treated with acupuncture. One of the most popular examples is the use of heart and lung points on the ear for the relief of withdrawal symptoms due to termination of a habitual behavior such as drugs, overeating, or smoking. Unfortunately, some problems have received premature publicity via the mass media, thereby encouraging individuals to be unrealistically expectant of results. The most notable example is the experimental use of acupuncture in the relief of deafness. Results of this use of acupuncture are much too premature and lack the success rates which should merit such attention.

Naturally, the immense growth in the interest in the practice of acupuncture has steadily required the increased involvement on the part of practicing nurses, both as assistants and then actually administering acupuncture, as well as sources of information to the public and colleagues regarding their many questions about acupuncture. There is an increasing need for nurses to be informed in order to convey information correctly and responsibly. Potential and actual recipients of acupuncture need a good deal of teaching regarding the appropriate uses of acupuncture, how to select an acupuncturist (whether physician or nonphysician), incidence and nature of side effects, and responses which can be expected, as well as the details of the appropriate expectations of the treatments.

Nursing educators need to continue to assess the need for information about acupuncture in nursing curricula. Whether acupuncture is legal or illegal is irrelevant in many states since as students and eventually as graduates, nurses are stimulating acupuncture points in regular nursing procedures. In addition, acupuncture is practiced in nearly every state, legally or "underground," resulting in the need for nurses to be informed in order to convey information to colleagues and the public alike. Fortunately, a few new texts in nursing have begun to include sections on the implications of acupuncture.

One can readily see that activities in all realms have increased phenomenally in regard to the potential uses and implications of acupuncture. Additional information regarding the theoretical basis and appropriate clinical applications of acupuncture is now becoming more readily available. As responsible health professionals, we must keep informed and make responsible decisions regarding our practice and education and research activities related to new developments which may influence patient care.

References

1. Acupuncture Anesthesia Research Group. The relation between acupuncture analgesia and neuro-transmitters in rabbit brain. *Chin. Med. J.* 8:478, 1973.
2. *Acupuncture Directory*. Los Angeles: Chan's Books, 1975.
3. Chan, P. *Finger Acupressure*. Los Angeles: Price/Stern/Sloan Publishers, Inc., 1975.
4. Chew, E. C., and Plummer, J. P. Connective tissue, Masson's trichrome stain

and acupuncture loci. The Third World Symposium on Acupuncture and Chinese Medicine. *Am. J. Chin. Med.* 3(2):26, 1975.

5. Katz, R. L., Kao, C. Y., Spiegal, H., and Katz, G. J. Pain, acupuncture, hypnosis. In Bonica, J. J., ed., *Advances in Neurology* (Vol. 4). New York: Raven Press, 1974, pp. 819–826.

6. Myer, S. Attitude about and Knowledge of Acupuncture. Master's essay, University of Rochester, 1974.

9

Narcotic and Nonnarcotic Analgesics for Relief of Pain

Gerald F. Gebhart

Agents employed for relief from pain are the most widely used of all pharmacological classes of drugs and are of undeniable importance to man. In this chapter, the structurally diverse group of compounds comprising the broad class analgesics will be discussed. For this purpose, analgesia is defined as relief from the sensation of pain, in the broadest meaning of that concept, without loss of consciousness. Differentiation between pain as a specific sensation associated with certain anatomically delineated pathways and anatomical structures, and pain as suffering (i.e., culturally associated, learned reactions to pain, etc.) will not be addressed directly. The latter aspect of the pain experience is adequately discussed elsewhere in this book while presentation of the former, the neural basis of pain, appears in this as well as many other sources [6, 8].

Various remedies have been employed for a multitude of pain-associated conditions throughout recorded history. Many of these remedies were opium-containing products and, as such, contained the active analgesic principle morphine. Over-the-counter analgesic preparations, which no longer contain morphine, are today heavily advertised and extensively used by a large segment of the population for a variety of conditions (e.g., headache, arthritis, muscle pain, etc.). Many compounds having a variety of effects, including that of a placebo, are employed as analgesic agents. Usually, this structurally heterogeneous group of analgesia-producing compounds is classed into narcotic and nonnarcotic agents. While other classification schemes are sometimes employed (e.g., strong/weak analgesics, narcotic/antipyretic analgesics, addictive/nonaddictive analgesics), the narcotic/nonnarcotic classification scheme has the greatest pharmacological utility and is the classification scheme that will be employed throughout this chapter.

The narcotic analgesics (also referred to as the opioids) are structurally homogeneous, more so than are the nonnarcotic analgesic agents. The most distinguishing characteristics of the narcotic analgesics are (1) the development of tolerance to their analgesic effect (as well as other effects) and (2) the development of physical dependence. Associated with physical dependence, of course, is the development of a withdrawal or abstinence syndrome on discontinuance of narcotic administration or on administration of a narcotic antagonist (i.e., precipitated withdrawal). Neither tolerance nor physical dependence, however, is associated with the nonnarcotic analgesic agents. Another important difference between these two classes of analgesic agents is their analgesic efficacy; that is, the nature and severity of pain that they are capable of relieving significantly differ. The narcotic analgesics have a greater efficacy (i.e., can relieve pain of a more severe nature) than nonnarcotic analgesic agents. This difference in analgesic efficacy (not to be confused with potency, a dose characteristic) is in part the basis of the strong/weak analgesic classification scheme previously mentioned. The efficacy of the narcotic analgesic agents is such that in sufficient dosage they are considered capable of relieving virtually every nature of pain. Nonnarcotic analgesics, while capable of significant relief of pain, are limited to relief from mild to moderate pain (e.g., headache, muscle and joint pain) regardless of the dose administered.

The final two important differences between narcotic and nonnarcotic classes of analgesic agents relate to the sites and mechanisms of action responsible for their production of analgesia. It has long been held that the narcotic analgesic agents produce analgesia by central nervous system (i.e., brain and spinal cord) mechanisms whereas the nonnarcotic analgesic agents are effective by virtue of peripheral mechanisms outside of the central nervous system. There is considerable evidence supporting central nervous system loci of action for narcotic analgesics as well as reliable data supporting loci of action outside the central nervous system for nonnarcotic analgesic agents. There is, in addition, some evidence suggesting a central nervous system contribution to analgesia produced by nonnarcotic analgesics. As is generally the case regarding identification of drug loci of action, considerable work is necessary to satisfactorily demonstrate analgesic loci of action related to analgesia induced by both narcotic and nonnarcotic analgesics. Regarding their mechanisms of analgesia production, the evidence is less compelling than for their loci of action. A large number of hypotheses have been advanced regarding the mechanism(s) of narcotic-induced analgesia, but none yet satisfactorily accommodate all of the available data. A confounding aspect of determination of the mechanism(s) of action of narcotic analgesic agents relates to the attendant tolerance and physical dependence associated with their repeated use. Regarding the nonnarcotic analgesic agents, data is rapidly accumulating that support the hypothesis that many of the agents so classed act via interference with the biosynthesis of prostaglandins. Additional information is discussed later in this chapter relative to both loci and mechanisms of analgesia production by both narcotic and nonnarcotic agents.

The generalized differences, then, between the narcotic and nonnarcotic analgesic agents relate to: (1) development of tolerance and physical dependence; (2) analgesic efficacy; (3) site of analgesic effect; and (4) mechanisms of analgesic effect. Narcotic and nonnarcotic analgesic agents also differ in other aspects of their pharmacology (e.g., so-called side effects, toxicity, and oral efficacy), but these are not general bases upon which categorization is usefully effected. The remainder of this chapter will be devoted to discussions of selected narcotic and nonnarcotic analgesic agents and their respective associated important pharmacology. Where appropriate, important differences between specific agents within each class are emphasized as well as particular applications for specific conditions.

The Narcotic Analgesics (Opioids)

Opium is a product of the poppy plant, *Papaver somniferum*. The unripe seed capsules are incised and the exudate collected, dried, and powdered. Opium powder contains many alkaloids, but only morphine, codeine, and papaverine among them are medically useful—morphine and codeine primarily as analgesics and papaverine as a smooth-muscle relaxant (antispasmodic).

First knowledge of opium is often erroneously credited to mankind's first civilization, Sumeria. There is no evidence that the Sumerians knew of opium, but written descriptions of *Papaver somniferum* do appear in the Ebers papyrus (1552 B.C.) of the ancient Egyptian civilization [73]. Other sources credit the Greek philosopher Theophrastus with providing the first undisputed written reference to the uses of opium in the third century B.C. [47]. Regardless, it was not until 1803 that the German pharmacist, Sertürner, isolated and named as "morphine" the important analgesic alkaloid from opium. Since then, many semisynthetic derivatives made by modification of the morphine molecule (e.g., heroin, hydromorphone [Dilaudid], oxymorphone [Numorphan], hydrocodone [contained in Hycodan], and oxycodone [contained in Percodan]) and many entirely synthetic compounds (e.g., meperidine [Demerol], fentanyl [Sublimaze], methadone [Dolophine], and propoxyphene [Darvon]) have been introduced into medicine. These structurally diverse compounds all share with morphine the ability to produce analgesia, respiratory depression, gastrointestinal spasm, and physical dependence. None, however, have yet been demonstrated as significantly different from or superior to the prototypical narcotic analgesic, morphine, with respect to their important pharmacology. Morphine, consequently, will be discussed in greater detail than any other agents with which we will be concerned. It will, however, be understood that what is discussed about morphine applies in general to all narcotic analgesics. The incidence of untoward effects and the intensity of action of the opioids as a group are essentially similar and differ but little when compared at equi-analgesic doses. The frequent use of the terms "opioid(s)," "narcotic analgesics" and "morphine and its congeners" will serve to reemphasize this throughout the chapter. Significant differences between morphine and semisynthetic and synthetic morphine analogues will be indicated when the individual agent is discussed.

Morphine

Despite the long-standing application of the opioids as analgesics, the mechanism by which, and the central nervous system site(s) at which, these agents act are poorly understood. Recently, several independent avenues of research have implicated the periaqueductal central gray matter in the brainstem as being important to analgesic mechanisms per se as well as being at least one central locus where morphine exerts an analgesic effect. Reynolds [70] initially implicated the periaqueductal central gray matter as a pain or nociception-relevant central locus when he demonstrated that electrical stimulation of that brain area induced an analgesic state sufficient to perform laparotomies in experimental animals. Many workers since then, Liebeskind's group prominent among them [30, 52, 53, 58, 59], have elaborated on the analgesic efficacy of focal brain stimulation of the periaqueductal gray matter. These data have subsequently been extended to man. Richardson and Akil [71] have reported significant pain relief in patients suffering from chronic pain after electrical stimulation of the medial brainstem. Additional converging data relative to analgesic brain loci are provided by demonstration of regional localization within the brain of an "opiate receptor." Several workers [37, 49, 56, 69] have, by evaluating stereospecific narcotic binding to fractions of brain protein, implicated areas of the brain limbic system as well as the periventricular-periaqueductal area of the brainstem. It is not clear at present whether there is only a single opiate receptor for all opioid effects or multiple opiate receptors, one each for the many actions of the opioids. Moreover, it remains yet to demonstrate pharmacological relevance of these receptors. Most recently, Hughes [40] reported the isolation of an endogenous compound from the brain having pharmacological properties similar to morphine. This morphinelike substance is unevenly distributed in the brain; the highest concentrations were found in the striatum, midbrain, pons, and medulla. It has been suggested that this compound forms part of a central nervous system pain-suppression system, but evidence is currently lacking. Further investigation, however, will eventually reveal this compound's relevance to pain perception as well as stimulation-produced and narcotic-induced analgesia.

The relationship of various brain sites to narcotic-induced analgesia has been evaluated by the injection of narcotic analgesics directly into the brain —initially into the ventricular system [34, 35] and more recently directly into specific brain sites. Herz's group was able to localize effective narcotic analgesic brain sites to the gray areas surrounding the cerebral aqueduct and structures on the floor of the fourth ventricle by intraventricular injection techniques in experimental animals. Subsequently, other workers [43, 44, 51] injected minute amounts of narcotic analgesics directly into the periaqueductal gray matter as well as other, opiate receptor–rich brain areas and demonstrated significant analgesic efficacy. With respect to the periaqueductal gray matter, the microinjection of other, nonanalgesic agents was without effect [51], thus establishing both site and drug specificity for this brain area.

While research has been primarily directed toward elucidation of brain sites relevant to the analgesic effects of the opioids, considerable evidence has also accumulated for brain sites associated with the respiratory depressant, hypothermic, and nauseant/emetic effects of the narcotic analgesics [47, 55, 74]. In addition to the search for brain sites related to opioid effects, an extensive body of literature has been generated concerning the role various putative central neurotransmitters (e.g., norepinephrine, dopamine, acetylcholine, serotonin, glutamate, and gamma-aminobutyric acid) play in the actions of the narcotic analgesics. There is reliable data that the opioids interact with several neurotransmitters, but the literature is often contradictory. Since the opioids exert many effects on the central nervous system and because neurotransmitters do not act alone, but in concert, it is not possible at present to associate any single neurotransmitter with any particular opioid effect. It is probable that one transmitter is related to one opioid effect more than to another, but revelation of those associations awaits refined research efforts [33, 83].

Our limited knowledge regarding the site(s) and mechanism(s) of action of the narcotic analgesics notwithstanding, the pharmacology and our basic understanding of the nature of their effects are extensive.

Morphine is the prototypical narcotic analgesic and the single agent about which most is known. Morphine and its congeners primarily exert their effects on the smooth muscle of the gastrointestinal tract and the central nervous system. Indeed, the use of opium (which contains approximately 10 percent morphine) for relief of diarrhea and dysentery antedated by centuries its use as an analgesic. The central nervous system effects of morphine are expressed as a combination of overt stimulation and depression and include analgesia, dysphoria/euphoria, drowsiness, respiratory depression, depression of the cough reflex, miosis, inhibition of ACTH and gonadotropin release, increased antidiuretic hormone release, and initial stimulation of the medullary chemoreceptor trigger zone for emesis followed by depression of the vomiting center.

As previously defined, opioid-induced analgesia occurs without loss of consciousness. The narcotic analgesics, it must be emphasized, when administered for relief from pain (or cough or diarrhea, for that matter) provide only symptomatic relief without removing or altering the cause for pain. In therapeutic analgesic doses there is a drowsiness from which the patient is relatively easily aroused and a "tranquilization" produced by morphine and its congeners. The first recorded use of the term tranquilization in conjunction with opioid use appears in the writings of Thomas DeQuincy, the English philosopher and author of *The Confessions of an English Opium-Eater* (1822). There is without doubt a significant antianxiety or "tranquilizing" contribution to the analgesic effect of the narcotic analgesics. Moreover, an often overlooked and underemphasized reason for abusing narcotics relates to their "tranquilizing" action; the orgasmic "rush" being overemphasized by nonabusers. There is, undeniably, a euphoria often experienced by the patient in pain after the administration of a narcotic analgesic. Paradoxically, perhaps, a dysphoria characterized by mild anxiety often results after the same analgesic dose in the pain-free patient. These subjective effects of morphine and its congeners are dose-related. As the dose is increased, drowsiness becomes more pronounced and sleep ensues; the euphoric or dysphoric effects will also be accentuated at increased doses. The analgesic effect of the narcotic analgesics is also enhanced as the dose is increased (i.e., pain of a more severe nature will be relieved) as is the degree of respiratory depression and the incidence of nausea and vomiting.

ANALGESIA   As previously indicated, the site(s) and mechanism(s) of opioid-induced analgesia are incompletely understood at present. It is generally accepted that morphine and its congeners raise the threshold for pain perception as well as alter the reaction to pain. The experimental data on these points, particularly with respect to pain threshold, are not consistent. The earlier literature does not agree with later reports regarding morphine's ability to elevate the pain threshold; more recent investigations emphasize morphine's predominant effect on the affective component of the pain experience. As in all studies of analgesic efficacy, the discrepancies regarding these two aspects of opioid-induced analgesia relates in part to the inherent difference between experimentally induced pain and pathological or clinical pain (attended, as it may be, by fear, anxiety, suffering, etc.). A relatively new experimental approach may help clarify our understanding of the nature of opioid-induced analgesia. Signal detection theory [31, 75, 77] is a psychophysical procedure by which the subject's ability to sense or discriminate a signal (e.g., pain) can be separated from his willingness to respond to that signal (e.g., capacity to tolerate experimentally-induced pain). This approach has been applied in the analysis of response to noxious stimulation in humans [14], in the evaluation of the analgesic effect of nitrous oxide [11], and in the study of acupuncture analgesia [15], verbal suggestion, and placebo effects [14, 23]. At this writing, a signal detection theory analysis of opioid-induced analgesia has not yet appeared in the scientific literature. The expectation is that such an experimental approach and analysis would be useful.

The analgesia induced by morphine and its congeners is considered to be selective in nature in that other sensory modalities (i.e., vision, audition, etc.) are unaffected at therapeutic dosages. In fact, identification of the pain itself may be affected but little. A common report from the patient in pain is that the pain is still present, but is no longer discomforting or intolerable. These clinical impressions and patients' reports argue for a predominant action by the narcotic analgesics against the motivational/affective component of the pain experience, presumably effected via opioid action within the brain's limbic system. Nonetheless, carefully conceived and executed experimental studies also reveal an opioid action on the sensory discriminative component of pain perception. It would appear, however, that in man this is of secondary significance. An additional important aspect of the analgesia produced by the narcotic analgesics is that they are generally considered to be more effective against continuous dull pain than sharp intermittent pain [47]. Nevertheless, the narcotic analgesics are the most efficacious pain-relievers known to man; they are without peer and are capable of relieving virtually every nature of pain. The standard analgesic dose of morphine is 10 mg per 70 kg of body weight, given parenterally. This dose is considered near optimal and in the majority of patients will relieve moderate-to-severe pain.

Morphine, and indeed most narcotic analgesics, are not nearly as efficacious when given orally in the same dose as when given parenterally. Consequently, the oral dose must often be substantially increased to provide the desired degree of pain relief. For morphine, oral administration is approximately one-sixth as effective as parenteral administration [61]. A final consideration regarding the analgesic effect of the narcotic analgesics relates to the patient's age. It has long been appreciated that some opioids (e.g., morphine) gain more rapid access to the brain in the newborn due to the immature status of the blood-brain barrier [82], resulting in altered sensitivity to opioid action. Other workers [3] have also found that increasing chronological age is highly correlated with pain sensitivity and pain relief afforded by narcotic analgesics; pain sensitivity decreases with age and pain relief is enhanced with age.

RESPIRATION   Morphine and its congeners depress respiration in a dose-related fashion. The respiratory depression attendant to opioid use is discernible even in therapeutic doses and is the primary undesirable aspect of their pharmacological effects. The narcotic analgesics are capable of depressing all phases of respiration: rate, minute volume, and tidal exchange. Irregular rhythms and periodic breathing are not uncommon manifestations of the narcotic analgesics. The mechanisms by which these agents affect respiration relates to an initial decreased responsiveness of brainstem respiratory centers to CO_2 circulating in the blood. The opioids also directly depress pontine and medullary centers regulating respiratory rhythm. The respiratory rate may be altered from the normal 18 to 20 per minute to as low as 4 to 5 per minute after toxic doses of morphine or its congeners. It is essential to indicate at this point that all narcotic analgesics, semisynthetic and wholly synthetic alike, are capable of depressing respiration to the same extent when administered in equi-analgesic doses. That is, there is little quantitative difference among the opioid group as a whole with respect to their respiratory depressant effect following doses of equivalent analgesia-inducing ability. In man, acute intoxication by morphine or its congeners results in life-threatening respiratory depression. In fact, death from poisoning by these agents is virtually always a result of respiration depressed beyond life-sustaining capability. Fortunately, opioid antagonists (e.g., naloxone) are available, which rapidly and reliably reverse the respiratory depression. These agents will be discussed later in this chapter. One should not, however, assume that respiratory depression is always the cause of death in chronic user "overdose" (e.g., heroin overdose). The term "overdose" is used with reservations since there are, in addition to respiratory depression, other possible causes for death in these individuals (e.g., contaminants contained in the illicit preparation, an immunologic-based phenomenon, and the conjoint use of other psychoactive drugs [7]).

COUGH SUPPRESSION   Morphine and its congeners are effective cough suppressants (antitussives) and some (e.g., codeine) are widely employed for this purpose. The central nervous system site of their antitussive action is located in the brainstem, as are respiratory centers that are, as previously indicated, affected by the opioids. While the brain sites for the respiratory depressant and antitussive actions of the opioids are anatomically nearby, there is no apparent relationship between depression of one and depression of the other since nonanalgesic, nonrespiratory depressant opioid analogues (e.g., dextromethorphan) are efficacious antitussives [12]. Further, suppression of the cough reflex apparently requires opioid doses lower than those necessary to produce an analgesic effect or respiratory depression.

PUPILLARY REACTION   Morphine and most, but not all, of its congeners produce a pupillary constriction (miosis) in man at therapeutic dose levels. The emphasis on man in this instance is significant since in some species where the opioids exert primarily an excitatory effect, the pupils are dilated instead (e.g., cats). As with the other opioid effects discussed thus far, miosis results from a central nervous system effect (the oculomotor nerve) and not via a direct effect on the circular or radial muscle fibers of the iris as might be assumed. The occurrence of pinpoint pupils, or miosis, in conjunction with depressed respiration is characteristic following toxic doses of morphine. In the asphyxiated individual, however, a pupillary dilation (mydriasis) will supervene. The immediate administration of an opioid antagonist will dramatically reverse either sign if the intoxicant was an opioid. Consideration of tolerance (a reduced effect with subsequent drug administration) to the opioids has yet to be discussed, but it is instructive at this juncture to indicate that tolerance to the miotic effect of morphine and some other opioids does not develop to any appreciable extent (methadone is a notable exception). Consequently, chronic users of morphine and heroin, for example, continue to have constricted pupils, although tolerance to many other opioid effects will have developed to a significant degree.

NAUSEA AND VOMITING   As indicated earlier, the opioids directly stimulate the medullary chemoreceptor trigger zone and are capable of producing nausea and vomiting. In addition to directly stimulating the medullary chemoreceptor trigger zone, morphine and its congeners subsequently depress the medullary center in the brain for vomiting. The subsequent depression, even after therapeutic doses of the opioids, is virtually total; other narcotic analgesics or emesis-inducing agents administered at this time are generally ineffective. The nausea and vomiting elicited by morphine and its congeners occur with greater frequency in ambulatory than in recumbent patients, indicating contribution of a vestibular component to the nausea and vomiting. Often, opioid-induced nausea can be attenuated in these patients by concurrent administration of agents employed to prevent motion sickness.

CARDIOVASCULAR SYSTEM   In therapeutic doses, the effects of morphine and its congeners on blood pressure, heart rate, and heart work are unremarkable. The vasomotor center of the medulla is relatively unaffected by the narcotic analgesics; normal blood pressure is well maintained even after toxic doses until hypoxia resulting from respiratory depression induces a fall. The effect of the opioids on the peripheral vasculature is not completely understood. Morphine and most other opioids release histamine, producing a vasodilation in the cutaneous vasculature that often results in an overall feeling of warmth or itching of the face and nose. This effect is local and not central in origin. There appears, however, also to be a central nervous system contribution to the peripheral vasodilation observed after opioid administration. Regardless, peripheral vasodilation is the primary cause of the orthostatic hypotension and fainting that occurs in some recumbent patients when the head-up position is suddenly assumed.

The opioids are without direct effect on the vasculature and circulation of the brain, but cerebral vasodilation is not an uncommon result of opioid administration. The cerebral vasodilation is, however, secondary to the respiratory depression and retention of circulating CO_2 in the blood. The net result is an increase in cerebrospinal fluid pressure which may prevent opioid use in those cases of cranial trauma and head injury where cerebrospinal fluid pressure may already be elevated. A final, significant cardiopulmonary effect of morphine relates to its effective use in the treatment of pulmonary edema. The mechanism by which morphine exerts this beneficial action is unclear, but morphine appears to function as a surrogate adrenergic blocking agent promoting a redistribution of blood to the periphery and reducing pressure in the pulmonary veins and capillaries without concomitant reduction of the systemic arterial pressure [81].

GASTROINTESTINAL TRACT   The opioids exert significant effects along the smooth muscle of the entire gastrointestinal tract. The overall action is constipative and this effect has been long appreciated and therapeutically useful. Morphine and its congeners increase muscle tone and decrease motility throughout the gastrointestinal tract. This constipative action produces its most significant delay in gastrointestinal emptying at the stomach/duodenum. Opioid effects on the smooth muscle of the small intestine do not contribute to the delayed gastrointestinal emptying to the same extent as they do in the stomach/duodenum. In the large intestine, however, the tone and nonpropulsive contractions of the musculature may increase markedly to the point where muscle spasm results. Spasm of the smooth muscle of the biliary tract also occurs after administration of morphine and some of its congeners and may be quite severe and painful. Biliary tract spasm, while not a consistent opioid effect, can occur even at therapeutic doses. The spasm prevents bile emptying, resulting in a sharp rise in the intraductal pressure to as much as ten times normal common bile duct pressures.

ACUTE OPIOID INTOXICATION   As indicated previously in the discussion of opioid effects on respiration, death from poisoning by these agents is most frequently a result of profound, direct respiratory depression. The signs of opioid intoxication are an extension of the pharmacology of these agents as previously discussed. The intoxicated individual is stuporous or asleep with constricted, pinpoint pupils and depressed respiration. As the state of intoxication deepens, coma ensues and the blood pressure, initially maintained near normal, will steadily fall if the hypoxia associated with the depressed respiration is unchecked. If remedial measures are not instituted to support respiration, pupillary dilation and shock, both due to persistent hypoxia, precede death. It is difficult to indicate reliably a toxic or lethal dose for morphine since many different factors contribute to the effects of the opioids (e.g., the presence of pain or tolerance due to prior usage) and the figures that have been reported show wide variation. Best estimations indicate, however, that serious life-threatening toxicity is not likely to result following doses of less than 120 to 150 mg of morphine taken orally or 30 to 40 mg of morphine given parenterally to the pain-free, opioid-naive individual. Significant individual variation in sensitivity to these agents exists, however, and patients administered relatively large doses of an opioid must be carefully monitored.

The essential principle of treatment of opioid intoxication is restoration of adequate ventilation. This is rapidly and dramatically achieved by administration of a narcotic antagonist such as naloxone (Narcan), the current narcotic antagonist of choice. If naloxone or other narcotic antagonists are unavailable, the method of treatment changes but the principle does not. Establishment of a patent airway and restoration of efficient pulmonary gas exchange, by tracheostomy and artificial respiration if necessary, will prevent the cardiovascular hypoxic sequelae of opioid intoxication. Two notes of caution are necessary, however, regarding the use of a narcotic antagonist in cases of opioid intoxication. First, the duration of action of most narcotic antagonists is shorter than that of most narcotic analgesics (which, moreover, have been given or taken in excess). Thus, the intoxicated patient requires continued monitoring and readministration of additional narcotic antagonist as necessary to prevent lapsing into coma. Second, administration of a narcotic antagonist to an acutely intoxicated, opioid-dependent individual (i.e., an "addict") must be initiated very carefully. Narcotic antagonists administered to opioid-dependent individuals, whether intoxicated or not, can precipitate a withdrawal syndrome of such severity that it cannot be significantly attenuated during the period of action of the antagonist.

TOLERANCE AND PHYSICAL DEPENDENCE   Tolerance is defined as a decreased responsiveness to any pharmacological effect of a drug as a consequence of prior administration of the drug. Consequently, increasingly larger doses must be administered to produce an effect (e.g., analgesia) equivalent to that of the initial administration. As mentioned earlier, however, tolerance does not develop uniformly to all opioid effects. In general, tolerance develops to the depressant effects of the opioids but not to the stimulant effects. That is, tolerance develops to opioid-induced analgesia, euphoria, drowsiness, and respiratory depression. Tolerance does not develop to any appreciable extent to opioid effects on the gastrointestinal tract or the eye (miosis). Consequently, the chronic opioid user will continue to experience the constipative and miotic opioid effects although significant, but not absolute, tolerance will have developed to the other, depressant opioid effects. In the therapeutic situation, the initial indication that tolerance to the analgesic effect of an opioid has developed to any appreciable extent will be reflected in the patient as a shortened duration or reduced efficacy of analgesic effect. These patients become "clock-watchers" in anticipation of the next scheduled dose of narcotic analgesic or they complain of pain and request the next dose of narcotic analgesic sooner than scheduled and often in greater amount (i.e., increased dose).

Experiments in animals reveal that tolerance (as well as physical dependence) is demonstrable after a single dose of opioid. The relevance of those data to the clinical situation, however, is not clear since it is not possible to demonstrate tolerance to the analgesic effect of the opioids in man after a single therapeutic dose by the methods of assessment presently employed. Houde [39] has stated that a patient receiving 60 mg of morphine intramuscularly (or its equivalent) per day over a two-week period will require about half again as much (i.e., 90 mg) to produce the same analgesic effect in the third week. This information serves only as a rough guide; it is not possible to provide a hard-and-fast rule that would reliably predict the rate of tolerance development to opioid effects. It is only possible at present to indicate that the rate at which tolerance to the analgesic effect of the opioids develops is a function of the dose and the frequency of administration as well as perhaps other, nonpharmacological, factors. Regardless of the possible contribution of these other factors, the greater the opioid dose and the shorter the interval between doses, the more rapid is the development of tolerance to any of the opioid effects.

Tolerance to the opioids can develop to such an extent that the lethal dose is increased significantly. For example, in two different cases morphine has been reported to have been taken in doses as high as 5 gm per day and 2 gm intravenously over a two-and-one-half-hour period without adverse effect [46]. These individuals were, of course, chronic abusers in whom significant tolerance to morphine-induced respiratory depression had developed. It bears reemphasizing, however, that tolerance is not absolute; there always exists an opioid dose capable of producing death via respiratory depression regardless of the extent to which tolerance has developed. As is the case regarding the mechanism of opioid-induced analgesia, the mechanism(s) underlying development of tolerance to opioid effects is unknown.

Physical dependence refers to an abnormal physiological state produced by repeated administration of a drug (in this instance an opioid), which then makes necessary the continued use of that drug to prevent the appearance of a withdrawal or abstinence syndrome. Another type of dependence associated with the opioids and many other commonly abused drugs (e.g., alcohol, amphetamines, and barbiturates) is referred to as a psychological dependence or "habituation." This concept is introduced at this point to help clarify a frequently misstated consequence of opioid use. Nurses and physicians often express concern regarding the continued administration of opioids for relief from pain and, in fact, may at times withhold opioid administration for fear of "addicting" the patient. Addiction is a frequently used but vague term having different connotations among various groups. The term addiction represents the extreme of a combination of physical and psychological dependencies manifested as a behavioral pattern of compulsive drug use. Consequently, iatrogenically induced physical dependence in a patient is not correctly identified as addiction nor the patient as an "addict." The question arises, naturally, regarding the extent to which opioids can be administered for pain relief before physical dependence is apparent. Of primary concern is the comfort and well-being of the patient; the development of or presence of physical dependence is of secondary importance. The specter of physical dependence upon the opioids should not be allowed to interfere with provision of the best possible care for the patient, and comfort for the patient in pain is a significant aspect of that care. After the cause or source of the pain has been removed or acceptably attenuated, physical dependence can be appropriately treated as a second, independent medical problem. This will be briefly touched upon later in this chapter.

Regarding the amount of morphine required to produce physical dependence, the available information is not extensive. It has been stated that anyone who takes as much as 60 mg of morphine in the course of postoperative care will have developed some degree of physical dependence [39]. The degree of physical dependence is, however, very low and is detectable only after administration of an opioid antagonist (i.e., the withdrawal must be "precipitated"). Other reports indicate that mild withdrawal symptomatology is apparent in patients who have received therapeutic doses of morphine several times a day for one or two weeks [46]. These withdrawal manifestations may not, however, be recognized as such by the patient since the symptoms are often not dissimilar from those associated with the common cold. Further, if the opioid employed is one that is biotransformed and eliminated relatively slowly (e.g., methadone), the symptoms will be even less pronounced.

Experimentally, physical dependence in man has been demonstrated (i.e., precipitated) by administration of an opioid antagonist following 120 mg of morphine given over a three-day period, 40 mg of methadone over a three-day period, and 60 mg of heroin over a two-day period [84]. However, while physical dependence can be demonstrated even after a therapeutic dosage regimen of opioids, its relevance to the therapeutic situation is uncertain since the withdrawal symptoms must be precipitated by an opioid antagonist. Moreover, the withdrawal symptomatology in the above instances would most likely have been mild or even unnoticed had an opioid antagonist not been employed. Definitive studies in man have not been done (for obviously good reasons) demonstrating an opioid dosage level which, when administered for some duration, produces easily recognized withdrawal symptomatology upon discontinuance. Consequently, as previously indicated regarding the rate of tolerance development, no easy guidelines can be presented to gauge either the rate of development or the degree of physical dependence upon the opioids. It is appreciated that the extent to which physical dependence upon the opioids develops is dose-related. The greater the opioid dose and the longer the duration of administration, the greater the degree of physical dependence, and the more intense the withdrawal syndrome. However, regardless of the potential degree to which physical dependence may develop, opioid administration should not be discontinued nor other, nonanalgesic agents (e.g., tranquilizers or sedatives) administered in their place for fear of "addicting" the patient in pain or, even worse, in the already opioid-dependent patient.

The opioids are far from being the panaceas they once were considered to be. While tolerance, physical dependence, and other undesirable effects (e.g., nausea and vomiting, respiratory depression, constipation) are drawbacks to opioid use, the opioids undeniably provide a combination of most desirable effects (e.g., analgesia, "tranquilization," sedation, and euphoria) for relief from chronic pain and should be employed without hesitation prior to other, perhaps irreversible or ineffective (or both irreversible and ineffective) approaches to pain-relief.

THERAPEUTIC APPLICATIONS   The narcotic analgesics (opioids) are employed primarily for relief from pain. The nature of the analgesia and other therapeutically useful effects produced by these agents and the risks inherent in their use have already been discussed. Although emphasized in previous discussion regarding opioid analgesia, the fact that they provide only symptomatic relief without action against the underlying cause of the pain must be clearly restated. Further, a clear distinction between their use in acute or short-lived pain problems and their use in the treatment of chronic conditions has not yet been made. In the preceding discussion of opioid physical dependence, almost by definition the discussion related to repeated opioid administration for chronic pain, since physical dependence is not of great concern in relatively short-term situations. The narcotic analgesics are commonly employed to control postoperative pain and comfort the patient. Since pain per se is also an important symptom, the opioids must be used somewhat cautiously lest the surgical outcome and the patient's recovery be compromised. As the course of recovery progresses, the patient may be switched from a parenteral to an oral form of opioid (e.g., codeine).

The narcotic analgesics are commonly employed for obstetrical analgesia. While the mother's comfort naturally is of concern, so too are the effects of the opioid on the fetus—particularly the respiratory depressant effect, to which the fetus is apparently more sensitive than the mother. When administered in equi-analgesic doses, all opioids will produce an equivalent degree of respiratory depression in the mother as well as approximately the same incidence and degree of untoward effects. However, it appears that the respiratory depressant effect of meperidine (Demerol) is less to the fetus than that of either morphine or methadone [9, 20]. Regardless of which agent is employed for obstetrical analgesia, opioid-induced respiratory depression in the newborn is rapidly reversible by administration of a narcotic antagonist (e.g., naloxone). Narcotic antagonist administration in the case of the newborn of an opioid-dependent mother, however, could have severe consequences depending upon the extent of maternal opioid dependence (i.e., precipitated withdrawal in the newborn). Further discussion of opioid-dependence in the newborn is well beyond the scope of this chapter, although it is of enough importance that the issue be raised; the interested reader is referred to other sources for detailed information [27, 87].

The narcotic analgesics are also employed along with many other, often nonanalgesic, agents in the treatment of pain associated with terminal illness. In these cases, the fact that morphine and the other narcotic analgesics are capable of inducing some degree of euphoria and enhanced well-being is significant. Suffice it to say that in cases of painful terminal illness, the primary obligation to the patient is to provide comfort, and at no time should an effective dose of opioid be withheld. The only consideration in these cases relates to continued analgesic efficacy should the course of the illness be prolonged. The general approach is to provide relief from pain with oral narcotic and nonnarcotic analgesic agents prior to utilizing more efficacious parenteral opioids. If the course of the illness is so long as to render the patient virtually completely tolerant to opioid analgesia, or should the pain be so severe that it is not attenuated by the opioids, other pain-relieving manipulations must be instituted.

The opioids are also useful in inducing sleep, providing the sleeplessness is due to pain or coughing. In these instances, oral codeine is often quite satisfactory. The opioids are the most efficacious antitussive agents available, and as indicated earlier, this effect is demonstrable at doses lower than that required for analgesia. For example, a 15 mg oral dose of codeine is an effective antitussive but generally an ineffective or low analgesic dose.

Aside from application for pain relief, sedation and sleep (when prevented by pain), and cough suppression, the opioids are very effective agents for treating diarrhea. This particular opioid application is outside of the context of this book, but is of importance because constipation in the patient given opioids for relief from pain can be a further complication one should be aware of. As indicated for the antitussive effect of the opioids, the constipative effect of these agents occurs at doses lower than those required to produce analgesia. That is, opioid effects on the gastrointestinal tract are more pronounced than analgesic effects at low dosages.

Codeine

Codeine, like morphine, is a naturally occurring alkaloid. Unlike morphine, codeine retains significant efficacy when administered orally and is thus employed as an orally administered analgesic and antitussive. As with all narcotic analgesics, the analgesic and antitussive actions of codeine (as well as respiratory depression, sedation, etc.) are central in origin. However, codeine and opioid central nervous system sites of action are incompletely understood and the mechanism(s) of action not at all understood at present.

Because codeine is used orally for treating various types of mild and moderate pain (often in outpatients), and because the untoward effects of codeine when used as such are few, codeine is customarily classified along with aspirin as a "mild" analgesic having an analgesic efficacy significantly below morphine. That codeine is a mild analgesic incapable of providing analgesia equivalent to morphine is a widespread, but erroneous, clinical impression. Morphine is, in fact, 12 to 13 times more potent than codeine (both drugs given intramuscularly), which simply means that approximately 120 mg of codeine is required to produce an analgesic effect equivalent to 10 mg of morphine [61]. Regardless of the dose required, morphine and codeine are both narcotic analgesics capable of producing significant analgesia. At present, however, doses of codeine greater than 65 mg (orally) are not commonly used and, moreover, are not recognized as safe and effective by the federal Food and Drug Administration. Hence, the impression that codeine has limited analgesic efficacy and that doses of codeine greater than 65 mg orally do not provide greater analgesia is supported by legal regulations, notwithstanding clinical evaluations to the contrary [10, 38, 80].

The recommended effective antitussive dose of codeine is 15 to 20 mg (orally); the recommended effective analgesic dose is 30 to 65 mg (orally). In these therapeutic doses, the side effects of codeine are few and seldom serious; nausea, constipation, dizziness, and sedation are the reactions most commonly seen. Codeine, as previously indicated, is widely employed for pain that is considered mild to moderate, often in the ambulatory individual. Codeine is suitable for this purpose since it is orally effective, it can provide significant analgesia and relief from dull continuous pain, and can be taken for long periods of time with little risk of significant dependence. The use of 65 mg of codeine every four to six hours for several months is not associated with a significant risk of opioid physical dependence. Tolerance to the analgesic effect will develop over a time, however, and the analgesic dose must therefore be gradually increased. Codeine's demonstrated usefulness in dental, postoperative, and postpartum and other pains that show little response to less efficacious, nonnarcotic analgesics make codeine the drug of choice over newer, untested analgesics promoted for use in the same pain states.

Meperidine

Meperidine (Demerol, pethidine) is a wholly synthetic agent structurally dissimilar to morphine. Meperidine was introduced as an analgesic, sedative, and spasmolytic (antispasmodic) agent effective against most types of pain and supposedly free of many of morphine's undesirable properties. In fact, meperidine does not significantly differ from morphine in its important pharmacology and in therapeutic doses (80 to 100 mg parenterally) produces analgesia, sedation, and respiratory depression as well as the other central nervous system actions common to the narcotic analgesics as a class. Moreover, meperidine is not the spasmolytic it was once believed to be. Like other narcotic analgesics, meperidine is spasmogenic to the smooth muscle of the gastrointestinal tract. Regarding its supposed lack of undesirable properties, it is important to indicate that meperidine is the narcotic most commonly abused by health professionals who still mistakenly believe that meperidine has a lower dependence liability and is easier to stop using than morphine. In fact, meperidine abuse and dependence have been widely documented since it was first introduced, and it is now recognized that meperidine differs little from morphine with respect to its potential for abuse and dependence.

Morphine is eight to ten times more potent than meperidine and when given parenterally in equi-analgesic doses, the degree of sedation and respiratory depression is the same for both agents. Meperidine is approximately one-fourth as efficacious orally as parenterally (i.e., four times the dose must be given orally to produce analgesia equivalent to that achieved with parenteral meperidine administration). While morphine and meperidine are equally efficacious analgesics, there are some important differences between morphine and meperidine. The duration of action of meperidine is shorter than morphine's, thus necessitating shorter intervals and more frequent administration of the drug for relief from continuing pain. As indicated previously, meperidine reportedly is less depressant to the fetal respiration than either morphine or methadone and thus may be a better choice than morphine for obstetrical analgesia. The effects of toxic doses of meperidine and morphine may also differ. Meperidine sometimes causes central nervous system excitation, manifest as tremors and convulsions, instead of the profound narcosis and coma usually associated with narcotic analgesic intoxication. A final difference between meperidine and morphine relates to their effect on the smooth muscle of the gastrointestinal tract. While their effects are generally considered to be qualitatively similar, meperidine is only moderately spasmogenic and at equi-analgesic doses produces less effect on the gastrointestinal musculature than does morphine. Thus, meperidine is not useful in the treatment of diarrhea. A meperidine congener, however, is widely used in the treatment of diarrhea. Diphenoxylate, in combination with atropine, is available as Lomotil. Diphenoxylate is capable of producing typical opioid-like subjective effects and has been proposed as a maintenance drug in the treatment of opioid dependence. However, as available in combination with atropine, the only recognized use of diphenoxylate at present is in the treatment of diarrhea.

Methadone

Methadone (Dolophine) is a synthetic narcotic analgesic qualitatively similar to morphine in its important pharmacology. Methadone produces analgesia, sedation, respiratory depression, miosis, and antitussive effects, as well as subjective effects similar to those of morphine. Methadone is approximately equipotent to morphine, but is significantly more efficacious when given orally than is morphine when given orally. The duration of action of methadone is similar to morphine's after a single administration; however, repeated methadone doses provide a cumulative effect, thus effectively increasing methadone's duration of action.

While methadone is a potent, orally effective analgesic agent, its availability for use even as an analgesic has been restricted by government regulations to prevent uncontrolled, widespread methadone use for detoxification or in maintenance programs. Methadone's primary use at present is not as an analgesic per se, but rather as an opioid replacement for heroin in treating heroin addiction. Several of methadone's properties make it useful in treating heroin addicts in methadone maintenance programs: oral efficacy, long duration of action in suppressing withdrawal symptoms in opioid-dependent individuals, and relatively long half-life in the body. Thus, the need for less frequent administration provides practical conveniences in maintenance programs, and methadone's oral efficacy eliminates those potentially serious medical problems associated with repeated intravenous administrations.

Unfortunately, the term "blockade" was employed when the utility of methadone in maintenance programs for heroin addicts was initially demonstrated. Dole and Nyswander [16, 17, 18] administered relatively high doses of methadone (80 to 120 mg) to heroin addicts and reported a "blockade" of the effects of heroin and a disappearance of "drug hunger." Their choice of the term blockade is unfortunate since it has been misinterpreted by many to be the equivalent of antagonism, thus bestowing upon methadone a pharmacological property it does not possess. Methadone is not a narcotic antagonist; methadone is a narcotic agonist as are morphine, codeine, fentanyl, and meperidine. The utility of methadone in maintenance programs relates to opioid cross-tolerance and cross-dependence and not to some unique ability of methadone to "block" heroin's euphorigenic effect. Opioid cross-tolerance relates to the fact that if a person has become tolerant to the effects of one opioid (morphine, for example), that person will also show tolerance to the effects of other opioids (e.g., codeine, meperidine, heroin, and fentanyl).

Opioid cross-dependence relates to the fact that if a person is physically dependent upon one opioid (morphine, for example), that person will also be dependent upon other opioids. Stated differently, opioid cross-dependence means that in the absence of the opioid upon which a person is dependent, the administration of another opioid will suppress or prevent the appearance of a withdrawal syndrome. These are statements of general principles that apply to the opioids as a class. In practice, the cross-tolerance and cross-dependence among the opioids (as well as among other drug classes) is not complete. Thus, as used in maintenance programs, methadone simply represents the substitution of one opioid (methadone) for another (heroin). Methadone is used rather than other opioids because of its superior properties (as previously indicated) compared to other opioids.

Propoxyphene

Propoxyphene (Darvon) is a synthetic agent structurally related to methadone. When initially introduced, propoxyphene was classed (legally) as a "nonnarcotic." At present, it is not "scheduled" within the Controlled Substances Act (1970) whereas codeine, the agent to which propoxyphene is most frequently compared, is controlled (Schedule II). Its legal status notwithstanding, propoxyphene is subject to abuse and physical dependence can develop during high-dose, chronic use [13, 22, 72, 85]. In fact, its dependence liability is considered to be nearly equivalent to or somewhat less than codeine's. In addition, neonatal withdrawal symptoms have been reported to be associated with maternal use of propoxyphene [78], and further, propoxyphene (as the napsylate salt, Darvon-N) has been successfully tested as a heroin substitute in a Darvon-N maintenance program [42]. Thus, physical dependence is demonstrable with propoxyphene and cross-dependence is evident between propoxyphene and other opioids. Consequently, while propoxyphene has never been subjected to strict, legal narcotic controls, it is nevertheless appropriately classed pharmacologically as an opioid.

Use of the term analgesic in conjunction with propoxyphene has been avoided thus far in the consideration of the pharmacology of propoxyphene. The analgesic efficacy of propoxyphene has been debated and contested for almost two decades. Undeniably, propoxyphene produces central nervous system effects qualitatively similar to those of codeine and other opioids. However, whether significant analgesia is one of those central actions produced by propoxyphene (at doses commonly employed) is not universally agreed upon. In a critical review of the published literature on propoxyphene by Miller and his colleagues [63], and in later comparative evaluations of analgesic drugs by other workers [64], propoxyphene was judged to be no more effective an analgesic than aspirin or codeine and perhaps to be even inferior to those analgesics. The dosage levels employed, the nature of the pain against which the agents are evaluated (e.g., postpartum or dental), single-dose versus repeated administration, combination with other agents (e.g., aspirin and caffeine), and many other factors all contribute to the difficulty in comparative evaluations of oral analgesics. The literature is far too extensive and beyond the scope of this chapter to review, but the general dose equivalency for relief from mild-to-moderate pain that can be extracted from this literature indicates that approximately 65 mg of propoxyphene hydrochloride (Darvon) or 100 mg of propoxyphene napsylate (Darvon-N) is equivalent in analgesic efficacy to 65 mg of codeine. The analgesic efficacy of these doses of propoxyphene and codeine is approximately equivalent, in turn, to 650 mg of the nonnarcotic oral analgesics, aspirin and acetaminophen. It is important not to misinterpret these narcotic versus non-narcotic analgesic dose equivalencies. At the doses indicated, all four agents provide approximately equivalent relief from mild-to-moderate pain. The efficacy of the nonnarcotic analgesic agents is limited to mild-to-moderate pain, however, whereas increased doses of codeine or propoxyphene are capable of producing greater analgesia; that is, codeine and propoxyphene have greater efficacy. At these higher doses, of course, codeine and propoxyphene will also produce a greater incidence of untoward effects; constipation, nausea, and dizziness are among the more common complaints. Toxic doses of propoxyphene can produce central nervous system and respiratory depression, confusion, hallucinations, and occasionally convulsions [1].

Propoxyphene is widely prescribed and has largely supplanted codeine as the "nonnarcotic" oral analgesic of choice for relief from mild-to-moderate pain. This has occurred primarily due to unjustified overconcern with codeine's dependence liability and the initial promotion of propoxyphene as being "nonaddicting." In fact, there is no great difference between the dependence liabilities of codeine and propoxyphene.

Fentanyl

Fentanyl (Sublimaze) is a relatively new, very potent, synthetic opioid employed (at present) only as an anesthetic supplement. Fentanyl is approximately 80 times more potent than morphine; its duration of action is approximately one-half to one-third that of morphine's. Fentanyl in combination with droperidol is available as Innovar and is employed for neuroleptanalgesia—a method of anesthesia for major surgery that obviates the use of inhalation anesthetic agents.

Other Agents

Many other narcotic analgesics which have not been discussed (see Table 9-1) are available for relief from pain. The agents that were discussed were selected on the basis of their importance in therapy and frequency of use. The agents that were not discussed (not all of which appear in Table 9-1) possess no superiority over morphine that would warrant their inclusion in this chapter. They are opioids and as such do not significantly differ qualitatively from morphine or other opioids.

Table 9-1 Comparison of opioid analgesics

Analgesic	Usual Therapeutic Dose (mg)	Potency (IM) (morphine = 1)	Duration (hours)	Respiratory Depression (as compared to morphine at equi-analgesic doses)
Morphine	10–15 (IM)	1	4–5	1.0
Heroin	3–5 (IM)	2–4	3–4.5	1.0
Codeine	30–60 (Oral)	0.16–0.33	4–6	1.0
Oxymorphone (Numorphan)	1.0–1.5 (IM) 10 (Oral)	10 1	4–6	1.5
Dihydromorphinone (Dilaudid)	2 (IM) 2–3 (Oral)	5	3–4	1.0
Meperidine (Demerol)	50–100 (IM) 50–100 (Oral) [a]	0.1 0.05–0.1	2–4	1.0
Anileridine (Leritine)	25–50 (IM) 25–50 (Oral)	0.2–0.4	2–3	1.0
Alphaprodine (Nisentil)	40–60 (SC)	0.16–0.25	2–3	1.0
Methadone (Dolophine)	7.5–10 (IM) 10–15 (Oral)	1.0–1.3	6–8	1.0–1.2
Levorphanol (Levo-Dromoran)	2–3 (SC) 2–3 (Oral)	3.3–5.0	4–7	0.9–1.0
Piminodine (Alvodine)	7.5–10 (IM) 25–50 (Oral)	1.0–1.3	2–5	0.8
Phenazocine (Prinadol)	0.5–2.5 (IM)	4–20	2–4	1.0–1.2
Fentanyl (Sublimaze)	0.05–0.1 (IM) 0.05–0.1 (IV every 2–3 min) [b]	100–200	10–15	1.0–1.2
Pentazocine (Talwin)	30 (IM) 50 (Oral)	0.33	3–5	1.0
Propoxyphene (Darvon)	30–60 (Oral) [a]	0.16–0.33	2–4	0.5 (?)

Note: Estimates of potency and respiratory depression are based on the latest information available in the literature and do not pretend to be definitive.
[a] The efficacy of oral meperidine and propoxyphene is a matter of controversy.
[b] For use in induction and maintenance of anesthesia.

Source: Reproduced (with permission) from "Synthetic Substitutes for Opiate Alkaloids," J. Cochin and L. Harris, Drug Abuse Council, Inc., 1975, p. 34.

The Narcotic Antagonists

While agents classed as "narcotic antagonists" are at present not generally employed as analgesics per se, most agents in this class do possess analgesic efficacy. That is, most have both narcotic agonist and narcotic antagonist properties and are therefore more appropriately classed as mixed agonists/antagonists. One notable exception, naloxone (Narcan), is considered to be a "pure" narcotic antagonist. That is, it lacks opioidlike actions. Their inclusion in this chapter is appropriate, since one agent that possesses antagonist efficacy (pentazocine) is widely employed as an oral analgesic, and further, an understanding of the pharmacology of narcotic antagonists is important to those who might at some time be confronted with an instance of opioid overdose or intoxication.

The number of narcotic antagonists or mixed agonists/antagonists has grown considerably since the initial demonstration that appropriate chemical manipulation of the opioid structure produced a compound that possessed most actions of the opioids, but was also capable of reversing or antagonizing the actions of the opioids when given concomitantly with them. The search for such agents is an active area of research at present, since it is expected that agents with the appropriate balance of agonist/antagonist properties would provide a better analgesia to side-effect-to-physical-dependence ratio and would also be useful in the treatment of heroin addiction [21]. Since most narcotic antagonists possess analgesic efficacy and because it is expected that these agents have a low dependence liability as well as utility in the treatment of heroin addiction, an obvious question arises: Why are these agents not used as analgesics in place of the opioids, which have considerable dependence liability? The primary reason why they are not widely used as analgesics or for the treatment of heroin addiction is due to the undesirable subjective effects they produce in an unacceptably high percentage of individuals. The undesirable effects range from dizziness, headaches, and anxiety through dysphoria and hallucinations.

As indicated in the preceding section of this chapter, morphine is the prototypical narcotic analgesic. All of its actions—analgesic, respiratory depressant, gastrointestinal, etc.—are agonist effects. Most agents in the class "narcotic antagonists" (e.g., nalorphine [Nalline], levallorphan [Lorfan], pentazocine [Talwin], and cyclazocin) possess both agonist and antagonist efficacy. When administered in the absence of an opioid, narcotic antagonists produce analgesia, respiratory depression, etc., which are agonist effects. When administered in the presence of an opioid, however, narcotic antagonists will: (1) antagonize the opioid's effects if given just prior to or at the same time as the opioid; (2) reverse the opioid's effects if given after the opioid has been administered (e.g., opioid intoxication); or (3) precipitate a withdrawal syndrome almost instantly in the opioid-dependent individual. As indicated previously, however, not all narcotic antagonists possess agonistic properties; naloxone is virtually devoid of agonistic action and naltrexone, a new agent, has only slight opioid agonist efficacy.

The primary therapeutic application of the narcotic antagonists is in the treatment of opioid-induced respiratory depression. For this purpose, the narcotics are antagonist-specific and virtually instantly reverse the depressed respiration of the opioid-intoxicated individual. The narcotic antagonists are not, as is often misconstrued, general respiratory stimulants. The opioid antagonists will not alter the respiratory depressant effects of other drugs (e.g., barbiturates and alcohol), and in fact may worsen the respiratory depression associated with these other central nervous system depressants because of their own opioid agonistic effect on respiration. Naloxone, the pure antagonist among the group of opioid antagonists, is the only antagonist currently available that will not further embarrass respiration in such a situation. The narcotic antagonists are also employed in the diagnosis of opioid physical dependence and have also been evaluated in the treatment of heroin addiction.

Nalorphine

In man, nalorphine (Nalline) is equipotent to morphine as an analgesic and also has agonistic actions on the gastrointestinal tract (i.e., constipation) and respiration. As a narcotic antagonist, nalorphine is the agent within the class against which all other agents are compared. Nalorphine will antagonize most of the central nervous system and gastrointestinal effects of the opioids; sedation is the only notable opioid effect not completely reversed. Nalorphine will reverse even profound opioid-induced respiratory depression within minutes after intravenous administration of an appropriate dose (5 to 10 mg). Depending upon the severity of the respiratory depression and the dose of nalorphine administered, nalorphine's duration of action will last one to four hours, emphasizing again the generally shorter duration of action of antagonists compared to agonists and the need to readminister the antagonist frequently in cases of acute opioid intoxication.

The use of nalorphine to diagnose opioid physical dependence was once a standard procedure called the "Nalline Test." Because nalorphine has agonistic efficacy, it will constrict the pupils (miosis) in an opioid-free individual. If nalorphine is given within 48 to 72 hours of the last dose of an opioid in an opioid-dependent individual, however, a mydriasis or pupillary dilation will occur instead. The dose of nalorphine, of course, must be appropriately small (e.g., 2 mg subcutaneously) lest serious withdrawal manifestation be precipitated in the opioid-dependent individual.

Levallorphan

Levallorphan (Lorfan) is an agonist/antagonist approximately seven to ten times more potent an opioid antagonist than nalorphine. At usual respiratory-depression-antagonizing doses, however, levallorphan exhibits negligible analgesic efficacy. While levallorphan has a greater antagonist-to-agonist balance than nalorphine, it is otherwise similar in onset and duration of effect to nalorphine and offers little advantage over nalorphine as a narcotic antagonist.

Naloxone

Naloxone (Narcan) is regarded as a pure narcotic antagonist because it is essentially devoid of agonistic actions except at very high doses. Naloxone is approximately seven to eight times more potent an opioid antagonist than nalorphine. Naloxone is not only capable of antagonizing the effects of the opioids, but can also antagonize the agonistic effects of other antagonists as well. This is of some significance, since the respiratory depression produced by pentazocine (an agonist with antagonistic efficacy) is reversible by naloxone but not by nalorphine. In addition to this advantageous aspect of naloxone's actions, the fact that naloxone virtually lacks agonistic effects is also advantageous when one is confronted with respiratory depression of unknown etiology; naloxone will not further compromise the respiratory status of the individual if the intoxicant was not an opioid. Like nalorphine and levallorphan, the duration of action of naloxone is between one and four hours. Further, none of these three agents possess oral efficacy; all must be administered parenterally.

Naltrexone

Naltrexone is not yet commercially available, but is similar to naloxone in that it too is a virtually pure opioid antagonist. Its advantage over naloxone is its oral effectiveness and longer duration of action, thus enhancing its potential usefulness in the treatment of heroin addiction. Moreover, naltrexone is twice as potent as naloxone, or approximately 17 times as potent an opioid antagonist as nalorphine.

Cyclazocine

Cyclazocine is an orally effective opioid agonist/antagonist having an exceedingly long duration of action (up to 24 hours). Cyclazocine is approximately five times as potent an analgesic as morphine, but like most other agonist/antagonists, is not useful as an analgesic per se because of unpleasant side effects (dizziness, headaches, and hallucinations). Cyclazocine has been evaluated in the treatment of heroin addiction [45, 57], but because these initial unpleasant effects are intensified as the dose is increased to levels appropriate for treatment of heroin addiction and may reappear when cyclazocine use is discontinued, cyclazocine may not be as useful as was once thought. Cyclazocine is not commercially available at present.

Pentazocine

Pentazocine (Talwin) is an opioid agonist with weak opioid antagonist activity; it is approximately one-fiftieth as potent an antagonist as nalorphine. It is somewhat of an anomaly and can neither be classed with the other narcotic antagonists nor appropriately classed as a morphinelike opioid, in both instances because of its low opioid antagonistic potency. Pentazocine represents the product of considerable (and continuing) effort to develop an efficacious analgesic agent without abuse liability. However, while pentazocine will not substitute for other opioids in the opioid-dependent individual as other opioids can, pentazocine itself is abused and physical dependence can be a consequence of chronic use. Indeed, pentazocine administration (in sufficient doses) to the opioid-dependent individual can precipitate a withdrawal syndrome even though pentazocine's antagonistic effects are weak.

On the other hand, although pentazocine has antagonistic efficacy, it will not effectively antagonize the respiratory depression produced by other opioids. Thus, the residual opioid antagonistic efficacy of pentazocine neither prohibits its abuse nor is of value in reversing opioid-induced respiratory depression.

Pentazocine is primarily employed as an analgesic in much the same manner as is codeine for relief of mild-to-moderate pain, often in the ambulatory patient. Oral doses of 50 mg of pentazocine are approximately equivalent to 60 mg of codeine, but like codeine, pentazocine's ability to relieve pain at higher doses is comparable to that of morphine (i.e., they have approximately equivalent efficacy). When used parenterally as an analgesic, pentazocine is approximately one-fourth as potent as morphine. The central nervous system and gastrointestinal effects of pentazocine are qualitatively similar to those of morphine and the other opioids. Unlike other opioids, however, pentazocine will increase both the heart rate and blood pressure. At doses in the therapeutic range, dizziness, nausea, and sedation can occur. In high or toxic doses, pentazocine can produce nalorphinelike dysphoric effects as well as characteristic opioidlike respiratory depression. As previously mentioned, however, of the various narcotic antagonists only naloxone can counteract the agonistic effects of pentazocine [68].

Reemphasizing pentazocine's weak antagonistic efficacy, one final caution regarding pentazocine's use as an analgesic is necessary. Pentazocine should be used cautiously in patients who have been regularly using other opioid analgesics. Depending upon the doses of the opioid and of pentazocine, withdrawal manifestations may be precipitated.

Nonnarcotic Analgesics

Agents classed as nonnarcotic analgesics comprise a large, structurally heterogeneous group of compounds far too extensive to adequately address within the limitations of this chapter. Therefore, only selected agents, those that are widely used and those with potentially unique application in pain states, will be discussed. The interested reader is directed to any of several fine pharmacology texts for discussions of agents not included in this chapter as well as for comprehensive information regarding the toxicity of agents that are discussed here. The toxicity of these agents is often underestimated and understated, and space permits only superficial treatment of this important aspect of their pharmacology.

The historical antecedents of the nonnarcotic class of analgesic agents are closely related to the early belief that relief from fever was in itself curative. Various natural products were widely employed in febrile individuals and highly regarded as antipyretics. It eventually came to be realized, however, that fever was only symptomatic of some underlying, more fundamental condition. Consequently, interest in some of these preparations waned. It was noted with other of the antipyretic preparations, however, that relief from minor aches and pains was associated with their use—hence the some-time classification of these agents as the antipyretic analgesics. Historically, the salicylates (salicylic acid, methyl salicylate, and acetylsalicylic acid) and para-aminophenol derivatives (phenacetin and acetaminophen) were among the first of the group of nonnarcotic analgesic-antipyretic agents to receive widespread application. Today, these "older" agents as well as many newer agents are primarily employed as analgesics, notwithstanding the fact that many are also efficacious antipyretic or anti-inflammatory agents, or both. That antipyresis and anti-inflammation are often associated with analgesia in these compounds is today explainable on the basis of the relationship of all three of these effects to interference with prostaglandin biosynthesis, as will be discussed below.

Aspirin

Aspirin (acetylsalicylic acid) is the most effective and important of the analgesics classed as nonnarcotic and, moreover, is the single most widely used of all the analgesics—narcotic and nonnarcotic alike. Unfortunately, because aspirin is so readily available and "common," it is not generally credited with the analgesic efficacy it in fact possesses. In addition to being an effective analgesic, aspirin also possesses antipyretic and anti-inflammatory efficacy. Moreover, compared to other oral analgesics, aspirin is inexpensive and has a relatively low incidence of side effects.

ANALGESIA   Aspirin, as well as all other nonnarcotic agents, has lower analgesic efficacy than the opioid analgesics. That is, aspirin has a lower maximal analgesic effect than codeine and the other opioids. As indicated previously, 650 mg of aspirin produces relief from pain equivalent to or superior than 65 mg of either codeine or propoxyphene [63, 64]. Doses of aspirin exceeding 650 mg, however, do not increase peak analgesia (although the duration of effect may be prolonged) whereas increased doses of codeine, for example, will provide a greater analgesia. Aspirin alleviates pain by both a peripheral and a central action, the mechanism(s) of which are not fully understood at present. Aspirin and many of the other nonnarcotic analgesic/anti-inflammatory agents inhibit the synthesis of prostaglandins [28, 79], and it is hypothesized that blockade of local generation of prostaglandins explains the peripheral analgesic action of aspirin [25]. It has been further suggested that prostaglandins (probably of the E series) actually act as pain mediators and are responsible for sensitizing peripheral pain receptors [24]. Aspirin and other agents that inhibit the enzyme prostaglandin synthetase, and thereby the synthesis of prostaglandins, are thus analgesic by virtue of indirectly preventing sensitization of pain receptors. The evidence regarding the mechanism of aspirin's central nervous system analgesic action is less compelling, however [19]. There is a suggestion that aspirin exerts its central analgesic action via the hypothalamus, the same central locus where aspirin's antipyresis is effected, but convincing evidence is lacking.

AND ANTI-INFLAMMATION Aspirin lowers body temperature in ⌐viduals but not in individuals with normal body temperature. ⌐ antipyretic effect is exerted at the locus of the anterior hypothala- ⌐the brain, the central nervous system area that regulates the set point ⌐ch body temperature is maintained [65]. There is now considerable ev⌐ence that prostaglandins (probably of the E series) mediate the fever response to pyrogens, which increase the synthesis and subsequent release of prostaglandins at the thermoregulatory centers of the hypothalamus as well as throughout the brain. Antipyretics like aspirin and acetaminophen reduce an elevated body temperature indirectly by interfering with prostaglandin synthesis and thus with the pyrogen-mediated pyretic response [29].

The anti-inflammatory action of aspirin, as well as other nonsteroidal anti-inflammatory agents (e.g., indomethacin [Indocin] and phenylbutazone [Butazolidin]), can be readily explained by interference with the prosta-glandin-mediated inflammatory response. These agents will reduce the pain, redness, and swelling of inflammation in joint tissues and surrounding struc-tures. Prostaglandins are present in inflammatory exudates, and aspirin and these other agents are anti-inflammatory by virtue of their ability to inhibit the biosynthesis of prostaglandins [26].

TOXICITY Aspirin is widely, but often indiscriminately, employed for vir-tually all kinds of aches and pains. Because it is low in cost and readily avail-able, aspirin is also erroneously considered by the laity to be safe and free of serious toxicity. Aspirin intoxication, however, can result in death, and as-pirin in fact is a common and sometimes fatal intoxicant in young children. Acute aspirin intoxication comprises a complex series of events that can culminate in deranged acid-balance, dehydration, hyperthermia, coma, and death [86]. Fortunately, most cases of acute aspirin intoxication are not life-threatening.

Aspirin, and the other anti-inflammatory agents previously mentioned, are locally irritating and injurious to gastric mucosal cells. Use of these agents may result in epigastric distress, nausea, and vomiting, as well as exacerbation of peptic ulcer symptoms. Chronic use of these agents is ulcero-genic and sometimes results in painless gastrointestinal bleeding. Mild intoxi-cation associated with chronic aspirin use is termed salicylism. The signs and symptoms of salicylism include headache, dizziness, tinnitus (ringing in the ears), mental confusion, drowsiness, sweating, thirst, nausea, and vomiting. More serious chronic aspirin intoxication can result, in addition, in hyper-ventilation, alterations of acid-base balance, delirium, hallucinations, and convulsions. The acid-base disturbances are the most significant aspect of as-pirin intoxication; plasma aspirin and electrolyte values should be determined regularly to monitor the severity of intoxication and indicate the nature and progress of treatment.

THERAPEUTIC APPLICATIONS Aspirin is employed primarily as an analgesic for relief of mild-to-moderate pain (i.e., that of "low intensity") and is the standard against which new oral analgesics are compared. Aspirin is recommended for use against headache and aches arising from muscle, joints, and bone, whether well localized or widespread in nature (e.g., arthritis, dysmenorrhea, tendonitis, bursitis, and neuralgias). The recommended analgesic as well as antipyretic dose of aspirin is 325 mg to 650 mg orally every four hours. Doses greater than 650 mg do not produce an enhanced analgesia, but do increase the incidence of side effects. Since high local concentrations of aspirin are irritating to the gastric mucosa, it is recommended that the particle size for oral ingestion be reduced (i.e., the tablet should be crushed) and a generous quantity of water taken with the aspirin; both measures will reduce the local gastric aspirin concentration as well as promote drug dissolution and absorption.

There is no tolerance or physical dependence associated with the use of aspirin or any of the nonnarcotic analgesic agents, although they are widely abused (in the strict sense of the term). Consequently, these agents can be employed for the long-term treatment of chronic pain such as that associated with rheumatoid arthritis (where they exert a beneficial anti-inflammatory effect) without fear of "addicting" the patient. There is no single, recommended aspirin dose for anti-inflammation/analgesia in the treatment of inflammatory joint diseases (of which rheumatoid arthritis is the most prominent) as there is for analgesia alone. Fairly large doses of aspirin ranging between 3.6 gm and 6.0 gm daily are commonly employed. The patient taking aspirin at the high end of this dose range should be carefully watched for early signs of salicylism. Aspirin doses of approximately 6.0 gm daily are associated with ringing in the ears, an early indication of salicylism [86].

COMBINATION PREPARATIONS　Aspirin is frequently employed in fixed-dose combination with other analgesic as well as nonanalgesic compounds. Among the many aspirin-analgesic combinations available, the only valid and documented claim for superior analgesic relief is associated with aspirin in combination with the opioid codeine. This combination is appropriate since both agents are unquestionably efficacious and are possessed of different mechanisms as well as loci of analgesic action. Other common mixtures, even the once-popular APC (aspirin, phenacetin, and caffeine), have not been reliably demonstrated to provide either greater analgesic relief or fewer adverse effects than an equivalent dose of aspirin given alone [64]. Consequently, the only rational manner in which to give aspirin in combination with other analgesic or nonanalgesic agents—when therapeutically indicated—is to administer the agents separately in appropriate dosage.

Acetaminophen

Acetaminophen (Tylenol, Datril, Tempra, Liquiprin, and others) is approximately equipotent to aspirin as an analgesic and antipyretic. It is recommended for headache, arthralgia, myalgia, etc., and has an onset and duration of action similar to aspirin. Acetaminophen, however, has only weak anti-inflammatory properties and thus is less efficacious than aspirin in the treatment of inflammatory disorders (e.g., rheumatoid arthritis). In recommended therapeutic dosages of 325 mg to 625 mg orally, acetaminophen is well tolerated. It lacks the gastric mucosal irritating effect and bleeding common with aspirin, and moreover in high doses does not produce the acid-base disturbance that aspirin does. However, acute intoxication of acetaminophen is associated with methemoglobinemia and a potentially fatal hepatic necrosis. Chronic use of acetaminophen (as well as other nonnarcotic analgesic mixtures, including those with aspirin) is associated with an analgesic nephropathy characterized by papillary necrosis and nephritis.

Acetaminophen is thus recommended as an analgesic and antipyretic substitute for aspirin, particularly in individuals allergic to aspirin or when aspirin is contraindicated (i.e., in patients with peptic ulcer). Acetaminophen self-medication, however, is not recommended for a period of time greater than ten days or in a total daily dosage exceeding 1.2 gm in older children or 2.5 gm in adults except upon advice of a physician [86].

Phenylbutazone

Phenylbutazone (Butazolidin) is analgesic, antipyretic, and anti-inflammatory, but its anti-inflammatory effect predominates and it therefore is used primarily as such. Phenylbutazone's anti-inflammatory efficacy is due to its ability to inhibit prostaglandin synthesis; in inflammatory joint diseases, for example, its ability to relieve pain is due primarily to that anti-inflammatory action. Phenylbutazone, however, is associated with a high incidence of serious toxicity—nausea, vomiting, and epigastric distress are common; vertigo, nervousness, blurred vision, and insomnia can also occur; and agranulocytosis and aplastic anemia have resulted in deaths. Consequently, if phenylbutazone is employed for treatment of acute tendinitis, bursitis, gout, rheumatoid arthritis, and related disorders, close medical supervision of the patient and periodic hematological evaluation is required. At present, the use of phenylbutazone is restricted to short-term treatment periods not greater than seven days' duration. Other efficacious nonsteroidal anti-inflammatory agents are presently available for chronic use in the treatment of inflammatory disorders; phenylbutazone use is justified only in the event that less toxic agents are ineffective.

Indomethacin

Indomethacin (Indocin) is analgesic, antipyretic, and anti-inflammatory and, like phenylbutazone, is used virtually exclusively as an anti-inflammatory agent for treatment of rheumatoid arthritis, osteoarthritis, and acute attacks of gout. Like phenylbutazone, the use of indomethacin is associated with a high incidence of adverse effects; approximately 20 percent of patients taking therapeutic doses of indomethacin must discontinue the drug due to gastrointestinal and central nervous system side effects. As an analgesic, 50 mg of indomethacin is reportedly equivalent to 600 mg of aspirin [32], but indomethacin's use should be restricted to anti-inflammatory therapy, and then only if aspirin is ineffective or not tolerated.

Ibuprofen

Ibuprofen (Motrin) is a newer analgesic/anti-inflammatory agent employed in the treatment of rheumatoid arthritis and osteoarthritis. Promoted as a replacement for aspirin in the treatment of rheumatoid arthritis because it supposedly produces less gastrointestinal distress and occult bleeding, ibuprofen (at recommended dosage levels) also appears to be inferior to usual doses of aspirin as an anti-inflammatory agent [60]. Ibuprofen is, however, an efficacious analgesic [4] and can also be an effective anti-inflammatory agent equal to aspirin in efficacy, but only at doses of ibuprofen higher than recommended. The toxicity and safety of higher dose, long-term ibuprofen use relative to aspirin has not yet been established.

Fenoprofen

Fenoprofen (Nalfon) is a compound with analgesic, anti-inflammatory, and antipyretic properties. Fenoprofen is structurally related to ibuprofen and, like ibuprofen, is recommended as useful for patients who cannot tolerate aspirin or other, more toxic anti-inflammatory agents, or whose disease is not of sufficient severity to justify their use. Fenoprofen and ibuprofen, however, significantly differ from other anti-inflammatory agents, exemplified by aspirin, indomethacin, and phenylbutazone, that reduce the interphalangeal joint size as one aspect of their effect [5]. Fenbuprofen and ibuprofen do not reduce joint size and perhaps are more appropriately categorized as efficacious analgesics with minor anti-inflammatory properties [41]. Fenbuprofen and ibuprofen, moreover, are reportedly well tolerated and produce fewer side effects (e.g., abdominal distress, nausea, and vomiting) than aspirin. These agents are being promoted as particularly useful when aspirin or other anti-inflammatory agents cannot be tolerated and in less severe cases of rheumatoid arthritis and minor musculoskeletal disorders where the risk of the potential toxicity of aspirin, indomethacin, or phenylbutazone is not justified. Promotions aside, these agents are significantly more expensive than aspirin and high-dose, long-term evaluations that demonstrate superiority over aspirin have yet to be carried out. Until superiority is demonstrated, aspirin will remain the treatment of choice in rheumatoid arthritis, as well as the standard of comparison.

Methotrimeprazine

Methotrimeprazine (Levoprome) is a phenothiazine derivative structurally related to the antipsychotic chlorpromazine (Thorazine). Methotrimeprazine reportedly is an efficacious analgesic (20 mg methotrimeprazine is equivalent to 10 mg of morphine [2]), but lacks anti-inflammatory or antipyretic efficacy. As one might expect, this agent will produce significant sedation and also possesses antiemetic efficacy, but lacks dependence liability. The principle disadvantage to methotrimeprazine use is orthostatic hypotension, which limits its usefulness in ambulatory patients. Methotrimeprazine does not depress respiration (as opioids do) and may be useful in some cases of terminal malignancy.

Carbamazepine

Carbamazepine (Tegretol) is structurally related to the tricyclic antidepressants and pharmacologically related to the anticonvulsants. While carbamazepine is an efficacious antiepileptic agent (temporal lobe epilepsy), its interest here is its novel usefulness in the treatment of trigeminal and glossopharyngeal neuralgias. Carbamazepine is not an analgesic per se and should not be employed except in specified cases of central neuralgias [54]. Carbamazepine is a potentially valuable agent, but serious adverse effects (i.e., aplastic anemia and cardiovascular effects) require regular monitoring of the patient. In cases where carbamazepine is not well tolerated or ineffective, phenytoin (Dilantin), another antiepileptic, has proven useful.

Delta-9-Tetrahydrocannabinol, LSD, and DOET

Delta-9-tetrahydrocannabinol (THC), lysergic acid diethylamide (LSD), and dimethoxy ethylamphetamine (DOET) are all psychoactive agents. None are presently available or approved for use for relief from pain. THC and LSD, however, have both been critically evaluated in pain states and judged to be potentially useful; DOET has not yet been evaluated but might also be potentially useful in certain instances.

Delta-9-tetrahydrocannabinol (THC) is the psychoactive ingredient in marijuana (*Cannabis sativa*). Marijuana has been used for centuries for relief from the pain of dysmenorrhea, migraine, and terminal illness [62]. Despite enthusiastic support, it has been only recently that marijuana or its constituents have been critically evaluated for analgesic efficacy. In one study where marijuana was smoked [36], the findings suggest that marijuana failed to elevate sensation and pain thresholds; instead, marijuana may actually have increased sensitivity to the stimuli. In studies on the analgesic properties of THC in advanced cancer patients with continuous pain of moderate severity, 10 mg of THC was found to be similar to 60 mg of codeine and 600 mg of aspirin (all administered orally) in pain relief [67]. At a higher THC dose (20 mg), the pain relief and pain reduction was reported to be equivalent to 120 mg of codeine, but undesirable side effects (e.g., dizziness, ataxia, and blurred vision) were also more prominent [66, 67]. The authors reported that 10 mg of THC in combination with 600 mg of aspirin provided the greatest pain relief and pain reduction and suggest that THC may prove useful in combination with other analgesic agents, particularly those whose mechanism of action differs from that of THC.

It appears that THC has analgesic efficacy; whether it relieves pain by altering the threshold of pain sensation or the reaction to pain, or both, is not known at present. Since THC is psychoactive, its potential future usefulness may relate more to its ability to improve the depressed nature of the terminally ill than to analgesia per se.

A more potent psychoactive agent, LSD, has been evaluated in terminal cancer patients in great pain and was reported as effective as the opioids in relieving that pain. Moreover, LSD's palliative effect was much longer lasting, often outlasting the "trip" itself. More remarkable still, many patients retained their equanimity even after the pain returned; they no longer considered the pain important [48, 50].

Another potentially useful psychoactive agent is DOET. It has not yet been evaluated in painful terminal illness, but it would appear to be potentially useful since it produces a euphoria in the absence of hallucinogenic or psychotomimetic effects [76], whereas LSD does not.

As the reports for LSD indicate, there may be a place in the treatment of painful terminal illness for agents with psychoactive properties that are not analgesics per se, but instead improve other aspects of terminal illness that may be just as important or perhaps more so than the pain itself. Certainly, considerable effort would be required to evaluate agents of this nature objectively and critically, but it should be recalled that a significant aspect of opioid relief from pain is the euphoric state or sense of well-being the opioids induce and the potential utility of agents with this property should not be dismissed out of hand.

Summary

There are scores of agents employed for relief from pain, certainly many more than were discussed here. How is one to choose from all of those available which ones are "best"? In reviewing the two classes of agents discussed, narcotic and nonnarcotic, the differences between them should be reemphasized. Analgesics classed as narcotic differ from those classed as nonnarcotic in that tolerance and physical dependence develop upon repeated use of narcotic analgesics. However, the narcotic analgesics are significantly more efficacious analgesic agents than are the nonnarcotic analgesics. Hence, when confronted with significant pain, the choice is not between narcotic and nonnarcotic analgesic agents but between several of the narcotic agents. In most cases, morphine is the narcotic analgesic of choice. Its pharmacology is well understood, and it is the standard of comparison among the narcotic analgesic agents. In obstetrical analgesia where narcotic-induced respiratory depression of the fetus is important, meperidine may be the more appropriate narcotic analgesic to use. When oral administration of a narcotic analgesic is indicated, meperidine, however, is not a wise selection because it is only approximately one-fourth as efficacious orally as parenterally. The recommended oral meperidine dose (50 to 100 mg) does not provide analgesic relief significantly different from 650 mg of aspirin. The oral dose of meperidine must be raised above that recommended and at higher dose levels cost becomes an important consideration. Methadone would be the narcotic analgesic of choice for oral administration were it not for the current restrictions against its use as such. Codeine, propoxyphene, and pentazocine remain available for use orally; of the three, codeine is the best choice. Recall that pentazocine retains some narcotic antagonist efficacy and patients should not be abruptly switched from morphine or meperidine to pentazocine.

Regarding the nonnarcotic analgesic agents, aspirin remains the most effective agent for general application against mild-to-moderate pain. Acetaminophen is an excellent alternative to aspirin as an analgesic or antipyretic, but because of its potential for serious adverse effects is not recommended for long-term use. Acetaminophen, however, is not a particularly efficacious anti-inflammatory agent. The other nonnarcotic analgesics are widely promoted for specific conditions, usually those associated with inflammatory disorders. None has been reliably demonstrated as superior to aspirin despite advertising claims to the contrary. Although several of these agents might be useful when aspirin is not tolerated (e.g., ibuprofen), their long-term efficacy and safety have not yet been established.

While there is, then, no "best" agent but instead several from among which to choose, morphine and aspirin remain, respectively, the preeminent narcotic and nonnarcotic analgesic agents.

References

1. Beaver, W. T. Mild analgesics: A review of their clinical pharmacology. *Am. J. Med. Sci.* 250:577, 1965.
2. Beaver, W. T., Wallenstein, S. L., Houde, R. W., and Rogers, A. A comparison of the analgesic effects of methotrimeprazine and morphine in patients with cancer. *Clin. Pharmacol. Ther.* 7:436, 1966.
3. Bellville, J. W., Forrest, W. H., Jr., Miller, E., and Brown, B. W., Jr. Influence of age on pain relief from analgesics. *JAMA* 217:1835, 1971.
4. Bloomfield, S. S., Barden, T. P., and Mitchell, J. Comparative efficacy of ibuprofen and aspirin in episiotomy pain. *Clin. Pharmacol. Ther.* 15:565, 1974.
5. Boardman, P. L., and Hart, E. D. Clinical measurement of the anti-inflammatory effects of salicylates in rheumatoid arthritis. *Br. Med. J.* 4:264, 1967.
6. Bonica, J. J., ed. *Advances in Neurology* (Vol. 4). New York: Raven Press, 1974.
7. Brecher, E. M., and the Editors of *Consumer Reports. Licit and Illicit Drugs.* Boston: Little, Brown and Company, 1972. Chapter 12.
8. Brodal, A. *Neurological Anatomy in Relation to Clinical Medicine,* 2d ed. New York: Oxford University Press, 1969.
9. Campbell, C., Phillips, O. C., and Frazier, T. M. Analgesia during labor: A comparison of pentobarbital, meperidine and morphine. *Obstet. Gynecol.* 17: 714, 1961.
10. Cass, L. J., and Frederik, W. S. Clinical comparison of the analgesic effects of dextro-propoxyphene and other analgesics. *Antibiot. Med. Clin. Ther.* 6:362, 1959.
11. Chapman, C. R., Murphy, T. M., and Butler, S. H. Analgesic strength of 33% nitrous oxide: A signal detection theory evaluation. *Science.* 179:1246, 1973.
12. Chou, D. T., and Wang, S. C. Studies on the localization of central cough

mechanism: Site of action of antitussive drugs. *J. Pharmacol. Exp. Ther.* 194: 499, 1975.

13. Claghorn, J. L., and Schoolar, J. C.   Propoxyphene hydrochloride: A drug of abuse. *JAMA* 196:1089, 1966.

14. Clark, W. C.   Pain sensitivity and the report of pain: An introduction to sensory decision theory. *Anesthesiology.* 40:272, 1974.

15. Clark, W. C., and Yang, J. C.   Acupunctural analgesia? Evaluation by signal detection theory. *Science.* 184:1096, 1974.

16. Dole, V. P., and Nyswander, M.   A medical treatment for diacetylmorphine (heroin) addiction. *JAMA* 193:646, 1965.

17. Dole, V. P., and Nyswander, M.   Heroin addiction: A metabolic disease. *Arch. Intern. Med.* 120:19, 1967.

18. Dole, V. P., and Nyswander, M.   Rehabilitation of heroin addicts after blockade with methadone. *NY State J. Med.* 66:2011, 1966.

19. Dubas, T. S., and Parker, J. M.   A central component in the analgesic action of sodium salicylate. *Arch. Int. Pharmacodyn. Ther.* 194:117, 1971.

20. Eddy, N. B., Halbach, H., and Braenden, O. J.   Synthetic substances with morphine-like effect. Clinical experience: Potency, side-effects, addiction liability. *Bull. WHO* 17:569, 1957.

21. Eddy, N. B.   Agonist-antagonists: An historical overview. In Kosterlitz, H. W., Collier, H. O. J., and Villarreal, J. E., eds., *Agonist and Antagonist Actions of Narcotic Analgesic Drugs.* Baltimore: University Park Press, 1973.

22. Elson, A., and Domino, E. F.   Dextro propoxyphene addiction: Observation of a case. *JAMA* 183:482, 1963.

23. Feather, B. W., Chapman, C. R., and Fisher, S. B.   The effect of a placebo on the perception of painful radiant heat stimuli. *Psychosom. Med.* 34:290, 1972.

24. Ferreira, S. H.   Prostaglandins, aspirin-like drugs and analgesia. *Nature [New Biol.]* 240:200, 1972.

25. Ferreira, S. H., Moncada, S., and Vane, J. R.   The blockade of local generation of prostaglandins explains the analgesic action of aspirin. *Agents Actions* 3:385, 1973.

26. Ferreira, S. H., and Vane, J. R.   New aspects of the mode of action of non-steroid anti-inflammatory drugs. *Annu. Rev. Pharmacol.* 14:57, 1974.

27. Finnegan, L. P., Connaughton, J. F., Emich, J. P., and Wieland, W. F.   Comprehensive care of the pregnant addict and its effect on maternal and infant outcome. *Contemp. Drug Probl.* 1:795, 1972.

28. Flower, R. J.   Drugs which inhibit prostaglandin biosynthesis. *Pharmacol. Rev.* 26:33, 1974.

29. Flower, R. J., and Vane, J. R.   Inhibition of prostaglandin synthetase in brain explains the anti-pyretic activity of paracetamol (4-acetamidophenol). *Nature [New Biol.]* 240:410, 1972.

30. Gebhart, G. F., and Toleikis, J. R.   Peri-aqueductal central gray (CG) focal brain stimulation (FSB)-induced analgesia evaluation in cats. *Fed. Proc.* 34: 439, 1975.

31. Green, D. M., and Swets, J. A.   *Signal Detection Theory and Psychophysics.* New York: John Wiley & Sons, Inc., 1966.

32. Halpern, L. M.   Analgesics and other drugs for relief of pain. *Postgrad. Med.* 53:91, 1973.

33. Harris, L. S.   Central neurohumoral systems involved with narcotic agonists and antagonists. *Fed. Proc.* 29:28, 1970.

34. Herz, A., Albus, K., Metys, J., Schubert, P., and Teschemacher, H. J.   On the central sites for the antinociceptive action of morphine and fentanyl. *Neuropharmacology* 9:539, 1970.

35. Herz, A., and Teschemacher, H. J.   Development of tolerance to the anti-

nociceptive effect of morphine after intraventricular injection. *Experientia* 29:64, 1973.

36. Hill, S. Y., Schwin, R., Goodwin, D. W., and Powell, B. J. Marihuana and pain. *J. Pharmacol. Exp. Ther.* 188:415, 1974.

37. Hiller, J. M., Pearson, J., and Simon, E. J. Distribution of stereospecific binding of the potent narcotic analgesic etorphine in the human brain: Predominance in the limbic system. *Res. Commun. Chem. Pathol. Pharmacol.* 6:1052, 1973.

38. Houde, R. W., Wallenstein, S. L., and Beaver, W. T. Clinical measurement of pain. In de Stevens, G., ed., *Analgetics*. New York: Academic Press, Inc., 1965.

39. Houde, R. W. The use and misuse of narcotics in the treatment of chronic pain. In Bonica, J. J., ed., *Advances in Neurology* (Vol. 4). New York: Raven Press, 1974.

40. Hughes, J. Isolation of an endogenous compound from the brain with pharmacological properties similar to morphine. *Brain Res.* 88:295, 1975.

41. Huskisson, E. C., Wojtulewski, J. A., Berry, H., Scott, J., Hart, F. D., and Balme, H. W. Treatment of rheumatoid arthritis with fenoprofen: Comparison with aspirin. *Br. Med. J.* 11:176, 1974.

42. Inaba, D. S., Gay, G. R., Whitehead, C. A., and Newmeyer, J. A. The use of propoxyphene napsylate in the treatment of heroin and methadone addiction. *West. J. Med.* 121:106, 1974.

43. Jacquet, Y. F., and Lajtha, A. Morphine action at central nervous system sites in rat: Analgesia or hyperanalgesia depending on site and dose. *Science* 182:490, 1973.

44. Jacquet, Y. F., and Lajtha, A. Paradoxical effects after microinjection of morphine in the periaqueductal gray matter in the rat. *Science* 185:1055, 1974.

45. Jaffe, J. H., and Brill, L. Cyclazocine, a long acting narcotic antagonist: Its voluntary acceptance as a treatment modality by narcotics addicts. *Int. J. Addict.* 1:99, 1966.

46. Jaffe, J. H. Drug addiction and drug abuse. In Goodman, L. S., and Gilman, A., eds., *The Pharmacological Basis of Therapeutics*, 5th ed. New York: Macmillan, Inc., 1975.

47. Jaffe, J. H., and Martin, W. R. Narcotic analgesics and antagonists. In Goodman, L. S., and Gilman, A., eds., *The Pharmacological Basis of Therapeutics*, 5th ed. New York: Macmillan, Inc., 1975.

48. Kast, E. C. Pain and LSD-25: A theory of attenuation of anticipation. In Solomon, D., ed., *LSD: The Consciousness Expanding Drug*. New York: G. P. Putnam & Sons, 1964.

49. Kuhar, M. J., Pert, C. B., and Snyder, S. H. Regional distribution of opiate receptors in monkey and human brain. *Nature* 245:447, 1973.

50. Kurland, A. A. The therapeutic potential of LSD in medicine. In De Bold, R. C., and Leaf, R. C., eds., *LSD, Man and Society*. Middletown, Conn.: Wesleyan University Press, 1967.

51. Lewis, V. A., and Gebhart, G. F. Evaluation of the periaqueductal central gray (PAG) as a morphine specific locus of action and examination of morphine-induced and stimulation-produced analgesia at coincident PAG loci. *Brain Res.*, in press.

52. Liebeskind, J. C., Guilbaud, G., Besson, J. M., and Oliveras, J. L. Analgesia from electrical stimulation of the periaqueductal gray matter in the cat: Behavioral observations and inhibitory effects on spinal cord interneurons. *Brain Res.* 50:441, 1973.

53. Liebeskind, J. C., Mayer, D. J., and Akil, H. In Bonica, J. J., ed., *Advances in Neurology* (Vol. 4). New York: Raven Press, 1974.

54. Loeser, J. D.   Neuralgia. *Postgrad. Med.* 53:207, 1973.
55. Lomax, P., and Kirkpatrick, W. E.   The effect of n-allynormorphine on the development of acute tolerance to the analgesic and hypothermic effects of morphine in the rat. *Med. Pharmacol. Exp.* 16:165, 1967.
56. Lowney, L. I., Schulz, K., Lowery, P. J., and Goldstein, A.   Partial purification of an opiate receptor from mouse brain. *Science* 183:749, 1974.
57. Martin, W. R., and Gorodetzky, C. W.   Cyclazocine, an adjunct in the treatment of narcotic addiction. *Int. J. Addict.* 2:85, 1967.
58. Mayer, D. J., Wolfle, T. L., Akil, H., Carder, B., and Liebeskind, J. C.   Analgesia from electrical stimulation in the brainstem of the rat. *Science* 174: 1351, 1971.
59. Mayer, D. J., and Liebeskind, J. C.   Pain reduction by focal electrical stimulation of the brain: An anatomical and behavioral analysis. *Brain Res.* 68:73, 1974.
60. *Medical Letter.*   Ibuprofen (Motrin)—A new drug for arthritis. 16:109, 1974.
61. Medical Literature Department, Merck, Sharp and Dohme Research Laboratories.   *Codeine and Certain Other Analgesic and Antitussive Agents.* Rahway, N.J.: Merck and Co., 1970.
62. Mikuriya, T. H.   Historical aspects of cannabis sativa in western medicine. *New Physician* 18:902, 1969.
63. Miller, R. R., Feingold, A., and Paxinos, J.   Propoxyphene hydrochloride: A critical review. *JAMA* 213:996, 1970.
64. Moertel, C. G., Ahmann, D. L., Taylor, W. F., and Schwartau, N.   A comparative evaluation of marketed analgesic drugs. *N. Engl. J. Med.* 286:813, 1972.
65. Myers, R. D.   Temperature regulation. In Myers, R. D., ed., *Drug and Chemical Stimulation of the Brain.* New York: Van Nostrand Reinhold Company, 1974.
66. Noyes, R., Jr., Brunk, S. F., Baram, D. S., and Canter, A.   Analgesic effect of delta-9-tetrahydrocannabinal. *J. Clin. Pharmacol.* 15:134, 1975.
67. Noyes, R., Jr., Brunk, S. F., Avery, D. H., and Canter, A.   The analgesic properties of delta-9-tetrahydrocannabinol and codeine. *Clin. Pharmacol. Ther.* 18:84, 1975.
68. Payne, J. P.   The clinical pharmacology of pentazocine. *Drugs* 5:1, 1973.
69. Pert, C. B., and Snyder, S. H.   Opiate receptor: Demonstration in nervous tissue. *Science* 179:1011, 1973.
70. Reynolds, D. V.   Surgery in the rat during electrical analgesia induced by focal brain stimulation. *Science* 164:444, 1969.
71. Richardson, D. E., and Akil, H.   *Abstr. 7th Annu. Meeting Neuroelectric Soc.,* 1974.
72. Salguero, C. H., Villarreal, J. E., and Hug, C. C., Jr.   Propoxyphene dependence. *JAMA* 210:135, 1969.
73. Sapira, J. D.   Speculations concerning opium abuse and world history. *Perspect. Biol. Med.* 18:379, 1975.
74. Sherman, A. D., and Gebhart, G. F.   Morphine and pain: Effects on aspartate, GABA and glutamate in four discrete areas of mouse brain. *Brain Res.* 110: 273, 1976.
75. Snodgrass, J. G., ed.   *Theory and Experimentation in Signal Detection.* Baldwin, N.Y.: Life Sciences Associates, 1972.
76. Snyder, S. H., Weingartner, H., and Faillace, L. A.   DOET (2,5-dimethoxy-4-ethylamphetamine) and DOM (STP) (2,5-dimethoxy-4-methylamphetamine), new psychotropic drugs. In Efron, D. H., ed., *Psychotomimetic Drugs.* New York: Raven Press, 1970.

77. Swets, J. A., ed. *Signal Detection and Recognition by Human Observers.* New York: John Wiley & Sons, Inc., 1964.
78. Tyson, H. K. Neonatal withdrawal symptoms associated with maternal use of propoxyphene hydrochloride (Darvon). *Pediatr. Pharmacol. Ther.* 85:684, 1974.
79. Vane, J. R. Inhibition of prostaglandin synthesis as a mechanism of action for aspirin-like drugs. *Nature [New Biol.]* 231:232, 1971.
80. Wallenstein, S. L., Houde, R. W., and Bellville, J. W. Relative potency and effectiveness of codeine and morphine. *Fed. Proc.* 20:311, 1961.
81. Ward, J. M., McGrath, R. L., and Weil, J. V. Effects of morphine on peripheral vascular response to sympathetic stimulation. *Am. J. Cardiol.* 29:659, 1972.
82. Way, W. L., Costley, E. C., and Way, E. L. Respiratory sensitivity of the newborn infant to meperidine and morphine. *Clin. Pharmacol. Ther.* 6:454, 1965.
83. Way, E. L., and Shen, F. H. Effects of narcotic analgesic drugs on specific systems: Catecholamines and 5-hydroxytryptamine. In Clouet, D., ed., *Narcotic Drugs: Biochemical Pharmacology.* New York: Plenum Publishing Corporation, 1971.
84. Wikler, A., Fraser, H. F., and Isbell, H. N-allylnormorphine: Effects of single doses and precipitation of "abstinence syndrome" during addiction to morphine, methadone or heroin in man (post-addicts). *J. Phamacol. Exp. Ther.* 109:8, 1953.
85. Wolfe, R. C., Reidenberg, M., and Vispo, R. H. Propoxyphene (Darvon) addiction and withdrawal syndrome. *Ann. Intern. Med.* 70:773, 1969.
86. Woodburg, D. M., and Fingl, E. Analgesic-antipyretics, anti-inflammatory agents, and drugs employed in the therapy of gout. In Goodman, L. S., and Gilman, A., eds., *The Pharmacological Basis of Therapeutics,* 5th ed. New York: Macmillan, Inc., 1975.
87. Zelson, C. Infant of the addicted mother. *N. Engl. J. Med.* 288:1393, 1973.

10

Clinical Hypnosis in Problems of Pain

Harold B. Crasilneck and J. A. Hall

Management of pain problems is one of the oldest and most enduring uses of hypnosis in clinical practice. Removal of pain with hypnosis should be done with care by persons aware of the diagnostic and treatment problems of organic illness. Although there are various psychological and physiological theories of hypnosis, some clinical observations suggest a significant neurophysiological component in hypnotic analgesia. These observations include hypnotic analgesia in (a) naive children, (b) culturally unsophisticated subjects not acquainted with the expectations of the hypnotist, and (c) those clinically sophisticated subjects who have experienced hypnosis for pain relief and have described it as similar to "cortical inhibition." Used properly, hypnosis can alleviate much otherwise inapproachable pain and can help maintain the functional ability and dignity of many patients otherwise dependent on large quantities of medication with possible dulling of consciousness.

Hypnosis has been used for the control of organic pain since the time of Mesmer and Esdaile. Many theories have been advanced to explain this effectiveness, ranging from cortical inhibitions to role-playing. Some have even suggested that such reports are fraudulent, or that the supposed hypnotic anesthesia was actually due to surgical shock. Perhaps the only conclusion on which all authorities agree is that we do not know how or why hypnosis controls organic pain. The late Milton Marmer wrote in 1959 [12]:

The nature of the actual mechanisms by means of which chemical anesthetics produce their effect on the central nervous system is still unknown. All answers are hypothetical and theoretical. Many of the mechanisms of normal sleep are not well understood. Fortunately, this has never interfered with the clinical progress of anesthesiology. We all have learned how the drugs we use work clinically, even though we may not understand completely by what mechanism. So it is with hypnosis.

One of the first attempts to perform surgery under hypnosis occurred in France in 1821; eight years later Dr. Jules Cloquet removed the breast of a

Reprinted from *The American Journal of Clinical Hypnosis* 15(3):153, 1973, by permission.

64-year-old female while she was mesmerized. Surgery took 12 minutes without incident in terms of movement or complaints of pain. In 1842, M. Squire Ward, an English surgeon, performed a mid-thigh amputation while the patient was hypnotized. By 1851 Esdaile had performed many thousand minor surgeries and approximately 300 major surgeries in which the only anesthetic used was hypnosis. In 1880 J. Milner Bromwell gave a demonstration of hypnotic anesthesia to a group of physicians at Leeds, England.

Much later, in 1932, Sears [17] in the United States demonstrated that hypnotized subjects manifested less reaction to painful stimuli than did a non-hypnotized control group.

Barber and Hahn [1] are probably representative of those who feel that subjects who fail to respond to pain while in "hypnosis" are engaged in a form of role-playing. More specifically, Barber's many carefully designed laboratory studies have tended to emphasize antecedent variables that in his opinion account for the "hypnotic" phenomena observed. Barber has consistently argued against the concept of the hypnotic "state" as an explanatory principle.

The reality of hypnotic analgesia, however, seems firmly demonstrated by the prize-winning work of Hilgard [9, 10]. In Hilgard's study, those subjects who were highly responsive to hypnosis were able to block ischemic pain for 18 to 45 minutes. They also showed increased tolerance for the pain of immersing an arm in cold water. It was interesting that the mere induction of hypnosis alone, without suggestions for analgesia, did not significantly increase pain tolerance. This is the state that we have termed "neutral hypnosis," when a hypnotic trance has been induced but no specific suggestions have as yet been given for pain relief, or for any other alteration from the normal waking state [3].

McGlashan, Evans, and Orne [14] demonstrated, in a carefully controlled experiment, that the pain relief obtained with hypnosis was conceptually distinguishable from the mere placebo response. Their results "support the hypothesis that there are two components involved in hypnotic analgesia," these being identified as non-specific placebo effects and ". . . a distortion of perception specifically induced during deep hypnosis."

Evans and Paul [7] have reported that suggestion, rather than hypnotic induction procedures, produced a decrease in the subject's report of pain, although neither suggestions nor hypnotic induction procedures decreased certain physiological responses.

Hilgard is in agreement with Evans and Paul that the laboratory studies have not as yet produced a sufficient theoretical and experimental framework for the striking pain relief achieved by clinical hypnosis, as, for example, by Erickson [6], Cheek [2], Sarcedote [16], Wolberg [19], and Spiegel [18]. Hilgard [9] states that "Clinicians are at present far ahead of our laboratories in the hypnotic reduction of pain," while Evans and Paul [7] conclude that "an adequate evaluation of hypnotic analgesia as used clinically has not yet been undertaken."

Although numerous theories have been formulated concerning why hypnosis blocks the perception of pain, they generally can be grouped in three categories—those emphasizing (a) psychological mechanisms, (b) physiological mechanisms, or (c) a combination of the two mechanisms.

It is difficult to compare the psychological and physiological mechanisms that may be involved in clinical hypnosis. This is partly attributable to the unreality of separating "psychological" and "physiological," since no psychological subjective state ever occurs except in an intact organism that is functioning physiologically. In some ways "psychological" is a way of speaking about neurophysiology in action. In any case, they always occur together and can be separated only in a conceptual way.

The psychological theories of hypnotic analgesia are well supported by laboratory experimentation, notably that of Hilgard, Evans, McGlashan, Barber, and Orne. But the observations that suggest a possible physiological basis for hypnotic relief of clinical pain are more impressionistic and based on both repeated clinical observation and upon rare individual cases, which are not always replicable.

Psychological theories are often presented, while the observations suggestive of a physiological change in hypnosis are rarely discussed in print, with the exception of the Russian literature, where hypnotic experimentation is often couched in Pavlovian terminology.

Still, one finds repeated assertions by experienced clinicians suggesting some physiological or neural mechanism for hypnosis. The late Henry Guze wrote [8]:

It seems to me that hypnosis is a phenomenon which involves the reticular system and is manifest in the sensory motor effect which expresses itself in imagery and bodily experience. The activation period extends from deep sleep at the low activation level to excited at the high activation level. Activation depends upon cortical bombardment. The greater the bombardment from the ascending reticular activating system, the higher the activation.

Reyher [15] has considered a phylogenetic model of hypnosis:

When the induction procedure (which is really sensory restriction or a kind of sensory deprivation) succeeds, the phylogenetically older structures of the brain, which are now in control of overall brain functioning, are able to mediate behavior that is difficult or impossible to produce in the waking state. The compulsive quality of suggestions indicates that the operator has assumed the ego-function of analyzing and integrating sensory input. He has become the subject's eyes and ears, and his suggestions act in the same way as spontaneous impulses in the subject. These older structures (maybe the anterior cingulate gyrus) are known to have connections with many parts of the brain and to have inhibitory and exitatory influence over these areas.

A possible neurophysiological basis for hypnosis, rather than purely a role-playing or psychological mechanism, is strongly suggested by clinical reports of (a) an unusual response during brain surgery under hypnosis, (b) the success of hypnosis in naive children and in (c) persons not culturally acquainted with "how a hypnotized person is supposed to behave," and (d) the verbal reports of subjects who are clinically sophisticated. Each of these types is illustrated by case reports in the present paper. These observations do not *require* a physiological rather than a psychological explanation; they do raise in our minds the need to consider more carefully the physiological theories.

A review of the literature reveals that our group first used hypnosis during brain surgery [3]. This was done for a number of reasons, but primarily in order that certain neurological examinations could be done during surgery without the general anesthetic obscuring necessary psychological observations. Also, it offered a possibility of learning more about the neurophysiology of hypnosis.

Case 1

This case, previously reported, illustrates an unusual response that strongly suggests that hypnosis may have a neurophysiological basis [4].

A 14-year-old girl had developed epileptic convulsions after a head injury four and one-half years prior to her admission to the hospital. The convulsions occurred at the rate of two or three per day and were usually preceded by an aura consisting of a "tingling sensation in the fingers of both hands" and a loss of consciousness of from 30 to 60 seconds. Electroencephalographic studies revealed a focal discharge in the right temporal lobe. Anticonvulsive medication was successful only to the extent of reducing the number of daily seizures.

Since conservative treatment was not considered adequate and since there was a temporal focus, it was decided to perform a temporal lobectomy with electroencephalographic monitoring. It became necessary to consider the effects of anesthetic agents given by inhalation or intravenously upon the encephalographic patterns. Since it seems well established that there are no alterations in the brain wave patterns in even the deepest state of hypnosis [13], the method of anesthesia chosen was hypnosis together with infiltration of the scalp with procaine. The possibility of using hypnosis was discussed with the patient. She proved to be an excellent hypnotic subject and was hypnotized four times to condition her to enter the somnambulistic state required for the proposed surgery.

Prior to the surgery she was hypnotized, entering a state of somnambulism, at which time the scalp line of incision was injected with 2% solution of procaine and the surgical procedure was started. During most of the operation, the patient was relaxed and comfortable. She did, however, complain of a mild pain while the dura was being separated from the bone. Twice during the nine hour procedure it was necessary to inject the scalp with additional anesthetic because of the patient's perception of pain, especially upon forceful retraction of the scalp margin. The abnormal spiking electrical focus was confirmed by electroencephalographic tracings, and the proposed excision of the focus was performed. The patient did not complain of pain during this excision except on one noteworthy occasion, when, as a blood vessel in the hippocampal region was being coagulated, the patient suddenly awoke from the hypnotic trance looking startled. She said nothing, and did not appear in pain, although trance was momentarily interrupted. She was immediately and easily rehypnotized and was able again to enter a deep state of somnambulism. The surgeon then purposefully restimulated the same region of the hippocampus—once again the patient abruptly awakened from trance, but was quickly rehypnotized. The final electroencephalograms were completed, and the patient was given 100 mg. of thiopental sodium intravenously. She remained in excellent condition throughout the procedure. Upon completion of the operation, she was able to answer questions but was amnesic concerning the surgery because of a posthypnotic suggestion given prior to awakening. She had also been given a posthypnotic suggestion that she would experience a prolonged sleep, which she did for six hours without further sedation. The postoperative course was very satisfactory and free of complications.

The fact that the patient awakened twice from the hypnotic state when the hippocampus was stimulated has led to considerable interest and speculation on our part as to the neurophysiology of hypnosis.

We have used hypnosis in conjunction with a localized chemical anesthesia of the scalp in many other cases where various parts of the brain were operated, but at no other time did the patient awaken. This unique observation, though an isolated instance, opens another avenue for investigation.

Case 2

A second case illustrates hypnotic response in a naive subject.

A four-year-old child with inoperable brain cancer was referred for hypnosis to help control his discomfort. The child was in continual pain, refused to eat, cried constantly, and demanded that the mother remain with him most of the time. It was necessary that he be given narcotics several times daily for his pain. He had a special nurse during the day and the pediatrician saw him at least five times a week. Frequently he would cry out in agonizing pain. The mother and father could scarcely bear to see their son's continued suffering. At this time the pediatrician requested that the child be seen for possible hypnotherapy.

The mother and father were specifically asked if the child had ever heard of hypnosis. To their knowledge he had no idea of the concept. When first seen he was lying in bed crying and holding his head. When he learned another doctor was to see him he literally became hysterical with fright. But when left alone with the therapist for about ten minutes his crying stopped. He then tearfully asked if he were going to get "medicine or a shot." The therapist assured him that he would not get a shot and asked if he knew what hypnosis meant. The child was completely puzzled and knew nothing of the concept. He was then asked to stare at a cigarette lighter and within 15 minutes was in a state of somnambulism. Then he was given the sugestion that he would have much less pain, would eat better, would sleep well, and would enjoy T.V. and magazines. Soon it was possible to reduce narcotic injections from five or six daily to only a minimal amount of demerol. He ate considerably better, was able to take naps mornings and afternoons, enjoyed watching certain T.V. programs, would look at pictures with interest, and was much more cooperative. He was seen daily the first month, three times a week the second month.

His last appointment for hypnosis came at 7:00 A.M. during the first week of the third month after hypnotic treatment began. He smiled when the therapist entered the room. When asked how he felt, he replied "pretty good, but I have a headache." Under hypnotic suggestion most of the pain was removed and the patient responded well. After his lunch that day, he took a nap and sometime during this period he expired. He died peacefully, not addicted, not in constant pain.

This naive child had never heard of hypnosis, yet responded with almost total relief of pain in spite of the fact that he did not know how a hypnotized person was supposed to respond.

Case 3

Hypnosis is also effective in subjects who cannot be shown to have preconceived ideas of the behavior expected of them.

A 43-year-old housewife of very meager socioeconomic and educational background had been admitted to the hospital because of acute discomfort in both eyes. Examination and review of her history by the ophthalmologist revealed that she had corneal dystrophy. She had previously had two corneal transplants in her right eye, one in May of 1963 and one in February of 1964. Results were disappointing, and she was discharged as incurable. The left eye developed Fuch's endothelial erosion. Her vision was reduced to noting gross hand movements with the right eye, and to 20/40 vision in the left eye. Another corneal transplant was recommended. The patient at this time required heavy doses of narcotics for pain relief. Because of extreme discomort and the possibility of additional chronic and acute pain associated with further surgery, psychiatric consultation was requested. The psychiatrist saw the patient for two weeks of extensive treatment, but felt that he could offer little help. The psychiatric report suggested that any psychological problems were a secondary response to the severe organic pain. In addition, the patient had a very limited intelligence. Hypnosis for pain control was then considered.

At the first interview the patient appeared to be quite weak and in pain. She was crying pitifully and begging for narcotics. She apparently did not comprehend an explanation that an attempt would be made to hypnotize her. She was requested to close her eyes, which she finally did. This woman responded in an excellent manner, with deep somnambulism evident in about ten minutes, as judged by the ability to open her eyes while remaining in trance. She was given the suggestion that she would have "much less pain in your eyes . . . you will more easily tolerate discomfort in your eyes . . . you will not require a great amount of medicine and you will be much more relaxed." Following the first hypnotic suggestion she did not request narcotics again. She reported "a little hurt in the eyes, but sorta like a headache." Her previously described regression was replaced by a feeling of definite hope and cooperation.

Surgery was performed with excellent results. The patient did not ask nor require post-operative narcotics, but only aspirin on three occasions. The patient was dismissed one month later with good visual acuity.

It was our definite opinion that although this patient was never really cognizant of the meaning of "hypnosis" nor had any insight into its use, she nevertheless responded in a maximum fashion.

Case 4

Reports by clinically sophisticated patients of their experiences under hypnosis may suggest similarity to chemical analgesia.

A 32-year-old physician who had had two previous pregnancies asked if we would use hypnosis during her third pregnancy. Her obstetrician was in agreement, as her first two pregnancies were marked by prolonged labor of about 18 hours accompanied by much distress and pain. She responded well to hypnosis and was seen once a week during her pregnancy. Her labor started at 9:00 A.M. and hypnosis was induced immediately. Three hours later she delivered a normal 7½ pound male child. Some of her recorded comments were "I feel relaxed—no tension, no fears, no anxieties . . . I know the pain perception should be pretty rough at this point . . . but I am comfortable . . . very comfortable . . . just a dull pain . . . like having a period and yet I normally have a low pain tolerance . . . I should be perceiving pain, but I'm not . . . I almost feel like the 3+ drunk, relaxed, lethargic, but my brain is functioning so clearly, only a tight band around my abdomen occasionally . . . I just don't give a damn!"

She did not require nor was she given any anesthetic other than hypnosis during labor and the repair of the episiotomy. Her final comment was "No one could ask for an experience in which the pain was so intense during my first two deliveries and yet completely blocked this time. From the way I felt it must be some kind of psycho-physiological cortical lobotomy."

These last three cases clearly illustrate the clinical effectiveness and similarity of hypnosis for pain relief in patients who are (a) naive children, (b) culturally unaware of the meaning of hypnosis, or (c) who are highly sophisticated and intelligent in reporting their experience while under hypnotic analgesia.

These presentations may help to highlight the differences between pain which originates in the laboratory as opposed to the severe pain perceived, perhaps over the months or years, by a patient with an organic disorder. It seems questionable that the experience of pain that is induced in a laboratory experiment can be compared directly to the pain manifested by patients with metastatic tumor, or with thermal injury covering over one-half of the body surface [5], or even with patients with rheumatoid arthritis.

Several years ago a number of senior medical students volunteered as subjects for the demonstration of hypnosis. One of the students who frequently smiled throughout the procedure later admitted to role-playing, confessing that he was trying to please the experimenter by seeming to go along with the procedure. His resistance was evident, and he dropped out of the demonstration. But a number of years later this same man, now a practicing physician, developed a severe form of arthritis and was referred for hypnosis to help control his pain. He had suffered for several months, with his practice seriously affected, and his family was under severe economic pressure. The patient entered a state of somnambulism within five minutes after trance induction. His pain easily came under control and he was taught to use self-hypnosis. In a short time he was able to work half days and eventually resumed his full practice.

Our own observations suggest that there is some central inhibition of pain perception, perhaps analogous to that obtained when psycho-surgery is done for relief of intractable pain. In some cases, according to Kalinowsky and Hoch [11]:

. . . . there is no actual loss of sensory perception in any particular area of distribution of sensory pathways. What is impaired is a more complicated and not yet fully understood mental process of attachment or detachment which modifies the primary sensory perception into a secondary awareness of caring or not caring. . . . It may be mentioned that in lobotomized patients the perception of pain, for example in the usual sensitivity test to a needle, is not only preserved but the reaction of the patient to painful stimuli is even accented.

In contrast to this, however, the hypnotized patient seems to be able to block pain that is felt to occur in specified body areas. This can lead to complications if the hypnotist is not fully aware of the limits of anesthesia induced. Hypnosis has been successful for example, in decreasing post-operative pain of defecation following hemorrhoidectomy. In such cases it is important to limit the suggested analgesia to the anal area rather than inducing anesthesia "below the waist." If such a broad analgesia were inappropriately induced, the patient might not be aware, for example, of a need to urinate.

We were among the first to report the clinical observation that patients with organic pain were unusually good subjects, seemingly because of a greater motivation and need for relief. Also, in cases seen for pain relief there seems to be a greater correlation between depth of trance and effectiveness of suggestions than in such motivational uses of hypnosis as reinforcing a desire to diet. Although depth of hypnosis does not generally correlate with the effectiveness of suggestions, in the case of severe organic pain, it has seemed to us that the greater the depth of trance, the more likely it is that the suggestions for pain relief will be successful.

Hypnosis may at times be useful in aiding the differential diagnosis of organic or functional pain. Although suggestions for relief may be effective in pain of either type, we have *usually* found that the pain of organic origin tends to return more rapidly, usually within several hours after the first successful hypnotic induction. Thus, the hypnotic analgesia seems to abate at about the same rate as chemical analgesics such as morphine or meperidine. In contrast, pain of a functional origin may be relieved for days or weeks, even after the first few inductions. With repeated hypnosis, the length of effectiveness *may* dramatically increase in either organic or functional pain. If this differential response to suggestion for pain relief is to be used to decide between these two types of pain, the distinction must be based on the length of response to the first few successful treatments. Once the patient's pain relief is hypnotically reinforced on several occasions, both organic and functional pain may be relieved for equal periods of time. (This observation is at variance with the opinion of our late colleague and friend Milton Marmer.)

The following case illustrates the fashion in which the patient's response to hypnotic suggestions for pain relief may aid in deciding whether the pain is of organic origin.

Case 5

A woman hospitalized for diagnosis of an unusual pain in the left upper quadrant of the abdomen was seen in consultation after usual x-ray and laboratory procedures had failed to establish an unambiguous diagnosis. We were simply asked to give an opinion as to whether the pain was likely to be functional in nature. After the first hypnotic induction she obtained good relief for about four hours, after which the pain returned. She was again hypnotized and once more pain was greatly diminished, the effect again decaying in a few hours. On the basis of this observation, she was considered to have most probably pain of organic origin, which was confirmed when a later exploratory laparatomy revealed an unexpected tumor. Although decisions about surgical exploration should not be made on the basis of such response alone, the evidence of a differential response to hypnosis can be a useful clinical observation to aid in difficult and crucial choices.

In most cases of chronic organic pain, we have been careful to phrase suggestions in such a manner that not all perception of pain is blocked. For example, the subject might be told that "the pain will grow much less, but there will be some remnant of pain left, although the majority of the excruciating, tormenting pain will reduce itself considerably and you will be aware of only the slightest degree of discomfort." It is obviously important, from a medical standpoint, to leave sufficient perception of pain so that any change in the course of the organic illness will be detectable in clinical signs and symptoms.

A type of chronic pain problem seen by us several times a year is that of the orthopedic patient who has had repeated surgery for a herniated "disc," usually having had one or two unsuccessful attempts at fusion of the lower back to produce stabilization and reduce pain. Hypnosis has usually produced diminution of pain by 80 or 90 percent (based on patient's verbal estimates), lasting in most cases for several weeks, but requiring periodic reinforcement.

It is obvious that in such an orthopedic patient, it would be unwise to remove all pain, since a further herniation might occur at an intervertebral space different from those previously treated. If all pain were removed by hypnosis, an important diagnostic clue might be obscured, and there would be greater danger of increased impairment.

There are cases in which such considerations are not important, notably in terminal cancer patients for whom hypnotic analgesia may allow a decreased amount of narcotic and a clearer, more lucid mind during their last days. Even in these cases, however, some residual amount of pain perception may be desirable as an indicator of treatable complications.

In responsive subjects all pain can be removed hypnotically for a controlled period of time, as in surgery, tooth extractions, or delivery. In these instances the patient would otherwise be under chemical anesthesia and, in either case, will be closely monitored for signs of change in physiological functioning. When all pain is removed for such procedures, it will return during the immediate post-operative period, when it will again be important in monitoring the patient's condition.

Headache is an excellent example of how hypnosis can be used for pain relief. It should be remembered, however, that headache can mask organic problems, even brain tumor. It is our practice, therefore, to accept for hypnotic treatment only those cases of headache where thorough medical work-up has been done by a competent physician. There are often cases of several years duration in which many treatments have usually been tried with only transient relief.

In screening interview and initial hypnotic sessions it is not always possible to define a psychological dynamic behind the headache pain. In such cases, symptom suppression may be tried, but the therapist must continually strive for glimpses of hidden emotional meaning which may not become apparent until the pain has begun to diminish. Almost without exception, we have eventually found some emotional "pain" which seemed to lend a dynamism and impetus to the headache. This has frequently been some hidden feeling of guilt, as in one middle-aged husband who had developed headache after breaking off an extramarital affair that had continued for almost a year. Headaches may function in an interpersonal way as attention-getting devices, or as a means of controlling a relationship. At times the roots lie in childhood, perhaps from identification with a parent or other significant adult who also suffered from head pain.

Summary

Management of pain problems remains one of the first and most enduring uses of hypnosis. It should be used with care by persons aware of the diagnostic and treatment problems of organic illness. In proper perspective, hypnosis can alleviate much otherwise inapproachable pain and can help maintain the functional ability and dignity of many patients otherwise dependent on large quantities of medication.

References

1. Barber, T. X., and Hahn, K. W. Psychological and subjective responses to pain producing stimulation under hypnotically-suggested and waking-imagined "analgesia." *J. Abnorm. Psychol.* 65:411, 1962.
2. Cheek, D. B. Therapy of persistent pain states: Part I, Neck and shoulder pain of five years duration. *Am. J. Clin. Hypn.* 8:281, 1966.
3. Crasilneck, H. B., and Hall, J. A. Psychological changes associated with hypnosis: A review of the literature since 1948. *Int. J. Clin. Exp. Hypn.* 9:50, 1959.
4. Crasilneck, H. B., McCranie, E. J., and Jenkins, M. T. Special indications for hypnosis as a method of anesthesia. *JAMA* 162:1606, 1956.
5. Crasilneck, H. B., Stirman, J. A., Wilson, B. J., McCranie, E. J., and Fogelman, M. J. Use of hypnosis in the management of patients with burns. *JAMA* 158:103, 1955.
6. Erickson, M. H. The interspersal hypnotic technique for symptom correction and pain control. *Am. J. Clin. Hypn.* 8:198, 1966.
7. Evans, M. B., and Paul, G. Effects of hypnotically suggested analgesia on physiological and subjective responses to cold stress. *J. Consult. Clin. Psychol.* 35:362, 1970.
8. Guze, H. Psychological theories of hypnosis. In Kline, M. V., ed., *The Nature of Hypnosis.* New York: Institute for Research in Hypnosis, 1961.
9. Hilgard, E. R. Pain as a puzzle for psychology and physiology. *Am. Psychol.* 24:103, 1969.
10. Hilgard, E. R. Pain: Its reduction and production under hypnosis. *Proc. Am. Philosoph. Soc.* 115(6):470, 1971.
11. Kalinowsky, L. B., and Hoch, P. H. *Somatic Treatments in Psychiatry.* New York and London: Grune & Stratton, Inc., 1961.
12. Marmer, M. J. *Hypnosis and Anesthesia.* Springfield, Ill.: Charles C Thomas, Publisher, 1959.
13. McCranie, E. J., and Crasilneck, H. B. The electroencephalogram in hypnotic age regression. *Psychiatr. Q.* 29:85, 1955.
14. McGlashan, T. H., Evans, F. J., and Orne, M. T. The nature of hypnotic analgesia and placebo response to experimental pain. *Psychosom. Med.* 31:227, 1969.

15. Reyher, J.   Hypnosis. In Vernon, J., ed., *Introduction to Psychology: A Self-Selection Textbook*. Dubuque, Iowa: William C. Brown Company, Publishers, 1968.
16. Sarcedote, P.   The place of hypnosis in the relief of severe protracted pain. *Am. J. Clin. Hypn.* 4(3):150, 1962.
17. Sears, R.   An experimental study of hypnotic anesthesia. *J. Exp. Psychol.* 15:1, 1932.
18. Spiegel, H.   Hypnosis: An adjunct to psychotherapy. Section 34.4. In Freedman, A. H., and Kaplan, H. I., eds., *Comprehensive Textbook of Psychiatry*. Baltimore: The Williams & Wilkins Company, 1967.
19. Wolberg, L.   *Medical Hypnosis*, Vol. I. New York: Grune & Stratton, Inc., 1948.

11

Operant Conditioning:
An Approach to Chronic Pain

Wilbert E. Fordyce

Introduction

It is time to take another look at the problem of chronic pain. What we have been doing about it has helped many patients but there is still a large group of suffering, impaired, and unproductive people who have not responded to conventional treatment. And it is probably the exceptional physician whose caseload does not include more than one patient with chronic back pain, or some other nagging pain problem, for whom all treatment has failed. The frequent failure of traditional perspectives on chronic pain to lead us to the solutions for these problems is reason enough to take another look.

Typically, pain is seen as a disease state—an automatic response to the stimulus of a pathogenic factor peripheral to the central nervous system. If there is a stimulus (pathologic or organic factor), there will be a response: pain. If there is the response of pain, it must have been preceded by the pathogenic stimulus. Thus diagnosis is usually geared to finding that stimulus so that it can be eliminated or reduced, thereby alleviating the pain.

The Gate Control Theory of pain advanced by Melzack and Wall aims, in part, at explaining why peripheral stimuli may not always result in pain responses. Their work also calls attention to the large role central nervous system factors may play in pain. What we propose here (without challenging or minimizing the Gate Control Theory) is to consider the possibility that a patient's display or expression of pain *need not involve a peripheral nociceptive stimulus*, related and, to some degree, proportional to the pain response. Of course, a pain patient may raise a pain signal because there is indeed a peripheral nociceptive stimulus to which he is responding appropriately. But a second, equally logical possibility, is that the pain signal (the actions or behaviors in which he engages and which serve to inform others that there is a pain problem) is a pattern of conduct which like most of the rest of his be-

Reprinted from *Current Concepts of Pain and Analgesia.* New York: Current Concepts, Inc., 1974, by permission.

havior, is controlled by external consequences of that behavior. In other words, it is learned behavior which occurs (at least in part) because of environmental consequences that follow often enough to maintain the pattern.

When the chronic pain patient signals that he is in distress, he is displaying a complex set of behaviors which he has been displaying (one could say, rehearsing) for a long time and which by their very nature are influenced by learned factors in the form of systematic behavior-consequence relationships.

If, when you examine the chronic pain patient, you find an organic factor which accounts for the pain behaviors being displayed, your treatment may well solve the problem. But what if the pain behaviors persist, or diagnosis is indefinite, and treatments fail? If the physician sticks solely to a Disease Model perspective, he might well begin to consider that the patient's "disease" was mental: perhaps a case of conversion reaction or psychogenic pain.*

How Learning Influences Pain

How might "learning" influence behavior in this situation? One significant learning influence is the way people who are important to the patient react to his pain behaviors. If they are solicitous and concerned, if they direct special attention toward him when he hurts, they are making some elements of their behavior contingent on his being in pain. For example, the husband or wife may step in to help. The physician may give the patient extra time and attention, and prescribe rest and medications. These are environmental consequences of his being in pain. They happen if he hurts and they don't happen, or happen less frequently, if he doesn't. Such a set of systematic environmental consequences to pain behavior may serve to maintain it even after the original pathogenic factor is gone. Under such conditions you might say that the patient has developed a *pain habit* in much the same way that he develops a smoking habit. Reaching-for-a-cigarette behavior persists long after the original reasons to begin smoking have disappeared. But this does not surprise us, nor do we attribute to the smoker a "psychogenic pain" for a cigarette. The "habit" is real and is readily accounted for by learning or conditioning. The key point here is that environmental consequences which are

---

* There are two problems with the psychiatric illness approach to chronic pain. One is very pragmatic. Treatment of the alleged mental or personality disturbance purported to account for the pain is often ineffective, and the results of psychotherapy for chronic pain are unimpressive. The second reason for questioning the psychogenic or conversion reaction (or psycho-physiologic musculo-skeletal response, or hypochondriasis, or passive-dependent personality, etc.) notion is that it assumes, since there appears to be a discrepancy between pain behavior and identifiable organic stimulus, that there is a personality problem which has a causal relationship to the pain. Careful analysis of this notion shows that the evidence for the "personality problem" often rests solely on the failure of physical findings to account for the pain, a behavior or characteristic of the evaluator, not the patient. Even when there are personality problems or traits leading to the label of hysteric, or whatever, there is often failure to show a clear relationship to the pain problem. The major exception is in regard to secondary gain—which will be discussed later.

favorable—have positive value—will tend to increase and maintain the behavior they systematically follow, whether the person wants this to happen or not. When pain behavior is systematically followed by positive reinforcement in the form of favorable environmental consequences, it can be expected to recur with increasing consistency even without organic stimulus.

Avoidance and Pain Behavior

There is a second and probably even more important way in which learning factors can promote and maintain a pain habit (that is, learned or "operant" pain). When the consequences of a particular behavior are likely to be aversive, most people will do something else instead—they will try to avoid the aversive consequence. *What* they do do, the avoidance behavior, is thereby reinforced because it successfully prevented the expected aversive consequences. All of us have many "stock" avoidance behaviors: driving within (or near) the speed limit because to do so successfully avoids aversive speeding tickets; being polite and sensitive to the feelings of others because, among other things, it avoids the aversive consequences of social rejection; perhaps some people mow their lawns primarily because it successfully avoids scornful comments from neighbors. These avoidance behaviors, so long as they are successful in avoiding or minimizing the anticipated aversive consequences, are reinforced each time they occur.

On reflection we can see that the "guarding" motions of chronic pain patients are avoidance behaviors. The limp, compensatory posturing, the voluntary limitations of motion or activity, are all designed to avoid or minimize the aversive consequence: pain. A limp which doesn't do the job is quickly changed to another, more effective motion. That modified limp, if effective, is rapidly reinforced and quickly becomes established.

The interesting thing is that once these avoidance behaviors are established, they are very resistant to change because they are reinforced essentially by the *absence* of something—an aversive consequence—and not by the presence of something. All that is needed to reinforce avoidance behavior is for the aversive consequence not to occur or to occur with diminished frequency or intensity. Note that the avoidance behavior does not have to be successful every time. As long as it works some of the time it is intermittently reinforced. Intermittently reinforced behavior is very persistent. This point is so important in the context of chronic pain that it is worth illustrating. Many drivers have had the experience of being caught in a police radar "speed trap" while they were exceeding the speed limit. Thereafter, they may either change their driving routes to avoid the spot altogether or be extra careful not to speed as they pass the area. These changes in driving behavior may persist indefinitely. Notice that the aversive consequence need not be present for the avoidance behavior to occur, it must only have been present at some time in the past for its effects to linger on long after the aversive consequence itself is gone.

Recognizing many pain behaviors (limping, compensatory posturing, asking for medication to prevent an expected pain episode, and so on) as avoidance behaviors has most important diagnostic implications. First of all, when a pain patient displays pain behaviors it does not mean that he is experiencing pain. Of course, he *may* be in pain. On the other hand, the pain behaviors may occur because at some time in the past they successfully avoided or minimized pain. And they may continue to occur even when current nociceptive stimuli from the original site of tissue defect are mostly or totally absent.

The reinforcing characteristics of avoidance behavior relate to chronic pain in still another way. When a person's normal function is limited because of pain, the activities which he would otherwise be engaged in are avoided. If some of these normal activities are quite aversive, the occurrence of pain and associated pain behavior will be reinforced because they avoid unpleasant activities. This will quickly be seen as a sort of secondary gain. That is, pain behavior may, in a sense, "buy time out" from some activity the patient finds aversive. As a result the pain behavior may persist in the absence of diagnostic evidence of a continuation of the original pathogenic factor. Perhaps one of the most commonly seen examples is that of the middle-aged man with a limited education, limited skills, and limited intelligence who works as a heavy laborer until he sustains a back injury which, among other things, leads to time out from a low-paying, injury-threatening, unpleasant job—that is, successful avoidance of aversive consequences of normal activity. Another typical example is the wife who finds intercourse aversive and who may display lower abdominal pain long after some painful gastrointestinal or genito-urinary illness has abated because her pain behaviors buy her time out from intercourse.

In considering the potential role of these learning factors in chronic pain, it is important to keep in mind that learning or conditioning is something that occurs automatically if the conditions for its occurrence are favorable. It is *not* something we decide to do—or undo. On the other hand, if conditions are unfavorable, learning will not occur, no matter how much we want it to. Thus what we want to happen will play a role only in the sense of assisting us to get into or out of situations in which learning or conditioning can occur.

What all of this comes down to is that the process of evaluating chronic pain needs to take into account two sets of factors: the "organic" factors, where traditional Disease Model perspectives are used for diagnosis, and learning or conditioning factors.

Learning factors are evaluated or diagnosed by analysing the systematic consequences to pain and well behavior. This process, which is called a behavioral analysis, should consider what the consequences are to pain behavior. Does pain behavior systematically yield what appear to be positive consequences or reinforcers? Or does pain behavior yield "time out" from either anticipated (though perhaps not present) or sure-to-occur aversive consequences? In short, what happens if the patient engages in pain behavior? Equally important, what happens if he engages in well behavior? Do the systematic (that is, occurring with some frequency) consequences to either type of behavior promote learning or conditioning? If any of those combinations occur, it is possible that some or all of the patient's pain behaviors have come under control of environmental consequences. If this is the case, then a learning-based treatment strategy is probably indicated.

In patients who display significant learned or operant pain, the pain problem almost always starts with a tissue defect, or some type of organic pathogenic factor, and persists after the organic factor has diminished or disappeared.

Approaching the Patient

Chronic pain patients are often bitter and disappointed over the failure of the health care system to make them comfortable. Moreover, they will often have been informed directly or by innuendo of the suspicion that their pain is "all in the head"—imaginary, hysterical, etc., etc. This kind of feedback from the health care system puts the patient in an untenable position. On the one hand, if he is in pain, he can neither get help nor appeal to another health care system for a different answer. Frequently the patient tries to get help by consulting other physicians, but other physicians are not likely to provide significantly different answers. On the other hand, like smoking or drinking, pain behavior, no matter how much it is controlled by learning factors, is not something the patient can change by fiat or personal resolve.

How then can you convey to such patients that you feel he or she has a significant amount of operant or learned pain? Pointing out that pain can be influenced by learning, and that learning is automatic if conditions have been favorable, is a good way to start. Any implication that the patient's pain is unreal or imaginary is nonsense and shows misunderstanding of the nature of pain. The proper question is not, "Is your pain real?" But rather, "What factors influence or control your pain?" The patient should then be told that almost everyone who has had a pain problem for more than a few weeks will display some degree of operant or learned pain, no matter how much or how little the original organic "cause" is present and active. Moreover, the learned pain exists because of the automatic effects of learning, not because of any wish on the part of the patient. It can be reduced only by following a systematic learning or "unlearning" process, not by deciding to make it go away. Finally, since these concepts are new to patients, it may help to point out that the role learning or conditioning plays on basic body processes such as pain, blood pressure, heart rate, etc., has come to be understood only in the past few years. Learning-based programs to change body processes are even newer.

The Operant Treatment Approach

The program elements described here may be used in part on an out-patient or office practice basis or they may require a period of in-patient care, depending upon the resourcefulness of the patient's family unit and the amount of program surveillance the office practitioner can provide. References to more detailed discussions of the operant approach and to variations which may be used in it appear at the end of the article.

Program Objectives

The operant program does not "cure" pain. It is designed to help patients reduce the frequency and intensity of pain behaviors. To the extent that those pain behaviors are the result of environmental consequences and not organic factors, the pain problem can perhaps be reduced or eliminated. The program is not likely to help people whose pain behaviors are almost totally controlled by currently active organic factors.

The basic objectives are to: (1) reduce pain behavior by withdrawing positive reinforcement from such behavior; (2) at the same time, to increase activity or well behavior by programming positive reinforcement contingent upon increasing activity and exercise; (3) retrain the family unit in how to reinforce well behavior or activity, while avoiding reinforcement of pain behavior; and (4) modify (or refer for appropriate specialized help, as needed) the deficiencies of those patients who, when no longer limited by pain, would be limited by other functional impairments.

Every element of the program should be explained to patient and spouse before proceeding.

Medication Management

Traditional prescriptions of analgesics on a take-as-needed basis serve to make medication contingent upon pain. That arrangement can be expected, if continued for long intervals, to increase the chances of habituation or addiction. The remedy lies first in identifying (by in-hospital observation and/ or by having the patient or a reliable family member carefully record) what pain medications are taken, in what amounts, and at what time intervals. Usually 3 to 7 days of these baseline observations will suffice. All pain medications are to be taken orally during the baseline period.

The "Pain Cocktail" and Decreasing Medication

When the information seems clear as to current medication needs, all pain medications are incorporated into a single "pain cocktail." The pain cocktail consists of whatever combination of pain medications (with due regard for avoiding potentiating mixes) a patient is presently taking, plus a color-and-taste-masking vehicle (for example, cherry syrup) in volume sufficient to yield a 10 ml total amount per dose. The "cocktail" should be given on a fixed, 24-hour schedule at intervals which are the same as or slightly less than the average baseline intervals.

Active agents in the pain cocktail are gradually reduced without disclosing to the patient at what dates reductions occur—although he has already been told before beginning the program that this procedure would be followed. Active agents are reduced to zero or to the lowest level which does not result in consistent increases in pain behaviors. The reducing or fading process may also include any night-time doses (which the patient was awakened to receive) if the patient indicates that he is ready to eliminate this disturbance to his sleep. In the later stages of "fading," intervals between doses may also be lengthened. The key element is that medication is given on a set schedule independently of whether the patient feels he needs it. Fading should extend over 7 to 10 weeks or more.

If sleep medications are needed, they should be incorporated into the bedtime cocktail only. As fading occurs, increasing amounts of the vehicle are added to maintain a 10 ml total volume per dose.

Exercise and Activity Quotas

Most people with chronic pain do as much work as they can tolerate. They move about until they either feel the pain, or until it reaches a point at which they cannot continue with whatever they have been doing. Working-to-tolerance has the effect of making rest (for most pain patients a very potent reinforcer or positive consequence) contingent on hurting. If there is pain, it is systematically followed by rest. If there is no pain, activity continues. This arrangement directly reinforces pain behavior and (as in avoidance learning) means that stopping to rest will prove reinforcing because it eases the pain.

Treatment follows the same pattern as medication management. Baseline trials of prescribed exercises (for example, twice a day for 3 to 7 days) are conducted during which the patient works to tolerance without interruption within each exercise, and then carefully records how many times he could repeat the exercise before he felt the need to stop. Next, baseline performances are examined and quotas are set for each exercise. Each quota should be less than the average baseline number of repetitions. The key element is to insure that the patient is certain he can meet the first quota. When in doubt, set a low quota. Quotas are then increased at some pre-determined rate; for example, one per day or one per each four sessions. The rate of increment should reflect your level of confidence in the patient. If you are pessimistic, set a low increment rate. Once the quota is set, however, the end of any given session on any given exercise must be contingent upon reaching the quota without pause for rest. A patient's failure to meet quotas is ignored because you must, at all costs, avoid any effort to exhort or encourage the patient. Quotas continue to increase at the pre-set rate. If the patient fails several consecutive trials, he should be told that he will get another opportunity to "rebuild" by starting back at a lower level than the one at which he is presently failing. The increment rate is then re-instituted from that point. If he fails at the same point as before, his top for that exercise has probably been reached. Care must be taken to set upper limits to exercises, both as to how high quotas may climb, and so that, during any given trial, the patient does not exceed the quota.

The Family's Role in Operant Conditioning

The family training part of the program is more difficult to spell out concretely because many variations are often indicated. The key elements, in their approximate optimal sequence, are first, to have the spouse count precisely the number of times per 20 minutes of a visit that the patient displays one or more (in any combination) of the behaviors by which the husband or wife knows that the patient is experiencing pain, or pain-related functional impairment. This step is necessary to be sure the spouse will be able to modify his or her responses to all of the pain behaviors. Second, the spouse, while continuing to make covert counts of pain behaviors, observes and reports precisely his or her own behavior immediately after the patient's pain behavior. Once these are identified concretely and precisely ("I didn't do anything" will not suffice), it becomes a matter of judgment as to which of these responses to pain behavior needs to be changed.

A few sessions with the patient should be enough to try out the alternative responses which the trainer and spouse agree upon. Common examples include breaking eye contact ("look at the right shoulder"), pausing a second or two without doing or saying anything and then asking a question about some activity in which the patient has engaged ("How may laps did you walk in P.T. today?"), or, if the patient's pain behaviors are frequent or intense, interrupting the visit until the patient feels better ("It seems like you are quite uncomfortable now so I'll leave. I'll go have a cup of coffee and come back in 20 minutes or so to see if you are feeling well enough to visit."). Thirdly, the spouse will probably need practice at encouraging or reinforcing activity and well behavior. This can usually be done easily by having the spouse stop counting pain behaviors and start counting the number of times he or she makes some reinforcing comment about the patient's activity ("You look great." "It's good to see you walking so freely." "I'm glad we can go out to dinner together." "Thanks for ironing that shirt."). Sometimes it helps to ask the patient to also count the number of times the spouse reinforces activity or well behavior. Keep in mind that all elements of the program are explained to both patient and spouse before the program is begun.

Post-Treatment Activity

Most long-standing pain problems include some ineffective well behaviors. The secondary gains described above (for example, pain buys time out from a poor job, etc.) may remain problems and require treatment. In addition, any patient who has been functionally limited by pain or illness for a long time will find his re-entry into normal activities difficult, even threatening, after having been on the sidelines so long. Gradual re-introduction by slowly increasing amounts of exposure will usually work where these problems are not severe. Finally, it is not feasible or appropriate for many patients to return to work, and these people will need help finding activities which are suitable to their physical condition, interests, and skills.

The problems of post-treatment activity cannot be ignored. If they are, the gains the patient has made during the relatively intensive performance-monitoring regimens will quickly deteriorate. Here the physician must judge carefully whether he can handle the situation directly or whether the patient should be referred for specialized help.

In Conclusion

Many of the patients with significantly operant chronic pain can be recognized and treated using the above as a guide. However, there are many patients with operant or learned pain whose problems are so formidable that a trial of office treatment, or even treatment in hospitals only marginally trained in these procedures, is not indicated. In these cases, the physician now has the option of referring these patients to one of the increasing number of programs in the United States which are now developing the ability to apply operant-based methods.

Again, the methods described here are not likely to be of much help to pain patients for whom the current and active organic factor is substantial, and/or accounts for virtually all of their pain behaviors. In short, operant treatment of chronic pain is for operant pain.

References

1. Berni, R., and Fordyce, W. *Behavior Modification and the Nursing Process.* St. Louis: The C. V. Mosby Company, 1973.
2. Bonica, J., Clawson, D., and Fordyce, W. Management of Chronic orthopedic pain problems. *American Academy of Orthopedic Surgeons Instructional Core Course* (Vol. 21), November, 1972.
3. Fordyce, W. An operant conditioning method for managing chronic pain. *Postgrad. Med.* 53:123, 1973.
4. Fordyce, W., Fowler, R., and DeLateur, B. An application of behavior modification technique to a problem of chronic pain. *Behav. Res. Ther.* 6:105, 1968.

5. Fordyce, W., Fowler, R., Lehmann, J., and DeLateur, B.   Some implications of learning in problems of chronic pain. *J. Chronic Dis.* 21:179, 1968.
6. Fordyce, W., Fowler, R., Lehmann, J., DeLateur, B., Sand, P., and Trieschmann, R.   Operant conditioning in the treatment of chronic clinical pain. *Arch. Phys. Med. Rehabil.* 54:399, 1973.

12

Biofeedback Procedures in the Clinic

Thomas H. Budzynski

A host of researchers and clinicians are exploring the clinical possibilities of biofeedback techniques. However, unwarranted claims and expectations, as well as strong placebo effects, render a proper evaluation of these procedures somewhat difficult. Nevertheless, certain approaches would appear to be quite effective. Applications to tension and migraine headache, anxiety, and insomnia can now be described. There is a suggestion that biofeedback training may be helpful as a preventive program with regard to stress-related disorders.

The clinical application of biofeedback is such a rapidly evolving field that the techniques described in this paper may well be revised beyond recognition before another 12 months have passed. However, if this flurry of activity could be "frozen" at this time, one would no doubt find a continuum of emphasis on biofeedback in clinical settings that ranged from heavy to none at all. The fact that biofeedback in general has captured the imagination of both the layman and the professional has made a determination of its efficacy quite difficult. Preliminary research results, often amplified in significance by the popular press, become "fact" before being tested in the crucible of professional criticism. Poorly designed biofeedback equipment and quality units misused by inexperienced but eager clinicians have contributed to the confusion regarding the effectiveness of these procedures. And, finally, it is getting more difficult to find naïve subjects who do not bring a host of expectations to each biofeedback study, thus contributing to strong placebo effects.

Even though unrealistic expectations and inadequate or misused equipment continue to cloud the picture somewhat, it is possible nevertheless to point out several bright spots in the application of biofeedback to clinical disorders. For example, normative data slowly are becoming more available as system parameters are standardized. Certain types of biofeedback appear to be more useful than others. Clinicians are discovering how to use biofeedback in the context of existing therapies. Reliable equipment manufacturers are responding to the needs of both researcher and clinician in providing systems that

Reprinted from *Seminars in Psychiatry* 5 (4):537, 1973, by permission.

vary in complexity, yet give accurate quantified results as well as precise information feedback. In addition, it is a fact that biofeedback procedures are being explored in a variety of clinical settings including medical centers, hospitals, mental health clinics, behavior therapy clinics, private practice, and a few professionally staffed clinics specializing in biofeedback therapy.

What Can Biofeedback Provide in a Clinical Setting?

Biofeedback training essentially has three main goals: (1) the development of increased awareness of the relevant internal physiologic functions or events; (2) the establishment of control over those functions; and (3) the transfer or generalization of that control from the training site to other areas of one's life.

Awareness of the Event

Before voluntary control can be established over some aspect of one's physiology that ordinarily functions below the level of awareness, relevant knowledge of the event must be made known to the subject. Relevant knowledge may include the presence or absence of the event, as is the case with some EEG feedback systems, or an indication of the level of the event, as is the case with EMG; or both, as provided by certain sophisticated EEG feedback systems. Thus, the tracking system should be sensitive, accurate, artifact-free, and it must provide meaningful information feedback.

Voluntary Control Over the Function

Gradually, through a process of trial and error and hypothesis testing, the patient evolves strategies for controlling the feedback and thus the response. As he becomes more successful he learns to associate certain thoughts, as well as proprioceptive and interoceptive sensations, however subtle, with changes in the feedback. It is an interesting fact nevertheless, that a patient may develop some degree of control even before he is able to verbalize what it is that he is, or is not, doing. With continued training he is able to express what he is *not* doing, and finally, what he *is* doing, e.g., producing sensations of floating, or heaviness, or warmth in his limbs, and excluding certain thoughts.

Transfer of Control

The ability to verbalize control strategies enhances transfer from the clinic or laboratory to "real life." Therefore, the patient should be encouraged during the training phase to describe his sensations, as well as his successful and unsuccessful strategies. Often the patient will use a phrase or series of phrases that will become conditioned to the desired physiologic pattern. The autogenic training formulae of Schultz and Luthe [17] are very useful for this purpose. In fact, Green et al. [8] were the first experimenters to combine autogenic training phraseology and biofeedback. Other researchers who have employed autogenic-type phrases to enhance biofeedback learning and transfer are Budzynski and Stoyva [2] and Love [13].

Jacobson's progressive relaxation exercises [9] are also helpful in the initial stages of biofeedback training. These exercises, along with certain of the autogenic formulae, and other specialized instructions, can be placed on cassette tapes for use in the clinical setting, as well as for home practice. For the past 8 months we have used clinic and home practice cassette tapes at the Applied Biofeedback Institute. They are now an integral part of the therapy programs. It appears that a patient is more inclined to do the home practicing if he can listen to a tape recording. The patient's progress from one tape to another is based on his ability to demonstrate a certain level of control over a particular function. Home practice cassettes also ease the transition of the patient away from the biofeedback equipment. Of course, the transfer is never completed until the patient can successfully demonstrate his newly developed ability under real-life aversive conditions.

Self-Perceived Progress

If the successful pursuance of the three goals can be implemented, then biofeedback training can be of great value in clinical settings. For example, the use of feedback equipment with adequate quantification capability allows the therapist to specify target behaviors in terms of desired physiologic parameters at each stage of training. Thus, the patient perceives that he is progressing as he meets each criterion in turn.

Moment-to-moment knowledge of results provided by the feedback, as well as charts and graphs illustrating longer-term changes, provide objective evidence of progress. The confidence gained from this illustration of increasing control seems to generalize to other areas of the patient's life. Leitenberg et al [12], for example, have shown that providing a subject with information about his performance has therapeutic effects.

What Biofeedback Cannot Provide in a Clinical Setting

Although biofeedback training alone can result in positive change, it may be made more effective when used in conjunction with other therapy procedures. This is especially true if factors in the patient's environment appear to be contributing to his problem. These trouble areas of the patient's day-to-day existence may never be brought to light if he interacts only with a biofeedback machine. It is true that biofeedback training alone may help him to cope with these difficulties; however, the problems themselves can act to prevent progress with the training. The patient may find himself dwelling on problem-related thoughts during the training sessions, or he may find it difficult to practice at home.

A more troublesome situation for the therapist occurs when the patient is getting positively reinforced for maintaining his maladaptive behavior, or when he uses his symptoms to avoid certain feared situations. This may also manifest itself as an inability to progress in training and/or a reluctance to practice at home. A good relationship between therapist and patient can reduce, or at least help uncover, some of these motivational problems.

In short, biofeedback is simply a mirror reflecting some aspect of physiology. The patient really must want to learn to use the mirror in developing control over this response. An important part of the therapist's task is to maintain this motivation.

Specific Biofeedback Therapy Procedures

Since biofeedback is useful for altering and bringing under control physiologic responses, this training would seem to be particularly suited to disorders characterized by maladaptive physiologic patterns such as are evident in cases of tension and migraine headaches, essential hypertension, certain types of epilepsy, Raynaud's disease and cardiac arrhythmias. However, only a few of the possible clinical applications have been adequately researched. Requirements such as lengthy base lines, proper control conditions to guard against habituation and placebo effects, control of medication, and meaningful evaluation procedures render such research with humans a gruelling and time-consuming task.

With equipment design and training procedures evolving at a rapid rate, it is often difficult for the researcher to "freeze" design and training for the length of time it takes to complete an adequate experiment. For example, the tension headache studies carried out at the University of Colorado Medical Center [4, 5] involved a "bare bones" procedure. Patients in the second of these two studies were given only EMG (electromyographic) feedback from the forehead musculature for 16 sessions of 20 minutes each. They were asked to practice relaxing twice a day at home but were told only to do what they had learned in the training sessions. In spite of this simplified procedure approximately 70% of the patients showed significant reductions in headache activity.

Following the completion of the study, the control group patients were offered the real training. In this instance the "bare bones" procedure was augmented by cassette tape relaxation instructions, as well as portable EMG feedback units for home use. These additional measures seem to provide a greater incentive for practicing outside the laboratory.

The transfer of control to real life is enhanced not only by the daily home practice periods but also by reminding the patient to make frequent checks of his general tension level during the day. If he found himself tense, he was to attempt to relax for a short period (30 sec. to 3 min.). This practice can be implemented by placing a small sliver of brightly colored tape on the wrist watch dial. Thus, each time the patient looks at his watch the tape reminds him to scan around for tension spots. Incidentally, we have found that the color and shape of the tape reminder should be changed at least once a week; otherwise, people tend to habituate and subsequently ignore it.

Since we ask our tension headache patients to chart headache intensity every hour, the wrist watch tape serves also as a reminder to complete this task.

Clinical Procedures for Headache Conditions

One of the more interesting conclusions arising from the work with tension headache at the University of Colorado Medical Center and the study of migraine headache at the Menninger Clinic [16] is that EMG feedback alone is quite effective for tension headache but not for migraine, whereas peripheral temperature feedback is effective for migraine but not for tension headache. Consequently, a careful differential diagnosis should be made prior to biofeedback training. Following this, an attempt should be made to determine the circumstances associated with the onset of the headaches as well as the present environmental contingencies that may be maintaining the headaches. The patient is told that he will have to maintain an hourly (if he has tension headaches) or daily (if he has migraine headaches) record of the headache intensity. He is also told that he must practice relaxing at home or at work twice daily, and that the degree of relaxation for each of these sessions must be charted. The patient is taught also to record the type and amount of medication on the headache intensity chart.

It is very important to ascertain from the patient when during the day he feels he can take time to relax. Although most patients will have agreed to follow all the instructions to this point, some patients balk when asked to be specific about home practice times. The therapist may have to review with the patient each day's activities, hour by hour, in order to find appropriate times for the relaxation practice. The patient is also instructed to inform his immediate family of the necessity for privacy and quiet during the home practice periods. If he has a private office at work he is told to have his secretary hold all calls and visitors during the 20-minute practice periods.

In most instances a 2-week base line of charting headaches and medication is taken before training is begun. Following the base-line period, training is initiated with twice-a-week sessions. An abbreviated form of Jacobson's tense-relax procedure is used during the first two or three sessions in order to provide the patient with at least a gross awareness of differing levels of tension in his muscles. A measure of arm and frontalis EMG levels is taken before and after each session. The patient is given a cassette tape with tense-relax instructions for home use. He is told to practice twice a day and to rate the degree of relaxation achieved on a scale of 0 to 5.

The next phase of training involves EMG biofeedback from the forearm extensor. Autogenic-type phrases are coupled with the physiologic changes resulting from the feedback training. These auto-suggestive phrases also help to bring about the desired changes signalled by feelings of heaviness and warmth in the limbs. A cassette tape with the autogenic formulae allows the patient to practice at producing the changes outside the clinic.

When the patient can maintain his forearm tension below a certain level $(3\mu V)$, and when he can feel the heaviness and warmth sensations in his limbs, the feedback can be transferred to the forehead. Surface bioelectric activity in the forehead area is reflective of not only frontalis tension but jaw (masseter and temporalis) muscle tension, eye movements, and eye muscle tension. The diminution of all these signals contributes to a general decrease in arousal level [7, 9]. A third cassette tape, building on the prior learning, is used for home practice during the forehead-training phase.

Eventually, the patient learns to reduce forehead bioelectric activity below $3\mu V$ while sustaining the warmth and heaviness sensations in his limbs. The patient then practices at keeping the forehead EMG low with his eyes open in an upright sitting posture. The feedback can be withdrawn gradually at this point to check the patient's ability to maintain relaxation in the absence of feedback.

A final phase of the biofeedback training for tension headache involves a "stress management" procedure. While receiving forehead EMG feedback, the patient visualizes, as vividly as possible, a variety of stressful situations. While doing so, he attempts to maintain relaxation, or at least to recover quickly if aroused momentarily. As in the prior phase of training the feedback is gradually removed as the patient learns to sustain a relaxed physiology in the presence of stressful thoughts. At this point, the patient is encouraged to attempt to maintain an *optimal* arousal level in the face of real life stressors, and to try relaxing *after* the stressful situation is over (see Stoyva and Budzynski [19]). Typically, the duration of training to this point is approximately 15 1-hour sessions or 8 weeks.

Migraine patients receive training similar to those with tension headaches except that peripheral temperature feedback is introduced after the EMG feedback training. It has been our experience at the clinic that migraine patients quite often have cold hands (70°–80°F). They also tend to have somewhat lower forehead EMG levels than tension headache patients. Consequently, a shorter EMG training period is required before temperature feedback is initiated. The rationale for the EMG training with migraine cases is that the response of painfully dilated blood vessels in the head represents a rebound phenomenon occurring as a result of an initial over-reaction to stress. If this initial response to the stressor can be modified through relaxation training, then perhaps the rebound response will be weaker. Feedback of temperature information from the hand, a technique pioneered by Sargent et al [16] appears to be effective in the postponement, alleviation, or prevention of migraine headaches.

For this phase of training, the patient hears an auditory analog of the skin temperature of the hand. When he can maintain regularly a temperature greater than 90°F, the patient is asked to do this with visual feedback only. He will next attempt to do so without feedback. A final phase of training for migraine patients involves the same stress management procedure as employed with the tension headache patients, except that finger temperature is used as the feedback information source.

Biofeedback Used to Facilitate Behavior Therapy (Systematic Desensitization)

Drug Dependency Problems (with Migraine Patients)

Even after they have learned to control their muscle tension and temperature responses, some migraine patients find it all but impossible to give up or even decrease their daily drug intake. These are patients who tend to have particularly severe headaches if they fail to take rather large amounts of drugs, such as three to four Cafergot suppositories, some Valium, and a number of aspirin each day. Rather than risk getting an extremely painful headache, these patients begin taking their medication at the first sign of such an event. Some patients maintain a daily prophylactic dosage and then augment this with additional amounts as a headache seems imminent. Unfortunately, through the years many events become conditioned to the headache pain. Thus, a heightened irritability, a slight feeling of depression, a tense neck musculature, a weather change, an argument with a friend or relative, or a party can signal the onslaught. The response of taking large amounts of medication at this point avoids the headache pain and thus strengthens the response. When asked to give up their medication (even a little at a time), and substitute their newly developed ability to control peripheral warmth, these patients may become very anxious, and therefore, more disposed to headaches.

Consequently, a period of systematic desensitization is required to reduce this anxiety before the medication reduction can begin. The desensitization hierarchy includes scenes in which the patient visualizes himself giving up a progressively greater amount of medication. Upon completion of the hierarchy, the patient is encouraged to begin a very gradual withdrawal from his medication.

Eventually, migraine patients find they can exist without medication except in extreme circumstances or in cases of menstrual cycle headaches that occur once or twice each cycle. Typically, the patients find that they can accomplish the hand-warming in the face of headache onset cues. However, if they are unable to accomplish this warming in 15 minutes, it is an indication that the headache onset has progressed too far and they will need some medication. This procedure gives the patient a chance to try altering his physiology before giving in to medication. In three cases of menstrual cycle migraine headaches, the hand-warming was difficult to accomplish and the patients usually resorted to medication at these times. . . . [pages 543–546 of original article have been omitted. *Ed.*]

Concluding Remarks

An accumulating body of clinical and research evidence suggests that biofeedback represents a relatively effective technique for the shaping of self-control over certain physiologic events. These events are usually autonomous in that they tend to occur automatically and below the level of awareness. When these internal events fall outside the normal range of functioning, they constitute maladaptive behaviors that can lead to feelings of anxiety, or the appearance of such stress-related disorders as migraine and tension headaches, certain cardiovascular problems, and sleep-onset insomnia, to name a few. Through biofeedback training, patients learn to maintain their physiology within a normal range of functioning.

In addition to the alleviation or elimination of the symptoms of stress-related disorders, biofeedback training could constitute a preventive technique to enable individuals to better cope with the stress of a "future shock" environment. Furthermore, the development of self-control of internal functions at an early age might represent one of the most effective programs for the prevention of those disorders that produce the highest incidences of morbidity and mortality in our industrialized, fast-paced culture.

References

1. Budzynski, T. Some applications of biofeedback-produced twilight states. *Fields Within Fields . . . Within Fields* 5:105, 1972. Republished in Shapiro, D., et al., eds., *Biofeedback and Self-Control.* Chicago: Aldine-Atherton, 1972.
2. Budzynski, T., and Stoyva, J. Biofeedback techniques in behavior therapy. In Birbaumer, N., ed., *The Mastery of Anxiety. Contribution of Neuropsychology to Anxiety Research.* Reihe Fortschritte der Klinischen Psychologie, Bd. 4, Munchen, Wein: Verlag, Urban & Schwarzenberg, 1973, in press. English version republished in Shapiro, D., et al., eds., *Biofeedback and Self-Control.* Chicago: Aldine-Atherton, 1972.
3. Budzynski, T., and Stoyva, J. EMG biofeedback and behavior therapy. In Jurjevich, R., ed., *Direct Psychotherapy,* Vol. 3: *International Developments.* Coral Gables, Fla.: University of Miami Press. In press.
4. Budzynski, T., Stoyva, J., and Adler, C. Feedback-induced relaxation: Application to tension headache. *J. Behav. Ther. Exp. Psychiatry* 1:205, 1970.
5. Budzynski, T., Stoyva, J., Adler, C., et al. EMG biofeedback and tension headache: A controlled outcome study. *Psychosom. Med.* In press.
6. Engel, B. T. Response specificity. In Greenfield, N., and Sternbach, R., eds., *Handbook of Psychophysiology.* New York: Holt, Rinehart and Winston, 1972. P. 571.
7. Gellhorn, E. Motion and emotion. *Psychol. Rev.* 71:457, 1964.
8. Green, E., Green, A., and Walters, E. Voluntary control of internal states: Psychological and physiological. *J. Transpersonal Psychol.* 2:1, 1970.
9. Jacobson, E. *Progressive Relaxation,* 2d ed. Chicago: University of Chicago Press, 1938.
10. Lader, M. H., and Mathews, A. M. A physiological model of phobic anxiety and desensitization. *Behav. Res. Ther.* 6:411, 1968.
11. Lader, M. H., and Wing, L. *Physiological Measures, Sedative Drugs, and Morbid Anxiety.* London: University of Oxford Press, 1966.
12. Leitenberg, H., Agras, W., Thompson, L., et al. Feedback in behavior modification: An experimental analysis in two phobic cases. *J. Appl. Behav. Anal.* 1:131, 1968.
13. Love, W. A. Problems in Therapeutic Application of EMG Feedback. Pre-

sented at the Annual Meeting of the Biofeedback Research Society, Boston, 1972. Unpublished data.

14. Marks, I. M. *Fears and Phobias.* New York: Academic Press, Inc., 1969. P. 207.

15. Raskin, M., Johnson, G., and Rondestvedt, T. Chronic anxiety treated by feedback-induced muscle relaxation. *Arch. Gen. Psychiatry* 28:263, 1973.

16. Sargent, J., Green, E., and Walters, E. Preliminary report on the use of autogenic feedback techniques in the treatment of migraine and tension headaches. *Psychosom. Med.* 35:129, 1973.

17. Schultz, J., and Luthe, W. *Autogenic Training.* New York: Grune & Stratton, Inc., 1959.

18. Sittenfeld, P., Budzynski, T., and Stoyva, J. Feedback Control of the EEG Theta Rhythm. Presented at the American Psychological Association Meeting, Honolulu, 1972.

19. Stoyva, J., and Budzynski, T. Cultivated low arousal—An anti-stress response? In DiCara, L. V., ed., *Recent Advances in Limbic and Autonomic Nervous System Research.* New York: Plenum Publishing Corporation. In press.

20. Wickramasekera, I. Instructions and EMG feedback in systematic desensitization: A case report. *Behav. Ther.* 3:460, 1972.

13

Conjoint Treatment of Chronic Pain

Jerry H. Greenhoot and Richard A. Sternbach

Patients with severe "benign" pain of long duration, no matter what the etiology, develop significant and persistent psychological problems [1, 2, 3]. These problems often obscure the complaint of pain, and lead to lengthy considerations of whether or not the pain is "organic" or "psychogenic" in nature. This consideration, which plagues the surgeon, serves only to confuse the real issue, namely, "Is the pain medically or surgically *treatable?*"

We have found that many of these patients cannot be categorized conveniently. Their problems do not respond to standard psychotherapeutic approaches [4, 5]. However, without the resolution of these problems, appropriate and well-planned neurosurgical intervention often fails to provide the expected rehabilitation. The patients either do not gain adequate pain relief or, following relief of pain, they remain so miserable that they do not return to adequate social function [6].

We have learned that the only adequate measure of success or failure of pain relief is the patient's behavior. A patient who has no pain, but who does not function adequately, has had a "bad result," whereas another with complaints of pain, but who lives well, has been rehabilitated.

The Pain Unit

In an attempt to deal better with the complexities of the chronic pain patient, we have established a Pain Unit at the Veterans Administration Hospital under the joint direction of the neurosurgeon and psychologist. The sequential outpatient approach has been abandoned, and replaced by an entire spectrum of techniques—physiological, pharmacological, and psychological—for the simultaneous treatment of all patients in an inpatient setting.

The Pain Unit is an integral part of the Neurosurgical Service and utilizes the same facilities and staff as the remainder of the service. Patients accepted for treatment are those with complaints of pain which are accompanied by

Reprinted from J. J. Bonica, ed., *Pain: Advances in Neurology*, Volume 4, © Raven Press, 1974. Used by permission.

at least some minimal physical findings which may be corrected by medical or surgical treatment; no patients with "garden variety" emotional disorders are admitted, and those found clearly to be malingering or hysterical are discharged or transferred to the Psychiatry Service.

Patients who have been treated include those with causalgia, anesthesia dolorosa following cerebral infarction, thalamic pain syndrome, brachial plexus avulsion, and cervical and lumbar disc syndromes. Patients are first seen in the outpatient department and are told that the Unit utilizes both medical-surgical and psychological approaches simultaneously, and that they will be expected to participate in both. This includes all patients, including those most well adjusted to their pain state. We have found that no useful purpose is served by separating organic from functional pain, even where it is possible, and, therefore, all patients are *evaluated and treated in parallel* for both aspects of the syndrome.

The Assessment Process

On admission to the Pain Unit, patients are evaluated medically in the usual manner and special tests such as X-rays, brain scan, EEG, myelograms, electromyography, and nerve conduction studies are obtained, as indicated by the specific problem. Simultaneously, all patients undergo a psychological evaluation, including the Minnesota Multiphasic Personality Inventory (MMPI), a Health Index [7], and an ischemic pain test [8] for estimating clinical pain levels and relating this to their maximal tolerance of this type of pain—a useful measure of the severity of the clinical pain.

With this information, the psychologist interviews the patient, taking a brief history, explaining the details of the program, and making a treatment plan which sets realistic goals for behavioral improvement in life style, consistent with the underlying disability [9]. This plan, or "contract," is specified in writing, and serves as a bridge between the diagnostic and therapeutic processes. It assists in confirming or modifying the psychological formulation, and ensures the patient's active participation in the subsequent program, rather than his passive acquiescence in allowing us to "fix" him. By specifying the details and expectations of this program, and what the patients are expected to do in order to "get well," vagueness and uncertainty for the patient are reduced and a clear direction is provided for the staff.

Usually, two or three behavioral goals emerge from this process. One is a specific kind of work, or occupational goal; another is a recreational goal; and a third is some improvement in family or personal relationships. The achievement of these goals represents getting well, and all activities of both staff and patients are subsequently directed to their fulfillment.

Patients are instructed to maintain daily records of their estimated clinical pain on a scale of 0 to 100; an accurate record of their own activities, both pain-compatible (e.g., lying down) and pain-incompatible (e.g., exercising, working at jobs on the ward or elsewhere in the hospital); and at least one behavior which the patient wishes to achieve as a goal of therapy. We realize that patients' estimates of pain are inexact, but they are one important index of success or failure, and we have found them to vary appropriately in direction with changes in medication, psychological setbacks, and after surgical pain relief.

The psychological evaluation is usually completed more quickly than the neurosurgical one, although it continues to be modified by observations of behavior on the ward. This evaluation is considered by the neurosurgeon, along with radiological and other clinical findings in making a decision about the possibility of surgery. The decision as to whether or not surgery is feasible is made by the surgeon. The decision as to whether or not surgery will be performed is made jointly by the surgeon and the patient after consideration of risks, potential gains, severity of the pain, and progress toward resolution of psychological problems.

For many patients who enter the program, surgery is not deemed feasible. The remainder of the program for these patients is to help them find more satisfying lives in spite of their pain. This requires reduction of pain-related behavior which is inimical to a satisfying life—invalidism, chronic dependency and the use of the pain against family members in a myriad of "pain games."

The Treatment Program

For purposes of description, it is convenient to discuss treatment separately. In actual fact, however, treatment begins as soon as the patient enters the program. All treated patients have undergone some adjustment as a result of their participation in the program. This adjustment usually begins with the formulation of the "contract" specifying goals to be achieved. An extraordinary number of patients have literally never considered the possibility that they may have to adjust to their pain. It is as if time spent with the pain has been suspended, as if it "doesn't count" in one's life, and that when relieved these patients expect to start again in life where they were suspended, despite the fact that many years have usually elapsed since they were pain free. The introduction of real goals and a plan in case surgery cannot be done (or if it is unsuccessful) is often the first therapy on the Unit. Patients who will have successful surgery must prepare to return to a life which may have become foreign to them. Those for whom surgical pain relief is impossible must plan to re-enter their lives in spite of their pain.

It is not our purpose here to review the nature or results of surgical treatments; these will be the subject of subsequent communications. The types of procedures done include cordotomy, rhizotomy, neurolysis, transcutaneous stimulation and implantation of spinal dorsal column stimulators, and stereotaxic electrode implantation and thalamotomy.

The decision about surgery is made after thorough evaluation, and usually about the second or third week of hospitalization. We have learned that this decision is absolutely critical to the psychological aspect of the treatment program. Until the decision is made, and the reasons for or against it discussed by the surgeon, patients go through the proper motions of participating in the program but have obvious reservations about the psychological approach. They are interested in showing how much they suffer and need surgery, and many cling to thoughts that no real change in their life is needed as they may soon expect to be made whole again. At the time of the decision, the program becomes more meaningful. Either the surgery will not be done, in which case they must learn to live with their pain and make the best of it, or they will have surgery, and they can give up their reservations and get to work on their psychological problems.

We have learned that the most critical point of the program is the explanation *by the senior surgeon* to the patient of his physical *and* psychological status, and the feasibility of surgery. Until patients have accepted the importance of psychological rehabilitation, only the surgeon carries sufficient credibility to force a confrontation of these emotional factors in chronic pain. Since surgery is performed to reward progress in solving psychological problems, the surgeon must be abreast of this progress and for this reason he participates in at least one group therapy meeting per week.

The goals of therapy differ for each patient and many aspects of the program are tailored to specific needs. Some patients need vocational retraining or educational assistance; some need financial assistance. The facilities and staff of the institution include vocational rehabilitation and educational counselors and social workers who are incorporated into the program as needed. Many patients have had interpersonal or family difficulties which require special counseling. These problems have responded to directive therapy, usually behavioral in nature, in two or three private sessions with the psychologist. We have learned that most pain patients are not psychologically minded, and nondirective therapy or psychodynamic interpretations are less useful than a directive and behavioral approach.

In addition to individualized programs, each patient participates in therapies common to all. These consist primarily of a specialized form of group therapy [10] and behavior modification techniques practiced by the nursing staff [11].

The group therapy session is held daily for an hour and is attended by all patients, the psychologist, and nurses. On at least one occasion per week, the surgeon attends as well. The therapy consists of frank discussions of "pain games," of their use by patients in pain, and the ways in which they interfere with rehabilitation. The games represent behavior which is useful to patients in manipulating others, using pain in the service of the interpersonal manipulation. The number of these "games" and their variants is truly amazing. We have seen patients, for whom fear overrides reality, exaggerate their complaints in order to convince the surgeon that he should worry about them as much as they do. We have seen patients lie about the results of placebo anesthetic blocks in order to convince the surgeon that he should do what they know correctly from previous blocks should be done. We have seen patients use their pain as retaliation against a spouse in a marriage that both parties wished dissolved long ago.

These games obviously confuse the surgical management of pain, as surgery will not relieve fear or an unhappy marriage. The exaggerated complaint may lead the surgeon to a diagnosis of malingering or hysteria and away from further investigation or surgery which should be done, thus depriving the patient of what he truly needs. Patients who need their pain as weapons cannot afford rehabilitation even after an organic lesion has been corrected. The chief function of the group therapy is to expose these games, and, by making them explicit, to stop them. The goal is to direct patients' behavior back to a real-world evaluation of their pain, their lives, and the interrelationships of the two.

Some emphasis is given to the role of "pay-off" such as sympathy, narcotics, financial compensation, or admiration for bravery. Many games and pay-offs are not consciously conceived of by patients, and their exposure *by other patients*, who have participated in the same type of game-playing, is frequently more effective than when done by the staff. The value of this group process cannot be overestimated. Patients may deceive themselves or the staff, but they do not long deceive other patients with whom they live, and the games are soon stopped. The exposure of the game, and its pay-off, to a spouse who has suffered from its impact, is an important aspect in preventing recurrence or preventing the development of new games.

Patients have felt so strongly the benefit of this program that they continue these discussions among themselves on the ward, and many discharged patients return to the hospital to attend meetings on the days of their outpatient follow-up visits.

Apart from the formal therapy, nurses and staff practice a form of behavior modification based upon experimental operant conditioning [11]. The purpose of this is to modify pain behavior and to shape pain-incompatible behavior. This requires abandoning the traditional offering of sympathy and concern to patients in pain, and the substitution of rewards for healthy behavior such as productive activity directed toward achievement of goals set upon admission. The essence of the technique is to ignore pain and complaints of pain, so as to not reinforce it with attention, and to reinforce desired behavior (e.g., walking, socializing) with compliments and favorable attention. Medications are given on a schedule, not on demand, so as to separate the reinforcing power of the drugs from the complaint of pain.

We have seen this operant conditioning procedure alone cause a bedfast patient to walk, unaided, more than 1 mile per day after only 3 days in the program. Patients' activity logs and graphs of estimated pain levels reflect these changes and give the staff an additional opportunity to reward improvement.

The result of these therapeutic programs is that after a few weeks, patients are engaged in nearly a full day's work, or in goal-directed, pain-incompatible behavior. This is important in the change of patients' self-concepts. When working a full day, one cannot long think of oneself as a chronic invalid. Thus, patients for whom surgical pain relief is possible maximize the usefulness of their pain relief, and those for whom it is not possible soon learn that they are capable of significant, if not normal, function in spite of their pain.

Preliminary Results

At this writing, 54 patients have been through the program. It is too early to have long-term follow-up data in significant numbers. We are following these discharged patients in the outpatient clinic, and thus far their improvement seems to be holding up.

Figure 13-1 shows the improvements in the total patient group. From left to right, top to bottom, the graphs represent:

Weekly averages of patients' subjective pain estimates. This estimate is made daily by each patient, on a scale of 0 to 100, for which 0 represents "no pain at all" and 100 means pain "so severe it results in suicide in a minute or two." Such psychophysical scaling methods as magnitude production, which this is, and magnitude matching (below) are quite consistent and show lawful behavior [8]. These data show a decrease in pain from 65 to 45 over the duration of stay, despite decreases in analgesic intake and increases in activity.

Weekly averages of patients' maximum ischemic pain tolerance levels (top) and the point at which the pain equals their clinical pain levels in severity (bottom). Maximum tolerance time shows a decrease from about 8 min. to about 5 min. due to the reduction in analgesics. The clinical pain levels show a similar decrease, from about 6 min. to 3 min. and 20 sec. This parallels and tends to confirm the decrease in pain reflected in the pain estimates.

The remaining graphs show the marked increase in activity levels: the average daily time spent walking increased from $3\frac{1}{2}$ to $4\frac{1}{3}$ hr; the number of "laps" walked (30 laps = 1 mile) increased so that patients averaged $1\frac{1}{2}$ miles per day by discharge; numbers of exercises increased dramatically; and amount of time in goal-related activities increased to the maximum (limited by shop schedules) of about 2 hr. per day.

Of this initial patient group, less than half received surgery (21 of 54 patients). Nevertheless, our findings suggest that all chronic pain patients may show decreased levels of pain, despite reductions of analgesics and markedly increased activity levels.

Figure 13-2 shows the classic psychophysiological MMPI profile of these patients, and the improvement with treatment. The decrease in hypochondriasis (Scale 1) approaches significance, $p < .10$. The decrease in depression (Scale 2) is significant, $p < .02$. The decrease in hysteria (Scale 3) is significant, $p < .05$. And the decrease in anxiety (Scale 7) is significant, $p < .01$. Thus psychological improvement parallels behavioral improvement.

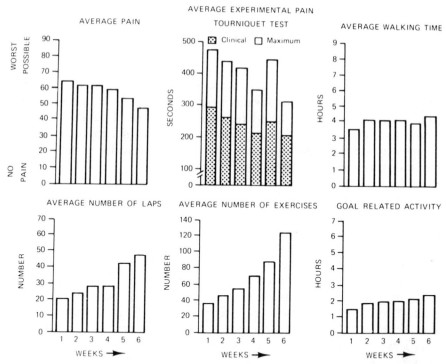

Figure 13-1 Progress of patients in Pain Unit. A. Patients' estimates of the severity of their clinical pain. B. Weekly ischemic pain test showing maximum tolerance and match to clinical pain levels. C. Amount of time "up" (on feet). D. Distance walked. E. Physical therapy exercises. F. Time spent on individual goal activity (usually shop work). Total number of patients = 54.

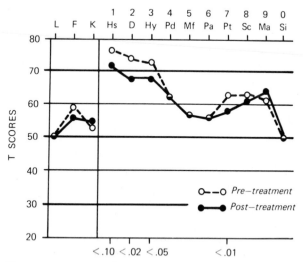

Figure 13-2 Pretreatment and post-treatment MMPI profiles. Scales 1, 2, and 3 are typically elevated in chronic illness, and represent the "neurotic triad" of hypochondriasis, depression, and hysteria (denial of emotional problems). Scale 7, psychasthenia, is primarily a measure of anxiety; improvement in Scale 1 approaches significance; in Scales 2, 3, and 7, it reaches significance. Total number of patients = 54.

Summary

Patients with chronic pain of long duration do not uniformly benefit from surgery. An important reason for this is that patients with intractable organic pain develop emotional problems very similar to those of patients with primarily psychogenic pain. These emotional problems of chronic invalidism, compensation neurosis, drug dependence, etc., are typically unresponsive to traditional psychiatric approaches. In recognition of these difficulties, and the failure of the usual pain clinic approach to resolve them, we have developed an inpatient Pain Unit.

In the Pain Unit, psychological assessment is performed in parallel with the neurosurgical evaluation. This permits an evaluation of the relative proportion of organic and emotional causes of the pain. It is done by psychodiagnostic testing, testing of pain thresholds, and by observation of ward behavior, while patients are receiving diagnostic blocks, radiological procedures, etc. When the psychological problems have been identified, these are treated by a specialized form of group therapy, and by behavior modification techniques practiced by the nursing staff. This produces a decrease in pain levels, despite a decrease in analgesic intake and a marked increase in activity levels. It is then possible for the surgeon and the patient to decide if surgery is feasible and warranted, or if the patient can live with his pain. With this conjoint treatment program, the surgeon can also be confident that his surgical intervention will not be sabotaged by patients' psychological problems.

Acknowledgment

We thank Gretchen Timmermans, M.S., for the data analysis.

References

1. Bond, M. R. *Br. J. Psychiatry* 119:671, 1971.
2. Sternbach, R. A., Wolf, S. R., Murphy, R. W., and Akeson, W. H. *Psychosomatics* 14:226, 1973.
3. Woodforde, J. M., and Merskey, H. *J. Psychosom. Res.* 16:173, 1972.
4. Tinling, D. C., and Klein, R. F. *Psychosom. Med.* 28:766, 1966.
5. Szasz, T. S. *Pain.* New York: Academic Press, 1968. P. 93.
6. Penman, J. *Lancet.* 1:633, 1954.
7. Sternbach, R. A., Wolf, S. R., Murphy, R. W., and Adeson, W. H. *Psychosomatics* 14:52, 1973.
8. Sternbach, R. A., Murphy, R. W., Timmermans, G., Greenhoot, J. H., and Akeson, W. H. In Bonica, J. J., ed. *Advances in Neurology* (Vol. 4): *Pain.* New York: Raven, 1974.
9. Sternbach, R. A., and Rusk, T. N. *Psychother. Theory Res. & Pract.* In press.
10. Berne, E. *Games People Play.* New York: Grove Press, Inc., 1964.
11. Fordyce, W. E., Fowler, R. S., Jr., Lehmann, J. F., and LeLateur, B. J. *J. Chronic Dis.* 21:179, 1968.

III

Pain and Its Alleviation in Specific Groups

14

Pain Associated with Neurological Conditions

Sandra S. Sweeney, Marion Johnson, and Joann M. Eland

Pain, regardless of its origin, is received, perceived, and communicated by an intact nervous system. Pain is rarely, if ever, a pleasant sensation, but the pain associated with pathological conditions of the nervous system is particularly severe in its onset and course. The nervous system has three major divisions involved in stimulus-response behavior—the peripheral nervous system, the central nervous system, and the autonomic nervous system. Pain originating from sources outside the nervous system such as body organs or tissues, or both, is frequently amenable to relief by pharmacological, surgical, or medical interventions, or all three of these. Pain arising from within the nervous system, however, is less amenable to treatment and, in some instances, suicide has become the final means of escape for patients suffering from pain of neurological origin.

The nervous system is a complex entity. While science has made considerable advances in identifying its structural components and physiological functions, much remains unknown. Its complexity is increased all the more by the innumerable relationships and interdependent roles that exist between its structural and functional qualities. Much of the research that focuses on various structural and functional components has been done on animals as compared to human subjects. Application of animal study findings to human subjects is frequently not feasible. The human subject's ability to perceive, combined with the cognitive skills of interpretation, places him in a higher category than animal subjects, and predictions regarding human behavior become increasingly difficult to determine. It is not uncommon to treat successfully patient A's neurological pain on one day and to fail to treat patient B's neurological pain the next day—even when both cases are assumed to be almost identical and receive the same treatment.

Research on the nervous system often yields confusing results and contradictory evidence. Results of one study frequently dispute the results of other similar studies. Debates flourish as to what actually initiates pain-receptor activity, the modes of conduction, tracts employed in the transmission of impulses, the systems affected, the spinal cord levels at which impulses may cross, and where the sensation of pain is actually perceived. Knowledge of the concepts of specificity, summation, divergence, convergence, patterning, inhibition, excitation, intensity, and threshold and their roles in the overall function of the nervous system is essential. These concepts are commonly encountered in discussions focusing on attempts to explain the structural and functional relationship of the nervous system.

Causal Mechanisms of Neurological Pain

Causal mechanisms serving as stimuli for and eliciting responses from the nervous system are similar to mechanisms causing pain as a result of pathological processes elsewhere in the body. Mechanical causal mechanisms include compression, pressure, obstruction, edema, trauma such as severing, inflammatory processes, infection, and vascular changes. Chemical causal mechanisms are also important factors to consider when discussing pain of neurological origin. Damage to nerve cells produces and releases chemical secretory substances with pain-producing capabilities similar to effects of cellular damage elsewhere in the body. Potassium, acetylcholine, serotonin, histamine, and plasma kinins can be effective pain-producing substances in the correct environment. The effects caused by the secretion or excretion (or both) of these substances are discussed in greater depth in other chapters of this source book. The reader is referred to discussions in Chapters 2 and 15 for a more detailed presentation of these underlying causal mechanisms.

Wall categorizes causal mechanisms responsible for initiating the sensation of neurological pain in the following framework:

(1) primary afferent signals with sudden onset that trigger pain, including: stimulation of terminals by pressure, temperature, and chemical agents; stimulation of axons by pressure, transection, chemical agents, and electric current; and, block of axons; (2) afferent signals with delayed onset after injury that trigger pain, including: stimulation of terminals by sensitization and inflammation; disorders of axons by complete transection or partial destruction; (3) secondary effects of tissue destruction which affect pain, including: reflex muscle contraction, referred pain, autonomic reflexes, and antidromic impulses; and (4) spinal cord mechanisms receiving afferents which trigger pain [34].

There is evidence to support another theory about a causative mechanism of pain that incorporates the concepts of stimulation, convergence, and inhibition. Research documented by several authors and summarized by Fields et al [4] suggests that afferent neurons that are specifically sensitive to noxious stimuli have small diameters. Stimulation of these small-diameter neurons is generally responsible for producing sensations of pain. This is in contrast to stimulation of larger-diameter afferents, which do not generally produce pain. In fact, increasing the activity of the larger-diameter afferent fibers may serve to block the transmission of pain sensations by smaller-diameter afferent fibers via inhibition. It seems as though certain procedures designed to increase large-diameter afferent activity may either elevate the pain threshold or inhibit the smaller-diameter afferent fiber input and thus decrease the transmission of pain sensations. Research findings have demonstrated also that selective blocking of large-diameter afferents can increase and prolong pain sensations being mediated by smaller-diameter afferents [4]. Melzack and Wall's gate control theory is based largely upon these concepts [21].

A specific anatomical location for inhibitory function by larger-diameter afferents has yet to be identified. It has been predicted that the selective loss of the large-diameter nerve fibers would subsequently result in the occurrence of pain, but such predictions have not been substantiated. Rather, in cases of human neuropathy, the loss of large afferent fibers has not been consistently or predictably associated or correlated with painfulness [31]. So the problem remains unresolved. This means then, that the presence of large-diameter afferent nerves can inhibit pain impulses from smaller-diameter afferents or elevate the pain threshold; but the loss of larger afferents does not necessarily produce pain per se. Some theorize that the occurrence of pain may not be related to the degeneration of either the small or large afferent nerves, but rather may result from other factors such as (1) the nature of the fiber degeneration, (2) the rate of fiber degeneration, or (3) other as yet unknown factors.

The possibility remains, however, that destruction of the larger, unmyelinated fibers may destroy the pain-inhibitory qualities possessed by these fibers, thus allowing the smaller myelinated fibers to conduct their impulses and pain sensations freely over the nervous system to the higher centers of interpretation and perception. If this hypothesis is indeed true, then nursing and medical interventions designed to increase large-fiber input will attempt to activate the inhibitory qualities possessed by these fibers, thus decreasing and preventing the smaller myelinated fibers from conducting impulses and pain sensations freely over the nervous system to the higher centers of interpretation and perception to decrease pain.

Types of Neurological Pain

A review of the literature suggests numerous typologies for describing and organizing pain of neurological origin. The pain of neurological origin is generally discussed from two primary perspectives—peripheral and central. Upon close examination, it is apparent that there is considerable variation in the definitions and pathological conditions ascribed to the two terms. It is becoming increasingly difficult to distinguish what is defined as peripheral from that which is defined as central when discussing neurological pain.

Until recently, the consensus of researchers using the term "central pain" seemed to follow the traditional definition of Riddoch [25], i.e., limiting the definition of "central pain" to the generally accepted components of the central nervous system, i.e., the brain and spinal cord [18]. Pagni [23] defines "central pain" as that pain which can "arise as a result of lesions of the first-, second-, or third-order neurons of specific pain pathways"; but his concept of central pain remains consistent with traditional definitions. Recently, however, there have been attempts by some researchers to enlarge the definition of "central pain" to include sensations of pain arising from within the nervous system itself, regardless of the location. Noordenbos [22] credits Goodly as being responsible for this extended definition of "central pain" which includes "all lesions central to the nerve endings." This extended definition, therefore, includes the following conditions within his definition of central pain: tic douloureux, multiple sclerosis, the causalgias, the neuralgias, phantom limb, thalamic syndrome, peripheral neuropathies, postparaplegic pain, and so forth. The phenomenon of phantom pain is an excellent example of the problems involved in attempting to define pain of neurological origin as being either peripheral or central.

The causal mechanism of phantom pain has not been successfully clarified. Irritation of the peripheral nerves, sympathetic activity, and psychological factors have all been implicated as causative factors [19]. Theories explaining phantom pain include the peripheral definition of causation—pain resulting from persisting sensations of the stump; and the central definition of causation—phantom pains are the result of conscious processes that need not be dependent upon sensations [5]. Others have theorized that phantom pain results from self-sustaining activity throughout the neural circuits [20]. At this time, none of the models have been accepted as an adequate explanation of phantom pain, and the difficulties in distinguishing between present definitions of peripheral versus central neurological pain are readily demonstrated.

Characteristics of Neurological Pain

The traditional categories of acute and chronic pain have also been used to refer to pain of neurological origin. Talbott [30] associates peripheral pain generally with being acute while chronic pain may be associated with either central or peripheral sources. Acute pain usually results from traumatic injuries or tissue damage or both, and is viewed as being of short duration. Chronic pain syndromes, however, are much more complex, involving numerous pathological processes; they are long in duration, occasionally persisting throughout one's life.

For purposes of this chapter, the more extensive definition of central pain will be utilized in describing the pain of neurological origin. Peripheral and central will be associated with anatomical locations rather than characteristics of pain. Lesions causing pain of neurological origin have many commonalities in clinical symptomatology as is readily seen in the text below.

Neurological pain tends to be spontaneous and severe, that is, it occurs without any apparent cause or stimulation of the area in which the pain may be localized. The usual sequence of steps between stimulus and response no longer exists. These unusual characteristics lead Noordenbos [22] to suggest that the pain of neurological origin results from the faulty transmission of impulses between reception of the stimulus and perception and reaction to the stimulus. Patients examined do demonstrate evidence of damage to the afferent pathways. "There is often a distinct delay before the stimulus is felt, the various stimuli are incorrectly identified, and localization is faulty" [22].

Loeser [14] likewise subscribes to the extended definition of central pain (i.e., pain associated with diseases or injuries, or both, affecting the neurons, their processes, and synapses) and describes the characteristics of central pain according to two categories—episodic central pain versus constant central pain.

Central pain syndromes characterized by episodic pain include the conditions of: tic douloureux, tabes dorsalis, and some types of multiple sclerosis and postparaplegic pain. The pain accompanying these diseases is described as being electric-shocklike, shooting, or lancinating, or all three. Trigger areas in which light stimulation precipitates an attack are present in these cases. The trigger area may or may not be in the exact area of pain but is generally located quite near it. The pain is dermatomal in distribution and does not involve a large area of the body. The location of the pain remains constant [14, 22].

Central pain presenting a constant pain picture is associated with the following conditions: postherpetic neuralgia, atypical facial pain, the thalamic syndrome, causalgias, anesthesia dolorosa, phantom limb, and some types of peripheral neuropathies, multiple sclerosis, and postparaplegic pain. Peripheral nerve damage that has altered or reduced the amount of sensory input accompanies most of these conditions. Patients describe these pains as being cold, burning, crawling, itching, pins and needles, numbness, or grabbing. The severity of the pain experienced has a wide range, but it does not fluctuate within a given condition or patient state. This type of constant pain is perceived over wide areas of the body and may follow either a peripheral nerve distribution or body region of involvement [14, 22].

The pain of phantom limb is a frequently encountered example of constant central pain. Phantom pain can be described as "that phenomenon occurring after the healing phase of an amputation or an extensive avulsion, which is described as a cyclic pain that is perceived as being in the vicinity of the absent body part, the usual case being an extremity" [5]. Nonpainful phantom sensations are reported by most amputees after loss of an arm or leg. The limb is usually described as having a tingling feeling, warmth or coldness, heaviness, a definite shape, and the ability to move [19, 20]. About five to ten percent of amputees develop severe pain which may become progressively worse [19]. Phantom pain is described as twisting, cramping, shooting, and crushing [5, 19]. It frequently occurs in the same location as the phantom limb and may even be described as resulting from activity, such as a tightly clenched fist that cannot be relaxed.

Melzack has identified four characteristics of phantom pain as found in the literature [20]. These are: (1) The pain endures after healing of the tissue and may persist for years. (2) Pain may be caused by stimulation of trigger zones or pain at another site. (3) Phantom pain is more common in individuals who have suffered pain in a limb prior to amputation, and it may resemble that pain. (4) Pain may be abolished by changes in somatic input. Some of these characteristics might be used to describe other types of constant central pain.

The term "peripheral" as it is used in this chapter refers to the outermost parts of the body. The traditional neurological approach defines the peripheral nervous system as being composed of the cranial and spinal nerves with their associated ganglia [9]. Descriptions of neurological pain in peripheral locations are varied and can include any of the adjectives listed previously under central pain of either episodic or constant typologies, depending upon the location and type of pathology involved.

Headache, frequently associated with neurological disorders, can manifest itself either in episodic or constant patterns of pain. While common, headache is rarely discussed in literature dealing with pain. Therefore, a special section of this chapter has been devoted to the mechanism of headache and its nursing management.

Headache

Head pain may originate in (1) tissues covering the cranium, (2) cranial periosteum, and (3) certain intracranial structures [27]. The intracranial structures that are sensitive to pain include the blood vessels and venous sinuses, the cranial nerves with sensory fibers, the first three cervical nerves, and the dura at the base of the brain. Structures that are insensitive to pain include the cranium, the brain, most of the dura and the pia-arachnoid, the choroid plexus, and the ependymal linings of the ventricles.

Blood vessels are the most frequent source of head pain. Vasodilation, displacement of the vessels, or traction on the vessel can stimulate nerve endings in the immediate area of the vessel walls and result in pain. Migraine headache is an excellent example of pain resulting from vasodilation. Displacement of vessels and traction on vessels can be caused by any space-occupying lesion—tumor, hematoma, enlarged ventricles, or cerebral edema—or by rapid changes in cerebrospinal fluid pressure. Pain arising in vessels can be transmitted along the sensitive cranial or cervical nerves with typical pain patterns emerging. In general, pain arising from pain-sensitive intracranial structures above the tentorium is transmitted by the trigeminal nerve and is readily referred to the eye and forehead of the same side [13]. Pain arising from structures below the tentorium is transmitted by the glossopharyngeal nerve, the vagus, and the first three cervical nerves [11] and is referred to the back of the head and the upper part of the neck. Pain arising from extracranial arteries is usually localized in the area of the affected vessel. Headache of vascular origin will tend to throb with the pulse wave and can be made worse with exertion, coughing, and straining. Friedman [8] has estimated that in cases of chronic recurrent headache, 85 to 90 percent are vascular headaches of the migraine type, muscle-contraction headaches, or a combination of these two.

Pain can arise directly from nerve endings or nerve fibers. Pressure on a nerve, inflammation of the nerve or nerve sheath, or abnormal transmission of impulses, whether due to chemical abnormalities or tissue injury, can account for pain. Pressure can be exerted on intracranial nerves by any of the space-occupying lesions noted before. Herpes is a common example of pain due to inflammation of a nerve. Pain of neuralgias, such as tic douloureux, may be due to abnormalities in transmission. The pain will radiate along the nerve fiber and may occur as headache or as facial pain, depending upon the distribution of the stimulated nerves. This type of pain is often described as an intense burning or shooting pain.

Headache literally means a pain in the head and is one of the most common complaints of man. The degree to which headache will be incapacitating to an individual is determined by the frequency and severity of the attacks. As with any pain, headache is a symptom; it may be a symptom of intracranial or systemic disease, or it may be symptomatic of a stress reaction. As progress has been made in understanding the pathophysiology of headache, various classification systems based on this knowledge have emerged. Categories that are common to many of these systems include: (1) vascular headache of the migraine type, (2) muscle-contraction headache, (3) headache of nasal vasomotor reaction, (4) psychogenic headache, (5) traction headache, (6) headache due to disease of cranial or neck structures.

The large majority of persons treated for headache will be followed on an outpatient basis. Some may be seen in pain clinics or headache clinics, and a few will be hospitalized for diagnostic tests if intracranial or systemic disease is suspected. The diagnosis and management of headache falls within the purview of medical practice; however, nurses may assume increasing responsibility for history taking and patient teaching in many outpatient settings. During a period of hospitalization, the nurse will administer prescribed medical care or nursing care to alleviate the discomfort of headache.

A brief description of pathology and symptoms of some common headaches will be given. Medical therapy and nursing management pertinent to the maintenance of comfort and relief of pain will be discussed later in the chapter.

Vascular Headache of Migraine

Vascular headaches of the migraine type have been described for centuries. Within the last few decades, they have been the focus of many studies, but the etiology of migraine is still not definitely established. There is agreement that a phase of intracranial arterial constriction occurs, which is followed by a period of vasodilation of extracranial origin [8]. It is during the period of vasodilation that the attack of pain occurs.

Migraine is characterized by recurrent attacks of headache which may vary in intensity, frequency, and duration. It occurs more frequently in women, and, in 25 percent of the cases, the first attack occurs at age 10 or younger [13]. The classic migraine and the common or nonclassic migraine are the most frequently occurring types of migraine. These two painful varieties of migraine headache are differentiated on the basis of symptoms, both prodromal and during the attack.

Classic migraine is preceded by symptoms of sharply defined neurological disturbances referred to as the aura. The focal neurological symptoms can include various types of visual disturbances, abnormal sensations, or distorted sensory perceptions, and, on occasion, muscle weakness. In contrast, the prodromal symptoms of common migraine may be vague and include such signs as mood changes, gastrointestinal disturbances, and disturbances in fluid balance. They may precede the attack by hours or days. Nausea and sometimes vomiting may be associated with both types during the attack. Attacks are commonly unilateral, although the involved side may alternate from one attack to another. The pain may be located in the frontal and temporal regions, may be felt behind the eye, or it may extend over the entire head [13]. It is frequently described as a throbbing, pulsating pain. As the vessel wall becomes edematous and loses its resiliency, the pain will change to a constant ache [26]. The pain of common migraine is frequently of longer duration than that of classic migraine. Patten [24] has described a type of atypical migraine in which the pain is located behind one eye and is of a stabbing or bursting quality but rarely pulsating. The pain is typically of severe intensity.

A number of factors have been implicated as precipitating causes. In women, the attacks may be consistently related to the menstrual cycle, occurring just prior to or during menses. Tyramine and monosodium glutamate ingested in foods, fatigue, glaring lights, vasodilating drugs, and contraceptive drugs have all been shown to trigger migraine in some individuals. Stress and personality characteristics have been emphasized as factors in migraine. Some authors refer to a "migraine personality"; the characteristics generally identified are compulsiveness, perfectionism, rigidity, sensitivity to criticism, and overconscientiousness. This description of "migraine personalities" has been difficult to substantiate, since many studies have lacked appropriate control groups for purposes of comparison. Stress does seem to be implicated as a precipitating factor in some attacks, but it is often not the amount of stress as much as the significance of the stressful event that is important [8]. The headache will frequently occur following the stressful event rather than during the event.

Muscle-Contraction Headache

Muscle-contraction headache refers to tension, psychogenic, or nervous headache [8]. It is associated with and results from sustained contraction of muscles in the face, scalp, neck, and shoulders. This contraction can be emotionally induced (the typical tension headache) or can be secondary to underlying structural problems in joints and muscles [6]. The development of the headache frequently coincides with periods of tension, worry, or emotional stress, but, unlike migraine which occurs after the stressful event, muscle-contraction headache often accompanies the stressful period [7].

The pain of muscle-contraction headache is frequently suboccipital with the center of discomfort in the back of the head and the neck. However, the pain may involve other areas of the face and head, and if so, most often will be lateral. It is described as a constant or steady pain, frequently as an ache or a sensation of tightness, pressure, or constriction. It does not have the throbbing quality of migraine and is generally not as intense as migraine. The headache may be associated with a general feeling of fatigue, depression, or tension. Infrequently, it may be accompanied by nausea and vomiting. The muscle-contraction headache is not characterized by any periodic pattern of occurrence; it can remain almost constant for weeks or even months. It may alternate with migraine in certain individuals [8].

Personality factors may be of importance as causative factors with this type of headache when it is not secondary to structural pathology. Anxiety, tension, or intrapsychic conflicts are almost always present with the primary muscle-contraction headache [17]. These factors must be considered when pain management is undertaken.

Headache of Systemic or Intracranial Origin

Headache can be symptomatic of intracranial vascular disease. According to Dinsdale [2], "the headache of sub-arachnoid hemorrhage is one of the most excruciating pains experienced by man." The onset is sudden, and the pain is intense. It initially may be localized before spreading over the head and neck. Transient loss of consciousness may occur with the onset, and rigidity of the neck occurs as the meninges become irritated. Intense focal headaches may have preceded an actual bleed, having occurred in the area of an aneurysm or arteriovenous malformation. The focal headaches or the actual bleed is often preceded by some type of physical exertion. Any headache that is intermittent and consistently in the same location should always be taken seriously, and the individual should seek medical care. Although headache may occur with other cerebrovascular accidents, both hemorrhagic and ischemic, the headache assumes importance because of the resulting discomfort caused if the patient is alert rather than as a diagnostic symptom when other neurological deficits are present. Headache may occur with systemic disease, such as hypertension; one author estimates that it occurs in about 50 percent of the cases of essential hypertension [12]. It may be described as throbbing [7] or dull and generalized [12]. It tends to occur upon awakening and to disappear as the individual is up and around.

Cerebral edema and space-occupying lesions can cause headache by increasing intracranial pressure as well as by traction on pain-sensitive structures. Headaches of this type frequently have a constant, deep, aching quality and are generalized. If due to a tumor, the headache may be intermittent early in the disease and later become more frequent and of longer duration. The headache may be mild or severe but tends to become more intense as the tumor progresses [32]. These headaches may occur at night and awaken the individual [7]. The headache may be associated with a variety of symptoms indicating interference with neurological functioning, e.g., memory loss, personality change, and altered levels of consciousness. Tenderness of the skull as well as nausea and vomiting may also accompany the headache [32].

This has been a brief description of the common types of headaches that are most likely to confront the nurse. Table 14-1 presents a summary of characteristics most often associated with the headaches that have been discussed. There are a number of other conditions in which one of the symptoms can be headache; for further discussion of headache, the reader is referred to items in the Reference section.

Table 14-1 Typical characteristics of pain associated with headaches caused by different pathological conditions

Condition	Location	Intensity	Quality	Duration/ frequency	Associated factors
Migraine	Usually unilateral	Severe	Throbbing	Few hours to days/varies	Prodromal symptoms ("triggering factors") may exist. Nausea and vomiting may occur.
Muscle-contraction	Usually bilateral Frequently suboccipital	Mild to severe	Constricting, tightness, constant ache	Hours to weeks/varies	Tension may accompany. Muscles of neck frequently contracted.
Subarachnoid hemorrhage	Initially may be localized, then become general	Excruciating	Intense, constant ache	Days/occurs following bleeding	Physical exertion may precede. May be accompanied by L.O.C. and neck pain/stiffness.
Hypertension	Generalized	Mild to moderate	Throbbing or dull	Few hours/ daily in mornings	Will disappear when patient up and about.

Nursing Interventions for Patients with Neurological Pain

Neurological Pain–Peripheral Locations

In general, neurological pain in peripheral locations usually results from traumatic incidents, vascular disturbances, neoplasms, or degenerative disorders; infectious processes may also serve as pathophysiological causes. Treatment of neurological pain in peripheral locations usually involves surgical intervention or subsequent degrees of immobilization, or both.

Nursing care for this group of patients, therefore, tends to be primarily supportive with the nurse taking care to ensure maintenance of correct limb alignment, position, and prevention of additional complications. There may be need for patient education regarding what, if any, motor or sensory dysfunction (or a combination of both) may exist to ensure adaptation of the patient to his or her particular condition. In general, nursing interventions associated with the care of patients experiencing peripheral nerve dysfunctions depend on the type, location, and extent of injury or involvement.

Neurological Pain–Central Locations

Nursing management and interventions for this group of patients must focus on supportive and adaptive mechanisms. The pain associated with pathological processes of the central nervous system is severe and excruciating. It is often the most difficult kind of pain for health professionals to comprehend.

Once, in talking with a nurse colleague who was experiencing post-herpetic pain, I asked her to describe her pain in such a way that I could begin to appreciate the degree or level of severity of the pain she was experiencing. She could not do this. I asked if she was ever pain-free, and she responded, "No." Then I asked her to describe the least amount of pain she ever experienced with her condition. She replied that the least amount of pain she has ever experienced would be comparable to the severe, excruciating headache that a person occasionally experiences, which is located behind the eyes and which becomes more painful when one tries to move one's eyes in any direction.

An excruciating headache is frequently incapacitating for most people, and yet, it is the least amount of pain experienced by others, all of whom must continue to function or to cease existing. It is small wonder that persons with post-herpetic pain mount a never-ending search for relief.

Nurses can do little to offset or minimize pain of central origin. Interventions need to be directed toward supportive measures and attempts to assist patients in adapting to their condition. These patients need help in finding a coping mechanism for dealing with the pain. Coping mechanisms may be cognitive, such as distraction or dissociation therapies, or more assertive ones, such as the operant conditioning programs. The nurse can be instrumental in assisting the patient to consider transfer to one of the available pain clinics or in allowing the patient to verbalize about his pain and concerns for the future. Nurses must be knowledgeable about current therapies to treat pain—their advantages, disadvantages, and risks (pharmacological, surgical, and medical)—and use this information in answering each patient's questions about alternative methods of therapy that could be offered to him for the alleviation of his pain.

Patients receiving pharmacological agents need to be informed of the possible side effects and sensory alterations they might experience while taking drugs. Total relief of pain of neurological origin by pharmacological agents is rare, even with the administration of narcotics such as morphine.

The nursing care of patients undergoing surgical procedures designed to relieve pain of neurological origin or chronic pain syndromes, or both, is dependent upon the type of intervention being done. For example, the nursing care of a patient undergoing a cordotomy will vary depending on the method used to perform the cordotomy (surgical versus percutaneous technique) and the spinal cord level being severed (cervical level versus either the thoracic or lumbar areas). The reader is referred to Chapter 7 for an in-depth presentation of current therapies utilizing surgical approaches and the variety of locations at which surgical intervention is employed. These patients experience postoperative pain and discomfort that is similar to that which is experienced by any patient undergoing a surgical procedure. Care of postoperative pain is discussed in detail in Chapter 15.

In addition to postoperative pain and discomfort, however, these patients can experience a wide range of complications and disabilities subsequent to surgical interventions designed to alleviate pain. The specific type and extent of complication(s) are again dependent upon the level and extent of the procedure performed. For example, there may be some degree of neurological loss, or dysfunction or alterations in sensation, or both. It is not infrequent to find the pain recurring after a period of time or, even more distressing, the sensation of pain may be replaced by various peculiar sensory disturbances that may ultimately become more diffuse and severe than the original pain for which relief had been sought [16].

Patients experiencing the surgical procedure of cordotomy may experience complications such as respiratory distress and dysfunction, bowel and bladder dysfunction, hypotension, and motor weakness or paralysis. Complications such as these depend on the level of cord treated and appear less frequently with percutaneous techniques as compared to surgical methods [15].

Patients developing complications as a result of procedures designed to alleviate their pain present a nursing challenge from both physiological and psychological perspectives. Nursing observations with regard to motor and sensory function or dysfunction are very important. It is essential to maintain the patient's present capabilities and prevent additional complications such as pulmonary and urinary tract infections, skin breakdown and decubitus formation, and circulatory stasis. The patient needs support to accept and cope with the results of attempts to alleviate pain whether the results be positive or negative. Patients may require a program of rehabilitation and reeducation depending upon the success or failure of attempts to alleviate pain of neurological origin or chronic pain syndromes, or both.

Recent advances in the alleviation of pain employ techniques of electrical stimulation by placement of electrodes externally on or through the skin, stimulation of spinal cord or peripheral nerves, or stimulation of various areas of the brain [15]. Nursing care of these patients is a relatively new aspect and is given special attention and consideration at the end of this chapter.

Nursing Management of the Headache Patient

Management of migraine and muscle-contraction headache is directed toward preventive and symptomatic treatment. Preventive measures may include any combination of patient education, pharmacotherapy, and psychotherapy. The aspect of care with which the nurse will most likely be involved is patient education. Such education will include information concerning headache control and the medications that are prescribed.

The patient should be assisted in identifying and eliminating the precipitating factors that are present. If migraine attacks are precipitated by foods high in tyramine or monosodium glutamate, these foods should be eliminated from the diet. Foods to be avoided on a tyramine-restricted diet include beer, wine, and liquors; cheese; chicken livers; smoked or pickled fish; yogurt; and chocolate [29]. Monosodium glutamate is added to a number of foods during processing, and labels must be read to avoid this additive in the diet. Regular meals without excessive carbohydrates should be taken to avoid reactive hypoglycemia; fasting should also be avoided. Muscle-contraction headaches that are related to structural disease will be treated by the physician with methods aimed at correcting the underlying pathology; such treatment may eliminate the significant causative factor for these headaches. In the absence of pathology, the patient may benefit from education in techniques of voluntary muscle relaxation and correction of body posture [17].

Since stress may be a precipitating factor with both types of headache, the patient should be advised to distribute tasks in a manner that will eliminate as much as possible the pressure of deadlines and fatigue. Reviewing a typical day or week with the patient and assisting him to find a way to decrease periods of peak activity might prove beneficial. If migraine attacks are related to the menstrual cycle, it is especially important to prevent fatigue and unnecessary stress at this time. Counseling to assist the individual in rearranging the pressures of daily life may not be sufficient; if intensive psychotherapy is necessary, the patient should be referred to an appropriate therapist. The patient with emotionally induced muscle-contraction headache often will benefit from formal psychotherapy.

A variety of drugs may be prescribed in an attempt to eliminate attacks. Barbiturates, tranquilizers, and antidepressants may be helpful if there is a need to reduce anxiety or treat an underlying depression. Tranquilizers with muscle-relaxing properties, such as diazepam (Valium) or meprobamate (Miltown), may be prescribed with or without psychotherapy as prophylaxis for the patient with muscle-contraction headache [6]. Diphenylhydantoin (Dilantin), diuretics, histamine, and hormones are sometimes prescribed for migraine, but these compounds are not significantly more effective than placebos [8]. The drug that has been most effective for migraine prophylaxis is methysergide maleate (Sansert). It is indicated for patients with frequent (one or more per week) severe headaches, or headaches of such severity that acute attacks are difficult to control [8]. Unfortunately, serious adverse reactions—retroperitoneal fibrosis, pleuropulmonary fibrosis, and fibrotic thickening of the cardiac valves—may occur. Therefore, patients *must* remain under the supervision of the physician and *must* take the medication only as prescribed. The patient is generally on the medication for six months and off for two months, and he needs to understand the necessity for the rest period. Positive suggestion should be used with any of the medications prescribed for chronic headache; the patient should not be given the idea that the medication may not be effective or that other medication is readily available if the prescribed drug fails to control pain. As with any medication, patients should be told of any side effects that need to be observed and reported.

Symptomatic treatment of acute attacks includes the use of medication and comfort measures. Acute attacks of migraine may sometimes be controlled with acetylsalicylic acid (aspirin) if taken at or shortly before the onset of the headache; if not taken early, aspirin is not likely to be effective [3]. Ergotamine tartrate is the most effective drug for pain relief with migraine. It is important that the patient understand the correct amount and method of administration as well as the need to take the medication early in the attack. The medication should be carried at all times so it can be taken as soon as possible during the attack. Females should not take the drug if menses are late until the possibility of pregnancy has been ruled out.

For muscle-contraction headache, nonnarcotic analgesics and a tranquilizer with muscle-relaxing properties may be prescribed. The medication should be taken during the beginning stages of headache development before the pain becomes too severe. Rest is essential with both types of headache if the action of the medication is to be most effective. The patient needs to be told to slow down and assume a comfortable position after taking the drug if he is not in the habit of doing so. Narcotics, although effective in producing pain relief, are rarely prescribed because of the frequency with which they would need to be used and the possibility of addiction.

Other measures that may prove helpful in alleviating pain during an acute attack should be tried and evaluated. Many individuals find rest in a darkened room helpful for migraine. Cold compresses or gentle pressure to the painful area may provide relief for some individuals during an attack of migraine. In muscle-contraction headaches, relaxation of tense muscles may prove beneficial. Measures that can be used include hot packs to the neck or back of the head or immersion in warm water [8]. Gentle stroking massage may serve as an adjunct to the use of heat for relaxation of the neck and shoulder muscles [17].

New ideas in treatment are being evaluated with sufferers of migraine or muscle-contraction headaches. Autogenic feedback training, in which individuals learn to regulate temperature differences between the scalp and fingers by increasing blood flow to the hands, has been tested with both types of headache [19]. The improvement shown with some migraine sufferers may be due to redistribution of blood flow causing vasoconstriction (cooling) of the scalp. Training the patient in the use of relaxation techniques using electromyographic (EMG) feedback has proved beneficial in some initial studies for muscle-contraction headache [35]. Autohypnosis has been attempted but has not been evaluated with enough patients to determine the extent of its effectiveness. Until such time as these techniques are more fully evaluated, pharmacotherapy remains the most common method of treating migraine or muscle-contraction headache.

Medical management of headaches due to systemic or intracranial pathology will be directed toward the diagnosis and treatment of the underlying condition. Nursing management will consist of comfort measures, the appropriate administration of prescribed analgesics, and alleviation of tension and anxiety during this period of diagnosis and treatment. Measures pertinent to the treatment of the pathology may also be effective in providing pain relief. Although this kind of management sounds relatively easy, the ingenuity of the nurse may be taxed in finding the best method of providing comfort when headache pain is severe.

Nursing Care of the Patient with a Biostimulator

Recent advances in and increased use of biostimulators open wide areas of nursing care previously not known. Specific guidelines for care were developed by Joann Eland of the University of Iowa and are being used with her permission.

Electrical stimulation for the relief of chronic pain is not a new concept. Recent technological developments have brought about new devices and an increasing number of people, including neurologists, neurosurgeons, nurses, and patients, are finding themselves involved in one way or another with the concept of electrical stimulation.

Transcutaneous Nerve Stimulation (TNS)

Transcutaneous Nerve Stimulation (TNS) is one method of relieving chronic pain on a permanent basis. It can also be used to screen people for implantable devices such as dorsal column or peripheral nerve stimulators. A TNS system consists of two electrodes (one positive, one negative) that are attached by flexible wires to a battery pack. On the battery pack are two or three controls, depending on the make and model, that control the voltage, frequency, and pulse width. See page 324. The nurse must know about such factors as electrode placement, taping, conductive jelly, adjustment of the various controls, and the changing of batteries. In order for a patient to obtain maximum benefit from TNS, a program of patient education must be initiated by the nurse.

Electrode Placement

The placement of electrodes differs with each individual and is worked out empirically by physician and patient. Initially, electrodes are placed over an area where a nerve is relatively superficial and, therefore, more easily stimulated; for example, the ulnar nerve at the elbow for arm, shoulder, and chest pain, and the common peroneal nerve at the fibula head for hip and back pain. If this placement is not effective, then the electrodes are positioned close to the site of the pain, such as near a painful scar, or along the course of the involved nerve, the paraspinal region, or along the dermatome pattern of the painful area. If neither of these placements is successful, stimulation is then tried along the corresponding acupuncture meridians. Nurses may need to explain why the physician has placed the electrodes in a certain location. For example, a patient may not understand how an electrode along the paravertebral region could possibly help the pain in his leg.

Electrodes must be taped flat against the skin to provide maximum contact. The tape should be wide enough to secure maximum contact between the electrodes and the skin. Pieces of tape should be just long enough to anchor the electrodes securely because excessive tape pulls and irritates skin. Usually an inch of tape beyond the electrode on each end is adequate; however, different areas of the body may require methods other than taping for securing electrodes. At times, Ace wraps or antiembolism stockings are more suitable for securing electrodes to extremities.

There are two electrodes in a TNS system, one carrying a positive charge and one carrying a negative charge. Usually, the positive electrode produces a greater sensation of stimulation than does the negative, and patients frequently will feel that they are getting more of a sensation of stimulation from the positive electrode. The nurse can capitalize on this feeling of the patient in the placement of the electrodes. For example, if a patient were stimulating the ulnar nerve at the wrist, she could place the electrode that was giving the greater sensation of "power" over that area, and thus be delivering more sensation to the nerve itself. If the nurse has reapplied or retaped the electrodes and finds that the electrode delivering the power sensation is not the one she thought it was, she can change the polarity of the two electrodes by turning the stimulator off, unplugging them at the battery pack, and switching them at the battery pack as opposed to taking off the tape and reapplying the electrodes.

Conducting jelly is applied to the electrode in a thin coat, evenly spread over the surface of the electrode which, in turn, is placed next to the skin. Because electrode conductive jelly dries out and loses its contact every six to eight hours, the electrodes should be washed at these time intervals. The manufacturer's instructions regarding the cleaning of electrodes may vary slightly from model to model. The skin under the electrodes has a tendency to break down because it is constantly subjected to the electrode conductive jelly. Proper skin care is necessary so that the patient's problem will not be compounded. Some patients who have negative reactions to the electrode jelly can use hand cream, which also conducts electrical impulses and is less irritating than electrode jelly.

Adjustment of the Controls, Voltage, Frequency, and Pulse Width

The adjustment of the voltage (output), frequency (rate), and pulse width are very important. The settings of these three controls are different for each patient. Proper adjustment can make the difference between success and failure with the stimulator. It is absolutely imperative that the nurse and the patient work together to obtain the settings that are best for him and experiment with all conceivable combinations and settings. It may take several days to adjust the unit to its maximum efficiency. Patients need to be encouraged to experiment on their own with these controls.

After the electrodes are taped on and plugged into the battery pack, the patient can adjust the various controls. To begin with, all controls should be set at the lowest setting possible. The output, or voltage control, is adjusted first. The sensational electrical stimulation is sometimes described as "tingling, buzzing, prickly, or warm-feeling." The output control is turned on until the patient begins to feel the sensation of stimulation. Patients frequently make the mistake of thinking that the more voltage they can endure, the more relief they will obtain; this is simply not true. Therefore, when the patient begins to feel the sensation of stimulation, the voltage adjustment should be stopped and other controls adjusted. It is possible that the patient may require more voltage after the other controls are adjusted. The nurse and patient must remember that a biostimulator improperly used can create pain or make existing pain worse.

The rate control regulates how many impulses per second are delivered through the electrodes to the skin. As with the output control, the rate is also highly individualized. It is sometimes hard for a patient to decide what the appropriate rate control setting should be for him. Whatever the setting, it should not be unpleasant nor should it cause any twitching of muscles.

The pulse-width control is not present on all makes and models of stimulators. It is mentioned here to assist nurses and patients who use stimulators with this specific control. The description of the sensation caused by the pulse-width control is elusive. Some patients feel it is of absolutely no value, while others feel it is as valuable as the other two controls. Patients who do find it valuable say that the pulse-width control regulates the depth of penetration of the electrical stimulus. The use of pulse-width control is a fairly new development in electrical stimulation, and time is needed to evaluate it effectively.

After all controls are set, providing the sensation is *not* unpleasant, they should be left alone for at least one half hour. At the end of one half hour, if relief is not being obtained, all the controls are left at their settings, and readjustment is begun in this sequence: voltage, rate, and pulse width. If the patient cannot tolerate an increase in voltage (i.e., if it causes pain or is unpleasant), then repeated attempts should be made to adjust the rate or the pulse width, or both.

The settings of all controls may vary with changes in body position, taping, the drying out of conductive jelly, and the decreasing output of batteries over time. Patience and perseverance on the part of the nurse and the patient are extremely important to obtain the settings that will best benefit the patient.

Batteries and Mechanical Failure

Usually the stimulators the nurse will use in a hospital setting will have fresh batteries. Obviously, a dead battery cannot stimulate. On occasion, batteries sit in factories or physicians' offices long enough to lose part of their charge. If a person is using the stimulator continuously, he can drain the batteries in as quickly as one to two weeks. When dead batteries are suspected, place the electrodes on a flat surface, put fingers of the same hand on both electrodes, and turn the unit on. If the electrical tingling sensation is felt, the stimulator is working. If there is no sensation, new batteries should be inserted, and the unit rechecked. Patients should be instructed to use alkaline batteries, which have much longer life with constant use than do ordinary batteries.

Caution should be used in handling any stimulator to avoid damage by banging or dropping it. Needless to say, the battery packs themselves should never be in water.

Because of the complexities involved, it may take a week or two for a person to obtain pain relief from a biostimulator. At times a patient's first comments may not appear to relate to pain relief. He may for example report that he is still experiencing pain but will relate a change in his sleeping patterns. (He may be sleeping longer or more soundly than he had been prior to stimulation.) The patient's comment may be coincidental or may reflect his learned pain behaviors. After many years of pain if the painful stimulus is removed a patient's reaction to painful stimuli may still be present. A patient who has used stimulation successfully for two years related that if she has pain upon awakening and turns on her stimulator her pain will stop immediately; however, it takes one to two hours for her anxiety and her generalized reaction to the stimulus to stop.

Many patients who are trying stimulation have had multiple hospitalizations, several surgeries, many medication experiences, and, in general, have tried everything imaginable to relieve their pain. It is imperative that they be encouraged to give stimulation a fair chance (at *least* one week or more of constant experimentation). Sometimes nurses need to insist that they try it for that period of time, despite protests. Electrical simulation is not for everyone, but it can provide pain relief for many people if it is used properly. It is also very important that nurses assume their responsibility in helping patients work through the initial difficulties they may encounter in using biostimulators effectively.

Peripheral Nerve Stimulators and Dorsal Column Stimulators

Because the underlying principles and nursing interventions are the same for Peripheral Nerve Stimulators (PNS) and Dorsal Column Stimulators (DCS), they will be discussed together. The electrodes and the specific surgical procedures for implantation are different for PNS and DCS. The chapter on Surgical and Electrical Stimulation Methods for Relief of Pain describes their individual differences.

Both PNS and DCS include an external battery pack that has the same patient controls as the TNS system. The battery pack is actually a miniature radio transmitter that sends a radio wave through an externally worn antenna to an internally implanted radio receiver. The radio receiver, somewhat smaller than a pocket watch, transforms the radio wave into electrical pulses that travel from the receiver through a subcutaneous wire to the electrode itself. See Figure 14-1.

After the electrode(s) and receiver are surgically implanted in the patient, the time between surgery and the activation of the system depends upon the surgeon involved. The only absolute requirement for activating the unit is that the patient must be alert. All dressings from the surgical procedure are left in place so there is minimal danger of contaminating the incisions. At the University of Iowa, patients are usually activated on the first day postoperatively if they are alert.

Implanting the units has some common aftereffects during the postoperative period. There will be pain from the wire, which is pushed subcutaneously, either with a Kelly clamp or uterine forceps, from the electrode to the radio receiver. As would be expected, wire tracking creates edema and fluid around the wires, making the area where they are passed rather painful in the immediate postoperative period. Another painful area is the subcutaneous pocket created by the surgeon where the radio receiver is placed. With both types of units, there will be incisional pain. The nurse needs to be aware of these various types of pain associated with implantation and needs to intervene with appropriate pain-relief measures. The reader is referred to Chapter 15 on surgical pain for nursing interventions concerning pain-relief measures.

To activate either a PNS or DCS, the center of the antenna, which is a round rubber disk about three inches in diameter, is placed over the center of the implanted receiver and taped in a way to maximize the contact be-

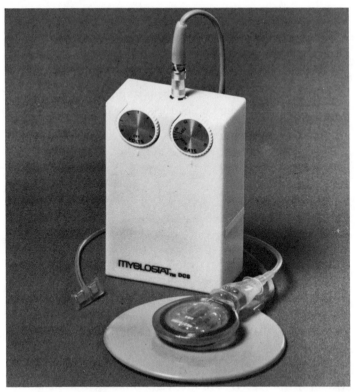

Figure 14-1 Myelostat–dorsal column stimulator. (Medtronic, Inc., 3055 Old Highway Eight, Minneapolis, Minn., 55418.)

tween the antenna and the skin. It has been our experience that three pieces of tape about five inches in length are sufficient to secure the antenna, if they are placed in a triangular configuration on the outside borders of the antenna. See Figure 14-2. After the antenna is secured to the skin, it is attached to the battery pack (transmitter), and the transmitter is then activated. The controls on the PNS and DCS are the same as the controls on the transcutaneous nerve stimulator and the reader is referred to the section on TNS for their adjustments. It is important to note that even if a person with a DCS or PNS has been using a TNS, he is now using a much more efficient system and the settings for the output (voltage), rate (frequency), and pulse width will be different. The patient will again go through an experimentation stage during which he will determine what settings are best for him. The nurse needs to be aware of this all-important stage of experimentation and may need to encourage the patient to continue to try to find the settings that will alleviate his pain.

There are some specific problems relating to the antennas and their receiving of radio waves by the implanted receiver. If the center of the an-

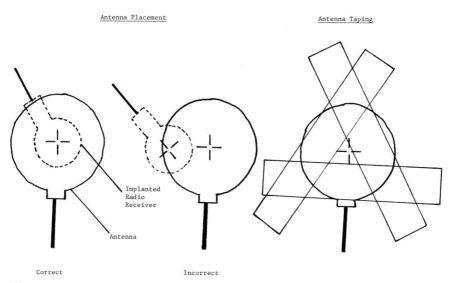

Antenna Placement

Antenna Taping

Implanted
Radio
Receiver

Antenna

Correct

Incorrect

Figure 14-2 Placement and taping of antenna for activation of PNS or DCS.

tenna is not over the center of the receiver, the patient will not receive maximum stimulation. If the tape that holds the antenna in place over the receiver becomes loose, the signal can be either decreased or stopped entirely. The obvious solution for both problems is retaping the antenna. Usually there is an incision and dressing near the receiver that was made when the subcutaneous pocket for the receiver was created. When the center of the antenna is centered over the receiver, a portion of the antenna may cover the dressing; the interference created by the dressing will prohibit effective transmission and reception of the radio signal. In addition, radio signals are not initially received at their maximum strength early in the postoperative stage due to the fluid and edema present around the receiver itself. Neither the patient nor the nurse can do anything specific about the last two problems but be aware of them. The nurse needs to reassure her patient that when the dressing is removed and the fluid and edema are decreased, his reception will be better.

Patients should keep an extra antenna on hand because the unit will stop working if an antenna breaks. If a unit is still malfunctioning after a new battery has been inserted, the most likely cause is a broken antenna.

The antenna can be washed using the manufacturer's suggested method. Care should be taken when cleaning an antenna to avoid getting the electrical connection that joins the antenna to the transmitter wet. A wet connection will cause the unit to malfunction and will probably necessitate the purchase of a new antenna.

Checking batteries with either DCS or PNS is easily accomplished. As earlier noted, the unit is a small radio station. All the patient needs to do is to place the antenna near an AM radio (preferably a transistor set at 540 kilocycles) and turn on the transmitter. If the transmitter and antenna are functioning, the radio will emit a buzzing or static sound. If no buzzing is heard, the battery should be replaced. If no buzzing is heard after the new battery is installed, the antenna should be replaced. If both of these measures fail, the physician should be notified.

As with the transcutaneous nerve stimulator, care should be taken to avoid banging or dropping the unit or submerging it in water.

There are some very distinct advantages to the implantable units. Certainly there is a more direct stimulation than with the transcutaneous unit because a patient is directly stimulating the involved nerves. In addition, the units themselves are smaller and weigh less than TNS units.

Not all patients will benefit from electrical stimulation, but a large part of success or failure is dependent upon the knowledge that both the nurse and the patient have at their disposal.

Summary

This chapter presented an overview of the types and causes of pain generally ascribed to neurological origin. Current theories and terminology relating to discussions of neurological pain were presented. It is difficult, if not impossible, to separate the pain of neurological origin from the pain of any origin because of the reception, transmission, and perception attributes of the neurological system.

Rather than duplicate material covered in other chapters, this chapter attempted to focus on aspects of pain not addressed in other sections of this source book. This accounts for the section dealing with the types, causes, and nursing management of patients with headache; and the section discussing the nursing management of patients with biostimulators.

Because pain of neurological origin is generally severe and frequently not amenable to treatment, the exploration of methods that best alleviate the suffering that must be endured by these individuals is an open arena for research. Nursing studies designed to meet the needs of these patients may provide a promise of hope for the numbers of patients experiencing excruciating pain.

References

1. Dalessio, D. J. Dietary migraine. *Am. Fam. Physician* 6:60, 1972.
2. Dinsdale, H. B. Headache in vascular disease and hypertension. *Headache* 13:85, 1972.
3. Edmeads, J. Management of the acute attack of migraine. *Headache* 13:91, 1973.
4. Fields, H. L., Adams, J. E., and Hosobuchi, Y. Peripheral nerve and cutaneous electrohypalgesia. In Bonica, J. J., ed., *Advances in Neurology* (Vol. 4). New York: Raven Press, 1974. Pp. 749–754.

5. Frazier, S. H., and Kolb, L. C. Psychiatric aspects of pain and the phantom limb. *Orthop. Clin. North Am.* 1:481, 1970.
6. Friedman, A. P. An overview of chronic recurring headache. *Wis. Med. J.* 71:110, 1972.
7. Friedman, A. P. The headache patient: Part I. Headache patterns in diagnosis. *Curr. Concepts Pain Analg.* 1:1, 1974.
8. Friedman, A. P. Headache. *Postgrad. Med.* 53:172, 1973.
9. Gatz, A. J. *Manters Essentials of Clinical Neuroanatomy and Neurophysiology*, 4th ed. Philadelphia: F. A. Davis Company, 1970.
10. Greenhoot, J. H. The management of intractable pain. *Va. Med. Mon.* 97:117, 1970.
11. Horton, B. T. Headache: Clinical varieties and therapeutic suggestions. *Med. Clin. North Am.* 33:973, 1949.
12. Kudrow, L. Systemic causes of headache. *Postgrad. Med.* 56:105, 1974.
13. Lance, J. W. *The Mechanism and Management of Headache*, 2d ed. London: Butterworth & Co., 1973.
14. Loeser, J. D. Central pains. *Clin. Med.* May, 1975.
15. Long, D. M. Recent advances in the management of pain. *Minn. Med.* September, 1974. Pp. 705–709.
16. Maspes, P. E., and Pagni, C. A. A critical appraisal of pain surgery and suggestions for improving treatment. In Bonica, J. J., Procacci, P., and Pagni, C. A., eds., *Recent Advances in Pain: Pathophysiological and Clinical Aspects.* Springfield, Ill.: Charles C Thomas, Publisher, 1974. Pp. 201–255.
17. Martin, M. J., and Kome, H. P. Muscle-contraction headache: Therapeutic aspects. In Friedman, A. P., ed., *Research and Clinical Studies in Headache* (Vol. 1). Baltimore: The Williams & Wilkins Company, 1967. Pp. 205–217.
18. Mehler, W. R. Central pain and the spinothalamic tract. In Bonica, J. J., ed., *Advances in Neurology* (Vol. 4). New York: Raven Press, 1974. Pp. 127–146.
19. Melzack, R. Phantom limb pain: Implications for treatment of pathologic pain. *Anesthesiology* 35:409, 1971.
20. Melzack, R. Central neural mechanisms in phantom limb pain. In Bonica, J. J., ed., *Advances in Neurology* (Vol. 4). New York: Raven Press, 1974. Pp. 319–326.
21. Melzack, R. *The Puzzle of Pain.* New York: Basic Books, Inc., 1973.
22. Noordenbos, W. Pathologic aspects of central pain states. In Bonica, J. J., ed., *Advances in Neurology* (Vol. 4). New York: Raven Press, 1974. Pp. 333–338.
23. Pagni, C. A. Pain due to central nervous system lesions: Physiopathological considerations and therapeutical implications. In Bonia, J. J., ed., *Advances in Neurology* (Vol. 4). New York: Raven Press, 1974. Pp. 339–348.
24. Patten, J. P. Atypical migraine. *The Practitioner* 211:304, 1973.
25. Riddoch, G. *Lancet* 234:1093, 1938.
26. Rubinowitz, M. J. Practical aspects of migraine. *Rocky Mt. Med. J.* 70:37, 1973.
27. Ryan, R. E. *Headache, Diagnosis and Treatment.* St. Louis: The C. V. Mosby Company, 1957.
28. Sargent, J. D., et al. The use of autogenic feedback training in a pilot study of migraine and tension headaches. *Headache* 12:120, 1972.
29. Staff of the Department of Nutrition, University of Iowa Hospitals and Clinics. *Recent Advances in Therapeutic Diets*, 2d ed. Ames, Iowa: Iowa State University Press, 1973.
30. Talbott, J. H. In Bonica, J. J., moderator. Attacking the puzzle of pain—Part I. Pain: Its definition, its effects, and its mechanisms. *Mod. Med.* 42(23):56, 1973.

31. Thomas, P. K.   The anatomical substratum of pain: Evidence derived from morphometric studies on peripheral nerves. *Can. J. Neurol. Sci.* 1(2):92, 1974.
32. von Storch, T. J. C.   Headache in intracranial disorders. In Friedman, A. P., and Merritt, H. H., eds., *Headache: Diagnosis and Treatment*. Philadelphia: F. A. Davis Company, 1959. Pp. 165–200.
33. Wall, P. D.   The mechanisms of pain associated with cervical vertebral disease. In Hirsch, C., and Zotterman, Y., eds., *Cervical Pain*. Oxford: Pergamon Press, Inc., 1972. Pp. 201–210.
34. Wall, P. D.   Physiological mechanisms involved in the production and relief of pain. In Bonica, J. J., Procacci, P., and Pagni, C. A., eds., *Recent Advances in Pain: Pathophysiology and Clinical Aspects*. Springfield, Ill.: Charles C Thomas, Publishers, 1974. P. 63.
35. Wickramasckera, I.   The application of verbal instructions and EMG feedback training to the management of tension headache—Preliminary observations. *Headache* 13:74, 1973.
36. Wilkins, R. H.   Neurosurgical relief of pain: Recent developments. *Tex. Med.* 70:53, 1974.

15

Pain Associated with Surgery

Sandra S. Sweeney

This chapter focuses on the characteristics of pain as they apply to the surgical postoperative patient. The characteristics and mechanisms underlying postoperative pain are presented; and discussion of the intensity, duration, quality, quantity, and meaning of the pain experienced emphasizes the need to individualize interventions on a situationally determined basis. The objective of the chapter is to convey the notion that caring for postoperative patients is a complex undertaking requiring and deserving considerable attention for patients to achieve optimum results with minimal complications.

Patients in the postoperative phase of their therapy comprise a unique group of individuals with particular needs and concerns—not the least of which includes the relief of pain. The nursing care and management of these patients is challenging and complex. While the nursing literature continues to emphasize the need for individualizing patient care, such specificity of care is rarely accorded the postoperative patient. Rather, the care of these patients tends to be given according to "familiar" preestablished standardized routines of care that are uniformly applied to all patients during the postoperative period. While many aspects of the standardized routines of care during both the pre- and postoperative phases of the surgical experience are essential, care must be exercised to preserve, protect, and promote the specific needs of this group of patients. Relief of postoperative pain is an example of such a need.

Pain is a personal and unique experience. Pain is a response by some one individual or thing to a particular noxious stimulus. The pain response possesses certain characteristics such as intensity, duration, quality, quantity, and meaning. The pain response is a complex entity further complicated by the subjectivity with which it is experienced, interpreted, reported, and evaluated.*

---

* Preceding chapters have discussed the characteristics of the pain experience in considerable detail. The reader is referred to previous discussions, especially Chapters 1, 2, and 3, for this information.

Incidence of Postoperative Pain

The degree to which a patient experiences pain in response to surgery is related to both physiological and psychological factors. Attempts to correlate incidence and severity of postoperative pain with numerous variables generally have been unsuccessful as evidenced in an early study by Keats, who attempted to determine whether or not relationships could be established between the severity of postoperative pain and age, sex, type and duration of anesthesia, previous surgical history and hospitalizations, incidence and severity of preoperative pain, and personality types or disorders [26]. Absence of associations between pain and any of the preceding variables prompted Keats to conclude that the incidence and severity of postoperative pain is randomly distributed among patients with regard to various patient characteristics. Beecher [1], likewise, was unable to determine any correlation between the incidence and severity of pain and the size of the wound, the patient's age, anesthetics used, or previous health histories of either acute or chronic conditions. While later studies suggest that there may be some relationship between severity of postoperative pain and personality characteristics such as neuroticism, dependence, and so forth [4, 36, 40, 43], such findings often are based on small samples of patients and are not reported consistently enough to allow for predictability. Confusion is also created when discussing the concepts of incidence and severity because of the closeness of their meanings and interpretation. Loan and Morrison [32] differentiate between the two concepts by associating incidence of postoperative pain with surgical sites and severity with the variables of personality, age, sex, physical status, surgical sites and management, environment, and preanesthetic medication and anesthesia. For purposes of this chapter, however, the two terms are viewed as being closely associated and therefore synonymous.

Postoperative pain as usually experienced by patients tends to be of short duration and acute in nature. One would expect to encounter few problems in studying it, but quite the reverse is true. Swerdlow [42] suggests two major problems that create difficulty in studying postoperative pain. The first problem he identifies is the lack of available knowledge regarding the natural course of postoperative pain, i.e., what occurs naturally—without benefit of drugs, anesthetics, and so forth—remains essentially unknown. The second problem relates to the fact that postoperative pain occurs against a constantly moving background. That is, patients in the initial phase of the postoperative period may be experiencing the effects of anesthesia and drugs that can create altered states of awareness. When the patient regains full consciousness, several modifying influences may affect the pain experience. Examples of modifying influences identified by Swerdlow are the significance of the operation, the awareness of other patients and health team members, the need to appear brave, and the need to receive comfort. In later recovery phases the level of pain diminishes in intensity and occurrence and patients experience difficulty in remembering their pain.

The surgical experience places formidable physiological and psychological demands on the human organism, frequently complicated by coexisting pathological processes. The patient's response to surgery and postoperative pain is the result of a lifetime of experience, cultural and religious influences, learned responses to pain, and resources for coping with life.

The psychological make-up of the patient is an important element to be considered, particularly in terms of his ability to respond and adapt to stress. There are some specific psychological concerns which the surgical experience creates for the individual. One is the nature and location of the operation and the meaning this has for the individual, that is, the emotional investment associated with the part of the body that is involved. Whether or not a surgical procedure is elective or exploratory, if an organ is retained or removed, if more than one incision is necessary, possible cosmetic effects, and whether or not a body part (arm, leg, breast, and so forth) is lost are all potential sources of concern to the patient.

The patient's psychological state during the actual pain experience also is important. Whether or not a patient is depressed, anxious, excited, or resistant will modify the effects of identical noxious stimuli. Another factor contributing to the patient's pain response is his level of awareness. The diffuse awareness of a patient who is barely awake will elicit a different response than will an emotional awareness that allows him to attribute either a good or bad value to a particular stimulus, or a higher level of intellectual awareness that provides for both temporal and spatial analysis of various stimuli [7].

The location of the surgery also has physiological implications for the degree of postoperative pain. Incisions involving the thoracic, upper abdominal, and abdominal cavities are reputed to produce the greatest amount of postoperative pain and related discomforts due to the proximity of the diaphragm and the respiratory function. Anorectal surgery is the next most painful type followed by operations involving the back. Pain associated with these surgeries is usually the result of muscle spasms [5].

Closely related to location and a definite factor in the production of postoperative pain is the extent of surgery. The extent to which the body is subjected to surgical trauma, the kind and amount of manipulation received by the internal organs, and the duration of the surgical procedure all influence the degree of postoperative pain from a physiological aspect.

Physiological and psychological aspects of the surgical experience act in combination to produce the postoperative patient's reaction and response. Quimby [39] illustrates the interrelatedness of these aspects when he suggests that it is easy to predict the site and intensity of physical pain but difficult to predict the psychological response. He states that incisional pain of the bunionectomy patient generally will not be as severe as incisional pain associated with either a thoracotomy or cholecystectomy, but asserts that the psychological reaction of a patient to pain associated with any surgical procedure will be the determining factor in the extent to which the patient will cooperate with the postoperative regimen of treatment. Knowledge of the influence that both physiological and psychological factors can exert on the postoperative phase of treatment can provide a baseline of information upon which the health professional can begin to plan postoperative care.

The wide variation in patients' response to surgical procedures also is evident in studies reporting on postoperative drug use. Keats [26] found that 21 percent of 104 patients having major abdominal surgery (gastrectomy or colectomy) received either one dose or no pain medication during their postoperative period. Papper and his group [35] found that 44 percent of 237 patients and Jaggard et al [20] reported that 36 percent of 1,005 postoperative patients received little or no pain-alleviating narcotics while recovering from surgery. Papper's study also included 108 patients with intraabdominal or intrathoracic procedures of which 27 percent recovered from surgery without complaints of postoperative pain and without receiving any medication. Parkhouse and his associates [37] sought to determine correlations between types of surgical procedures and the proportions of patients requiring postoperative analgesia. Data obtained from approximately 1,000 patients demonstrated the following results: cholecystectomy and gastric surgery, 95 percent; upper abdominal surgery, 82 percent; appendectomy, 75 percent; inguinal herniorrhaphy surgeries, 48 percent; neck and head (superficial) surgical procedures, 55 percent; and minor procedures of the chest wall and scrotal areas, 20 percent. Similar findings regarding associations between sites of surgical procedures and postoperative analgesia have been reported by Loan and Dundee [31] and Keats [26].

Results of these early studies are reinforced by later ones. Keats [27] has combined data from several sources. All categories of postoperative patient are included and the data obtained present an interesting summary of the variation in reports of postoperative pain experienced by patients. According to Keats, approximately 40 percent of all postoperative patients never complain of pain; an additional 20 percent report relief of pain with placebos; 20 percent are relieved of pain by receiving morphine doses of 10 mg or less; slightly more than 10 percent require more than 10 mg of morphine for relief of pain; and the remaining patients (slightly less than 10 percent) never achieve pain relief—even with the administration of narcotics. Bonica [5] supports these findings and comments that in general about one-third of all surgical patients do not experience postoperative pain, as evidenced either by a lack of complaint or by not actively seeking medication. He states that placebos are effective in alleviating pain in one-third to one-half of postoperative pain complaints.

Studies on the incidence of postoperative pain present provocative data for the clinician. It should be emphasized, however, that many of these studies have been conducted to determine the effectiveness of specific analgesic medications on postoperative pain and subsequently data collected may only reflect the patients' demand for such analgesic agents. This means, then, that pain is assumed to exist in those patients requesting medication and presumed absent in those patients not requesting medication. In the course of conducting a research program on pain, it became apparent that many postoperative patients actively deny the presence of pain, but admit to experiencing what they define as discomfort (see Chapters 3 and 5 of this book). Numerous patients stated, "No, I don't have any pain, I'm just uncomfortable." The question arises, then, as to how many patients reported in studies as not experiencing postoperative pain may have been unnecessarily uncomfortable because they were unable to communicate their discomfort within the framework of pain terminology commonly used by health professionals.

In general, patients expect some degree of pain as one of the consequences of surgery and accept this fact as a necessary means to recovery. Nurses and physicians usually anticipate patients' initial complaints of postoperative pain and willingly administer analgesic medications for the first 24 to 48 hours. Patients who conform to this general pattern of postoperative behavior rarely present assessment problems for the health professional charged with their care. Such problems tend to arise, however, with the patient who complains of little or no postoperative pain or, conversely, with the patient who reports severe postoperative pain and requests large doses of medication over prolonged periods of time. The clinician must make a judgment regarding the amount of pain the patient is experiencing, and such judgments often are difficult to make.

Patients experiencing postoperative pain should receive medication and whatever assistance they need to alleviate their pain. Administration of medication, however, should not be done indiscriminately during the postoperative period. Administration of narcotics to patients not complaining of pain may only complicate and further prolong their recovery period due to the depressant effects of narcotics [39]. Nurses and physicians need to have a sound understanding of pain assessment in order to be able to adapt their care according to the vast variation in postoperative pain. (See Chapter 6 on pain assessment in Part I of this book.)

Types and Causal Mechanisms of Postoperative Pain

The literature cites three types of pain as being most frequently experienced by postoperative patients: (1) incisional, (2) somatic, and (3) visceral. Causal mechanisms cited as responsible for producing pain in postoperative patients include both chemical and mechanical means of nociception, i.e., factors that are responsible for producing, interpreting, and transmitting painful sensations. Mechanical causal mechanisms that serve as stimuli for all three types of pain are: distention, spasm, obstruction, edema, traction and contraction, stretching and tearing, inflammation and infection, and pressure—either intra-abdominal or compressive [5, 11, 25, 41]. Chemical causal mechanisms that are generally associated with pain of incisional (i.e., cutaneous) and somatic origins include endogenous pain-producing and threshold-lowering chemical substances [16, 17].

In this chapter, the categories "type" and "causal mechanism" of postoperative pain are used to organize content related to caring for the postoperative patient. However, while certain characteristics concerning incisional pain, for example, can be described, incisional pain per se cannot be isolated from the total response of the person to painful stimuli. Numerous factors are involved in the postoperative patient's response to pain, the sum of which culminate in his response to the situation.

Causal Mechanisms of Postoperative Pain

Postoperative pain is the body's response to stimuli of both mechanical and chemical origin. No one causal mechanism is specific to any one type of pain (i.e., incisional/cutaneous, somatic, visceral), although the degree to which a causal mechanism is involved may be greater in one type of pain than in another. This overlap is one factor that makes pain so difficult to study and manage in postoperative patients.

Postoperative pain results from the stimulation of one or more of the modalities responsible for conveying various bodily sensations. Examples of these somatesthetic (i.e., bodily) modalities are: mechano- (touch and pressure), thermo- (cold and warmth), and chemosensations (ache and pain) [29]. These modalities are present in all three types of pain. In addition, the somatesthetic modality of proprioception (kinesthetic sense) is generally associated with pain of somatic origin. The adequate stimulus for producing pain is believed to be injury or nociception. In general, the cause-effect relationship between injury and pain remains the accepted explanation for a stimulus evoking the receptor mechanism that produces the subjective and objective manifestations of pain [14, 29]. Pain resulting from nociception, the perception of traumatic stimuli, produces impulses that are then transmitted and interpreted by an intact nervous system as pain [15].

Researchers have identified several different types of nerve fibers that are involved in the transmission of somatesthetic impulses throughout the body. Two groups of nerve fibers have been ascribed primary responsibility for the transmission of pain impulses originating in peripheral locations. These fibers are the type A and type C fibers [46]. The A group of fibers associated with the transmission of pain is further divided into A delta and A gamma types of fibers, which are myelinated and rapidly conduct impulses from the periphery to the central nervous system. The C group of fibers are unmyelinated and consequently conduct impulses more slowly. This distinction is important in understanding the differences in the quality and duration of postoperative pain. The fast, pricking type of pain—usually of short duration—is attributed to alpha fibers, while to the C fibers are ascribed the slow, burning types of pain of longer duration [5].

Postoperative pain is not limited to the excitation and response of only A delta, A gamma, and C fibers. Fibers representative of all types (A, B, and C) are involved to some degree in the body's response to noxious stimuli depending upon the type and location of the stimulus. Also, the number of fibers activated by a stimulus tends to increase with an associated increase in the intensity of the stimulus.

Melzack [34] reports that while some fibers have very specialized functions and important roles to play in the transmission of pain, it is highly unlikely that such fibers are specific for pain. Rather, noxious stimuli tend to excite receptor-fiber units across the entire range of fiber types. The total number of active fibers together with their rate of firing may be just as important in the determination of pain as any one particular group of fibers.

A related concept necessary for the clinician to understand is pain threshold, which refers to the point at which a stimulus is perceived as being painful. High-threshold pain receptors are commonly ascribed to the A delta and C fibers, while low-threshold fibers encompass all types of fibers. Mechanical forms of stimuli, such as pressure, initially excite low-threshold receptors with involvement of the higher-threshold units at a later time. Mild-to-moderate intensities of stimulation will receive responses from fibers throughout the remaining range of types of fibers. Increasing intensity serves to stimulate greater numbers of fibers, which ultimately continues to increase the input and connections with cells in the dorsal horn [16, 34].

Hardy [15] translates this information into a useful clinical format in the following way. He suggests that pain of high intensity must also be of short duration due to the rapid conduction of pain impulses and the rate of tissue injury and destruction associated with high-intensity pain. Operative procedures per se and childbirth are examples of high-intensity pain, both of which may require the administration of anesthetic and elimination of consciousness in order to achieve adequate pain control. Pain of moderate intensity is also short in duration. Pain encountered in the postoperative phase of treatment provides an example of this degree of intensity. It is important with these patients to abolish the pain quickly, thus preventing the establishment of bodily responses such as increased muscle tension and contraction that can serve as rebound sources of pain, thus perpetuating the pain cycle. Pain of long duration, therefore, must be of low intensity since the rates of tissue injury and repair seem to be compatible with the maintenance of tissue integrity. Hardy postulates that the pain of chronic illness is an example of low-intensity pain.

Considerable research demonstrates the pain-producing capabilities associated with various endogenous substances. Pain-producing substances are contained in physiological, secretory, and excretory body fluids, and normally are separated from the sensory nerve network via cellular membrane barriers. Injured or damaged tissue releases part or all of its chemical substances into the surrounding area, which serves as a stimulus for and elicits a pain response. Potassium (K^+) released from cells damaged by trauma can produce pain for varying intervals of time depending upon the amount of

K$^+$ released. Acetylcholine is believed to lower the threshold for other pain-producing substances; histamine has been shown to produce deep pain when applied to deeper layers of tissue or superficial pain when combined with other chemicals such as acetylcholine. Serotonin, released during blood coagulation and disintegration of thrombocytes, is an effective stimulator of sensitive peripheral structures [14, 44].

Plasma kinins (bradykinin, kallidin, and methionylkallidin) are pain-producing substances that develop in blood plasma at the site of injury. Injured tissue experiences an initial decrease in circulation, i.e., the capillary and venule circulation becomes slower either because of the injury per se or as a result of liberated substances such as histamine and serotonin. Components of the blood such as red and white corpuscles accumulate, break down, and create a climate conducive to the formation of the chemical substance—bradykinin. The plasma kinins theoretically initiate further vasodilation, and increase vascular permeability, edema, and pain [14, 44].

Kim and Guzmans's [14] studies emphasize that a variety of chemical agents can excite the pain receptor, that is, that excitation does not depend primarily on a specific chemical configuration.

The nonspecific character of the receptor and the nature of some of the algesic agents suggest that excitation may depend upon electrophilic attraction, assuming that the receptor sites are negatively charged or electron-rich and that algesic agents, or parts of their molecules, are positively charged or electron-deficient [14].

The role of chemosensitive receptors in the production, conduction, and perception of pain is of increasing importance in caring for and alleviating pain in postoperative patients. As will be seen later in the discussion of nursing interventions, many of the nonnarcotic antipyretic analgesics serve as antagonists to these algesic chemicals, thus blocking their pain-producing properties.

The preceding section focused on causal mechanical and chemical mechanisms involved in postoperative pain. The reader is referred to Chapter 2 for additional information related to the anatomical and physiological components of the pain experience. The relationship of causal mechanical and chemical mechanisms in each type of postoperative pain will now be presented.

Types of Pain

All three types of pain previously cited are commonly associated with the postoperative phase of care, i.e., incisional/cutaneous, somatic, and visceral. The characteristics generally ascribed to these types of pain relate to the intensity, duration, quality, quantity, and meaning of the situation to the patient. Responses to these characteristics are as varied as the number of patients, types of incisions made, and kinds of surgeries performed.

It must be emphasized again that while some comments may be made in reference to any one particular type of pain, there is considerable overlap among the types of pain and, therefore, some of the following discussion relates to all three types of pain.

Incisional Pain

Incisional pain (i.e., cutaneous or superficial) arises primarily from the skin and mucous membranes. Incisional/cutaneous pain is produced by both mechanical and chemical mechanisms via mechano-, thermo-, and chemosensitive modalities. Pain of incisional/cutaneous origin is conducted by fibers of all diameters but primarily by the A delta and C groups.

Incisional pain is an expected outcome of any surgical procedure, and generally is described by patients as being sharp, bright, prickling, cutting, tearing, stabbing, burning, and full of pressure.

As with all types of pain, it is difficult to distinguish between the effects of causal mechanical and chemical mechanisms associated with incisional/cutaneous pain. The incision itself is important to consider in discussing postoperative pain. The surgeon's scalpel severs, damages, and destroys cellular components of the skin, subcutaneous tissue, muscle, fascia, and viscera. While the destruction of tissue is inevitable and initiates both chemical and mechanical means of nociception, several factors can influence the degree of cellular damage. Incisions properly placed will require less traction for exposure, undergo less tension when closed, and produce fewer separations of layers than incisions made less carefully [10]. Incisions severing and damaging many nerves will produce more pain than those involving fewer nerves. Transverse incisions of the abdomen generally result in less postoperative pain than either vertical or diagonal incisions because of the decreased trauma and severance of nerves, muscles, and fascia [5, 12]. Prolonged exposure and/or retraction of open tissues increases cellular trauma and lysis due to traction, stretching, and aeration of internal tissues [9]. Thus, even if two incisions are similar in location and extent, a longer procedure usually will produce more pain.

Extensive surgeries involving considerable handling of tissues generally increase postoperative pain of visceral origin due to reflex inhibition. Reflex inhibition refers to the disturbance of gastrointestinal function that can lead to distention, nausea, vomiting, or inadequate digestion [5]. This response, if marked, can alter and increase the degree of incisional pain [5]. Suture material, placement, and tension can affect the degree of postoperative pain [9]. Material left in wounds will function as a foreign body, and may serve as a source of chemical or physical irritation or both [9]. Incisional pain also is influenced by the normal healing processes of edema, inflammation, and contraction as well as the abnormal appearance of such complications as: infection, hematomas, abscesses, and more serious inflammatory responses. While much of the preceding relates to factors primarily under control of the surgeon, the nurse who is aware of such factors can be prepared to implement a plan of care based on their consideration. Specific nursing interventions are discussed later in the chapter.

Somatic Pain

Pain of somatic origin is associated with muscles, tendons, ligaments, periosteum, cancellous bone, joints, and arteries [5]. Somatic pain is produced by both chemical and mechanical causal mechanisms with proprioception (specialized groups of nerve endings located primarily in muscles, tendons, and joints that respond to changes in muscle tension and give information regarding body movements and position), the somatesthetic modality generally associated with the structures listed above. Proprioceptors are activated by either stretching or contracting-type movements. The somatesthetic modalities, i.e., mechano-, thermo-, and chemosensations, discussed in the previous section also are involved with somatic pain, but to a lesser degree than proprioception [16]. Somatic pain is conducted by A, B, and C types of fibers, and is a common companion to surgical patients both pre- and postoperatively. Its appearance postoperatively is normal, particularly in patients undergoing abdominal or thoracic surgical procedures.

Words used by patients to describe somatic pain focus on its dull, aching quality [5]. Somatic pain is generally difficult for patients to localize, particularly when it involves the abdominal or thoracic regions. Somatic pain possesses a characteristic pattern of spread that results in descriptions by patients of pain that is very diffuse and "aching all over."

Somatic pain closely resembles visceral pain in many aspects but certain characteristics remain unique to this type of pain. Perhaps the most unique aspect of somatic pain is its tendency to spread and envelop wide areas of the body. Somatic pain can originate from either superficial or deeply located sources and differentiates itself in the degree of localization possible for patients to report. Generally, the more intense the stimulus, the greater in duration the stimulus, and the deeper the tissue affected, the more widespread and diffusely perceived the pain. This spread factor is of clinical importance because prompt and early relief of pain can prevent it from spreading to wider areas [5]. Thus, the early relief of pain is of crucial importance in postoperative patients. Unrelieved, the pain stimulus continues to stimulate affected nerves, gradually involving greater and greater areas.

Mechanical mechanisms that may cause somatic pain postoperatively include abdominal distention, edema of tissues injured or destroyed either by the operation or by the process of repair, traction or contraction as a sequalae of the surgical procedure or subsequent to wound healing (or both), muscle spasms or stretching resulting from the trauma of surgery or associated with position changes and movement postsurgery, and inflammatory changes—either as the normal response to healing or by the presence of a complication such as infection.

The interrelationship between chemical and mechanical causal mechanisms of pain is readily apparent in somatic pain, as illustrated in the pain associated with postoperative abdominal distention. Chemicals produce pain when released from mechanically damaged tissues. Muscle pain, for example, is not readily provoked by stretching or contracting-type activities under normal conditions. Ischemic muscle, however, is very susceptible to and manifests pain responses when stimulated. The pain-producing chemical substances in muscle can be dissipated in a very short time once adequate circulatory perfusion of the affected muscle tissue is reestablished [16].

Chemical mechanisms influential in the production of pain via endogenous substances include: lowered pH values subsequent to metabolic disturbances such as the accumulation of lactic acid or other acid substances associated with muscle ischemia, release of hydrogen ($H^{\pm}$) ion and K^+ ion from cells injured by either trauma or inflammation; release of histamine, serotonin, and plasma kinins from cellular dysfunction; and altered cellular permeability, all of which contribute to the production of pain. The body's response to the stress of surgery may also alter the amounts of acetylcholine, adrenin, and noradrenalin circulating in the body, which may in turn lower the threshold of pain receptors [14, 44]. Referred pain is frequently experienced as a sequelae to pain of somatic origin.

Visceral Pain

Visceral pain generally is associated with visceral organs and parietal peritoneum or pleura. Although there is controversy over whether or not visceral pain does in fact exist, most researchers accept visceral pain as a legitimate response to stimuli [5]. Visceral stimuli are conducted primarily by sympathetic nerves, except for the vagus nerve, and enter the spinal cord through the posterior spinal nerve roots [5, 11].

Kaplan [25] identifies the medullated fibers in visceral nerves as B fibers, and states that visceral and somatic fibers are basically similar except that visceral fibers have a more sparse distribution.

Descriptions of visceral pain have many similarities to those of somatic pain, and most probably both types of pain occur in combination rather than separately. Visceral pain, however, has different manifestations depending upon the intensity and duration of the pain stimulus. Initially, visceral pain of abdominal origin, for example, produces a vague, poorly localized, diffuse, dull aching type of pain. Later in the process, however, the visceral pain is of longer duration and greater intensity which produces a sharp, stabbinglike pain much easier to localize and in greater proximity to the diseased organ [5].

Visceral pain is produced by both mechanical and chemical stimuli but the stimuli are lesser in number than those associated with incisional/cutaneous or somatic types of pain. Factors most frequently associated with the production of visceral pain include the causal mechanisms of both chemical and mechanical origin. The chemical and mechanical mechanisms responsible for producing visceral pain include: distention, spasm, contraction, stretching, tearing, or ischemia of the gastrointestinal, genitourinary, or other visceral musculature such as the heart, and visceral organs such as the liver, spleen, and pancreas. Studies suggest that the adequate stimuli for activating visceral afferents arise from the afferents' own environment and activities [5]. In other words, the transmission of pain impulses by the visceral afferent nerves of the intestinal tract occurs secondary to an alteration of the intestine's internal environment per se. Perhaps peristalsis is slowed or an obstruction occurs, or both. The subsequent distention and ischemia processes initiate the pain stimuli from which impulses are then transmitted to the central nervous system for processing.

Visceral pain is readily produced by distention or contraction of the hollow viscera [16]. The chain of events created by ischemic processes within a distended colon; the sequelae associated with obstruction of the cystic or common bile duct; the processes associated with inflammation of the gallbladder, i.e., cholecystitis; and the effects of increased pressure in the sphincter of Oddi and in the pancreas all illustrate the effects of chemical and mechanical causal mechanisms in the production of pain [8, 28, 38, 45].

While a considerable amount of visceral pain may be experienced preoperatively as clinical evidence of a diseased organ, postoperative visceral pain is the body's response to the stretching or tearing of internal tissues during the surgery itself, and to abdominal distention due to reflex inhibition of gastrointestinal function. Prompt relief of visceral pain, as in somatic pain, is important in the care of postoperative patients. Visceral pain lasting prolonged periods of time initiates a series of reflexive-type responses that can, in turn, induce additional pain and discomfort. For example, prolonged noxious stimulation of the viscera may cause cutaneous tenderness and hyperalgesia in the region of the affected viscera, induce skeletal muscle contraction or spasms, and stimulate the autonomic nervous system. Once stimulated, these responses can serve as additional sources of noxious stimulation and pain. Once this type of cycle becomes established, the pain may be prolonged and exceed the period of stimulation. Visceral pain generally follows dermatomal and segmental distributions* [5, 15].

Specific sequelae of the chemical causal mechanisms responsible for producing painful stimuli involve endogenous substances similar to those mentioned in the discussions of incisional/cutaneous and somatic pain.

In summary, how a patient responds to the experience of postoperative pain is influenced by many physiological and psychological factors. There is little predictability with postsurgical pain and nursing interventions must be determined on an individual basis for maximum effectiveness.

Nursing Process and Postoperative Pain

It is difficult for nurses to accurately assess and for patients to readily distinguish the specific discomforts of incisional/cutaneous pain from those of somatic or visceral origin. This difficulty arises from the interrelated physiological effects of pain, cutaneovisceral reflex, and reflex inhibition of visceral functions—all of which contribute to the patient's postoperative behavioral

---

* For an expanded discussion of the characteristics of various types of pain, see Chapters 2 and 6.

response. Carefully conducted assessments of the postoperative patient's pain status should enable the nurse to assist the patient in making some distinctions between discomfort and pain and to initiate an appropriate plan of care.*

Postoperative patients experience pain and discomfort from the variety of sources described above. They need and require good nursing care. The reader may be disappointed to learn that this chapter does not produce a series of innovative nursing interventions designed to resolve the dilemma faced by thousands of postoperative patients each year. Such content is neither possible nor practical at this stage of nursing knowledge. What *is* practical is the challenge for nurses to put into practice that which is already known about the care of postoperative patients.

Experience with postoperative patients suggests that complaints of incisional/cutaneous pain are associated primarily with the activities of coughing, deep breathing, and movement—particularly the activities of getting in and out of bed and changing position.† The greatest number of references made by patients to activities causing incisional/cutaneous pain are associated with the two activities of coughing and movement.

As with every facet of pain, both physiological and psychological aspects contribute to the patient's pain experience. For example, coughing and deep-breathing exercises may be relatively successful initially, but once the patient experiences the sharp, ripping, pressure-packed, tearing-apart-like sensations associated with performing the exercises, the fear of pain and evisceration assumes paramount importance. Subsequently, the fear of pain and evisceration inhibits the patient's willingness to cooperate fully with the postoperative regimen. The patient should be helped to understand this fear, and to overcome it. He should be instructed in the correct technique of coughing, with assurance that the incision will not eviscerate. For the patient to acquire such understanding, this may require more than verbal descriptions from the nurse. Demonstrating the exercises, explaining the basis for the sensations, and remaining with the patient while he attempts to do the coughing and deep-breathing exercises are all useful. Johnson's research [21, 22, 23, 24] dealing with the importance of interpreting sensations to patients undergoing various diagnostic and surgical procedures supports the need to provide information to patients concerning expected sensations and to assist them in performing activities necessary to complete the task.

Some nursing textbooks suggest that applying pressure to the incision by placing a pillow over the patient's incision while he/she coughs is one way of decreasing incisional pain. Some patients find that bath blankets, bath towels, or most preferably, the direct placement of hands is more useful in decreasing incisional pain while coughing. Whereas the pillow seems to absorb and disseminate the applied pressure, use of the hands seems to concen-

---

* The reader is referred to Chapter 6 for a detailed discussion of pain assessment techniques.
† The reader is referred to Chapter 6 for elaboration of this point.

trate controlled pressure at the incisional site and is an effective means of achieving some control over the pain associated with coughing.

The pain associated with movement, i.e., getting in and out of bed or changing position, or both, is best controlled by minimizing the amount of stress, strain, traction, and pull on the incisional site. Taking the time to elevate the head of the bed to a Fowler's position, providing support for the upper torso, holding and supporting the lower extremities, and instructing patients to gradually ease their feet to the floor using siderails, small foot stools, or other types of equipment as stepping-stones along the way are effective ways to minimize incisional pain.

The development and presence of abdominal distention have implications for all three types of postoperative pain. For example, distention occurring as a consequence of reflex inhibition will produce pain of visceral origin. The subsequent accumulation of internal secretions and flatus compounds the problem, eventually increasing the patient's intra-abdominal pressure, which influences the degree of somatic pain. An increase in intra-abdominal pressure results in greater stress, pressure, and traction placed on abdominal tissues and muscles, and subsequently exerted on suture lines and incisions, which is reflected in expressions of incisional/cutaneous pain. Once abdominal distention exists, a pain cycle is established that must be interrupted if the pain is to be alleviated. Noting the presence of abdominal distention at its inception can enable actions that will prevent many of the sequelae. Early detection is possible by observing closely the abdominal area for signs of distention, noting expulsion of flatus, and taking and recording measurements of the abdominal girth when its presence is suspected. The importance of alleviating pain due to the incision or to the presence of abdominal distention cannot be overemphasized during the initial postoperative period.

The efficacious use of pharmacological agents is an important adjunct to the nurse's armamentarium of ministrations. Analgesic medications exert their pharmacological effects peripherally at the receptor site or centrally at either the spinal cord or cerebral levels. The actions of analgesics may occur singly or in combination depending upon which drug is chosen and its mode of action. Analgesics act in one or more of the following ways: (1) alter pain perception by elevating the pain threshold; (2) influence the reception and transmission of noxious stimuli by direct action either at the afferent nerve site or upon the central excitatory states at the segmental level; (3) alter the mood or attitude of the person experiencing pain; and (4) produce a state of sedation [15].*

Selection of analgesics to minimize or alleviate pain during the postoperative period is the responsibility of the physician. The decision as to which of the drugs ordered will be chosen for use and when the drug will be administered is usually at the discretion of the nurse. Therefore, nurses need to make

* Please refer to Chapter 9 for a detailed discussion on the use of drugs to relieve pain.

their decisions regarding the drug of use based on a sound knowledge of the patient's condition and pain status.

Assessment of the patient's pain is an essential element in the determination of any nursing decision and intervention. Postoperative patients may experience one or more types of pain and may have both oral and injectable pharmacological agents available to reduce their pain. The somatic and visceral types of pain are best alleviated by the administration of narcotic agents such as morphine, meperidine, and so forth. These drugs exhibit a wide range of effects including alteration of cerebral cognition. Incisional/cutaneous pain, however, may be effectively alleviated or controlled by the administration of some of the nonnarcotic antipyretic analgesics such as acetylsalicylic acid, Tylenol, sodium salicylate, and so forth. These drugs exert their analgesic actions by chemically antagonizing and blocking the effects of algesic agents such as bradykinin at the pain receptor sites [14]. This means, then, that perhaps specific medications should be chosen and administered according to the type of pain the patient is experiencing in order to achieve optimum results.

Narcotics are generally used to control and alleviate pain during the initial 48 hours postoperatively, after which oral analgesics are used. This standardization is unfortunate, since it does not always correspond to the patient's need for a particular type of drug. If each patient is to be considered individually then the generalizations commonly made with regard to the administration of pain-alleviating drugs should be reexamined.

Many complaints of postoperative "pain" or "discomfort" are associated with aspects of therapeutic management and care such as the maintenance of IV administration, the pressure of urinary catheters, drainage tubes, nasogastric suction, and large, bulky dressings that have been applied too tightly. Patients also comment on the discomfort associated with the presence of nasopharyngeal irritation, nausea, thirst, hunger, backache, fatigue, and trying to find a comfortable position while lying in bed. These discomforts enhance and become part of the patient's overall response to pain.

As noted earlier, Keats's studies [26] also indicate that 10 to 15 percent of all requests for medication to alleviate pain were due to the sources of discomfort described above. Keats's figures seem understated. In an attempt to alleviate pain, many patients' requests for pain medication are fulfilled, but without the nurse making a personal assessment and determination of the specific sources underlying the request. The patient's request for pain-alleviating medication may have been communicated to the nurse by a family member, auxiliary nursing personnel, other health care professionals, or staff members and the medication administered without the nurse making her own assessment. The need to combine assessment techniques with nursing approaches based upon a psychosomatic view of pain is reflected in studies indicating that such approaches are more effective than those that equate pain relief with the giving and receiving of medication only [33]. It seems apparent that many requests for pain medication may, in fact, be prevented, delayed, or alleviated by attentive nurses administering basic nursing care.

Much has been written regarding the importance of frequent turning, proper positioning, and provision of support for postoperative patients. Extremities receiving intravenous fluids should be elevated, supported, and positioned comfortably; medications infused intravenously are to be given slowly and carefully, and the site checked frequently to prevent or detect signs of infiltration, extravasation, or other complications. Emphasis is placed on the need to maintain accurate intake and output records, to observe the times and amounts of both urinary output and expulsion of flatus, and to note the presence or absence of abdominal distention. Special equipment requires careful attention to particular aspects of patient care. For example, the patency of tubes such as catheters, drainage tubes, nasogastric suction apparatus, and so forth, must be ensured. Care must be exercised to prevent placing traction on tubes at their site of entrance into the body, thus avoiding additional traction and tension of these areas. These aspects of nursing care are designed to promote comfort and minimize the pain and discomfort frequently associated with therapeutic measures. Perhaps comfort measures such as back rubs, once a familiar aspect of nursing care, and now a rare commodity, should be reinstituted on a regular schedule because of their beneficial physiological and psychological effects. How much of the discomfort currently expressed by patients and referred to as "backache" could be alleviated if back rubs were again given intermittently throughout the day? In short, nurses do have the means by which much of the pain and discomfort associated with the postoperative phase of surgical care can be alleviated. But the means are effective only when transformed into action; the care must be *given* in order to effectively alleviate pain.

Nurses must be cognizant of and concerned about meeting the comfort needs of the patient. An accurate assessment will provide the data necessary to formulate a plan of care and nursing intervention. Decisions regarding use of pharmacological agents should be carefully considered and used to complement and supplement the nursing care being given—not to replace it.

Implications for Research

There is a great need for nurses and other health professionals to conduct research on the alleviation of pain in the postoperative patient. Research in this area was popular during the late 1950s and continued through the latter part of the 1960s, but has diminished considerably since that time. The identification of techniques to minimize and control pain experienced postoperatively could have a major impact on the care of the thousands of people who undergo surgery each year.

Physiological research is needed to determine the normal course of postoperative pain, thus assisting the health professionals to intervene more effectively and appropriately.

Nurses need to devise tools that utilize and test the nursing process. Such tools eventually may provide the ability to predict patients' postoperative behavior and permit the initiation of a plan of care preoperatively. Descriptive research is needed to determine differences between discomfort and pain. Attention needs to be given to the determination of discomforts associated with treatment, e.g., nasopharyngeal irritation, and how best to minimize these discomforts.

Common nursing-care measures associated with basic principles of care and designed to minimize discomfort and pain should be given to test their effectiveness. Once this is done, more elaborately devised nursing interventions utilizing distraction, dissociation, suggestion, vibration, patient teaching, and relaxation techniques can then be added and tested systematically for their effect on discomfort or pain, or both.

Numerous questions arise with respect to the administration of pharmacological agents for the alleviation of patients' pain during the postoperative phase of care. For example, two areas for additional research might be: (1) to examine the relationship, if any, that exists between the type of anesthetic used, the initial request for pain medication, and subsequent analgesics given during the remainder of the postoperative period of care; and (2) to examine the effects of narcotic agents administered specifically for somatic and visceral pain and nonnarcotic agents for incisional/cutaneous pain.

Research possibilities and questions are unlimited. Nurses, in particular, have a wide range of research questions for which answers are needed in order to provide the best possible care for postoperative patients.

References

1. Beecher, H. K.   Pain in men wounded in battle. *Ann. Surg.* 123:96, 1946.
2. Beecher, H. K.   *Measurement of Subjective Responses: Quantitative Effects of Drugs.* New York: Oxford University Press, 1959.
3. Beecher, H. K.   The placebo effect as a non-specific force surrounding disease and the treatment of disease. In Janzen, R., Keidel, W., Herz, A., and Steichele, C., eds., *Pain: Basic Principles—Pharmacology—Therapy.* Baltimore: Williams & Wilkins Company, 1972. Pp. 175–180.
4. Bond, M. R.   Personality studies in patients with pain secondary to organic disease. *J. Psychosom. Res.* 17:257, 1973.
5. Bonica, J. J.   *The Management of Pain.* Philadelphia: Lea & Febiger, 1954. Pp. 90, 104, 108–115, 1240, 1243, 1244, 1392.
6. Bonica, J. J., Procacci, P., and Pagni, C. A., eds.   *Recent Advances in Pain: Pathophysiology and Clinical Aspects.* Springfield, Illinois: Charles C Thomas, 1974.
7. Charpentier, J.   Parameters of pain in man. In Janzen, R., Keidel, W., Herz, A., and Steichele, C., eds., *Pain: Basic Principles—Pharmacology—Therapy.* Baltimore: Williams & Wilkins Company, 1972. Pp. 28–33.

8. der Plessis, D. J., and Jersky, J. The management of acute cholecystitis. *Surg. Clin. North Am.* 53:1071, 1973.
9. De Vito, R. V. Healing of wounds. *Surg. Clin. North Am.* 45:441, 1965.
10. Ferguson, D. J. Advances in the management of surgical wounds. *Surg. Clin. North Am.* 51:49, 1971.
11. Finneson, B. E. *Diagnosis and Management of Pain Syndromes*. Philadelphia: W. B. Saunders Company, 1969. Pp. 4, 16–17, 250.
12. Gaster, J. *Hernia: One Day Repair*. Darien, Conn.: Hafner, 1970. P. 137.
13. Gildea, J. The relief of postoperative pain. *Med. Clin. North Am.* 52:81, 1968.
14. Guzman, F., and Kim, R. K. S. The mechanism of action of the nonnarcotic analgesics. *Med. Clin. North Am.* 52:3, 1968.
15. Hardy, J. D. The nature of pain. *J. Chronic Dis.* 4:22, 1956.
16. Iggo, A. The case for pain receptors. In Janzen, R., Keidel, W., Herz, A., and Steichele, C., eds., *Pain: Basic Principles—Pharmacology—Therapy*. Baltimore: Williams & Wilkins Company, 1972. Pp. 60–67.
17. Iggo, A. Pain receptors. In Bonica, J. J., Procacci, P., and Pagni, C. A., eds., *Recent Advances in Pain: Pathophysiology and Clinical Aspects*. Springfield, Illinois: Charles C Thomas, 1974. Pp. 3–35.
18. Jacox, A., and Stewart, M. *Psychosocial Contingencies of the Pain Experience*. Iowa City, Iowa: University of Iowa, 1973.
19. Jacox, A., Principal Investigator. *Pain Alleviation Through Nursing Intervention: Final Report*. NU00467–3. Pp. 34–37.
20. Jaggard, R. S., Zager, L. L., and Wilkins, D. S. Clinical evaluation of analgesic drugs: A comparison of NU-2206 and morphine sulfate administered to postoperative patients. *Arch. Surg.* 61:1073, 1950.
21. Johnson, J. E. Altering Patients' Responses to Threatening Events—Surgical Study I. Unpublished paper presented at the N.L.N. Convention, New Orleans, 1975.
22. Johnson, J. E., and Rice, V. Sensory and distress components of pain: Implications for the study of clinical pain. *Nurs. Res.* 23:203, 1974.
23. Johnson, J. E. Effects of accurate expectations about sensations on the sensory and distress components of pain. *J. Pers. Soc. Psychol.* 29:710, 1974.
24. Johnson, J. E., Morrissey, J. F., and Leventhal, A. Psychological preparation for an endoscopic examination. *Gastrointest. Endosc.* 19:180, 1973.
25. Kaplan, H. A. Applied anatomical aspects of pain. *J. Med. Soc. N.J.* 70:935, 1973.
26. Keats, A. S. Postoperative pain: Research and treatment. *J. Chronic Dis.* 4:72, 1956.
27. Keats, A. S. Use of analgesics at the bedside. In W. E. Leong, ed., *New Concepts in Pain and Its Clinical Management*. Philadelphia: F. A. Davis Company, 1967. Pp. 143–154.
28. Lahana, D., and Schoenfield, L. J. Progress in medical therapy of gallstones. *Surg. Clin. North Am.* 53:1053, 1973.
29. Lim, K. S. Cutaneous and visceral pain, and somesthetic chemoreceptors. In Kenshalo, D. R., ed., *The Skin Senses*. Springfield, Illinois: Charles C Thomas, 1966. Pp. 458–465.
30. Lim, R. K. S. Pharmacologic viewpoint of pain and analgesia. In W. E. Leong, ed., *New Concepts in Pain and Its Clinical Management*. Philadelphia: F. A. Davis Company, 1967. Pp. 33–47.
31. Loan, W. B., and Dundee, J. W. The clinical assessment of pain. *Practitioner* 198:759, 1967.
32. Loan, W. B., and Morrison, J. D. The incidence and severity of postopera-

tive pain. In Weisenberg, M., ed., *Pain: Clinical and Experimental Perspectives.* St. Louis: The C. V. Mosby Company, 1975. Pp. 286–290.

33. McBride, M. A.   Nursing approach, pain, and relief: An exploratory experiment. *Nurs. Res.* 16:337, 1967.
34. Melzack, R.   *The Puzzle of Pain.* New York: Basic Books, Inc., 1973.
35. Papper, E., Brodie, B. B., and Rovenstein, E. A.   Postoperative pain: Its use in the comparative evaluation of analgesics. *Surgery* 32:107, 1952.
36. Parbrook, G. D., Dalrymple, D. G., and Steel, D. F.   Personality assessment and postoperative pain and complications. *J. Psychosom. Res.* 17:277, 1973.
37. Parkhouse, J., Lambrechts, W., and Simpson, B. R. J.   The incidence of postoperative pain. *Br. J. Anaesth.* 33:345, 1961.
38. Puestow, C. B., and Gillesby, W. J.   Longitudinal pancreaticojejunostomy for chronic pancreatitis. *Surg. Proc.* 33:2, 1966.
39. Quimby, C. W., Jr.   Preoperative prophylaxis of postoperative pain. *Med. Clin. North Am.* 52:73, 1968.
40. Shapiro, A. K.   The placebo response. In Howells, J. G., ed., *Modern Perspectives in Psychiatry.* New York: Brunner Mazel, Inc., 1971. Pp. 596–619.
41. Stephen, C. R.   Drug management of the patient with pain: Pharmacologic considerations. *South. Med. J.* 66:1421, 1973.
42. Swerdlow, M.   Problems in the clinical evaluation of pain. In Janzen, R., Keidel, W., Herz, A., and Steichele, C., eds., *Pain: Basic Principles—Pharmacology—Therapy.* Baltimore: Williams & Wilkins Company, 1972. Pp. 49–51.
43. Walike, B. C., and Meyer, B.   Relations between placebo reactivity and selected personality factors. *Nurs. Res.* 15:119, 1966.
44. Werle, E.   On endogenous pain-producing substances with particular reference to plasmakinins. In Janzen, R., Keidel, W., Herz, A., and Steichele, C., eds., *Pain: Basic Principles—Pharmacology—Therapy.* Baltimore: Williams & Wilkins Company, 1972. Pp. 86–92.
45. Williams, S. W., Majewski, P. L., Norris, J. E. C., Cole, B. C., and Doohen, D. J.   Biliary decompression in the treatment of bilothorax. *Am. J. Surg.* 122:829, 1971.
46. Wilson, M. E.   The neurological mechanisms of pain. *Anesthesia* 29:407, 1974.

16

Pain Associated with Arthritis and Other Rheumatic Disorders

Ardis J. O'Dell

The rheumatic disorders are those conditions in which pain and stiffness of some portion of the musculoskeletal system are prominent. Arthritis is the general term used when the joints themselves are the major seat of the rheumatic disease. Arthritis and other rheumatic disorders of inflammatory, degenerative, traumatic, and infective nature comprise approximately 160 diseases that afflict the human with pain. Many of these diseases persist as chronic painful disorders that a person must learn to adapt to and live with. These diseases, as shown in the list given below, cover a large part of the field of medicine [22]. In some of the conditions in this list, rheumatic complaints in which pain is a part occur irregularly or constitute only a minor problem, whereas in others, joint disease may play a dominant role in the patient's illness. The classification and nomenclature of the conditions continue to change with the acquisition of knowledge. The common property shared by most of the diseases and syndromes included in the list is that of an involvement of the joints or surrounding tissue structure or both. Pain in and about the joints is one of the most common symptoms and chief concerns of the total population seeking medical help.

Classification of the Rheumatic Diseases

A. Polyarthritis of unknown etiology
   1. Rheumatoid arthritis
   2. Juvenile rheumatoid arthritis (including Still's disease)
   3. Ankylosing spondylitis
   4. Psoriatic arthritis
   5. Reiter's syndrome
   6. Others
B. "Connective tissue" disorders (acquired)
   1. Systemic lupus erythematosus
   2. Progressive systemic sclerosis (scleroderma)
   3. Polymyositis and dermatomyositis
   4. Necrotizing arteritis and other forms of vasculitis

     a. Polyarteritis nodosa
     b. Hypersensitivity angiitis
     c. Wegener's granulomatosis
     d. Takayasu's (pulseless) disease
     e. Cogan's syndrome
     f. Giant cell arteritis (including polymyalgia rheumatica)
   5. Amyloidosis
   6. Others
     (See also Rheumatoid arthritis, A. 1; Sjögren's syndrome, F. 7)
C. Rheumatic fever
D. Degenerative joint disease (osteoarthritis, osteoarthrosis)
   1. Primary
   2. Secondary
E. Nonarticular rheumatism
   1. Fibrositis
   2. Intervertebral disk and low back syndromes
   3. Myositis and myalgia
   4. Tendinitis and peritendinitis (bursitis)
   5. Tenosynovitis
   6. Fasciitis
   7. Carpal tunnel syndrome
   8. Others
     (See also Shoulder-hand syndrome, H. 3)
F. Diseases with which arthritis is frequently associated
   1. Sarcoidosis
   2. Relapsing polychondritis
   3. Schönlein-Henoch purpura
   4. Ulcerative colitis
   5. Regional enteritis
   6. Whipple's disease
   7. Sjögren's syndrome
   8. Familial Mediterranean fever
   9. Others
     (See also Psoriatic arthritis, A. 4)
G. Associated with known infectious agents
   1. Bacterial
     a. Gonococcus
     b. Meningococcus
     c. Pneumococcus
     d. Streptococcus
     e. Staphylococcus
     f. Salmonella
     g. Brucella
     h. Streptobacillus moniliformis (Haverhill fever)
     i. Mycobacterium tuberculosis
     j. Treponema pallidum (syphilis)
     k. Treponema pertenue (yaws)
     l. Others
       (See also Rheumatic fever, C)
   2. Rickettsial
   3. Viral
     a. Rubella
     b. Mumps
     c. Viral hepatitis

        d. Others
    4. Fungal
    5. Parasitic
H. Traumatic and/or neurogenic disorders
    1. Traumatic arthritis (the result of direct trauma)
    2. Neuropathic arthropathy (Charcot joints)
        a. Syphilis (tabes dorsalis)
        b. Diabetes mellitus (diabetic neuropathy)
        c. Syringomyelia
        d. Myelomeningocele
        e. Congenital insensitivity to pain (including familial dysautonomia)
        f. Others
    3. Shoulder-hand syndrome
    4. Mechanical derangement of joints
    5. Others
        (See also Degenerative joint disease, D; Carpal tunnel syndrome, E. 7)
I. Associated with known or strongly suspected biochemical or endocrine
   abnormalities
    1. Gout
    2. Chondrocalcinosis articularis (pseudogout)
    3. Alkaptonuria (ochronosis)
    4. Hemophilia
    5. Sickle cell disease and other hemoglobinopathies
    6. Agammaglobulinemia (hypogammaglobulinemia)
    7. Gaucher's disease
    8. Hyperparathyroidism
    9. Acromegaly
    10. Thyroid acropachy
    11. Hypothyroidism
    12. Scurvy (hypovitaminosis C)
    13. Hyperlipoproteinemia type II (xanthoma tuberosum and tendinosum)
    14. Fabry's disease (angiokeratoma corporis diffusum or glycolipid lipidosis)
    15. Hemochromatosis
    16. Others (See also Inherited and congenital disorders, L)
J. Neoplasms
    1. Synovioma
    2. Primary juxta-articular bone tumors
    3. Metastatic malignant tumors
    4. Leukemia
    5. Multiple myeloma
    6. Benign tumors of articular tissue
    7. Others (See also Hypertrophic osteoarthropathy, M. 9)
K. Allergy and drug reactions
    1. Arthritis due to specific allergens (e.g., serum sickness)
    2. Arthritis due to drugs
    3. Others
        (See also Systemic lupus erythematosus, B. 1, for drug-induced lupuslike
        syndromes, e.g., hydralazine and procainamide syndromes; and Hypersen-
        sitivity angiitis, B. 4. b).
L. Inherited and congenital disorders
    1. Marfan's syndrome
    2. Homocystinuria
    3. Ehlers-Danlos syndrome
    4. Osteogenesis imperfecta

5. Pseudoxanthoma elasticum
6. Cutis laxa
7. Mucopolysaccharidoses (including Hurler's syndrome)
8. Arthrogryposis multiplex congenita
9. Hypermobility syndromes
10. Myositis (or fibrodysplasia) ossificans progressiva
11. Tumoral calcinosis
12. Werner's syndrome
13. Congenital dysplasia of the hip
14. Others (See also Arthropathy associated with known biochemical or endocrine abnormalities, I)

M. Miscellaneous disorders
1. Pigmented villonodular synovitis and tenosynovitis
2. Behçet's syndrome
3. Erythema nodosum
4. Relapsing panniculitis (Weber-Christian disease)
5. Avascular necrosis of bone
6. Juvenile osteochondritis
7. Osteochondritis dissecans
8. Erythema multiforme (Stevens-Johnson syndrome)
9. Hypertrophic osteoarthropathy
10. Multicentric reticulohistiocytosis
11. Disseminated lipogranulomatosis (Ferber's disease)
12. Familial lipochrome pigmentary arthritis
13. Tietze's syndrome
14. Thrombotic thrombocytopenic purpura
15. Others

Source: Adapted from the 1963 ARA Nomenclature and Classification of Arthritis and Rheumatism (tentative).

According to the National Health Examination Survey (NHES) statistics, there are more than 16 million people in the United States with some form of arthritis [22]. The prevalence in persons less than 45 years of age was 15 per thousand, while in individuals 45 to 64, it was 154 per thousand. Women comprised two-thirds of the involved population, with prevalence rates for women higher than those for men at every age level. Higher prevalence rates were found for rural than for urban populations, in persons with lower incomes, and in the Northeast than in other geographic sections of the country. The most prevalent rheumatic diseases with troublesome pain are: degenerative joint disease, ankylosing spondylitis, gout, and rheumatoid arthritis.

Population studies show that the incidence of degenerative joint disease (osteoarthritis) steadily increases with age. Men and women are nearly equally affected. Although as many as 50 percent of abnormal joints may cause no symptoms, this disorder is a source of disability and chronic pain.

Ankylosing spondylitis, a chronic progressive form of arthritis affecting the joints of the vertebrae, is less common, with a prevalence of 0.5 per thousand. This disorder most often affects males between the ages of 15 and 40 and has a distinctive familial pattern of occurrence.

The prevalence of gout, a condition characterized by recurrent episodes of violent arthritis associated with metabolism of uric acid, is estimated at two or three individuals per thousand.

Rheumatoid arthritis, chronic inflammatory disease affecting the joints, was found in 3.2 percent of the population examined. Based on criteria defined by NHES, the disease was considered "classic" or definite in 30 percent of these persons and "probable" in the remainder. There was a ratio of nearly three females to one male.

The chronic disease process of arthritis with its pain and disability produces psychosocial and economic impact on both the patient and his family. Economic loss results both from costs incurred in treating the disease and from loss of gainful employment as the disease invades the joints and prevents the person from carrying out his usual activities. The rheumatic disorders cause more time off work and more disability than any other group of diseases. The disease creates many stresses on the patient and family, which cause them to seek continuous medical and emotional support. Yet, there is much frustration for the patient, family, and medical personnel when patients seek help, because the nature of pain and the etiology of arthritis remain mysteries. Arthritis is one of the oldest known, yet most neglected, illnesses.

Medical textbooks generally deal with pathogenesis, underlying pathophysiological mechanisms, and clinical aspects of the major rheumatic diseases with little emphasis on the pain experience. Even though relief of pain is the primary target of most therapy for arthritis, little attention is given in the literature to describing the many facets of pain, persons' feelings, and their responses to pain and to pain-relief measures. Perhaps this is one of the reasons why health professionals generally are unprepared to manage the complexity of the pain experience of these patients. With the many unanswered questions, it becomes a challenge to help these patients with their pain and with the anxiety, depression, disability, and suffering that accompany the disease.

To be effective in the management of the pain associated with arthritis and other rheumatic disorders it is essential to have a clear understanding of the pain experience and of the diseases themselves.

Pain and Innervation at the Joint

Sternbach [26] defines pain as "a concept which refers to (1) a personal, private sensation of hurt, (2) a harmful stimulus which signals current or impending tissue damage, (3) a pattern of responses which operate to protect the organism from harm." This definition encompasses the reception of the stimuli, the perception that brings about a personal sensation of hurt, and the response. Later sections of this chapter and other chapters in this book (Chaps. 3 and 4) deal with factors influencing perception of pain and response to it. The following discussion focuses on the pathophysiology of the disease to provide information about the stimuli that trigger the pain experience associated with rheumatic diseases. After considering the pathophysiology common to joint pain generally, several of the most common rheumatic diseases and their treatment will be described.

Joints are supplied by articular nerves, which carry fibers derived from several spinal nerves. The articular nerves vary in number and in course. When the nerve enters a joint, there is wide distribution to the ligaments, capsule, and synovial membrane, as Figure 16-1 illustrates.

The articular nerves carry autonomic fibers and sensory fibers of varying size. The larger sensory fibers form proprioceptive endings in the capsule and ligaments called Ruffini endings. These endings are sensitive to position and movement, and are concerned with the reflex control of position, with locomotion, and with the perception of position and movement. The smaller sensory fibers form free nerve endings in the capsule, the ligaments, and the

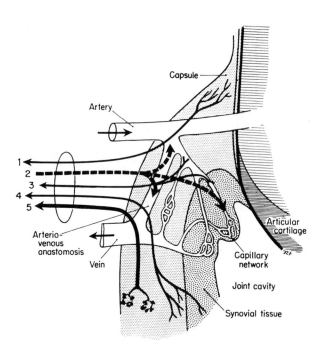

Figure 16-1 Schematic representation of blood and nerve supply of joints. The arterial supply to epiphysis, capsule, and synovial tissue is shown, as well as capillary networks, venous drainage, and an arteriovenous anastomosis. An articular nerve is shown enclosed by a circle. Such a nerve contains various fibers, indicated by numbers, with direction of conduction shown by arrows. 1. Afferent (pain) from the capsule. 2. Efferent (postganglionic sympathetic or vasomotor) to smooth muscle of blood vessels. 3. Afferent (pain) and others with unknown functions from adventitia of vessels. 4. Afferent (pain) from the capsule and synovial tissue. 5. Afferent (proprioceptive) from the capsule. (From E. D. Gardner, Instructional Course Lectures 10:251. Used by permission of the American Academy of Orthopaedic Surgeons.)

adventitia that transmit the feeling of pain. The most effective painful stimulus of the capsule and ligaments is twisting or stretching.

The autonomic fibers in joint nerves are vasomotor fibers that supply the blood vessels. No nerves are found in articular cartilage or in compact bone.

Periarticular tissues are abundantly innervated with nerve endings similar to those found in the joint capsule. The smaller nerve fibers from these various tissues form larger bundles, which become parts of the dorsal spinal nerve root of that segment. The constituent parts of these nerves synapse in similar spinal cord segments. This overlapping and joining of nerve endings explains why stimuli that originate in structures about the joints may produce a painful sensation mistakenly thought to originate in the joint tissue.

The capsule and ligaments are highly sensitive, whereas the synovial membrane is relatively insensitive [14]. Whether arising from the capsule or from the synovial membrane, joint pain is diffuse and poorly localized. (See Fig. 16-2.) Studies indicate that pain arising from a given structure is felt as either localized or as diffuse pain depending more on whether the location of the structure is superficial or deep than upon the nature of the tissue (periosteum, ligament, tendon, or fascia) [16]. If the involved tissue is deep, the pain will be experienced as diffuse. Moreover, joint pain is often referred, just as deep or visceral pain may be. In some hip disorders, for example, pain may be felt in an uninvolved knee. It is ordinarily believed that changes in temperature, humidity, and barometric pressure make joints more sensitive or painful [11].

When pain is severe it may be felt over much of the limb, especially dis-

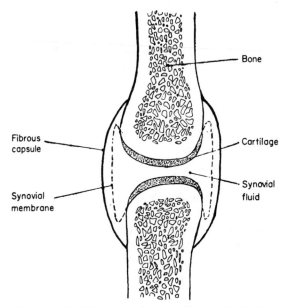

Figure 16-2   Gross anatomy of diarthrodial joint. (From J. A. Boyle and W. W. Buchanan, *Clinical Rheumatology*. Philadelphia: F. A. Davis. Used by permission.)

tally. When it is severe with sudden onset, there may be reflex reactions, including slowing of the pulse, fall in blood pressure, and nausea and vomiting. Joint pain commonly leads to reflex contractions of muscles, especially those that flex or adduct. These reflex contractions may take the form of spasm. Antagonistic muscles (extensor) may relax reflexly, to the extent that if pain continues for a period of time the extensor muscles may atrophy.

Experimentally induced pain in joints apparently is experienced in similar ways, regardless of the cause of the pain. Studies of Lennander [16], for example, have shown that the same type of pain results when tissues about the joints are stimulated by pinching, tearing, cauterizing by acid or heat, cutting, sticking, or use of electric currents. Lewis added to these observations by injection of chemical irritants to produce similar pain [15]. In the following sections, pain associated with specific rheumatic disorders will be discussed. The clinical features of the disease provide clues about the nature of pain experienced by the individual, methods of preventing additional discomfort and pain, and methods of controlling and relieving existing pain.

Rheumatoid Arthritis

Rheumatoid arthritis (RA) is a chronic inflammatory disease principally affecting the joints with swelling, pain, and deformity. It is a classic example of a chronic illness that manifests itself continuously in varying degrees of activity and subactivity, partial remission being followed by relapse and exacerbation. It is this course of the disease that causes the most persistent pain and suffering. Rheumatoid arthritis is the greatest problem of the rheumatic diseases from the standpoint of severity, prolonged disability, and pain. For this reason pathophysiology and psychosocial aspects are discussed first.

Pain in and about the joints is the first symptom and usually the chief complaint when a person seeks medical help. Pain usually persists throughout the active disease. In addition to joint pain, there may be pain in the ligaments, tendons, muscles, fascia, and in the periosteum. Usually there is symmetrical joint involvement. Any joint in the body may be affected including the temporomandibular and the cricoarytenoid joints of the larynx as shown in Figure 16-3.

The nature of the painful stimuli varies according to the inflammatory process and the destructive tissue changes in the joint. Most of the pathological changes of rheumatoid arthritis are nonspecific and produce a highly variable picture of pain.

The principal lesions of the systemic disease are found in the synovial joints. Present evidence indicates that joint changes begin in the synovial tissue. Microscopically, the synovial tissue appears highly variable, depending on the location, duration, and recurrent character of the inflammation. Three separate pathological processes occurring in joints are described, although they are integrally related and continuous [11]. Knowledge of these

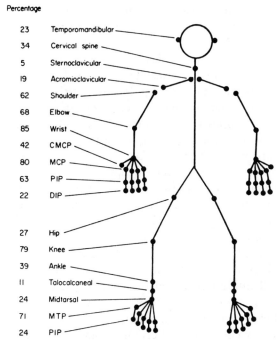

Percentage

23	Temporomandibular
34	Cervical spine
5	Sternoclavicular
19	Acromioclavicular
62	Shoulder
68	Elbow
85	Wrist
42	CMCP
80	MCP
63	PIP
22	DIP
27	Hip
79	Knee
39	Ankle
11	Talocalcaneal
24	Midtarsal
71	MTP
24	PIP

Figure 16-3 Incidence of joint involvement in 50 patients with rheumatoid arthritis. (From J. A. Boyle and W. W. Buchanan, *Clinical Rheumatology*. Philadelphia: F. A. Davis, 1971.)

processes is important to an understanding of the pain associated with rheumatoid arthritis.

The first process is exudation. Congestion and edema are most marked at the internal surface of the synovium, particularly close to the margins of the articular cartilage. In the remaining part there is effusion into the joint space. In focal areas of desquamation of synovial lining cells and of necrosis of the superficial synovial tissue, compact fibrin exudes onto the surface and into the swollen tissue.

The second process is cellular infiltration. Large numbers of polymorphonuclear leukocytes are present in acute inflammation. The principal infiltrating cells are lymphocytes and plasma cells that are distributed diffusely and in small nodular aggregates that may have germinal centers.

The third pathological process is formation of granulation tissue. There is proliferation of blood vessels and of synovial fibroblasts in the areas of cellular filtrations. The synovial lining, normally composed of an ill-defined, usually single layer of cells, becomes distinct and multicellular. In places, the lining cells become elongated and are in a closely arranged palisade perpendicular to the surface.

As a result of these three processes, the synovial tissue becomes grossly thickened. The hypertrophy has a villous character that is most marked near the joint cartilages. As the process progresses, the synovial tissue grows from the margin of the joint onto the surface of the articular cartilage or erodes between it and the bone. The granulation tissue that spreads as a carpet over the cartilage is referred to as pannus. The articular cartilage will disappear at the time of ingrowth of the pannus and subchondral granulation tissue. The precise mechanism is unknown, but enzymes derived from the synovial cells or infiltrating cells have been proposed for the process. The subchondral bone also can be eroded by invading pannus, and granulation tissue in the marrow spaces beneath the articular cortex can form fibrous cysts. The bones in the vicinity of the diseased joints become osteoporotic. Destruction of the articular cartilage and bone can progress to total destruction of the original joint surfaces. The granulation tissue may form adhesions and undergo changes leading to fibrous, cartilaginous, or bony ankyloses. These destructive changes in tissue and bone are sources of pain.

Periarticular tissues, notably tendons and tendon sheaths, show edema and cellular infiltration during periods of joint inflammation. Muscles show interstitial foci of mononuclear cell infiltration called lymphorrhages. Contractures of the capsule, ligaments, or muscle groups may occur with healing by scar formation particularly during periods of immobilization. The effort to move the contracted tissue, bear weight, and use crippled joints causes considerable pain.

Stiffness is perhaps the most constant symptom of the disease. Aside from pain, many persons complain of stiffness associated with arthritis. The stiffness of joints is caused by a "gelling" of the periarticular tissue following sleep. This makes morning the most uncomfortable time, for the arthritic person experiences both pain and stiffness. On first arising in the morning a period of a half hour to several hours is required to limber up and recover from the aggravation of pain and stiffness.

Since rheumatoid arthritis is a systemic disease, it manifests generalized feelings of discomfort. These symptoms are general malaise, unnatural fatigue, fever, tachycardia, and weakness producing a diffuse discomfort rather than pain. In addition to the primary polyarthritis from inflammation and dysfunction, ill health may be due to involvement of the lymphatic system, the cardiovascular system, or the pulmonary system, or to ocular or neural manifestations.

Two major conditions, Sjögrens syndrome and amyloidosis, and other extra-articular manifestations are considered as extensions of the disease rather than as complications [11]. Hospitalization may be required for treatment of extra-articular manifestations and iatrogenic conditions, resulting from reactions to drugs and drug interactions. In addition to pain and discomfort arising from articular structures, extra-articular problems, and systemic processes, there are psychological aspects to be considered in treating the total patient.

The pain and illness may become so overwhelming as to totally preoccupy a person. Bonica [1] suggests that patients with long-standing pain do not become accustomed to it, but seem to suffer more as time passes. He states that protracted pain produces physical and psychological depletions that vary widely from one person to another and may be evidence of basic personality differences. Bonica [1] asserts that chronic pain eventually produces an alteration in the person's attitude toward his environment and can become a "consuming problem which completely dominates his life."

Patients who have lived with the disease for a number of years usually can give detailed descriptions about the location, timing, quality, and quantity of their pain. This may be expected since there is constant awareness of pain; it is a part of their everyday activity, and it has been described many times before. Although experimental pain studies of joints indicate that various painful stimuli result in similar pain experiences, patients with rheumatoid arthritis use a wide variety of terms in describing pain. Some of the more common terms are sharp or dull, vague or intense, aching or gnawing, tearing or burning, and local or diffuse.

Common comments on their pain are:

"It is hard to describe."
"It changes—sometimes, it's severe and then it just aches."
"My shoulders are bothering me and I'm a little stiff all over."

A large percentage of patients with long-standing rheumatoid arthritis experience anxiety and depression at some time in the course of the disease [7]. The psychogenic factors are a grave concern and receive considerable attention in determining whether personality patterns and emotional states play significant parts in the etiology and clinical course of rheumatoid arthritis.

It has been postulated that premorbid, negative personality traits and linkage of emotional factors are related to the disease onset and exacerbations [4]. Cobb et al suggest that persons with certain personality characteristics when exposed to relevant environmental circumstances will have physiological responses that contribute to certain diseases but not to others. Their study and others show that when persons with rheumatoid arthritis are compared to nondiseased controls, those with rheumatoid arthritis tend to be more anxious and depressed and to exhibit conflicts in the expression of hostility. Further research has shown that individuals with arthritis manifest conflicts and deficits in the expression of autonomy, affiliation, anger and aggression, and sexuality [10].

Moldofsky and Chester [17] investigated the association between psychological and somatic factors in patients with rheumatoid arthritis. Two pain-mood patterns were defined: "a synchronous state, characterized by mood changes within an anxiety or hostility spectrum, either closely preceding or concomitant with joint tenderness; and a paradoxical state, characterized by an inverse relationship between intensity of joint tenderness and a sense of hopelessness." The subjects with synchronous pain-mood state appeared to have coped with their disease more easily, required less medical attention and more conservative treatment measures, continued with work and social involvement, and functioned better within the medically prescribed regime than the paradoxical pattern group. The conclusions are that there appears to be an association between emotional issues and articular pain as an index of rheumatoid arthritis inflammation activity. The pain-mood patterns may have prognostic significance.

Robinson et al [25] indicated an overall personality similarity between patients recently diagnosed and patients diagnosed more than three years earlier. These researchers also attempted to determine if any person who suffers from a chronically painful and disabling disease is likely to demonstrate the "RA personality" observed by so many investigators. They noted a tendency for any person who suffers from chronically painful and disabling disease to exhibit greater levels of anxiety and depression, thus demonstrating the RA personality. Further, Moos has observed that RA patients in general are characterized not so much by consistent patterns of personality traits that differ from nondiseased normals but by a greater variability of personality functioning than normals [18].

Review of studies that investigated psychological characteristics of individuals with rheumatoid arthritis indicates the complexity of the relationships. At the present time, for example, the psychological factors are considered by some to be a result of the disorder rather than a cause. The important point here is that anxiety and depression are integral parts of rheumatoid arthritis and the pain experience.

The diversity of research techniques, subject samples, and methodology seriously limit generalizations of the reported findings. However, it is provocative to identify (1) relevant psychological variables and their relationship to the disease, (2) whether or not they are present prior to the disease, (3) significant association between certain life experiences or psychological states (or both) and the onset of the disease, and (4) how psychological responses observed in persons with rheumatoid arthritis influence the course of the illness.

Treatment

Since there is no known cure and no completely predictable therapy that is effective for rheumatoid arthritis, management is the term of choice in discussing treatment. The primary objectives of the management are to reduce inflammation and pain, preserve function, and prevent deformity that leads to further pain. The foremost goal of the patient will be to have less pain or to be free of pain.

Table 16-1 diagrams the major modalities—education, rest, exercise, temperature application, drugs, and surgery—in the management of rheumatoid arthritis. Level I is the basic approach used with newly diagnosed rheumatoid

Table 16-1　Basic program for management of rheumatoid arthritis

Level I	Education of patient, family, and society	Application of heat or cold	Range-of-motion exercises	Emotional, joint, and systemic rest	Salicylates to tolerance (20–30 mg/ 100 ml)
Level II	Anti-inflammatory drugs	Analgesic-tranquilizer-relaxant (e.g., Darvon)	Intensive occupational and physical therapy	Intra-articular injection of steroids	Orthopedic devices (e.g., splints)
Level III	Steroids q.o.d.	Preventive surgery	Gold	Antimalarials	
Level IV	Steroids daily	Hospitalization	Rehabilitative surgery		
Level V	Immuno-suppressive drugs				

Source: From Godfrey, Robert G., 1973.

arthritis patients. Levels II through V are available treatment measures that may be effective for prevailing symptoms at different stages of the disease. In planning a management program for the patient with RA the following factors should be considered: (1) the status of joint function, particularly range of motion, with respect to the apparent duration of the disease; (2) the degree of disease activity, from slight, with mild complaints confined to a few joints, to most severe, with extra-articular manifestations; (3) the age, sex, occupation, and family responsibilities of the patient, and the patient's response to the disease, and (4) the results of previous treatment. Each patient is different and must have a customized individual plan. The prevailing view of experienced physicians is to use conservative measures at the outset of treatment and to continue these as long as indicated.

The keystone to effective treatment is education: of the patient, his family, the community, and health professionals. An understanding of the disease and what to expect can assist in gaining the cooperation of the patient and family to carry out and participate in the plan of care. When the patient is aware that there are no cures or measures of quick relief from pain, discouragement and disappointment may be avoided. Because rheumatoid arthritis is an unpredictable disease, the emotional state of the patient must be considered. Education of the patient and family at crucial and appropriate times in the management plan can alleviate certain psychosocial problems. This includes setting realistic goals for rest and activity during flare-ups, teaching the patient to anticipate pain, knowing measures to alleviate pain, and learning how to "live with" a modicum of discomfort.

Application of heat is used for analgesic action and to permit exercise with greater ease. The use of hot moist packs applied to involved joints before activity in the morning was tested with a sample of 12 patients to determine the relief of morning stiffness associated with rheumatoid arthritis [21]. It was found that moist heat was effective in modifying the morning stiffness by decreasing the duration and amount of stiffness and increasing the range of motion. In recent years patients with rheumatoid arthritis have been advised to use ice packs for swollen joints [20]. If a joint is tender and swollen the application of heat may provoke an increase of the blood supply and swelling, which aggravates the joint inflammation. Some patients have found ice more helpful than heat. Although applications of heat and cold are useful in relieving pain and have similar effects, the mechanism by which they produce analgesic action is not known.

Exercise and physical therapy are integral parts of the basic treatment program. Exercises should be prescribed to attain the goals of maintaining function and muscle strength and prevention of deformities. Range-of-motion exercises, both active and passive, are used, carefully tailored to fit each patient. Pain is used as a guide to controlling the amount of exercise. To relieve pain and stiffness, heat is frequently used before the exercises to enable the patient to participate more fully in the exercise program. Although there is pain associated with exercises, prevention of flexion contractures and of decreased range of motion alleviates the pain associated with deformity and immobility [5].

Adequate rest balanced with activity has been part of the basic program for treatment of rheumatoid arthritis for many years. The patient seems to require 8 to 12 hours of sleep each night and frequent rest periods during the day when the disease is more active. During acute flare-ups of the arthritis, several days of bed rest are helpful in reducing joint inflammation and systemic symptoms. Rest that also relieves emotional stress is desirable. However, complete inactivity for prolonged periods of time should be avoided since it leads to increased muscle weakness and limitation of joint motion. A controlled study of therapeutic bed rest in rheumatoid arthritis in which patients were kept in bed most of the time, compared to a control group of patients allowed up ad lib, showed no significant difference [20]. However, based on past experience, rest is still advocated and imposed on the patient by fatigue and pain from the disease process. Rest of an inflamed joint using splints and braces may relieve muscle spasm and pain, and insure correct position, especially at night.

The use of drugs in the treatment of rheumatoid arthritis is primarily to aid in the relief of pain. Many of the drugs have an anti-inflammatory action to suppress the inflammation that is the major cause of pain in active arthritis. Medications that have this effect include the salicylates, phenylbutazone, indomethacin, the antimalarial drugs chloroquine and hydroxychloroquine, gold, and the corticosteroids.

Aspirin is the best overall salicylate available. It is definitely helpful in the large majority of patients. In addition to the analgesic action, aspirin seems to have an antirheumatoid effect. Although there is not conclusive evidence, it is speculated that there is a difference in the way that nonrheumatoid persons and persons with rheumatoid arthritis metabolize aspirin [20]. It has been shown that when a patient with RA is given a measured amount of aspirin compared with the nonrheumatoid patient, there is a significant difference in plasma salicylate levels. It has been postulated that there is a difference in aspirin metabolism in the patient with rheumatoid arthritis because of hypoalbuminemia, owing to the binding of the drug between salicylate and protein.

Although the specific action of aspirin is not known, aspirin administered in regular, adequate doses can control pain associated with rheumatoid arthritis. Most patients require relatively large doses of aspirin, 0.6 to 1.5 gm four times daily on a regular schedule.

To facilitate a comprehensive management program that controls pain, it is necessary to use a team approach utilizing several health professionals, such as a physician, nurse, physical therapist, social worker, occupational therapist, and dietitian. Each member can contribute to overcome that aspect interfering with achieving the ultimate goal of controlling pain with optimal physical functioning.

Individualized Nursing Care

It is essential to have basic knowledge about the pathophysiology of rheumatoid arthritis and the noxious stimuli causing pain. To be effective in alleviating pain and promoting physical and emotional comfort it is necessary to assess the patient's pain and utilize measures to modify the noxious stimuli and perception of pain. In addition to the clinical assessment of pain described in Chapter 6 there are clinical features and factors to be considered in planning nursing intervention.

1. length of time coping with the disease
2. amount of pain endured with frequent or infrequent exacerbation
3. number of joints involved
4. duration of morning stiffness
5. fatigue and general malaise
6. anemia
7. degree of loss of range of motion
8. results of erythrocyte sedimentation rate (elevated indicates inflammatory activity)
9. extent of deformity (ankylosis)
10. extraarticular involvement
11. medical plan of treatment
12. goals of the patient

Making this kind of an assessment provides information on the current status of the patient's pain and physical functioning that can be used to evaluate the effectiveness of nursing interventions.

Beginning with education, the nurse can be instrumental in teaching the patient and family to understand the disease and develop a proper attitude toward it. For example, knowing that joint stiffness is more common in the morning and that fatigue and general malaise are a part of the disease process rather than "laziness" or a character defect is helpful. Equally important is for the patient and family to understand the purpose of the treatment measures. For example, aspirin is used to relieve inflammation and pain. This is useful so that the patient and family can help evaluate which treatment measure is beneficial. Also the patient and family become actively involved in complying with the treatment. Emphasis is being placed on teaching the family because they greatly affect how the patient interprets and responds to pain. Moral support is a very important aspect of treatment and can mean the difference in success or failure of the overall management program. A hopeless reaction with lack of motivation may be a major factor in causing disability. Failure to acknowledge the limitations placed on him by the disease can also cause the patient further stress and difficulty. The person needs help from the family and health professionals in adopting a realistic attitude toward his disease, learning to live within the limitations imposed by it, and following advice about treatment.

Many aspects of routine nursing care of patients hospitalized with rheumatoid arthritis need to be modified to fit the needs of the individual. It is an opportunity for the nurse to teach the patient about the disease and treatment; also the nurse must allow the patient to carry out certain activities he can do for himself. It may be necessary to give aspirin and medication at an early hour to relieve morning stiffness and pain when the patient wishes to start activities. Morning care or hygiene may need to be delayed due to the duration of morning stiffness. Astute assessment needs to be made of which activities the patient can perform for himself. He should be allowed to do these and be given assistance with activities he cannot perform. It requires ingenuity on the part of the nurse to suggest and devise methods that will assist the patient to perform activities by himself. Using long handles on utensils and easy fasteners on clothing, and finding simpler ways of performing "nimble finger" tasks will enable the patient to perform more easily and with less discomfort. Because movement of joints may be painful and difficult due to stiffness, most activity is performed slowly. The patient should proceed at his own pace and avoid hurrying. To hurry the patient in any activity will create anxiety and increase the amount of pain. The mere anticipation of pain is sufficient to intensify pain.

Safety measures should be employed in the hospital and the home to avoid potential injuries due to weakness or instability. Handrails conveniently located in bathrooms and a raised toilet seat may prevent falls. Precautions should be taken in using wheelchairs and other walking aids, such as canes and crutches, to prevent accidents.

There are other measures that will promote physical comfort. Generally the patient with rheumatoid arthritis is most comfortable when the body is warm. Cool drafts in rooms should be avoided. Lightweight bed clothing and wearing apparel are advisable to provide the warmth and allow easy movement of involved joints. Comfortable firm mattresses and pillows placed appropriately will help with positioning and in the prevention of deformities. A thin pillow under the head should be used to minimize flexion of the neck. Pillows should not be placed beneath the knees because this can lead to flexion contractions of the knees and hips. A pillow placed between the knees is definitely helpful in preventing adduction deformity of the hips. Encouraging the patient to rest with joints extended as far as comfortable and maintaining proper body alignment is helpful in preventing deformity.

The nurse has the responsibility to help the patient determine which measures are helpful and which measures have not been effective in promoting comfort. The answer may be more rest versus exercise, cold versus heat, a change in the dosage of aspirin, devising a new method to perform a task, or changing time schedules for the various measures.

Degenerative Joint Disease

Degenerative joint disease is an extremely common, noninflammatory, progressive disorder of movable joints, particularly weight-bearing joints. The more popular term, *osteoarthritis*, used interchangeably with *degenerative joint disease*, is inaccurate since it implies an inflammatory process. The disease is more common with the elderly and appears to be a part of the aging process. There are factors in addition to aging that influence the rate of cartilage degeneration and progression of the disease, such as a sequel to joint injury or other type of disease process involving the joint.

The condition is characterized by deterioration of articular cartilage and by formation of new bone in the subchondral areas and at the margins of the joint. Symptoms of degenerative joint disease are related to the particular joint involved (see Fig. 16-4). The common complaints are joint pain, particularly on weight bearing, stiffness after periods of rest, and aching at times of changes in weather. The amount of pain will vary from slight to extreme depending on the joint or number of joints involved, the degenerative pathological status of the joint, the degree of stiffness, and the extent of deformity. There is evidence that the structural changes as shown in radiological features do not predict the amount of pain, since one patient may have little or no pain whereas another patient may have considerable pain and discomfort.

Heberden's nodes are characteristic of degenerative joint disease. These consist of deforming bony protuberances at the margins and on the dorsal surface of the terminal interphalangeal joints of the fingers that are usually

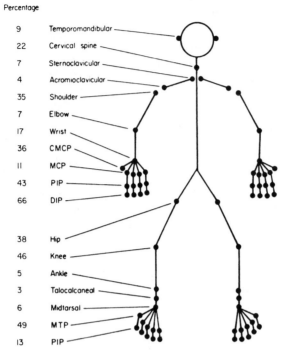

Percentage

9	Temporomandibular	
22	Cervical spine	
7	Sternoclavicular	
4	Acromioclavicular	
35	Shoulder	
7	Elbow	
17	Wrist	
36	CMCP	
11	MCP	
43	PIP	
66	DIP	
38	Hip	
46	Knee	
5	Ankle	
3	Talocalcaneal	
6	Midtarsal	
49	MTP	
13	PIP	

Figure 16-4 Prevalence of clinical joint involvement in a sample of 50 patients with primary osteoarthosis. (From J. A. Boyle and W. W. Buchanan, *Clinical Rheumatology.* Philadelphia: F. A. Davis, 1971.)

unsightly and awkward to use, but are seldom painful when fully developed. Local pain, tenderness to the touch, and the cardinal symptoms of inflammation may be present early in the course of their development. The cause of the painful inflammation appears to be the release of hyaluronic acid into the surrounding tissues from the degenerating cartilage [7].

Other causes of pain in more advanced degenerative joint disease are injury, small subluxations, and bruising of the involved joint.

Degenerative disease of the hip is the most disabling of the various joint problems. Pain on motion or weight bearing is the main complaint, and becomes progressively severe with the pain referred to the groin or medial side of the knee. Later the pain may become continuous and be especially difficult to tolerate at night. Degenerative disease of the knees is commonly observed in older women and is associated with loss of motion, crepitus, and flexion deformity.

The nature of the pain and symptoms will differ with factors that tend to ease or aggravate the joints for different persons. The joints involved—which

Table 16-2   Major differences between rheumatoid arthritis and osteoarthritis

Variable	Rheumatoid arthritis	Osteoarthritis
Age at onset	3rd and 4th decades	5th and 6th decades
Weight	normal or underweight	usually overweight
Constitutional manifestations	present	absent
Joints involved	any joint	mainly knees, spine and peripheral phalanges
Appearance of joint	soft tissue swelling	bony swelling
Special deformities	fusiform finger joint, ulnar deviation	Herberden's nodes
Subcutaneous nodules	present in 20 percent	never present
X-ray	osteoporosis, erosions	osteosclerosis, bony spurs
Joint fluid	increased cells, poor mucin	few cells, normal mucin
Rheumatoid factor	present in 85 to 90 percent	usually absent
Blood count	anemia, leukocytosis	normal
Course	generally progressive	stationary or very slowly progressive
Termination	ankylosis and deformity	no ankylosis
Complicating amyloidosis	15 to 25 percent	usually absent

Source: Robbins, Stanley L., *Pathologic Basis of Disease.* Philadelphia: W. B. Saunders Company.

may be cervical and lumbar spines, hips, knees, thumb bases, fingers or acromioclavicular joints—will produce a difference in the nature of the pain, and the joints will respond differently to various forms of treatment. Degenerative joint disease may be confused with rheumatoid arthritis although there are many differences in the two diseases. Table 16-2 summarizes these differences.

Treatment

The main objectives of therapy for degenerative joint disease are relief of pain, restoration of joint function, and prevention of avoidable disability or progression of the disease [2]. The modes of treatment are: (1) physical measures, (2) drug therapy, and (3) surgery.

General physical measures include a balance of rest and exercise. Daily periods of rest with support of the involved joint are essential and will avoid further aggravation. An acutely painful spondylosis will benefit from a firm mattress and an underlying board to support the spine. When weight-bearing joints are affected, local support is obtained with the use of canes, crutches, or other mechanical devices. Teaching the patient to use these methods of local support will promote greater ease of mobility and prevent further disability. Avoidance of unnecessary walking and stair climbing and wearing of proper or corrective shoes to shift the line of weight bearing often prove helpful.

Excessive rest may cause pain that can be relieved with exercise and change of position. This is most common in the knee and hip, where prolonged sitting with these joints in flexion to 90° or more after a period of 30 to 40 minutes of immobility produces pain. Relief of immobility pain can be obtained by extending the leg and walking. Exercises are essential to prevent contraction of the joint, which leads to further limitation of movement and pain. Assisting the patient to achieve a daily balance of rest and exercises and to perform activities that cause the least amount of physical stress can be effective in alleviating pain.

The use of heat and cold aids in the program of exercise, prevention of deformities and contractions, and maintenance of muscle tone. Various methods of applying heat such as heating pads, moist hot packs, or submerging the involved joint in warm water may be tried to determine which is the most effective in relieving the pain.

Traction is useful when there is muscle spasm, particularly for hip or cervical vertebral disease. Wearing a cervical collar often relieves discomfort when the cervical vertebrae are involved.

If the nurse knows the specific type of "arthritis" and the goal of the medical management, she can implement measures and modify them to be effective in relieving pain. Patients with degenerative joint disease should be reassured that the disease is likely to remain confined to a few joints, in contrast to the widespread disease so often pictured as "arthritis."

Pharmacological agents other than analgesics play a relatively minor role in the management of pain and the disease. Aspirin in moderate dosage (0.6 gm three to five times a day) is helpful in conjunction with rest and physical measures. Other anti-inflammatory agents and intra-articular injections may be tried to provide relief of pain, but often are inadequate in controlling the pain effectively and carry the risk of toxicity that is associated with the drug.

Surgical treatment is often necessary for the relief of persistent pain and correction of serious deformity. Surgical treatment of degenerative joint disease includes: (1) debridement, (2) arthrodesis (joint fusion), (3) arthroplasty (the formation of a prosthetic articulating surface), (4) osteotomy (section of bone to alter weight-bearing surfaces), and (5) total joint replacement. Recent developments in the procedures of arthroplasty and joint replacements for the knee and hip have resulted in pain relief with good stability and mobility [22].

The patient with degenerative joint disease who has surgical treatment requires diligent preoperative and postoperative care. The patient will need physical and psychological support to participate in exercises essential in the postoperative period to achieve desired outcomes for rehabilitation.

Ankylosing Spondylitis

Ankylosing spondylitis is a progressive form of arthritis distinguished by involvement of the sacroiliac joints, the spinal apophyseal (synovial) joints, and the paravertebral soft tissues. The disorder is also known as Marie-Strumpell arthritis and rheumatoid spondylitis. The cause is unknown.

The onset is usually in the second or third decade of life and is relatively uncommon after 30 years of age. Approximately 90 percent of the patients are males. The beginning is usually insidious, with episodes of aching referred to the low back, the sacroiliac areas, or the hips, or all three. In about 10 percent of patients, particularly in the early stage, pain may radiate along the course of the sciatic nerve. There is frequently well-defined morning stiffness of the back that is aggravated by immobility. These symptoms tend to grow progressively worse, and over a period of months or years they become associated with pain in the lumbar and dorsal spine, with restricted back motion. Complaints may be intermittent and progressive back limitation may develop with little or no pain.

Although these patients experience pain and painfully stiff joints in the mornings, as do patients with rheumatoid arthritis, there are a number of variables that make ankylosing spondylitis a different condition. Generally these patients are at their best when active and moving about. A study by Huskisson and Hart [12] found patients with spondylitic to have pain thresholds higher than those with rheumatoid arthritis. This group of patients are more active, take less analgesics, and have less time off work than the rheumatoid arthritics.

Patients with ankylosing spondylitis, particularly the young males, suffer less depression and emotional overtones than do the rheumatoids. The fact that their peripheral joints usually are normal enables them to lead more normal lives [7].

Treatment

Treatment consisting of full, regular doses of salicylates combined with physical therapy may prove sufficient for relief of pain and inflammation. In patients for whom this is not adequate, phenylbutazone, oxyphenbutazone, or indomethacin may be tried. These medications seem to be equally effective in appropriate doses and appear to be more helpful in ankylosing spondylitis than other anti-inflammatory drugs are.

Physical measures are used to maintain the best possible position of the vertebral column and to avoid flexion deformity of the spine. Proper positioning at rest is of paramount importance. Use of a firm mattress supported with a bed board is helpful. Regular daily exercises with emphasis on bodily activity rather than rest is encouraged.

Gout

Gout, a disease resulting from the abnormal metabolism of uric acid, is characterized by recurrent episodes causing violent pain in the affected joint. The typical acute attack of gout begins rather abruptly, with the affected area acutely inflamed, swollen, and tender. The usual attack lasts for 3 to 10 days when untreated. The large joint of the great toe is more commonly involved than any other joint, without any known reason. Other joints in the foot, the ankle, the knee, or any other joint in the body may be involved. In gout there is an increase in the amount of uric acid in the body which is evidenced by an increase in its concentration in the blood. In general, the higher the serum urate level, the earlier the appearance and development of tophi, deposits of uric acid, in various places of the body [22]. The presence of tophaceous deposits is associated with a tendency toward more frequent and severe episodes of acute gouty arthritis. Chronic gouty arthritis with deformity of the joints develops as a result of the erosion of cartilage and subchondral bone caused by the inflammatory reaction to deposits of tophi in the joints. The course of gout is quite variable, ranging from one or a few attacks to a progressively severe disease with marked crippling, when untreated, for some patients. Approximately 95 percent of the cases of gout are men and there is a heredity factor associated with the disease. There are no overtones of chronic anxiety or depression, but emotional feelings of frustration and annoyance to the point of rage occur.

Treatment

There are two main objectives in the treatment of gout. The first is the immediate control and prevention of the acute attack of gouty arthritis. The second is the long-term reduction of uric acid in the body to prevent formation of uric acid deposits and promote resolution of those tophi already present. It is possible to achieve both of these objectives in the majority of patients with the currently available medications. Colchicine, the traditional drug, phenylbutazone, oxyphenbutazone, and indomethacin are effective in the relief of acute gout. Probenecid (Benemid) and allopurinol are agents that must be taken regularly every day to control the amount of uric acid in the body. Early treatment with the appropriate drug seems to be the key to bringing the acute attack with the accompanying pain under control.

Summary

In order to help the individual who is suffering with pain associated with arthritis and other rheumatic disorders it is essential to know the source and nature of the pain. Both generalities and specifics of some of the rheumatic disorders and their treatment have been discussed to provide an understanding of the related pain and provide a basis for intervention to relieve and control pain. In addition to using the conventional modalities of treatment there should be an ongoing assessment to individualize care as the pain decreases or increases to help the patient.

References

1. Bonica, J. J. Management of intractable pain. In Way, E. W., ed., *New Concepts in Pain and Its Clinical Management*. Philadelphia: F. A. Davis Company, 1967.
2. Boyle, J. A., and Buchanan, W. W. *Clinical Rheumatology*. Philadelphia: F. A. Davis Company, 1971.
3. Cobb, S. Contained hostility in rheumatoid arthritis. *Arthritis Rheum.* 2:419, 1959.
4. Cobb, S., Schull, W., Harburg, E., and Kasl, S. V. The intra-familial transmission of rheumatoid arthritis VIII. Summary of findings. *J. Chronic Dis.* 22:295, 1969.
5. Glass, D. D. Physical measures in rheumatoid arthritis. *J. Albert Einstein Med. Center* 19 Spring, 1971.
6. Hart, F. D. Control of pain at night. *Nurs. Times*, March 3, 1973. P. 559.
7. Hart, F. D. *The Treatment of Chronic Pain*. London: Medical and Technical Publishing Co., Ltd., 1974. Chapter 3.
8. Hart, F. D., and Huskisson, E. C. Pain patterns in the rheumatic disorders. *Br. Med. J.* 4:213, 1972.
9. Heat and cold as analgesics. *Med. Lett. Drugs Ther.* 12:3, 1970.
10. Hoffman, A. L. Psychological factors associated with rheumatoid arthritis. *Nurs. Res.* 23:3, 1974.
11. Hollander, J. L., and McCarty, D. *Arthritis and Allied Conditions*. 8th ed. Philadelphia: Lea & Febiger, 1972.
12. Huskisson, E. C., and Hart, F. D. Pain threshold and arthritis. *Br. Med. J.* 4:193, 1972.
13. Jacox, A., and Stewart, M. *Psychosocial Contingencies of the Pain Experience*. Monograph. Iowa City: The University of Iowa, 1973.
14. Kellgren, J. H. Observations on referred pain arising from muscles. *Clin. Sci.* 351:175, 1938.
15. Lewis, T. *Pain*. New York: Macmillan, Inc., 1942.
16. MacBryde, C. M. *Signs and Symptoms*. 5th ed. Philadelphia: J. B. Lippincott Company. Chapter 3 and Chapter 12.
17. Moldofsky, H., and Chester, W. J. Pain and mood patterns in patients with rheumatoid arthritis. *Psychosom. Med.* 32:309, 1970.
18. Moos, R. H. Personality factors associated with rheumatoid arthritis: A review. *J. Chron. Dis.* 17:41, 1964.
19. Moskowitz, R. W. Psychosocial aspects of rheumatoid arthritis. *J. Albert Einstein Med. Center* 19:36, 1971.
20. Neustadt, D. H. Medical management of rheumatoid arthritis. *J. Albert Einstein Med. Center* 19:25, 1971.
21. O'Dell, A. J. Hot packs for morning joint stiffness. *Am. J. Nurs.* 75:986.
22. American Rheumatism Association Section of the Arthritis Foundation. Primer on the rheumatic diseases. *JAMA* 224:744, 1973.
23. Robbins, S. L. *Pathologic Basis of Disease*. Philadelphia: W. B. Saunders Company, 1974.
24. Robinson, H., Kirk, R. F., Frye, R. F., and Robertson, J. T. A psychological

study of patients with rheumatoid arthritis and other painful diseases. *J. Psychosom. Res.* 16:53, 1972.

25. Robinson, H., Kirk, R. F., and Frye, R. L. A psychological study of rheumatoid arthritis and selected controls. *J. Chronic Dis.* 23:791, 1971.

26. Sternbach, R. A. *Pain: A Psychophysiological Analysis.* New York: Academic Press, 1968.

17

Pain Associated with Cancer

Martha M. Shawver

Cancer pain is not a new problem or concern. For many people, the terms cancer and pain are synonymous. However, this close identification is not entirely based upon fact. If we consider pain to be primarily physical, it is not true that all those who suffer from cancer, suffer from pain. Although attempts have been made to convince people that physical pain does not always occur with cancer, these attempts, in the light of the ambiguities created by having a diagnosis of cancer, do little to eradicate the mental pain that accompanies the disease. Pain associated with cancer represents a wide gamut of experiences, sensations, types, and intensities. No two people with cancer suffer in the same way since each individual enters the situation with his or her own unique past experiences, his own set of coping behaviors, along with his own type of tumor. For some, a future of total pain relief is nonexistent. Thinking about this possibility can, in itself, be a devastating experience. The pain is always there and the only anticipated change is that it may get progressively worse. For others, there is no present pain, but always the fear that there can be in the future if the tumor gets out of control. The ambiguities and fear associated with cancer are present among health workers as well as among persons experiencing the cancer. Many nurses describe their feelings when caring for a patient who has cancer and pain as "helpless, frustrated, inadequate, drained, angry, anxious, confused, neglectful, and fearful."

When one speaks only of the pain associated with cancer, one deliberately fragments a discussion of the comprehensive care that is necessary for the person with cancer. It is evident, however, that to relieve or manage the pain adequately, if it exists, is to provide for a major aspect of the patient's care. This relief from pain allows the individual to use his energy to cope with the rest of his living experiences and, if necessary, to face his own death. Failure to relieve the pain adequately or to arrest the cancer can interrupt the life-style of the patient in such a way as to reduce him to a life of dependency and despair. It forces him to adapt to a repetitious, boring, and progressively less effective life-style. The nurse and physician are in excellent positions to interrupt this destructive process. Their effectiveness is determined in large part by their capacity to show a caring attitude that is manifested by their assertiveness in implementing pain-relief measures.

It should be remembered that the life of the patient with cancer did not begin with the onset of his illness. An assessment of the person's life-style and experiences before diagnosis will often provide insight into and understanding of the behavioral responses exhibited during his experience with cancer. It is important for the health worker to have some understanding about what having cancer means to an individual and his family. What, for example, does the loss or threatened loss of function or existence of a certain body part mean to the person? Such understanding requires that there be knowledge of the nature of cancer, as well as the nature of pain in order to see how the two interact to confront the individual with any number of stressors. Prolonged exposure to stressors can lead the person to a stage of both physical and mental exhaustion unless some attempt is made to reduce their impact.

Nature of Cancer

Cancer presents itself in an ambiguous, life-threatening manner. In the United States alone, it takes the lives of approximately 365,000 persons and another 665,000 are diagnosed yearly (this number excludes carcinoma-in-situ of the uterine cervix and nonmelanoma skin cancers [2]). While the incidence and end result—death—are somewhat consistent factors, cancer follows a highly unpredictable pattern of development. The numbers alone do not tell us how many people have suffered physical pain, how long they lived with their cancer, or how life-disrupting the experience was for them.

The term *cancer* refers not to one, but to a number of diseases. It is a common term used to refer to all malignant tumors, including leukemias and lymphomas; malignant tumors are also referred to as neoplasias. Neoplasia means "new growth" and the mass of cells that comprise the new growth is called a neoplasm. The abnormal masses of cells are purposeless in terms of function. They merely prey on the host and compete with normal cells for energy and nutrition. Cancer is characteristically a growing and spreading tumor. Most cancers grow rapidly, but follow an erratic course. Some cancers remain dormant for long periods of time while others experience an explosive enlargement. According to Robbins, the growth is "associated with the increased number of mitoses and growth rate of cells." This dissemination of cancer has been said to be its "most feared consequence" [13]. Dissemination or metastasis of cancer occurs by four major pathways: (1) seeding throughout the body cavities, (2) direct transplantation (the mechanical transport of tissue by instrumentation or gloved hand), (3) the lymphatic system, and (4) blood vessel embolization. These pathways of metastasis provide a basis for understanding some of the causes and sources of pain that will be described later in this chapter.

Oncologists are attempting to develop a common language in relation to the classification of cancers. Cancer is classified primarily according to its anatomical and histological association. Tumors are further classified according to their primary site or direct extension, the degree of advancing nodal disease, and the presence or absence of metastasis. A commonly referred to classification is the TNM classification. The three compartments are defined as T–primary tumor, N–regional lymph nodes, and M–metastasis. Further reference is made to staging of the illness. Staging attempts to define the extent of caner within each of the TNM compartments, with Stage 1 referring mainly to a mass limited to an organ of origin with 70 to 90 percent chance of survival and Stage IV (T_4N_3M+) indicating extensive metastasis beyond the original organ with little chance for survival [14].

The mode of spread and the site of probable metastasis are dependent upon the type of cancer and the tissue from which it arises. Cancer of the prostate commonly metastasizes to the bone. Osteogenic cancer may first show signs of metastasis in the lung. The lung is the most common site of metastasis. Other common sites are bone, liver, brain, and distant lymph nodes. Sites such as the genital and urologic organs, skin, and eye are less frequent targets [3].

The basic approaches used to treat cancer are surgery, radiation therapy, and chemotherapy, with some advances being made in immunotherapy. The selection and effectiveness of these approaches depend upon the stage, site, and histological nature of the cancer when it was first detected.

In summary, the nature of cancer is highly unpredictable and life-threatening. Its infiltrative and invasive characteristics present the person having cancer with continual physical and mental threats. The mode and manner of spread present are dependent upon the anatomical and histological origins of the cancer. The effectiveness of treatment is dependent upon when and where the cancer is detected.

The Nature of Pain

Pain has been described as a "disagreeable response to an awareness of a stimulus within or without the body" [12]. Earlier in this chapter pain was explained on a psychophysiological basis. Both neurological and cognitive-emotional systems of events were described as working together to create the experience known as pain. Chapter 2 described more extensively the pathophysiological mechanisms involved in the production of pain. Some of these mechanisms are more common than others and will be discussed in this chapter.

A discussion about pain can take many forms since there are many ways of categorizing pain. Maher [8] describes two basic categories of pain: (1) continuous and (2) incident. Incident pain is characteristically periodic. It is severe at onset but becomes less intense as time goes by. For example, incident pain can result from sudden hemorrhage, distention, and pressure caused by pathological fractures. The pain is usually exacerbated by movement and lessened by rest. Mehta states [9] that effective treatment of incident pain "consists of immobilization in the case of a fracture, drainage of an abscess or arrest of a hemorrhage. . . ." Continuous pain is characterized by a "constant unremitting sensation, often of such intensity that it dominates an individual's entire existence, disturbing sleep, thought and everyday activity" [9]. Continuous pain becomes an illness in itself. It no longer serves a useful purpose of alerting the individual to take action because little can be done except to try to reduce the effects of the pain. Continuous pain is not an extension of acute or incident pain; rather it carries with it its own set of characteristics that lead its host into feelings of despair and isolation.

Pain also can be described in terms of its types of sensation. The sensations are characteristically different, depending upon their origin. Deep somatic pain is generally experienced as a dull ache that is poorly localized. Deep somatic structures themselves vary in terms of their sensitivity to pain. Some of the more highly sensitive structures are the periosteum, ligaments, joint capsules, and deep fascia. Muscles, articular cartilage, and compact bone are thought to be less sensitive.

Visceral pain, originating from the abdominal, thoracic, and pelvic organs is usually poorly localized, dull, and aching. It is often accompanied by autonomic activity such as pallor, bradycardia, and hyperalgesia [9]. Visceral pain is frequently referred to areas remote from the diseased viscus.

Cutaneous pain, that which emanates from the skin, is usually biphasic in nature. In the initial phase, one senses a rapidly transmitted impulse, which is followed by another sensation often characterized as burning. The sensations are usually clearly localized and follow a dermatomal pattern [9].*

While physical pain can be enhanced by emotional or mental aspects, pain itself can be of a mental or psychogenic nature. Mental pain is usually the response to some kind of stress. It can be continuous or incidental in nature as it accompanies these categories of physical pain. Mental pain is characteristically overpowering; it creates feelings of powerlessness and loss of control. Mental as well as physical pain can produce fatigue and depression.

Mechanisms Causing Pain in Cancer

It is rare to find a primary tumor that creates a great deal of pain unless it is located near a highly sensitive structure. When pain does occur at a primary stage, it is often relieved after the tumor is surgically removed. When cancer is in the inoperable stage and pain is present, attempts to relieve the pain are generally aimed at reduction of the size or growth of the tumor. When tumor reduction is no longer possible, palliative ways of dealing with the symptoms of pain are introduced. This type of pain is termed *terminal* or *intractable* pain.

---

* Further discussion relating to deep somatic and cutaneous pain can be found in Chapters 6 and 15.

Bonica [1] describes some of the common mechanisms that cause terminal pain.

1. Compression of nerves by tumor or by metastatic fracture of bones adjacent to the nerves can produce pain typical of neuritis, which is characteristically a series of sharp, boring sensations of varying intensity. This mechanism is especially found at the nerve roots, a nerve plexus, or nerve trunk. Common areas in which this occurs are the lumbosacral plexus that is affected by pelvic tumors, bracial plexus affected by the superior sulcus tumors, and intercostal neuralgias often created by retroperitoneal or mediastinal tumors. This incident type of pain is also similarly experienced after "vertebral collapse, sudden massive hemorrhage, rapidly forming abscess, or pressure from other sources such as a large pleural effusion or localized edema" [9]. When compression of a nerve is secondary to one of these or to a pathological fracture, the pain is generally aggravated by movement and often is relieved by rest and immobilization of the body part.

2. Neoplastic infiltration of nerves, blood vessels, and other tissues gives rise to a continuous type of pain. The irritation of the nerve endings produces a stabbing, burning sensation and a relatively even level of pain intensity. The sensation is often accompanied by numbness. In breast cancer, pain often occurs in the upper extremities because of an infiltration of the plexus and the main nerves and blood vessels in the axilla. In cancer of the cervix and uterus, infiltration often occurs in the tissues of the pelvis and the lumbosacral plexus, creating pain in the lower extremities and back region.

3. Obstruction of a viscus such as the stomach, the colon, the rectum, and the gastrointestinal, urinary, and biliary tracts produce a visceral type of pain that is usually dull, diffuse, and poorly localized. This is mostly considered to be a continuous type of pain, especially once the obstruction is great enough to produce symptoms. Primary tumors located in or near these areas can produce this obstructive mechanism. Surgical removal of the tumor usually brings relief. This mechanism is often a complicating factor for those persons who have had irradiation near the viscus.

4. Vascular pain arises with an obstruction or occlusion of a blood vessel caused by pressure from an adjacent tumor. This incident type of pain can produce an ischemic, sudden, sharp, intermittent sensation. Occlusions of the subclavian vessels can produce upper extremity pain. Retroperitoneal tumors often produce pain in the perineal area and lower extremities by this mechanism. Active or passive contractions and torsions of blood vessels can cause these occlusions or obstructions that can lead to intense muscular contractions, giving the sensation of pain. Retroperitoneal and pelvic tumors often manifest this particular mechanism.

5. Infiltration, tumefaction, and swelling of the integument or capsule of hollow organs, periosteum, or fascia produce an incident type of pain that is usually severe and localized. This type of infiltration often occurs in the

uterosacral ligaments and lumbar root when cancer of the cervix is present.

6. Necrosis, infection, and inflammation produce severe and persistent pain of a continuous nature. These mechanisms can occur anywhere in the body. Pain in pelvic cancers commonly results from rupture of a hollow viscus, such as an ovarian cyst or abscess, caused by a tumor. Contamination of the peritoneal cavity can occur through such a rupture and can cause a severe, unrelenting pain. Other examples include larger lesions of the head and neck cancers that can produce erosions of underlying bone and periosteum.

By its very nature, a metastatic tumor spreads throughout various body parts. Because of this it should be understood that many of these mechanisms occur concurrently. This can cause pain of both an incident and continuous nature simultaneously.

Psychosocial Factors in Pain

There are many factors that cause pain on a psychosocial level. Cancer, a stressor in itself, is only complicated by a host of factors that can add to that experience and, in many cases, can increase or initiate the pain experience. Engel [5] has categorized groups of stressors that confront an individual. Three major categories are: (1) loss or threat of loss of a significant object, (2) injury or threat of injury, and (3) frustration of drives. A diagnosis of cancer accompanied by pain potentially can produce any one or all of these stressors.

Loss or threat of loss of a significant object or person is commonly exemplified in the life of one who has cancer. Cancer often creates a situation in which the person loses a particular body part or function. The mental pain associated with this loss is dependent upon how the person and society value that particular part or function. The loss of a breast or uterus may indicate to a woman that she is no longer needed or useful. Men who have had penilectomies often describe themselves as no longer being "a man."

Another loss often experienced as a threat is that of loss of roles previously assumed. Physical pain or weakness may mean that the person is no longer capable of holding his or her previous job. Along with this loss may come a change in relationships with friends. Working and social friendships are threatened because the person may feel too uncomfortable to meet the demands of maintaining friendships. Many times, the person with cancer experiences feelings of rejection because of the cycle of events.

The imbalance in supply and demand of energy leads to fatigue. Pain is often increased because of the loss of energy adequate to deal with the situation. Fatigue itself can create a vulnerable setting for mental pain to occur, as well as lowering the sufferer's resistance to persistent physical pain.

Injury or threat of injury to the body or mind is ever present. Cancer by nature is a perpetual assault on the body, since it saps the body for its own existence and nutrition. In addition, the treatments for cancer—surgery, radiotherapy, chemotherapy, and immunotherapy—are potential assaults because they create a system of reactions within the body that can affect not only tumor cells but normal, healthy cells as well. The body perceives these attacks as injury, and "inflammatory" response is evoked.

The fear of death and the fear of mutilation and suffering created by the metastatic nature of cancer are ever present in a devastating manner. The fear that physical pain will become uncontrollable at the end creates a kind of mental anguish with which the person must live. One person expressed it by saying, "Dying wouldn't be so bad if it weren't for the pain."

Frustration of drives, another category of stressors, is expressed in many ways. The patient with cancer lives with many ambiguities that can present problems to the individual and his family and caretakers. Will the cancer grow more? How far will it extend? How will it be treated? Will the treatment stop the growth? How will he feel when he is taking the treatment? These questions are faced every day and serve to depress the person. However, if he becomes depressed, others around him may try to cheer him to the point of denial of the frustrations that he is experiencing. Denial itself is looked upon as a negative type of behavior by many health workers.

Another point of frustration is the interruption of the individual's life-style. Dependency versus independency and integrity versus despair are conflicts continually faced in this change of life-style. Many fears override natural responses to everyday conflicts. Fear of abandonment often is expressed. Cancer induces both realistic and imaginary fears. Realistic fear is often easier to deal with because there is a known cause. Imaginary fears are uncontrollable because of their very nature and can perpetuate more fears if they are not interrupted in some manner. Senescu [15] claims, "the fearful individual also 'creates' dangers which then elicit more fear."

Decreased physical and emotional adaptability can cause the individual with cancer to experience a lack of gratification that leads to a reduced self-esteem. Senescu [15] states that "many patients with cancer who develop emotional complications are literally starved for gratification and pleasure." He describes pleasure as necessary to an individual since it has a buffering effect that serves to neutralize the pains and frustrations of life. Reduced gratification can result from no longer engaging in pleasurable activity. The satisfaction of sexual drive and the achievement of success often are not possible. Many times the pleasures of eating and socializing are lost because the individual loses his appetite, either from the cancer itself or from the therapy. Senescu states [15] that it is useful to explain to the patient that "the need for pleasure is as great as the need for food, and that a lack of gratification may be causing the pain and distress and feelings of hopelessness rather than being a result of them." This statement can be applied to all the categories of stress we have discussed. These factors can create pain as well as any physiological stimulus and the results can be equally intense. The feelings evoked by these stressors can be a cause as well as a result of pain and, therefore, must be recognized as important.

Assessment of Cancer Pain

A step essential to the adequate management of cancer pain is assessment. Much time is spent in verbalizing the importance of worthwhile assessment, yet too little time is spent in actually engaging in it. The executed sequence of behavior seems to be: (1) the patient must "complain of pain," then (2) the nurse prepares medication and administers it. The cycle is repeated every three to four hours. It varies little except for the patient experiencing severe pain who is not receiving adequate medication. In this case, there is usually included in that cycle a period of time during which the patient must battle with the nurse to convince her that he needs more pain medication "sooner." The fact that the patient is receiving his pain medication every three to four hours also creates within the nurse a feeling of concern that she is causing this patient to become an addict. The results of improper assessment are that only one method of pain relief is used, the administration of medication, and that continuous struggles and feelings of helplessness are generated on the part of both caretaker and patient. Real assessment of pain is also a beginning to the management of pain, because the patient gets the feeling that someone cares about him and is making an attempt to help him. This in itself can provide some relief from pain.

The person with cancer who is admitted to the hospital should be evaluated for pain upon admission. This evaluation provides base-line data for comparison with any changes that occur during his course of illness. If he has no pain on admission, he should be informed that if he does encounter pain with any of his treatments or diagnostic examinations, he should inform the nurse. This information should not be presented in a manner that is frightening but in a way that will aid the patient to recognize that these experiences sometimes do create distress and that there are means to relieve them. Most important is to establish an "open communication" relationship so that the patient is aware that he can talk to the nurse about his pain and that his responsibility is to do so. Too often, the nurse assumes that the patient will report pain, while the patient assumes that there is nothing ordered for his pain or the nurse would surely bring it. The end result is that the patient suffers and the nurse remains ignorant of his pain.

If in the initial visit to the patient the nurse finds that he is suffering pain, further assessment is necessary. This should include two major components— the nature of the pain and the effect of the pain upon the individual and his family.

Assessment of the nature of pain should provide information relating to the type of sensation and the location, intensity, and duration of the pain. The effect the pain has on the individual can be observed on both physiological and psychological levels. Observation of physiological signs, such as increased blood pressure, pulse changes, pallor, drawn face, clenched fist, restlessness, and fatigue, is an indication that a stressor is at work. The physical appearance of the patient who is having constant pain is often characterized by a dull glassy look in his eyes. Investigation of the patient's life-style changes, degree of mobility, and change of mobility patterns yields valuable information. Changes in disposition suggest that the individual is adapting to a new or stressing situation. The person in pain often focuses his major attention on his pain and on finding a means of relief for the pain.

Tools for Assessment

In order for the nurse to assess adequately a patient's pain experience, she must have some knowledge of the location, size, and extent of the tumor and the degree of metastasis. This step is essential in order to identify the source of the pain. A new location of pain may signal further metastasis or it may mean that another problem exists. Not every experience of pain is due to the malignant process, but a general understanding of the extent of malignancy gives the nurse a basis for further judgments.

In addition to a basic understanding of cancer and its presence in the patient being assessed, careful observation of the patient's verbal and nonverbal behavior is necessary. Astute listening is the most valuable tool the nurse can use to tap the richest source of information about the patient's personal pain experience—his own verbal descriptions. The patient's family can provide additional information about his change in disposition, activity level, and other aspects of his daily routine.

Assessment also is essential as a means to determine the effectiveness of nursing intervention directed at pain relief. Discussion and careful observation of the patient after the administration of medication or some other nursing measure will give the patient the freedom to report its effectiveness in the relief of pain. This exchange provides a basis for continuation, modification, or elimination of the method for future applications.

The patient with cancer pain often must live for many months with his pain. Reliance on medication as the only source of relief can reduce the person to a life of dependency upon medication. Accurate assessment to determine the severity sometimes can assist the patient in using measures that allow him some feeling of control over his situation. The patient can be taught to do an accurate self-assessment that in itself allows him some feeling of control. He no longer has to feel that all his pain is equal in nature or intensity, nor that all his pain is due to the malignant process. Self-assessment can be taught the patient by providing him with adequate information about pain and the extent of his disease. However, some individuals find this kind of control undesirable and frightening. For this reason, it is crucial that the nurse make an assessment of the patient's psychological characteristics so that a patient is not subjected to this kind of unwanted control.

Management of Cancer Pain

The nursing management of cancer pain requires an astute, sensitive, creative, and caring individual—one who is knowledgeable about cancer, pain, and the treatments for both. The nurse who is caring for the person with cancer must be able to deal therapeutically with her own reactions to cancer and death, as well as with the patient's reactions. Efforts to keep abreast of the continual findings from cancer research are representative of her interest in giving the patient the best care possible. Never should sight be lost of the individual and those immediate needs presented by his situation.

The medical management of cancer pain involves two major approaches that are somewhat related to the stage of the illness. The two approaches are: (1) tumor therapy to diminish or destroy the neoplasms, and (2) symptomatic therapy that does not affect the tumor but rather reduces the intensity of the symptoms associated with the tumor [11]. The first approach includes palliative tumor surgery, irradiation, hormonal therapy, ablation of endocrine glands, and the administration of anticarcinogenic agents. The second approach is aimed at reducing the symptoms of pain and discomfort. It includes the use of systemic analgesics, neurosurgery, nerve blocks, acupuncture, and biostimulation.

As noted earlier, the choice of approach depends greatly on the stage of cancer. In the early stages, cancer rarely creates significant pain. Pain and discomfort are more likely to be caused by the means used to treat the cancer, such as surgery. Many times the diagnostic procedures themselves create great discomfort. Medically, the treatment is usually simple analgesics for the few days of discomfort.

In later stages, radiotherapy or chemotherapy, or both, may have their effect on reducing the tumor size and, indirectly, reducing the pain. These treatments also can create further discomfort. Many sensations associated with radiation are said not to be painful but are described as discomforting. Patients describe cutaneous sensations associated with radiation as burning, itching, stinging, prickling, and dryness. Certain lanolin creams or lotions have been found effective in keeping the radiated area from becoming dry. Nausea associated with radiation therapy can be reduced by pretreatment injections of an antiemetic drug such as prochlorperazine or trimethobenzamide. The hard, flat x-ray table is a source of discomfort for many people. Assisting the patient to assume as comfortable a position as possible is helpful. Many patients benefit greatly from an analgesic injection one half hour before treatment. Pillows and other support devices are sometimes helpful.

The discomforting side effects associated with chemotherapy are varied. It is essential that the person administrating the medication be alert to the occurrence of potential side effects and prepare the patient in such a way as to minimize the distress they can cause. No attempts will be made here to describe the side effects of various chemotherapeutic agents. Let it suffice to say that the nurse working with these medications should be constantly aware of what she is giving and the effect it is having upon the particular patient. The patient's normal pattern of response and deviations to that response must be compared.

The neurosurgical and neurological block procedures done to relieve late-stage or intractable pain have been discussed in Chapter 7. The patient should be well informed of the risks and benefits of the procedure he undergoes. Many times, people become quite depressed to find that relief is incomplete after a procedure. Since the nurse's major role in caring for the patient is supportive, she should see that the patient is well informed and should carefully observe the patient's behavior for cues about his reactions. Observation and assessment after the procedure are most essential.

Most nursing approaches used to alleviate pain are directed at reducing the symptom. Occasionally, a source of incidental pain can be removed if it is caused by an extreme factor such as staying in one position for a prolonged time or pressure from a constricting garment. There are innumerable measures nurses can apply to aid in the relief of pain. Mehta states [9],

> . . . the value of other methods, such as encouragement of outside interests, spiritual help, tranquillizers and sedatives, should not be overlooked. Raising morale and elevating the threshold of conscious appreciation, lessen apprehension, diminish significance of the painful lesion and greatly facilitate general management of the case."

Management of chronic cancer pain is no easy task. It drains the energies of the sufferer and of the observer or one who is trying to find a means of relief. Often, the experience ends in bitter feelings with each placing the burden of guilt upon the other. The patient feels that if only those around him would take action, he would feel better. Those responsible for his care often tire of their lack of success in management and gradually withdraw from the scene, leaving the patient to suffer alone.

Pain associated with the early stages of cancer may be relatively mild and intermittent. Patients with cancer of the uterus or cervix may not suffer pain as much as they suffer from the discomfort of continuous vaginal bleeding. A cancerous lump in the breast is sometimes tender but not extremely painful. Whatever the site, tumors in early stages are rarely painful unless located near a highly neurosensitive area. If occasional pain occurs, mild analgesics often are taken to relieve the symptoms. Depending upon the nature of the person experiencing the pain, he may wish to use any number of independent techniques to eliminate it. Many persons have their own established means for dealing with minor pain, e.g., distraction, exercise, heat or cold, warm baths, and many others. The patient should be consulted about what means he has previously used and urged to continue using those that have proven effective.

When pain becomes more severe or more persistent, the patient usually turns to someone for help. The result of this appeal is usually a prescription for some type of drug.* The role of the nurse in delivering these medications to the patient will be discussed prior to discussing alternative methods of pain relief.

---

* Use of medication in alleviation of pain has been discussed in Chapter 9.

The Nurse's Role in Medication Administration

The most common method of pain relief has been the use of medication. It is the method that probably utilizes the least amount of time and effort and can, therefore, be considered to be the most efficient. On the other hand, analgesics have probably done for us what antibiotics have; that is, these medications helped us forget the alternative practices we once relied upon. While medications have done a great deal for patients, they may concurrently have made health professionals lazy and careless in their practices. Measures of pain alleviation could be more effective if the use of medication were combined with other creative and supportive relief approaches.

Administration of analgesics is no easy task if it is done appropriately. The person administrating the medication should be well informed of its onset, the peak and duration of action, its usual side and adverse effects, its interaction effects with other medications being administered, and the usual dosage range. The one administering medication should be able to distinguish between addiction, dependence, and tolerance so as not to label inaccurately the terminally ill patient in such a way that the drugs are withheld. Nurses seem to be entirely too concerned about addicting terminal patients. They show this concern by withholding medications because it is still "one-half to three-fourths of an hour early" before the four-hour interval between dosages expires. It seems paradoxical to think that nothing is done about the fact that the medication is not lasting the time interval indicated by the doctor's orders. Instead of evaluating the effectiveness of the current dosage and frequency, the battle goes on repeatedly with the patient complaining of pain two to three hours before the medication is given and the nurse insisting that the patient must wait because "it's not time yet." The patient becomes more irritable and anxious as his pain increases; meanwhile, the nurse becomes impatient and begins to believe the patient "just likes his shot" or is "addicted" to his medication. The drama is absurd and yet it is repeated over and over in many hospital settings.

The role of the person administering pain-relieving medication to the patient with cancer is quite crucial. It is imperative that the health professional know both the medication and the patient. Initial assessment of the patient's pain in relation to its nature and its effect upon the patient is necessary. The patient must be assessed in terms of his desire and ability to maintain activity as it is related to the progression of his tumor. Some patients prefer to tolerate some pain in order to be able to function with alertness. Others wish to be "put out" and totally relieved of pain, knowing that they will be in a drowsy state most of the time.

Another important step in giving medication is to inform the patient that medication is available. He should be told how he can acquire it, i.e., whether it will be delivered to him regularly or whether he must ask for it. Too often patients are not aware of this and endure pain for several days without reporting it. One patient described his pain as being like a knife stabbed into his chest. When asked if he had taken any medication for it, he replied, "No,

I figured they didn't want me to have any if they didn't bring it to me." Further investigation revealed that the nursing staff had not given him his analgesic because he had never requested it.

The patient should be included in deciding the time interval and dosage level. That is, he should be asked to report if it is effective and for how long it is effective. Time intervals are subject to change. Many times in well-planned medication regimens, the time interval can be lengthened after an initial testing of dosages is done to determine the dosage necessary to maintain a pain-free level. The aim should be to keep the patient free of pain so that he does not need to demonstrate pain behavior.

Often, medication is the only solution to pain that is offered. People in our society have been well socialized into taking medication for relief from its problems. There are, however, alternative routes to alleviation of pain that should be tried.

Suggestions for the management of pain will be focused in the physical and emotional areas. It is sometimes difficult to distinguish clearly between these two areas, since they are so intricately related. More research is necessary to determine which means is most appropriate for which type of pain so that less time is spent leaving the patient to suffer.

Physically Based Approaches

Nursing interventions that are physically based generally are aimed at reducing the painful stimulus or at reducing the perception of the painful stimulus through physical activity that can serve as distraction. It is important for the nurse to be aware toward which of these aims one's efforts are directed. If the painful stimulus is due to an enlarging tumor, then the focus of the nurse will be reducing the perception of the painful stimulus. If, however, the pain is due to an inability to move independently a lymphodemic arm, dyspnea, constriction of a garment, an inability to eliminate, or an obstruction, then the action taken is directed toward reducing the intensity of the stimulus or sensations associated with the stimulus.

Repositioning of a body part is often necessary in cases where edema is involved. The patient may have neither the strength nor the energy to move himself or a body part as often as is necessary to relieve the pressure that creates the pain when he remains in one position too long. Adequate support, such as pillows or a sling, many times is needed.

Immobility often is necessary to relieve severe incident pain due to pathological fractures. The patient often assumes this technique as a protective device to the point where other nursing care is sometimes made difficult. It seems highly unnecessary for nurses to create further pain by excessive amounts of movement when the person is in a great deal of discomfort. In the terminal stages, patients often request to be left alone, stating, "don't make me move, just let me be." The request should be granted to the extent that it does not interfere with essential care or contribute to other serious problems.

Applications of heat and cold can be used to alleviate pain, depending upon its source. Ice massages are sometimes effective in desensitizing a painful area for short periods of time. The patient often needs to be persuaded that an ice massage can make him feel better. Sitting in a tub of warm water, body massage, or vibration or manipulation of a body part adds additional sensory input that may reduce the sensations of pain for a period of time. These techniques often serve as forms of relaxing the body muscles as well as reducing the pain. Care must be exercised in applying techniques, and they should be discontinued if pain is increased by the intervention. Much research is necessary to determine under what circumstances these techniques help and why they sometimes create more pain rather than reduce it.

Reducing the perception of a painful stimulus is often accomplished through some method of distraction. This can be operationalized in many ways. Exercise, such as walking, swimming, sexual intercourse, and yoga, and carrying out activities of daily living, e.g., bathing, combing hair, and shopping, can serve as means of maintaining self-integrity and also as sources for gratification, and can assume the purpose of distraction in such a way that pain can be alleviated for a short period of time. Persons should be encouraged to engage in these activities as long as they are physically able. If exercise is undertaken, the patient should understand that it should be accompanied by adequate periods of rest.

Distraction also can be in the form of participating in social events, such as drinking coffee, tea, or liquor, visiting with family and friends, playing cards, attending church services, and any number of other social activities the patient may have enjoyed prior to diagnosis.

Cognitive and Emotionally Based Approaches

Most nursing interventions take into account the contributions of emotions to pain. Some of those techniques described above as physically based approaches to pain relief cannot be distinguished clearly from those discussed here.

A major aim in cognitive and emotionally oriented techniques is to reduce the degree and amount of anxiety associated with pain. Patients with cancer can suffer a great deal of mental pain as a result of ambiguities of prognosis and decisions relating to treatment. While the impact of these stimuli cannot be erased entirely, many attempts can be made to reduce them.

Reducing anxiety can be accomplished in two general ways: (1) support in coping behaviors that are already successful in reducing anxiety, and (2) providing the person with coping resources. Reduction of anxiety also will result in a decreased feeling of helplessness. With adequate coping resources, the patient will sense a greater degree of control over his situation.

Supporting and Providing Coping Resources

One way to help a patient to cope is to provide him with information about his plan of treatment. In a research study [6], patients who were interviewed about their knowledge regarding what to expect about radiation therapy reported that they knew very little. Patients reported concerns about some frightening aspects of radiation, such as not knowing they would be alone in the room, hearing the noise of the machine, assuming the uncomfortable positions necessary for proper exposure, and the fear that their hair would fall out. One could question how this enumeration of fears necessarily contributes to a discussion of pain. The answer is simply that while some of these fears do not involve physical pain, they lead to anxiety which makes the patient's general situation less bearable. One could argue that giving too much information or the wrong kind of information can be anxiety-producing. While this may be true sometimes, the error of health professionals probably lies more heavily in not giving enough information. Giving information about techniques and procedures without creating a great curtain of fear relating to possible side effects can probably do little more than satisfy the patient's curiosity. The most probable side effects should be discussed with the patient as matter-of-factly as possible. Patients seem to acquire a great deal of information from their neighbors or friends who have gone through similar experiences. Much of this information is not necessarily true. Therefore, it is crucial that health professionals deal honestly with the patient to dispel any myths that may be causing anxiety. Having adequate information can relieve the patient to deal with matters more important than worrying about his bone scan, radiation, or chemotherapy.

Muscle-relaxation training techniques have been found to decrease markedly a state anxiety situation. Johnson and Spielberger [7] studied the effects of relaxation training upon anxiety measures of 48 hospitalized psychiatric patients. State anxiety measures, defined as transitory measures that fluctuate over time, showed a significant decline in response to the relaxation training. State anxiety measures were systolic blood pressure, heart rate, and the Zuckerman Affect Adjective Check List, all of which were taken simultaneously. All measures were taken before and after the relaxation training during the first and second experimental day. An analysis of variance yielded significant relaxation effects on all three state anxiety measures.

If the patient with cancer pain is alert and willing to learn the muscle-relaxation techniques, he can acquire for himself a method of control over a potentially tense situation. The technique, if learned properly, can be used at times other than just during the training session and does not require the presence of the trainer. In a study using relaxation training with patients who had cancer, many who experienced the relaxation sessions expressed verbally their increased ability to relax systematically. Some expressed that it gave them the added energy and strength to cope with other activities of the day [6].

Therapeutic communication is another possible means of pain relief. Some nursing studies have focused on the effectiveness of communication in nurse-patient interactions as a means of pain relief. Diers, et al [4] found that nursing approaches that considered the "feeling" and "doing" components of a "whole" person were more effective than those that did not consider these aspects and that these nursing approaches were more effective than just giving medication alone.

Communication that offers the patient a chance to relate how he is feeling and allows him to have some control over his situation can provide relief of pain. Moss and Meyer [10] studied the nurse-patient interaction as a means of effecting attitude change in relation to pain relief. Nursing measures such as positioning, ambulating, and massage were suggested to the patient as possible means of relieving pain. Patients were allowed to choose what method of relief they wished. Twelve out of thirteen patients showed a change in their response by asking for some nursing measure instead of medication for relief of pain. These findings support the suggestion that patients should be given a choice in terms of method of relief of pain.

In addition to these forms of therapeutic communication, psychotherapy on a more formal level is sometimes useful. Many people with cancer suffer from various phobias; pain is one. Getting psychiatric consultation sometimes helps the patient to have a greater insight into what actually is happening. One patient with metastatic cancer of the breast developed pain on the extremities of one side a day before her intended dismissal. A psychiatric consultation, after diagnostic tests revealed no further metastasis to that area, helped the patient to understand that she had a fear of being discharged. This fear appeared to stem from her unresolved feelings of anger and nonacceptance of herself, which were expressed in feelings of being rejected by her husband. Being aware of what was happening helped the patient to work toward a resolution of her problem. Her pain was relieved and she was able to go home only a few days after her planned discharge.

Anticipatory guidance in preserving their energy for enjoyable activities also can be useful to patients in coping with their pain. Patients can be asked to evaluate their own pain patterns as to the times of day when the worst pain occurs and the kind of activity that precipitates pain. Assisting the patient toward an awareness of factors associated with his pain helps him to plan the activities he desires to carry out. Patients who must rely on pain medication or on some means of pain relief after being discharged from the hospital should be assisted to anticipate possible situations that may require more energy. They should be encouraged to plan for periods of rest and exercise. If holding a child is a desired yet painful activity, the patient should be helped to think of ways of engaging in physical contact that will provide the same benefit, yet with less pain.

Summary

Many people with cancer do not suffer physical pain, while others experience pain as a major focus of their illness. For the person with terminal pain, life is something to be endured. The continual presence of pain—either remaining constant or getting progressively worse—drains the individual of his energies to the point of exhaustion.

The existence of cancer pain is a long-standing problem. As research relating to cancer progresses, there is also a greater awareness of the mechanisms that cause cancer pain. Many approaches for reducing the pain are still in the trial-and-error stage. Considerable research is needed to determine what best will relieve pain of various origins and natures.

The nurse's role in research, clinical assessment, and care is crucial in interrupting a potentially devastating experience for the person with cancer. Her insight and contribution are essential to giving new hope for a more meaningful life to the person with cancer and pain.

References

1. Bonica, J. J. *The Management of Pain.* Chapter 40. Philadelphia: Lea & Febiger, 1954.
2. Cancer Statistics, 1975. *CA* 25:12, 1975.
3. DeWyes, W. Metastasis and disseminated cancer. In Rubin, P., ed., *Clinical Oncology*, 4th ed. Rochester: The University of Rochester, 1974.
4. Diers, D., Schmidt, R., McBride, M., Barron, A., and Davis, B. The effect of nursing interaction on patients in pain. *Nurs. Res.* 21:419, 1972.
5. Engel, G. *Psychological Development in Health and Disease.* Philadelphia: W. B. Saunders Company, 1962.
6. Jacox, A. Pain Alleviation Through Nursing Intervention. Unpublished findings, 1975.
7. Johnson, D., and Spielberger, C. The effects of relaxation training and the passage of time on measures of state and trait-anxiety. *J. Clin. Psychol.* 24:20, 1968.
8. Maher, R. M. Further experiences with intrathecal and subdural phenol: Observations on two forms of pain. *Lancet* 1:895, 1960.
9. Mehta, M. *Intractable Pain.* London: W. B. Saunders Company, 1973.
10. Moss, F., and Meyer, B. The effect of a nursing intervention on pain relief. *Nurs. Res.* 13:126, 1964.
11. Murphy, T. Cancer pain. *Postgrad. Med.* 53:187, 1973.
12. Perret, G. Management of pain in the patient with cancer. In Hickey, R., ed., *Palliative Care of the Cancer Patient.* Boston: Little, Brown and Company, 1967.
13. Robbins, S. *Pathological Basis of Disease.* Philadelphia: W. B. Saunders Company, 1974.
14. Rubin, P. *Clinical Oncology for Medical Students and Physicians: A Multidisciplinary Approach*, 5th ed. Rochester: The University of Rochester, 1974.
15. Senescu, R. The development of emotional complications in the patient with cancer. *J. Chronic Dis.* 16:813, 1963.

18

Pain and Nursing Care Associated with Burns

Mary Wagner

In 1968 approximately 100,000 persons were hospitalized for treatment of burns for a total of two million hospital days at a cost of one billion dollars [10]. The U.S. Department of Health, Education and Welfare stated that injuries involving flammable fabrics accounted for three to five thousand deaths and up to 250,000 injuries [9]. The National Safety Council statistics [7] listed a total of 6,718 persons dying as a result of fires. These statistics do not include burn deaths resulting from chemicals, electricity, scalds, or heat contact. The actual number of burn injuries and deaths resulting from burns is not known because of the lack of a standard reporting procedure.

Minor burns that cover small surface areas can be adequately treated in the physician's office or in an outpatient department. Treatment consists of cleansing and debridement, application of dressings, and tetanus prophylaxsis. The patient is instructed to return as needed. A major burn covering more than 20 percent body surface area and deep tissue injury requires hospitalization. Persons with deep facial burns and hand burns also should be hospitalized, due to the problems of infection and loss of function.

Major burn-injured patients are best handled in a burn unit where there is a multidisciplinary approach to handling the problem. The expenditure of time and energy required for handling major burn injuries is usually beyond the capabilities of small hospitals.

Although the literature on burn injury is very comprehensive in dealing with the pathophysiology and treatment of the burn injury, the pain suffered by a burn-injured patient has not been studied per se. There is, however, an increasing emphasis on the emotional impact of burns, and this usually deals with some aspect of pain. Fagerhaugh [3] has studied pain experienced by patients on a burn unit "from an organizational-work-interactional perspective"; this is the most recent nursing study. The first impression a nurse has when working with the burned patient is the horror of the injury and the amount of pain the patient must be suffering. The nurse must learn to control her reaction to the patient's pain and to channel her energies toward the medical goals, which are saving life and restoring integrity of the skin.

Nurses require many skills other than the purely technical ones. The nurse is a human being working and caring for another human. Allowing a patient to scream unrestrainedly when subjected to painful procedures exhausts the patient and the nurse mentally and physically. There must be control of pain, but drugs will not adequately control pain. Hence further efforts must be made to reduce the pain. How this control is achieved will depend on the patient and the nurse. The nurse must have support and help from the other members of the burn team. Care of the patient with major burns is not the specific province of either the physician or the nurse, but is the responsibility of a concerted multidisciplinary approach. This type of care can only be offered in a setting that is multifaceted, that is, a burn center.

The pathophysiological effects of the burn injury include both the direct effect of heat on the skin and systemic alterations. The skin has several functions that include temperature regulation, water and electrolyte balance, barrier against infection, tactile contact with the environment, and aesthetic value [6]. A burn injury can interfere with any or all of these functions. The disturbances resulting from the burn may be divided into three stages: (1) emergent, 0 to 72 hours postburn; (2) acute, 72 hours until complete skin coverage; and, (3) reconstructive, which is restoration of maximum function and appearance—a stage which may take years in a very severely burn-injured person (as defined by the National Burn Information Exchange). This chapter is organized according to the medical and nursing care associated with each stage of disturbance.

Emergent Stage

During the emergent phase of the injury, medical treatment is directed toward correcting the burn shock.

The major focus of care is: to maintain a patent airway for proper oxygenation by means of (1) nasal cannulas, (2) masks, (3) endotracheal tube, or (4) tracheostomy; to maintain circulation by meeting fluid losses and normal maintenance requirements; to prevent further microbial contamination by proper wound care and antimicrobial therapy; to maintain body heat by wet bulky dressings, coverings, protected heat lamps, and avoidance of drafts from air conditioners.

The heat injury to the blood vessels causes loss of capillary integrity and increased capillary permeability, which results in the loss of large amounts of fluid and protein from the intravascular space, leading to hypovolemic shock. The effects of the thermal injury on the skin involve loss of temperature regulation, which causes heat and water loss in proportion to the extent of deep-partial and full-thickness injury, which further depletes the total body water by vaporizational water loss. The loss of skin integrity opens the way for massive bacterial colonization of the wound.

Thus the task of the individual initially caring for the burn victim is to check the adequacy of the airway, to start an intravenous infusion of lactated Ringer's solution, to cover the wound with dressings moistened 0.9% saline in order to protect the wound from further contamination until definite wound care can be done, and to conserve body heat.

On admission, a patient with extensive partial-thickness injury may experience more pain than another patient who has sustained an extensive full-thickness burn. This is a result of the exposure of more free nerve endings in a partial-depth injury. A partial-thickness burn involves the epidermis and dermis, but the hair follicle and sweat glands are intact and can regenerate skin. (This is synonymous with *second degree*.) In full-thickness burns, all layers of the skin are involved and cannot close without grafting. (This is synonymous with *third degree*.) In a full-thickness injury it is postulated that nerve endings have been destroyed; therefore, the patient experiences less pain.

It is rather difficult to assess the depth of burn on admission since the pain the patient is experiencing can be exaggerated or minimized by the emotional and physical shock of the accident. If narcotics are used to control pain, the drug should be administered intravenously rather than intramuscularly because of microcirculatory stasis and stagnation. Intramuscular injections are not readily absorbed and may have a cumulative effect when remobilization of fluid occurs. An overdose may cause respiratory difficulty. Many patients have reported that pain was reduced when wet dressings were applied.

Within three to six hours following injury, edema is increasing. This edema formation is attributed to sodium flux into the burned tissue, capillary dilation, and increased capillary permeability [4]. The edema fluid is rich in protein and sodium while the systemic circulation is concomitantly depleted. The fluid resuscitation must be planned according to age, weight, and percentage of body surface area involvement in order to restore fluid balance. There are several formulas for calculation of fluid replacement, which can be obtained from most textbooks on surgery.

The edema formation may pose several problems; constriction (tourniquet effect) on extremities, impairment of ventilation from circumferential full-thickness burns of neck or thorax or both, and in the case of facial burns, swelling and eversion of the eyelids. With impairment of circulation and ventilation, escharotomies are likely to be necessary (escharotomies are incisions made through burned tissue). If the escharotomy is done properly, there should be little or no pain. The patient must be given an adequate explanation to help reduce anxiety. The patient needs to be observed frequently for bleeding from the sites. If bleeding occurs, the "bleeder" is cauterized or sutured. It is necessary to make sure that there is clot formation, since this bleeding may be a beginning sign of disseminated intravascular clotting.

Edema formation of the face and especially the eyelids may lead the patient to believe that his eyesight is impaired or destroyed [1]. Repeated explanations are mandatory that the eyesight is impaired at this time due to edema of the eyelids and that with proper eye care, vision will return.

During the emergent phase, the patient is in a state of emotional shock that may take two forms. Andreason et al. [2] reported that one form is a dream-like state in which the patient may talk lucidly but have no awareness later of the conversation. The second and more common response is termed an acute traumatic reaction. The symptoms include insomnia, emotional lability, exaggerated startle reflex, and nightmares. The nurse must remember to speak to the patient each time she enters the room and explain what she is doing. The patient during this period of time is being monitored hourly, with measurement of vital signs, fluid intake, urinary output, and other specific procedures being carried out. The explanations are especially important in view of the findings by Andreason and associates.

Diuresis and remobilization of fluid occurs forty-eight to seventy-two hours postburn. At this point the patient has usually recovered from the physiologic shock and the initial emotional shock.

Acute Stage

The patient then enters the acute phase of the burn injury. The major medical emphasis is restoration of the integument and control of burn-wound sepsis. It is in this period of time that patients suffer the most pain and the mortality rate is the highest.

In a survey of eighty-seven patients ranging in age from fifteen months to eighty-eight years, several categories of problems were elicited [13]. The activities and procedures that caused pain were:

1. Dressing changes
2. Tubbing (Hubbard tank)
3. Soaking of dressing with 0.5% silver nitrate solution
4. Piecemeal debridement
5. Active exercises
6. Preparation of donor sites
7. Excision of tissue from donor sites
8. Application of homografts and xenografts

These problem areas are used to organize the following discussion of nursing care.

The following glossary should assist in understanding the discussion.

debridement—process of removing eschar.
tubbing (tanking)—procedure of cleansing patient by immersion into a Hubbard tank.

donor sites—place from which skin was taken for autografting.
homografts—split thickness skin taken from a living or dead donor.
xenografts (heterografts)—animal skin used for biological dressing.
autograft—skin taken from one part of the body to cover a wound. Autografts
are never taken from face, hands or joints.

Dressing changes were most commonly cited as problems for the patients interviewed, with reactions varying from complete loss of control to
stoicism. In the hospital where the study was conducted, this procedure occurred at least twice a day. It is probably the most frustrating and grueling
experience for both patient and nurse—generally, staff and patient both
would like to withdraw from the stark reality of the situation.

One dressing technique is to employ bulky dressings saturated with 0.5%
silver nitrate solution, which is used as a method of topical antimicrobial therapy. The removal of dressings may be accompanied by tubbing, debridement, and exercise, making the duration of exposure to painful procedures
from forty-five to sixty minutes. One of the purposes of bulky dressing is to
assist in the removal of eschar. It is important that dressings are moist, not
dry, to accomplish this. If dressings are relatively dry, the patient seems to
experience much more pain, which is intensified as the open wound is exposed to the air. The pain is due to the exposed nerve endings. To minimize
pain, the patient may be given a mild analgesic or tranquilizer prior to the
dressing change. The medication should be given at least an hour before the
procedure so that the patient can receive the full benefit, but he should not
be asleep.

The method of doing dressing changes will depend on patient and staff.
However, a patient with a large surface area involvement (over 30 percent)
requires two or more persons to remove the dressings. As one seven-year-old
girl expressed it—"they [dressings] should be done fast, quick, and soft, with
no talking." At this point I would caution the neophyte burn nurse about
the use of diversional activity or conversation. It has been the author's experience that most patients in this situation do not want to talk, since they
are concentrating on maintaining control of themselves. While diversion
may be useful for patients, it is not universally so. Two or three experienced
burn-unit personnel can remove dressings deftly on a 70 percent burned patient in approximately fifteen minutes. It is important when more than one
person is working with a patient that directions to the patient should be
simple and not involve two or three persons talking at once.

Care should be taken that dressings are not pulled off, especially if they
are not sufficiently moist. Any dressing that adheres to the wound will need
to be soaked with 0.5% silver nitrate or allowed to "float" off in the tub.
The goal of care for dressing removal is to minimize pain because it is nearly
impossible to eliminiate it, short of using a general anesthesia, which is neither
desirable nor practical.

After dressings have been removed the patient is weighed and put into a
hydrotherapy tank (tub) that has been filled with warm water. Patients re-

port that the most comfortable water temperature is between 100 and 105 °F. The patient will experience stinging, which is most likely due to stimulation of exposed nerve endings. After two or three minutes the pain level decreases markedly while the patient is at rest. This respite from activity is not for long since the prolonged exposure in water leaches electrolyte and protein from the burn wound. Since the skin is destroyed, there is no mechanism for maintaining electrolyte balance and free diffusion occurs, causing water to be absorbed and electrolytes to leave the body through the burn wound. The greater surface area involved, the more rapidly this phenomenon occurs.

Piecemeal debridement is done at this time. This technique involves removal of all loosened eschar using scissors and hemostat. Any eschar that is adherent is left alone. If the patient complains of pain in the area in which the nurse is debriding, she stops and works in another area. Removal of eschar is a mandatory procedure since the major cause of death in extensive burns is infection. The eschar starts to separate by bacteriolysis in ten to twenty-one days postburn and if it is not removed, suppuration increases under the eschar leading to burn wound sepsis.

Piecemeal debridement is especially frightening to a child since he may perceive the procedure as a disruption of his body. The child may view procedures as punishment because he was bad, and his reaction may be out of proportion to the amount of pain being inflicted. Many times the staff will just battle and struggle with the child as seen in the following case.

J. T., a twelve-year-old male, was told to empty trash. He threw gasoline on it and lit the trash, catching his jeans on fire. He sustained a twelve percent full-thickness burn on his right leg. He was treated in a local hospital and then transferred two weeks later to a burn unit in a large university medical center. On admission he was febrile and had a flexion contracture of the knee. He shrieked when the nurse tried to remove the dressings while he was in the tub. Any attempt to remove these was met by screams and combative behavior. He was given sedation and the dressings were finally removed. The wound was debrided and AgNo₃ 0.5% dressings and a posterior splint were applied. His mother told the nurse that in the other hospital when he cried, the nursing staff would not change dressings or do his exercises. She stated that some of them cried in front of J. when he said that they hurt him. His mother was able to stay with him during hospitalization while at the university. Dressing change, tubbing, and other procedures became an ordeal for patient and staff.

Outside intervention in this situation was required since his behavior was disturbing to other patients and staff on the unit. The consultant learned that he had been told not to use gas on a fire and he felt he was being punished by everyone for being bad. The approach devised by the staff and consultant was to have him help in the procedures and allow him to make suggestions as to the best way to take off the dressings. He wanted to do it himself. The first time he took an hour and the staff finished the task, at which time he screamed. There was a time limit placed on J. to remove his dressings, bathe, and do his own piecemeal debridement with which he concurred, thus eliminating a great deal of strain on patient and nurse. He still resisted exercising and splinting, which were accomplished without his cooperation. Surgical debridement and grafting achieved sound closure and two weeks after surgery he was discharged.

It is well to keep in mind that a nurse, no matter how skilled, can lose sight of the underlying problem and react to overt behavior only. There is nothing that is going to make the experience of debridement pleasant. The adult can accept the reason that makes the procedure necessary, but should be allowed the choice as to where the process should start as well as trusting the personnel to stop when he feels an increase of pain at any given point. If the adult is able and is willing, he should be allowed to help debride. The explanation that may be helpful with the child, particularly of school age, is that the dead skin must come off so that new skin will grow, or in case of full-thickness burns, so that the doctor can put new skin on the area. Whenever there is evidence of reepithelialization, this should be pointed out to the patient, regardless of age, as tangible evidence of improvement.

Aside from the pain associated with changing dressings discussed earlier, the procedure of soaking dressings every three hours with 0.5% silver nitrate solution causes varying degrees of pain and discomfort. Some adult patients report no pain but discomfort or shivering when the solution is applied at room temperature. Other adult patients report that the room-temperature solution causes stinging and pain. Young children often cry or whimper when the cool solution is applied. Use of a warming oven to warm the solution to body temperature will decrease the shivering and thereby relieve one source of patient discomfort.

The choice of topical agents is up to the physician. Besides silver nitrate, other agents in use at the present for topical antimicrobial therapy include silver sulfadiazine and Sulfamylon Acetate in cream form. The experience of many burn nurses indicates that the Sulfamylon causes more pain than any other topical agent. Of the three major topical agents, silver sulfadiazine seems to cause the least pain on application according to nurses who have worked with all three agents. Methods of application to reduce patient pain and discomfort upon application must yet be devised.

Active range-of-motion exercises are another commonly reported source of pain. The necessity for such exercises is the possibility of contracture formation. Contractures are a major problem in the acute phase; if they are allowed to develop, loss of function will result. Various measures are useful in the prevention of contractures. Good body alignment is essential [11]. Splints and braces on affected parts are used when the patient is lying in bed, which can interfere with rest. Picture, for example, a patient with 70-percent body-surface burns encased in bulky dressings lying flat on his back, arms extended and abducted 90° from the body and splints on both upper and lower extremities. Is it any wonder that one patient, when asked how he was feeling, responded that he was being crucified?

These measures, combined with active range-of-motion exercises, can help in the prevention of contractures. The nurse's responsibility in regard to the exercises is to make sure they are carried out by the patient himself when the physical therapist is not on the unit. The specific program of exercises for the individual patient is determined by the physical therapist, who also designs and makes the necessary splints for each patient. A schedule of splinting and exercising is discussed with the nursing staff, patient, and family. The importance of these is explained to the patient, since failure to carry out the program will lead to stiffening of the joints and loss of function. Motion that is lost by not doing the exercises for one or two days can be regained but it is painful. Most patients will neglect the exercises if at all possible, but find to their extreme discomfort that pain is exacerbated. When possible, it is helpful to have a family member with the patient, since he can provide general support and encouragement in carrying out the exercises. The regimen of activity can be adapted to the patient's fatigue tolerance, since the family member can take the time necessary to see that the exercises are done properly. Thus the family can make an important contribution toward the goal of the patient's eventual recovery.

Activities that foster active use of joints are to be greatly encouraged for their therapeutic benefit as well as their psychological uplift. For children, games and toys that require arm and hand movement are helpful. A tricycle allows for leg, arm, and body movement. The tricycle should be of sturdy construction to provide stability and there should be no rough edges. The nursing staff and other persons in the burn unit should be cautioned against a hazardous driver on the loose!

During the acute stage, it is often necessary for the patient to be confined to his bed or room. If the patient is left alone without any contact other than painful stimuli, he suffers sensory deprivation, and some withdraw completely from reality. The use of the radio and television as a substitute for human contact may be just additional white noise unless there is also human contact. When the patient must be immobilized, every effort should be made to have a close family member with the patient. The family member should be allowed to stay with the patient from morning until evening. The only time the relative should not be there is during any painful procedure. This is especially true with children so that they do not associate the pain with the parent. This also saves the mother's feeling of helplessness when her child is being hurt and she is unable to help, even though she knows it is in the child's best interest. The relative can provide the warmth, love, and comfort the patient needs during this period of stress. The family is extremely important to the well-being of the patient, and should be encouraged to be with the patient whenever possible. The adult patient, when able to leave the unit, usually enjoys a walk outside, weather permitting. Care should be taken to protect the patient from direct sunlight and fatigue. All patients should be encouraged to feed themselves if at all possible. Patients with burns of the hands can have different types of spoons rigged, such as those used by other handicapped persons. Whatever individual hobbies and interests the patient has that can be utilized should be incorporated into the plan of care.

The final phase of the acute stage is successful wound coverage by autograft, a treatment that produces the remaining sources of pain previously identified by patients. An autograft is skin taken from uninjured parts of the body. Before the patient can receive autografts, the eschar must be removed and the wound surface made sterile. The eschar may be removed by piece-meal debridement or by surgical excision.

After the eschar has been removed, homografts or xenografts are used to protect the wound. Homograft skin is taken from a cadaver and xenograft is taken from an animal (porcine) under sterile conditions. These are called biological dressings, which implies that they are changed. The biological dressings cannot be left in place for more than four or five days, since they will adhere and later be rejected by the host, which causes many wound problems. The major benefits of biological dressings are that they prepare the wound for autografting by sterilizing the wound, acting as a test graft, preventing fluid and electrolyte loss, and most important to the patient, converting a painful wound to a painless one.

If there is still contamination in the wound, the xenograft will "float" off due to the accumulation of exudate. Fresh heterografts are applied on the unit after the patient is tubbed. The pain associated with this is again exposure of the wound to the air and the smoothing of the "skin" in place over the burn wound. When the porcine skin does not loosen, the wound is ready for autografts.

If surgical debridement has been performed in the operating room, tubbing is not done unless specifically ordered by the physician. If test grafting is successful, the patient is prepared for autografting. The donor site preparation includes cleansing and shaving the selected site. If the patient has been on 0.5% silver nitrate topical therapy, the silver chloride eschar must be removed. Care must be taken to prevent damage to the normal skin; vigorous scrubbing is to be avoided since this will damage the donor skin. The method that causes the least damage to the skin and least pain to the patient follows:

Purpose:　To prepare selected donor sites by removing silver eschar without damaging healthy skin.

Equipment:　1. pHisoHex in basin
　　　　　　　2. Topical saline solution in basin
　　　　　　　3. Unsterile 4 × 4 pad
　　　　　　　4. Blenderm tape

Procedure:　Explain to the patient what is going to be done. Donor sites will be designated by the physician. Screen patient, and remove any clothing or dressings around the donor site. Remove any loose debris by wiping off area with dry 4 × 4 pad. Wash area with pHisoHex, shave off hair and rinse well with saline solution. Apply long strips of tape overlapping ¼″ so that the entire donor site is covered with tape. After one hour, remove the tape with a rapid motion. Most of the silver eschar will come off. There may be a need for a second application of tape [12].

Any patient who must face surgery is apprehensive at the very least. The extensively burned patient will undergo repeated operations, and will require constant reassurance as to the success and progress he is making as a result. It is very important that there be a person who can function as liaison between the nursing staff of the burn unit and the operating room, with the goal of decreasing the patient's fear and anxiety. If at all possible, the same operating-room nurse should be there for each surgical procedure the patient must undergo. In this way, the patient has an individual whom he can identify as his operating-room nurse. This nurse should see the patient prior to surgery in order to get to know him, to describe the operating-room environment and procedures, and to elicit from the nursing staff on the burn unit any specific problems that may influence the patient during surgery.

Family members should be allowed to see the patient prior to surgery if at all possible. Children seem to evidence less fear when they are accompanied by parents to the operating-room elevator or door. If the child has a favorite toy, this item should be taken to the surgery with him. Lack of preparation for the surgery causes needless fear, as the following case illustrates.

A seven-year-old child who was 70 percent burned described her first surgical experience as being taken "to a green, cold, scary place. There were big green people who could talk but they had no noses and mouths." The child's eyes, as she described this episode two months after discharge, were wide open and the pupils were dilated.

This unfortunate situation could have been avoided with proper explanation to the child prior to her trip to the operating room.

The operating room should be warm, about 75°F., in order to prevent hypothermia when the burn wound is exposed. The patient's temperature is monitored carefully.

One method of dealing with the overall problems of the child's perception of what is happening to him throughout initial hospitalization was presented at the American Burn Association Meeting in March, 1975. Each child is given a doll that becomes the child's patient. The child is able to do to the doll what is being done to him [5]. This helps the child to act out his feelings since he may not have the vocabulary to express them. It also gives the nursing staff the opportunity to clarify misconceptions in the child's understanding of what is happening to him.

After autografting, the burn wound is painless but the donor sites are extremely painful. The pain is due to the removal of skin one-ten-thousandths to one-sixteen-thousandths of an inch thick. This skin removal is comparable to a partial-thickness burn. If porcine heterograft is not used as a biological dressing on the donor site, then the patient requires an analgesic. In extensively burned patients, the donor sites will be used repeatedly. It requires approximately twenty-one days for the donor site to heal. A donor site must be treated with the same care as any clean surgical wound.

Reconstructive Stage

The reconstructive phase of the burn injury is fraught with problems that are in proportion to the extent and depth of burn. Each individual patient requires a specific regimen of exercise, splinting, and pressure therapy to maintain function and prevent contracture. The scar resulting from the burn injury hypertrophies and forms unsightly ridges. The hypertrophic scar is inelastic and as it matures, it contracts causing changes in joint mobility and contours of the body. If the hypertrophic scarring is allowed to take place, the patient eventually must undergo many contracture releases. The site of surgical contracture release is usually determined by the physician and the patient's priority as to what is most important. For example:

A female who was 23 years old had sustained a 23 percent body-surface-area burn, which involved the face. As a result of the severe depth of burn, she lost most of her nose. Her priority in reconstruction was a "new" nose. This involved raising a full-thickness section of skin from her abdomen and three stages of pedicle transfer to her face. The amount of time involved was approximately six weeks. The patient experienced incisional pain and the discomfort of positioning as the pedicle was attached from abdomen to arm, from arm to forehead, until the pedicle was separated from the arm and the full-thickness skin was used for shaping her new nose.

A full discussion of the various techniques of reconstructive surgery is beyond the scope of this chapter. Many procedures may be necessary to obtain maximum function and cosmetic effect.

The relatives who stay with the patient require help to deal with the pain and discomfort that their loved one is suffering. Truthful and detailed explanations of what is happening to the patients must be given. This can be time-consuming, since giving detailed explanations often must be done on a one-to-one basis.

To help solve this problem in one hospital, the social worker and clinical nursing specialist designed a protocol for weekly group meetings with the relatives. The results of the first series of meetings showed that the family member was experiencing a variety of conflicts, emotions, and needs. The family member of a newly admitted burned patient in the emergent phase usually focused his or her concern on the threat to life, various aspects of the pathophysiology and treatment regime, and the possible loss of sight from edema formation. Fear about possible loss of limb was seen only in one person, whose husband had an electrical burn. Much time was spent in defining terms, which made the nurse aware of the need for a glossary, and this was subsequently attached to the "Burn Unit Information" sheet given to each family member on admission.

During the acute phase of the burn injury, the relatives' concerns were multiple. These were organized as follows:

1. Emotional response of the patient to the injury and relationship with the family

2. Family and patient relationship with the staff

3. Fears and concerns of the family in relation to the patient's condition

In dealing with the relative's ability to cope with the patient's emotional response, most relatives focused on the mood swing of the patient and when to stay with the patient. The persons involved wanted concrete information about what the relative could or could not do for the patient. There was evidence of concern about role changes in the family, such as the husband having to assume a dependent role. Rules about children visiting a parent or other siblings were questioned and answered by making arrangements for individual situations.

Having a child visiting a parent or sibling posed another problem, that of preparing the child for the appearance of the loved one. The request for a child visitor had to come from the patient before any arrangements were made by staff for a visit.

Family relationships with staff involved sensitivity to staff attitudes toward the patient and emerged as possible avoidance by the staff. This usually took place when the patient was not seriously ill and not receiving as much attention as he had when in the critical phase. Apparent lack of attention to the patient also cropped up when the burn unit census was exceptionally high (over 100 percent occupancy rate).

The other facet of staff-family relationship was that of the relative focusing all his anger and hostility on a specific staff person as a means of coping with emotional trauma. As the relative expressed his feelings, much of this behavior was decreased. Relatives had mood swings in which they picked up on the smallest change as an indicator that the patient's condition was improving or deteriorating. Many reported that they were afraid to show feelings of anxiety for fear of frightening the patient. The conflict of needing to be with the patient and needs in the home also became apparent. The family member seemed to be asking permission to leave.

The staff problems that caused sensitivity in the relatives were centered around the staff's feelings about dealing with seriously ill patients and not being assured that what they were doing was "right." Frustration of the staff was expressed when there were large numbers of severely burned patients, with staff attempting to do all of the necessary work and yet have time to talk with the patient and family. The occurrence of a death of a patient usually resulted in a depressed mood on the unit.

In order to help the staff cope with the multitude of problems identified above, weekly meetings were held with a member of the psychiatric team. At this time feedback from the relatives' group was introduced as appropriate to help reach a level of understanding of patient and family perceptions of the unit. These findings were substantiated in a subsequent series and reported at the Sixth Annual Meeting, American Burn Association [3].

The above discussion reports on the situation in one burn unit. A more detailed treatment of problems encountered by staff nurses has been reported by Quinby and Bernstein [8].

Summary

The reaction of health-care workers to the pain experienced by the patient varies from complete denial to oversolicitude. The act of inflicting pain is abhorrent to a person who sees herself as a caring and helping individual, and each individual who works on a burn unit must be able to resolve this conflict. There is no magic answer to this dilemma. Each nurse new to the burn team must work it through, and will require support from older members of the team and possibly help from psychiatric consultants.

Pain as experienced by the burn-injured patient has not been studied as a specific entity. Methods of dealing with the pain have been suggested that may help to minimize the pain experienced by the person who has suffered such a physical and psychological catastrophe.

References

1. Andreason, N. J. C., et al.   Incidence of Long-Term Psychiatric Complications in Severely Burned Adults. Unpublished paper, 1970.
2. Andreason, N. J. C., et al.   Management of emotional reactions in seriously burned adults. *N. Engl. J. Med.* 65:286, 1972.
3. Fagerhaugh, S. Y.   Pain expression and control on a burn unit. *Nurs. Outlook* 2:645, 1974.
4. Hartford, C. E.   The early treatment of burns. *Nurs. Clin. North Am.* 8:447, 1973.
5. McAfee, P. A.   Burn Injury as Interpreted by the Child and His Family. Unpublished paper, American Burn Association Meeting, March, 1975.
6. Montagna, W.   The skin. *Sci. Am.* 55:212, February 1965.
7. National Safety Council.   *Accident Facts.* Washington, 1974.
8. Quinby, S., and Bernstein, N.   Treatment problems with severely burned children—identity problems and adaptation of nurses, Part I. *Am. J. Psychiatry* 1:128, 1971.
9. U.S. Department of HEW.   Flammable Fabrics. DHEW (FDA) Publication No. 72–7013. Rockville, Maryland, 1971.
10. U.S. Department of HEW.   Home Burns and Fire Deaths and Injuries. DHEW Publication No. (HSM) 73–10001. Rockville, Maryland, 1972.
11. Wagner, M. M.   Position of burn patients. *Nurs. Care* 7:22, 1974.
12. Wagner, M. M.   Preparation of Donor Sites. American Burn Association Meeting, April, 1972.
13. Wagner, M. M.   Unpublished survey, 1969.

19

Pain in Cardiovascular Disease

Doris Houser

Pain is a subjective response most often associated with disturbed function or disrupted structural integrity of body tissues. Pain is nature's warning signal of tissue damage. After damage has occurred, pain generally is not felt [24]. Pain is a symptom of underlying pathology indicating the need for diagnosis and therapeutic management. This is particularly true as pain relates to the cardiovascular system, where the underlying pathology that may manifest itself with pain and discomfort has the potential for threatening the total well-being and life of the patient. With constant advances in medical therapy, appropriate care aimed at the origin of the pain has the potential of either restoring the patient's health status or significantly improving his functional status. It behooves the clinician to accurately evaluate the patient with presenting pain syndromes so that appropriate therapy may be instituted. In cardiovascular disorders the evaluation of pain as a symptom of underlying pathology is often a difficult process. The ability to evaluate pain and discomfort is an index of the clinician's expertise. The nurse as a member of the health team, by her assessment, can make a valuable contribution to this evaluative process.

Pain as a manifestation of cardiovascular pathology may be due to a variety of, or combination of, causes such as valvular heart disease, atherosclerosis, anemia, hypertension, cardiomyopathy, thromboembolic processes, metabolic-endocrine disturbances, or myocardial infarction. It may involve any part of the body from the head to the chest to the tip of one's toes. The most common cause for pain in disease of the circulatory system is cellular ischemia. Pain occurs when there is a discrepancy between cellular demand for oxygen and the oxygen supply provided by the circulation. The result is tissue hypoxia with altered cellular metabolism and a release of lactic acid and metabolites associated with the pain sensation [14, 44]. This may occur in the peripheral vascular tree, the heart, or both.

Trauma or inflammatory processes in the heart and vasculature may also induce pain by altering tissue tension or causing a release of chemical factors that stimulate the nerve endings or both [44]. Surgical trauma or pericarditis may be the stimulus for such pain.

Although cellular ischemia may be due to a variety of causes, alterations in blood flow to the cellular mass is most commonly due to atherosclerosis of the coronary or the peripheral vessels, or both. Atherosclerosis decreases the size of the vessel lumen, causing a decrease in blood supply and oxygen delivery to cells, which gives rise to pain and discomfort in accord with the location and extent of vascular insufficiency. Patients with coronary insufficiency may complain of varying patterns of chest pain; patients with arterial insufficiency in the legs may complain of leg cramps on walking (intermittent claudication); patients with intestinal arterial insufficiency may complain of abdominal pain following meals; patients with cerebral artery insufficiency may get transient episodes of neurological deficit (transient ischemic attacks); patients with venous insufficiency may complain of leg discomfort from their varicose veins.

The onset of severe, or the persistence of chronic, pain and discomfort is a disturbing and often terrifying experience for the patient. Associated symptoms of nausea, shortness of breath, weakness, and diaphoresis may accentuate the patient's concern that "something is wrong." Chest pain is a particularly frightening experience because a patient immediately considers the possibility of heart problems and the potential death or disability associated with heart disease.

Pain as a manifestation of heart pathology, particularly a myocardial infarction, is one of the most urgent concerns. This pain calls for immediate measures to relieve the pain and prevent additional myocardial work and stress that occur during the pain process. Associated with myocardial ischemia is sympathetic overactivity, manifested by a rise in heart rate and blood pressure. This mechanism increases the work of the heart and its oxygen consumption [44]. Sympathetic stimulation and endogenous catecholamine release may provoke serious ventricular arrhythmias and may also contribute to decompensation. The tachycardia and elevated arterial pressure may also induce parasympathetic stimulation, resulting in decreased heart rate and the possibility of cardiac asystole. Ischemia may not be associated with heart rate and blood pressure changes, but may accompany disorders of autoregulation of the coronary circulation. If this ischemia persists, myocardial necrosis with a functional deficit may occur [43]. Prompt pharmacologically induced relief of cardiac pain is essential in decreasing the patient's anxiety level, myocardial work, and subsequent release of catecholamines as well as further cellular ischemia and damage [27, 35, 47].

Management of the patient presenting with pain involves an initial assessment of the severity, location, and peculiar characteristics of the pain. Immediate therapy involves medication to relieve the pain, reassurance to decrease fear and anxiety, and placing the patient in a comfortable resting position, followed by a more probing evaluation to determine the underlying pathology causing the pain. Specific therapy to correct the etiology of the pain can then be instituted [46]. Cardiovascular pain involves the differential diagnosis and management of (1) chest pain, and (2) peripheral vascular pain.

Chest Pain

Chest pain has been termed a "haystack of diagnostic traps." Chest pain, particularly the visceral type, is often difficult to evaluate. Chest pain may be due to cardiovascular disease (myocardial infarction [MI], aortic aneurisms, angina, pericarditis), pleuropulmonary disease (pulmonary embolus, pleurisy, pneumonia), gastrointestinal disease (esophagitis, hiatal hernia, gallbladder, pancreatitis), neuromuscular-skeletal disease (spinal osteoarthritis, costal chondritis, gout, trauma), or psychosomatic conditions [18, 37, 46].

Patients with chest pain will present different symptoms of duration, onset, intensity, pattern of occurrence, or pathway. These differences in symptoms are related to: (1) site of pain origin, (2) degree of tissue ischemia at site, and (3) the degree of total functional interference the underlying pathology precipitates. Pain may come from several different sources. Pain from different organs in and adjacent to the chest area travels through different neuro pathways but enters the spinal cord to travel through the same pathway to the brain. The brain may have a difficult job in sorting out the source of the pain. Chest pain due to cardiac disease can occur within anatomical boundaries that other organs may also occupy in their pain mappings, as Figure 19-1 illustrates.

Pain in the chest may occur in the presence of local lesions of no serious consequence or may indicate significant somatic or visceral disease. The sudden, intense, and agonizing chest pain of a dissecting aortic aneurism is considered a medical emergency. This pain syndrome is the result of marked distention of the aorta as blood enters under pressure from the lumen and splits apart layers of the arterial wall. The intense distention of portions of the wall as blood flows in the false channel between the layers causes extreme "tearing" pain at the location of the dissection [9, 44]. The intense pain of a potential or documented myocardial infarction also warrants immediate concern and intervention. Pain also may be attributed to psychosomatic origin. This diagnosis must be made with extreme care and only after extensive evaluation.

Chest pain due to cardiovascular disease may or may not be due to occlusive vascular disease. Whether the etiology is small-vessel disease, abnormal blood-oxygen release mechanism, coronary vessel spasm, or atherosclerosis, tissue ischemia serves as the stimulus for pain and initiates the autonomic discharge. Myocardial ischemia and necrosis are the result of inadequate coronary blood flow or increased myocardial demand, or both. Ischemia produces an accumulation of metabolites in the tissue with widespread irritability of the pain nerve endings. Chemical factors and tissue tension from insufficient oxygen cause pain because of the accompanying tissue ischemia

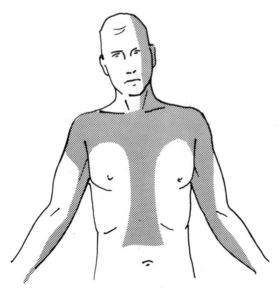

Figure 19-1 Anatomical areas of reference of cardiac pain.

[12, 44]. As mentioned earlier, ischemia is the underlying common denominator in cardiac and vascular pain.

Terminology

Attaching diagnostic labels to patients may be confusing, since nomenclature is not always definitive and standardized. We have become accustomed to using general terms to describe a group of clinical disorders associated with pain. Terms such as angina pectoris and coronary insufficiency have different meanings to different people. To avoid some of the pitfalls of inexact terminology, a clarification of some of the terms currently in use follows:

Myocardial Infarction—term implies that the myocardium has been deprived of blood supply or oxygenation, or both, long enough for myocardial cellular necrosis to occur. The term does not indicate the cause of the condition, which may or may not be due to occlusive disease [12]. Pain is a common manifestation of myocardial infarction. Classically, pain associated with myocardial infarction is intense, but characteristics differ and pain may be entirely absent.

Coronary Insufficiency—a confusing term that in the past referred to a type of chest pain that included several intermediate syndromes. The pain lasted longer and tended to be more intense than angina pectoris, but was not associated with death of heart muscle as in a myocardial infarction. It has also been called "pilot angina," "premonitory pain," "preinfarction angina," or "impending MI." Since many patients who are labeled coronary insufficiency actually have small infarctions, it is probably best to discard the use of this term. Coronary insufficiency is really a physiological term referring to a state of myocardial ischemia of various undetermined degrees and not a diagnostic category or an accurate descriptive category of cardiac pain [39].

Coronary Occlusion—term used to refer to a cause of ischemic heart disease or poor myocardial perfusion. It implies a diagnosis that cannot accurately be established without coronary angiography or autopsy [18]. Pain may be one of the manifestations of this disorder, but varies widely in character.

Angina Pectoris—Latin term for "chest pain." A clinical syndrome characterized by paroxysmal attacks of chest pain indicative of poor myocardial perfusion, but not the cause. Although angina may be present in occlusive coronary artery disease, it may also occur in the absence of occlusive disease, and is not necessarily a precedent to a myocardial infarction. There are different variations and causes for angina. Terminology refers to typical symptoms manifested [10, 12, 14, 15, 20, 28, 31, 39, 41, 43, 45, 49, 50].

a. *Angina decubitus* (recumbent angina)—chest pain that occurs in a recumbent position relieved by sitting or standing.

b. *Angina of effort*—chest pain precipitated by physical exertion.

c. *Status anginosis*—almost continuous chest pain at rest and not necessarily accompanied by any changes suggestive of an acute myocardial infarction. Also called "preinfarction angina."

d. *Nocturnal angina*—chest pain that occurs only at night and is not necessarily related to the recumbent position.

e. *Intractable angina*—chronic pain of varying degrees that is physically incapacitating. Like status anginosis except it occurs over a longer period of time.

f. *Prinzmetal (variant) angina*—form of angina described by Prinzmetal and associates in 1959 that is thought to be due to intermittent coronary artery spasm with or without underlying occlusive artery disease. It is characterized by ST segment elevation but no significant alteration in heart rate and blood pressure, can occur at rest but is not related to recumbent position, can occur during normal activity but is not particularly precipitated by exercise or emotion, and occurs in a cyclic pattern (occurs at same time of day or night).

g. *Classic angina*—broad category of variations first described by Heberden 200 years ago, due to myocardial ischemia from a variety of causes. It is characterized by ST segment depression and hemodynamic changes causing increased myocardial oxygen demand prior to onset of pain, precipitated by factors such as exertion, emotion, or cold weather, and relieved by a vasodilator (nitroglycerine) and rest. Classic angina tends to have a sudden onset, occurs in the anterior chest, is of short duration, and has a certain uniformity of specific aspects of each attack.

Assessment

Chest pain can be a great deceiver; the peculiar characteristics of the patient's complaints can mimic characteristics of a variety of disorders. A patient may complain of abdominal pain similar to peptic ulcer or gallbladder pain, and yet have coronary artery disease; another patient may complain of itching, which may be an atypical somatic expression of referred pain from coronary artery disease. A myriad of symptoms more typical of cardiac disease can be confusing to the clinician. Esophagitis often produces pain in the identical position (substernal) as angina or pericarditis. Nitroglycerine may relieve the pain of angina, but also relieve the pain associated with abnormal motor function of the esophagus, although for different reasons. Nitroglycerine relieves anginal pain by reducing the afterload, decreasing the left ventricular and diastolic pressure, and reducing myocardial work. It relieves esophagitis because of relaxation of spastic smooth muscle. Anginal pain may be worse in the recumbent position and relieved on sitting or standing. Symptoms such as bloating, fullness, and postprandial occurrence of pain can be present with both angina and hiatus hernia. If a hiatus hernia is documented, then all symptoms may be attributed to this cause, when in fact the patient may also have coronary artery disease with angina. The patient with cardiac disease and some gastrointestinal or pulmonary problems presents a particular problem in sorting out symptoms.

There are many diagnostic traps, and effective management is dependent upon a thorough evaluation of patient symptoms. The first step in assessment is identifying all the peculiar characteristics of the patient's pain syndrome. A good clinical history is essential. Depending upon the diagnostic impressions after this initial assessment, further and more definitive diagnostic tests may be made. Coronary angiography, chest films, ECG, enzyme levels, exercise stress testing are means the physician may utilize to diagnose the specific underlying etiology of the pain.

The patient's history can be decisive in making the proper diagnosis or it may be of little value if chest pain is the only presenting symptom. The nurse's role in compiling this information is valuable to the physician in eliciting as many details as possible in differential diagnoses of chest pain.

In taking a clinical history, the clinician must be careful not to provide misleading answers by inappropriately posed questions. For example, if you ask a patient if he has chest pain, he may say "no" because he may not be feeling what he calls "pain." If you ask, "Do you have any sensation of discomfort in your chest and can you describe it?" a more meaningful response may be obtained. It is helpful to communicate in terms that are meaningful to the patient in order to elicit significant facts. For example, if you ask the patient if his pain radiates, he may say "no" because he doesn't understand what you mean by "radiate." If you ask, "Does your pain 'travel' any place?" a more descriptive reply may be given. While one is getting the information from the patient, he may tend to ramble in his story. This is particularly true for older patients. Although the patient should be kept on the "communication track," he should not be hurried, since one may clip off the conversation just as a significant fact is about to emerge. For example, patients tend to forget past episodes of mild pain or chest discomfort, thinking that they were insignificant at the time they occurred. Sometimes, only by relating stories of their daily activities can the incidence of chest pain and the precipitating factors that preceded the onset of pain be recalled. It is helpful to remember that an elderly person does not always have as acute a sensation of pain as a younger one, and may not complain of "pain," but of symptoms such as "gas," "burning of chest," "overfatigue." These symptoms may be just as significant as frank pain.

If the patient complains of chest pain of increasing frequency, it is important to ascertain how the pain is affecting his functional status. Does it interfere with his daily life-style? Some patients may have difficulty relaying meaningful information about how their daily routine and activity level are affected. Posing the questions, "How far can you walk on level ground on a nice day?" and "How many steps can you slowly climb without any pain or shortness of breath?" is a way to identify functional class.

To get at more specific details of his pain syndrome, ask him to describe the pain. Chest pain of cardiac origin often tends to have a vague, all-encompassing character. Ask the patient if he can point to the pain with one finger. Cardiac, especially anginal, pain is almost never so sharply localized. Patients with cardiac pain tend to complain of a "viselike" or "squeezing" sensation and will tend to move their clenched fist to the site of the pain. This clenched fist over the substernal area is called the *Levine sign* and is a common way for patients to communicate chest pain that is cardiac in origin. Ask the patient if the pain is a deep or superficial sensation. Anginal pain is deep, although it may spread to involve the surface. It is almost never just superficial. Does body position or respiratory action and coughing relieve or aggravate the pain? In general, chest pain due to pleuropulmonary disorders tends to be aggravated by respirations and coughing while cardiac pain is not affected. Changing positions and muscular activity may aggravate the pain if it is due to a musculoskeletal disorder, but does not usually do so with a cardiac problem. The recumbent position versus the sitting position may affect chest pain in cardiac, pulmonary, and gastrointestinal disorders, and must be considered in association with the myriad of other presenting symptoms. Does rest in itself relieve the pain? Is rest in the sitting or lying position more helpful to the patient? Observation of what aggravates or relieves the chest pain or discomfort and how soon the discomfort subsides is a valuable diagnostic tool that the nurse should use and communicate to the physician.

Evaluation of what intervention relieves or lessens the pain and the time interval required for the pain to subside after intervention should be recorded. Do nitroglycerine or antacids relieve the pain? If an antacid relieves it, the chest pain may be due to a gastrointestinal disorder rather than to a cardiac problem. Is the pain so intense that a narcotic is necessary to relieve it? If so, this gives some clue to the severity of the situation. Is prompt relief achieved after narcotherapy or nitroglycerine? If so, then the underlying ischemia may not be as severe as one in which relief is difficult to obtain in spite of multiple interventions.

Although the patient's history can be important for diagnosis and subsequent treatment and a thorough history takes time, a patient in acute pain cannot relate a complete history until his acute episode has abated. In the situation of acute pain, only significant questions can be asked in a short time interval and immediate intervention for pain relief is necessary. For the patient whose pain pattern is familiar to the nurse, few questions are necessary prior to intervention. For the new and unfamiliar patient, a more thorough history can be taken after pain relief is obtained. An important part of the clinical picture is also what relieved the pain and the time interval involved. It is all part of the assessment process. The significant information to obtain from the patient is:

1. Where is the pain or discomfort? (location)
2. Describe the pain—what does it feel like? (severity, intensity)
3. How did it start? (onset)
4. Does your pain travel anywhere? (radiation)
5. Have you had the same or similar pain before? (pattern)
6. What other symptoms do you have with your pain? (Such as: shortness of breath, profuse sweating, nausea, etc.) (associated symptoms)
7. What usually relieves your pain? (relief)
8. How long did the pain last? (duration)
9. What brings on the pain? (precipitating factors)

The nurse as an evaluator of the chest pain syndrome must keep in mind not only such basic objective criteria as location, quality, duration, and so forth, but also the peculiar characteristics of the various causes of chest pain that can aid in the differential diagnosis. The majority of patients with chest pain will follow a characteristic pain pattern and accompanying symptoms, so that diagnosis is objective and straightforward. It is the atypical patient who presents the diagnostic dilemma for the physician; the nurse's assessment and documentation of patient symptoms is often invaluable to the physician in diagnosis and instituting subsequent therapy that is appropriate.

Table 19-1 identifies the common characteristics of chest pain according to etiology. A careful review of the table makes clear why differential diagnosis of chest pain can be so difficult.

When the patient is experiencing chest pain it is advisable to obtain vital signs and note any alterations in blood pressure, heart rate, and respiratory rate. This may or may not help in the diagnosis of the underlying cause of the pain. It does identify the patient's response to the pain and if he is physiologically compensating for the stress factor. If functional decompensation is occurring, such as a drastic fall in blood pressure, rapid shallow respirations, and a sudden rise or fall in heart rate, the physician should be notified at once and immediate measures instituted to prevent failure and shock. There will be some rise in heart rate, respiratory rate, and blood pressure as a normal compensatory response to pain. Except when there is a drastic and sudden change in vital signs, the blood pressure response will be a more reliable tool after the pain has subsided.

A 12-lead ECG during chest pain is helpful in determining if the pain is cardiac in origin, and the severity of the ischemia. A comparative ECG recording after the pain has subsided also should be made. If a 12-lead ECG recording is not immediately available, an ECG tracing per cardiac monitor should be obtained in lead II, AVF, or V_3 to V_6 [38, 40]. Analyze the ECG tracing and report for:

1. arrhythmias
2. displacement of the ST segments or changes in the T waves
3. abnormalities in the QRS morphology
4. changes in the polarity of the QRS complex [47]

An ECG tracing in the angina patient recorded before and after intervention (such as nitroglycerine) is often helpful in documenting the patient's response to the intervention.

Nursing assessment is helpful to the physician in determining the etiology of the chest pain and subsequent management, but it is also necessary before and after nursing intervention to relieve the pain. If the physician has left prn orders for nitroglycerine, a narcotic, and an antacid, the nurse must be able to determine which medication would be most beneficial to the patient. The nurse should document in the chart the patient's symptoms prior to administering the medication and his response to the medication.

Management of Chest Pain

Management of chest pain involves relief of pain at the time of occurrence, prevention of pain, and a thorough evaluation of the underlying pathology causing the pain. Chest pain due to ischemic heart disease may vary in forms of severity from the sudden intense pain of an acute myocardial infarction to the chronic less severe pain of angina pectoris. Chest pain after cardiac surgery may require some narcotics in the first 24 to 48 hours, but discomfort is usually relieved with milder analgesics (Darvon, Tylenol) during the remaining hospital course. This is particularly true with sternal incisions, which are less pain-producing than thoracotomies.* If the chest pain is due to a GI or pulmonary problem, the pain will vary in character and management is aimed at relief and altering the etiological factor.

The first step in pain management is pharmacological intervention to relieve the pain. Chest pain due to the GI problem may benefit from an antacid. The sudden occurrence of severe chest pain due to an acute myocardial infarction usually requires narcotics to relieve the pain. Many years ago, Thomas Sydenham stated "among the remedies which it has pleased the Almighty God to give to man to relieve his sufferings, none is so efficacious as opium" [46]. This still applies to the acute myocardial infarction patient who frequently requires morphine sulfate (MS). Although MS is contraindicated for some people, in the myocardial infarction patient it has the advantages not only of decreasing the pain but of inducing drowsiness and rest, and of clouding sensorium, which reduces the anxiety associated with chest pain. It also increases venous pooling, thus decreasing venous pressure and lowering myocardial oxygen demand [11, 27, 35, 46]. The usual dosage is 10 mg but some patients may require more because of very severe or persistent pain [46]. Narcotherapy in acute MI patients is unlike that of abdominal pain in which a narcotic may be withheld by physician's request to prevent masking

* See Chapter 15 on postoperative pain.

Table 19-1 Chest pain characteristics by etiological classification

Characteristics	Myocardial Infarction	Pericarditis	Angina	Pleuro-pulmonary	Esophageal-gastric	Musculo-skeletal	Psychosomatic
Onset	Sudden	Sudden	Build-up of intensity (crescendo), or sudden	Gradual or sudden	Gradual or sudden	Gradual or sudden	Gradual or sudden
Location	Substernal—anterior chest and midline	Substernal—to left of midline or precordial only	Substernal—not sharply localized; anterior chest	Over lung fields to side and back	Substernal—anterior chest; midline	To side of midline	Left chest or variable area
Radiation	Down one or both arms, to jaw, neck, or back	To back or left supraclavicular area	To back, neck, arms, jaws, and occasionally upper abdomen	Anterior chest, shoulder, neck	To upper abdomen, shoulder, or back		None—sharply localized
Duration	At least 30 min; usually 1-2 hrs Residual soreness 1-3 days	Continuous May last for days Residual soreness	Usually less than 15 min and not more than 30 min (average = 3 min)	Continuous for hours	Continuous for short or longer intervals or intermittent	Continuous or intermittent	1 min to several hours
Quality-intensity	Severe, stabbing, choking, burning, squeezing, viselike, intense pressure, deep sensation	Sharp, stabbing, knifelike; moderate to severe or only an "ache"; deep or superficial	Mild to moderate, heavy pressure—squeezing, viselike, vague, like weight on chest, uniform pattern of attacks, deep sensation, tightness	Sharp ache—not severe Knifelike shooting	Squeezing, heartburn	Soreness	Superficial, hyperesthesia of chest wall, dull ache to sharp, stabbing
Method of relief	Narcotics	Some relief with ASA, Tylenol	Relieved with rest and/or nitroglycerine or other vasodilators	Narcotics	Antacids—may be relieved with NTG	ASA, Tylenol, heat, immobilization	Rest and sedation

Associated symptoms	Apprehension, nausea, dyspnea, disphoresis, dizziness, weakness, pulmonary congestion, increased pulse, decreased BP, gallop heart sound	Precordial rub; muscle movement & inspiration cause increased pain. Pain decreased on sitting; increases when on left side, laughing, or coughing	Dyspnea, diaphoresis, nausea, desire to void. Associated with "belching," apprehension, or uneasiness	Dyspnea; tachycardia; apprehension; increased pain with coughing, on inspiration, and on movement; pain decreased on sitting. Pleural rub	Dysphagia, belching, diaphoresis, reflux esophagitis, pain decreased on sitting or standing, vomiting	Pain increased with movement	Fatigue, dyspnea, "sighing" respiration, palpitation, hyperventilation, dizzy spells, claustrophobia
Precipitating factors	Not necessarily anything. May occur at rest or with increased physical or emotional exertion	Not induced with effort	Classical: physical exercise, emotional stress, eating, cold or hot, humid weather, recumbency, micturition, or defecation. Variant: not necessarily related to any factors as exertion		Food intake, recumbency, alcohol ingestion, highly seasoned foods, history of GI problems	History of previous neck and arm pain	Fatigue, emotional stress, or none
Other diagnostic criteria	Elevated blood enzymes, ECG changes, positive cardiac scan	Chest x-ray—pericardial effusion; ST segment shifts opposite to myocardial ischemia	ST segment elevation or depression ECG changes with activity and during episode, treadmill test, cardiac arteriography	Chest x-ray Lung scan	GI series	X-ray	ECG normal

of symptoms indicative of further complications until the physician evaluates the etiology of the pain. Acute chest pain due to a possible MI calls for an agent that will relieve the pain and decrease the cyclic effects of pain and associated catecholamine release that can cause additional oxygen consumption, myocardial work, and stress-induced ischemia.

To relieve and prevent pain episodes, patients with angina may be placed on vasodilators such as nitroglycerine (NTG) or Isordil to decrease oxygen cellular demands and myocardial work. Patients with angina need to be properly instructed in the use of these drugs, taking them not only at the onset of pain but in the anticipation of discomfort. Some physicians prefer to have the angina patient on a fixed schedule of a long-acting vasodilator (Isordil) to prevent the occurrence of angina, while others prefer the prn use of a short-term vasodilator (NTG). Other patients may be placed on a beta-blocking agent (Inderal) to decrease myocardial work consistently and lessen the ischemia precipitating the angina. The selection of the proper agent is usually dependent upon the severity of the patient's disease and symptomatology. For the patient with occasional angina, the prn use of a vasodilator such as NTG usually works well. The patient should be instructed to take the medication at the first indication of pain for optimal results. Patients tend to resist taking the medication until the pain is more severe and difficult to relieve. This is because of: (1) the false belief that the less drug they take, the less severe the underlying disease, (2) the needless worry of habituation and loss of drug effectiveness with repeated use, and (3) the uncomfortable side effects of headache, dizziness, and flushing that they may feel are necessary if the drug is to be effective. If the patient is troubled with these side effects he should contact his physician so that reevaluation of dosage requirements for pain relief and the status of the underlying disease process can be made. Patients need to know they should: (1) keep the pills out of heat and light, (2) carry them on their person at all times, (3) renew the prescription approximately every three months or when they no longer feel a tingling sensation under their tongue (the pills lose their potency), and (4) call the physician if they cannot obtain pain relief after taking 3 to 4 tablets (one every 5 to 10 minutes) or if the pain increases in intensity and location. For the patient whose requirement for a prn vasodilator (NTG) increases to several times a day, a longer-acting vasodilator taken on a fixed schedule several times a day may be preferred. If this does not reduce the need for additional NTG, then a beta-blocking agent may be added to the regimen. The patient's response to medication should be evaluated and charted [14, 16, 22, 23].

Drugs are but one component in managing the chest pain of cardiac disease, particularly angina. The patient's life-style will need to be modified so that precipitating factors can be avoided. The well-informed patient can function more effectively if his environment is devoid of precipitating factors, and if he realizes that a medication such as NTG is an immediate antidote for pain and is within his reach. This enables him to feel more self-reliant about his management and furthers a more positive, less anxious attitude. An optimistic and confident attitude is an important factor in management of a long-lasting illness such as ischemic heart disease.

The primary care objective is to keep the patient with angina under control with a minimal modification of essential daily activities. The patient should be made to feel that with a few modifications, he can continue to be an independent and productive member of the community and family unit. The patient teaching program is essential in communicating the elements of the prescribed care regimen as well as an attitude of optimism and compliance with the regimen.

The patient with angina needs to be taught: (1) the names, action, dosage, and side effects of prescribed medications; (2) the symptoms of distress that warrant attention of a physician, such as increased intensity, frequency, and duration of the chest pain, symptoms of congestive heart failure, or a decrease in his functional ability to perform his daily activities; and (3) the avoidance of such risk factors as tobacco, obesity, extremes of hot and cold weather, excessive physical exertion (particularly activities with an isometric component, which imposes additional myocardial work demands), and emotional stress. The patient should be aware of the cumulative effect of several of these risk factors at a given period of time. Precipitating factors vary from patient to patient, but the long-standing angina patient is usually well aware of specific factors that bring on chest discomfort. Some patients find they need to avoid cool showers or swimming in a nonheated pool. Others suffer from postprandial angina and should avoid big meals and divide their total food intake into small frequent feedings. Patients who find a hot, humid environment difficult to tolerate may find a dehumidifier or air conditioner in the office or home helpful. Other patients may find that even cold bed sheets are a precipitating factor, which can be resolved by warming the bed with an electric blanket prior to retiring. Most patients find the tempo of their daily activities a decisive factor in provoking angina. "Beating the clock" and a "nonstop" round of physically and emotionally charged activities are patterns the patient has to avoid. The patient has to learn that by slowing the tempo of his activities he can still accomplish a great deal without incurring the disabling effects of chest pain or discomfort.

A physical conditioning or exercise program is an important part of the therapeutic regimen for some patients with ischemic heart disease. This may be for the post-myocardial-infarction patient or the angina sufferer. A program of controlled physical exercise has the beneficial effects of increasing collateral circulation and decreasing myocardial work with activity, both of which decrease the incidence of myocardial ischemia that is manifested in the form of pain. It is also believed that the hemoglobin-oxygen dissociation curve is altered to allow more oxygen to be released with exercise. This effect of enhancing myocardial oxygen delivery is similar to the action of beta-blocking agents [40, 51]. While a physical training program does increase exercise performance in selected patients, this type of therapy is not for all cardiac patients and may be contraindicated in patients with failure, hypertension, dangerous arrhythmias, or other debilitating diseases. A standardized exercise test on a treadmill is a necessary diagnostic tool to evaluate the patient's tolerance level so that an exercise program can be initiated that is within the individual's physical capacity. This exercise program should be well controlled and isometric exercises should be avoided. Bicycling, swimming, and walking are often beneficial. Regular walking as a means of maintaining or improving physical conditioning can be used with the least amount of special precautions or monitoring. Angina is one of the most chronic forms of chest pain for the cardiac and can be one of the most disabling. The properly managed patient, within his physical limitations, can generally maintain functional status within the normal range. If the patient fails to respond to conservative management, then medical reevaluation is warranted. Other approaches such as surgical bypass vein grafts may be needed to alleviate the ischemia and anginal symptoms.

Nursing Care Plan for Patient Presenting with Acute Chest Pain
The following is a step-by-step care plan in brief form:

1. Initially evaluate chest pain according to: location, quality/severity, duration, onset, its association with respiration and position change, precipitating factors, modes of relief, and other accompanying symptoms such as dyspnea, nausea, vomiting, diaphoresis
2. Obtain vital signs
3. Obtain sample ECG tracing
4. Administer prompt relief of pain
   a. medicate
   b. place patient in comfortable resting position
5. Reassure patient—stay with him until pain subsides if possible
6. Record on chart
   a. pain symptoms presented
   b. intervention for pain relief and effect
7. Report immediately any chest pain that is
   a. different from prior pain incidence
   b. accompanied by different symptoms
   c. accompanied by changes in ECG or vital signs
   d. increasing in frequency or severity, or both
   e. not completely relieved by usual mode of therapy or medication

Nursing Care of the Patient with Chronic Chest Pain
The patient with episodes of chest pain who is hospitalized for diagnostic studies to determine the pathology causing the pain needs:

1. Astute assessment of characteristics of pain when they occur. This involves symptoms, vital signs, ECG tracing, modes of relief, and so forth.
2. Record and report incidents and characteristics.
3. Reassure patient. Remember pain of unknown origin is often a fearful and frustrating phenomenon to the patient whether he verbally admits it or not. The patient may suspect the worst with chest pain. Remain calm yourself—overanxious nurses make overanxious patients.
4. After a diagnosis is made and communicated to the patient and a regimen of medical care identified, reinforce the physician's explanation to the patient. Repetition and reinforcement often are necessary whether dealing with chest pain due to an acute myocardial infarction, angina, ulcer, or pulled muscle. Patients subconsciously tend to diagnose their ailment before the physician does, and may disbelieve, deny, or resist the actual diagnosis. The close and sympathetic attention of the staff during this time is important in establishing a trusting relationship conducive to compliance with the prescribed care regimen.
5. Implement the patient teaching program specific to his prescribed care regimen. This involves things such as medication, diet, activity levels, avoidance of precipitating factors, recognizing symptoms of trouble requiring medical attention, and medical care follow-up plan.

Problems of Care for the Patient with Chest Pain due to Cardiac Disease

Patients with ischemic heart disease require long-term therapy with varying modifications according to the stage or degree of the disease process. You are not just dealing with chest pain as a separate entity, but a total patient with an underlying disease process who needs care. Even if myocardial ischemia is alleviated by bypass surgery, the underlying cause of the ischemia is still present, perhaps to cause problems even years later. Prevention of pain due to ischemia by avoiding risk factors and making modifications in the life-style that are conducive to the patient's physical limitations and yet enable him to maintain a fairly normal functional status is a basic goal. A trusting and open relationship among the patient, his family, and the clinical staff is a care factor conducive to positive counseling. Because each patient is an individual in a specific life situation, working with the patient-family unit often presents new and varied challenges. The counseling process is a time-consuming task, but a very important one if the goals of care are to be realized. Nurses need to be more cognizant of the preventive aspects of care in managing the patient with chest pain. The health team is caring for a patient with an underlying disease process, not just chest pain.

Patients with cardiac pain who have a history of myocardial infarction or angina, or both, may experience pain that is of a little different character than before, but is not severe. The patient may suspect something is different, but because it is not severe, or if the discomfort has subsided somewhat, the patient may not call a physician when in fact the patient may have an acute myocardial infarction. It is recognized that many patients do not see a physician for several hours after the onset of even rather intense pain, and especially if it is not severe in nature. It is because of this time lag prior to medical care that many needless deaths occur. Thus it is important for the patient to contact his physician with the onset of any new symptoms. Patients are reluctant to do this because: (1) they don't want to bother the busy physician needlessly, (2) they don't want to be labeled a "crock," (3) they don't believe it is anything serious, and (4) they have had previous "false alarms" and don't want another. The differentiation of significant from nonsignificant chest pain can be a diagnostic problem for the physician and thus it presents a unique dilemma for the patient. Although you don't want to make the patient overly conscious of every ache and discomfort, the properly instructed patient should be able to identify the most significant symptoms that will include the majority of the situations. The patients who walk the fine line in between present the greatest problems, but should be encouraged to seek medical help and not feel guilty if it turns out to be a "false alarm." This fact in itself is reassuring to the patient. For patients with known cardiac disease, it is often helpful if they have someone they can call on a 24-hour basis, who can substantiate their need for medical care and encourage them to seek this help. Then if it is a "false alarm," they don't feel guilty. This "crisis line" is one way of speeding necessary medical referrals for the reluctant cardiac patient with chest discomfort.

Vascular Pain

Pain attributed to pathology in the vascular system may be due to chronic occlusive arterial disease (arteriosclerosis obliterans), chronic venous insufficiency, trauma, or an inflammatory process. The common denominator of pain in the vascular tree is tissue ischemia. For the majority of patients, vascular pain is a result of peripheral vascular disease, but it may involve any portion of the vascular tree. Peripheral vascular disease is a term that encompasses a wide variety of conditions affecting arteries, veins, and lymphatic vessels of the extremities. Although peripheral vascular disease is not a synonym for chronic occlusive arterial disease (COAD) due to atherosclerosis of the aorta or its branches (or both) in the extremities, 95 percent of the cases are due to COAD [26]. Atherosclerosis behaves differently in different vascular beds, and the presenting symptoms vary in character depending upon the location of the tissues involved and the severity of the underlying disease process. Buerger's disease, Takayasu's disease, and some collagen disorders are other conditions with occlusive artery disease that involve some degree of mechanical obstruction of, or diminished blood flow through, the arterial vascular system. More commonly, the etiology of occlusive artery disease is primarily atherosclerotic, thrombotic, embolic, or a combination of these factors. Atherosclerotic plaques are more common at the bifurcation or branching of an artery because the arterial intima is subject to injury from the high pressure currents produced by major changes in direction of blood flow. Aneurisms of the arterial tree also may occur at these sites and may alter function or be subject to vascular rupture [9]. Most of these conditions manifest symptoms of decreased peripheral perfusion, particularly distal to the lesion site. Pain may or may not be a predominant symptom depending upon the extent of the underlying disease process and the tissues involved. The location of any presenting pain is a significant symptom as it aids in the diagnosis of the underlying pathology. Figure 19-2 identifies sites of vascular pathology and associated symptoms.

Chronic venous insufficiency is essentially the end result of incompetency of the valves of damaged veins and usually occurs in the lower extremities [26]. This may lead to conditions such as varicose veins and stasis skin ulcers. The extent of the disease and its interference with normal venous flow varies greatly, but in the more severe form pain and discomfort are predominant symptoms [26].

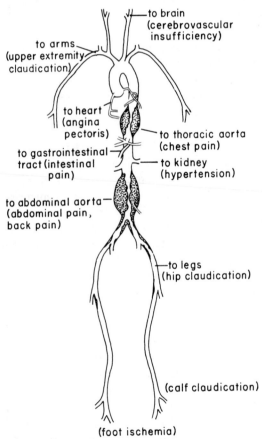

Figure 19-2 Common sites of occlusive disease and aneurismal formation and associated pain symptoms.

Assessment

Evaluation of the patient with vascular disease involves identification not only of pain characteristics but also of associated symptoms indicative of impaired blood flow or decreased peripheral perfusion. Associated symptoms such as numbness, muscle weakness, decreased or absent pulses of extremities, changes in color, changes in temperature of the part (cold), or edema are indicative of diminished blood flow. Because of the diminished blood flow, ischemia manifested by pain will result. Pain can take many forms from muscle cramps to aching to severe pain that may be continuous or intermittent in occurrence. The significant information to ask the patient is: Where is the pain or discomfort (location)? How did it start (onset)? Have you had the same or similar pain before (pattern)? Describe the pain (severity). How long does it last (duration)? What brings on (precipitates) the pain? What relieves the pain (relief)?

Identifying the location and severity of the pain is particularly important in the total evaluation of the patient. Intermittent claudication occurs when ischemic muscle is active and the pain or discomfort is relieved with rest. In the legs this may be manifested in the form of leg cramps, "charley horse," numbness, aching, or muscle weakness. Occlusive disease of the subclavian and axillary artery may cause cramping, aching, or numbness of the forearm muscles with activity such as typing, writing, or painting. Arterial or venous insufficiency severe enough to cause ulcers or gangrene of the part can cause severe pain at the site [26]. Pain associated with peripheral vascular disease varies: the pain of thromboembolism tends to be sudden and excruciating; the pain of progressive occlusion tends to be of an intermittent cramping character; the pain of varicose veins tends to be a "heavy," burning sensation; and the pain of gangrene is steady with a progression to numbness.

Pain associated with aneurisms varies according to the type of aneurism and its location. Aneurisms can occur in the heart (ventricle) and may or may not cause chest pain [7, 30]. These patients usually have some associated symptoms of failure or decreased functional status that identify the need for a complete diagnostic evaluation. Abdominal and aortic aneurisms may or may not produce pain, but the location of any presenting pain is a means to determine the site of the lesion [7, 9, 30, 44, 46]. Thoracic aortic aneurisms may cause chest pain; abdominal aneurisms may cause abdominal or back pain; a dissecting aortic aneurism is manifested by the sudden onset of extreme and agonizing "tearing" pain that warrants the immediate attention of the physician. A dissecting aneurism occurs from splitting of the intima when the high arterial pressure forces blood into a channel between an atheromatous plaque and the underlying intima. The result is intimal tearing as the blood burrows between the layers of the arterial wall. The false channel can extend either proximally or distally from the origin. The process can lead to death from rupture or ostial occlusion of a vital artery [9]. When the dissecting aneurism is confined to the aortic arch, the pain is substernal or radiates over the upper anterior chest and shoulders. As dissection progresses into the descending aorta, extreme pain along the base of the neck and in the back may occur [44]. Patients with a dissecting aneurism generally have a long history of hypertension [9, 44].

When assessing pain due to vascular disease, one must recognize that other conditions such as osteoarthritis, peripheral neuropathy, and degeneration of lumbar disks may occur concurrently and be contributing to the pain syndrome. These conditions along with occlusive vascular disease are more likely to occur in the over-fifty age group [26].

Assessment of pain characteristics and any presenting symptoms of impaired perfusion should be recorded and reported. More definitive diagnostic tests can be made by the use of (1) arteriography, and (2) equipment to detect arterial and venous blood flow such as the Doppler ultrasound stethoscope.

Management

Management of pain in vascular lesions involves: (1) analgesics for pain relief, and (2) treatment of the underlying lesion. Management, like symptomatology, varies according to the cause, location, and extent of the lesion. Analgesics such as morphine sulfate or Demerol may be given for patients experiencing severe pain, or milder preparations such as Tylenol or Darvon may suffice. One should be careful not to overmedicate (as with narcotics) so that significant pain symptoms of distress are masked. The treatment regimen may involve medical or surgical intervention, or both, aimed at treating the underlying pathology causing the pain. This may be: (1) resolution of a vascular inflammatory process by drug therapy, (2) resolution of a traumatic injury via vascular surgery, (3) resolution of a vascular stricture or aneurism via vascular surgery, or (4) control of diffuse peripheral occlusive disease via surgery, drug therapy, exercise, and so forth. The specific regimen of care varies but vascular surgery is being utilized as an effective means of controlling pain by removing or reducing the effect of the underlying disease process. Analgesics and an exercise program to improve peripheral perfusion help to reduce the discomfort in the postoperative period after vascular surgery (see Chapter 15).

Nursing Care Plan for Patient with Peripheral Vascular Pain

The following is a step-by-step care plan in brief form:

1. Initially evaluate the pain characteristics
2. Assess for any associated symptoms of impaired peripheral vascular perfusion
3. Relief of pain
   a. medicate
   b. place patient in a comfortable resting position conducive to optimum perfusion
4. Record on chart

a. pain symptoms presented
b. associated symptoms of status of peripheral perfusion
c. intervention for pain relief and effect
5. Report any pain that is different from past episodes, or that the usual modes of therapy do not relieve

In addition to care of the patient when pain is experienced, the nursing care plan should include aid in the prevention of pain by improving circulation. A few basic principles to be utilized during hospitalization and communicated to the patient in a home-care teaching program are:

1. Keep the affected part warm—warmth increases vasodilatation and thereby improves circulation.
2. Keep the affected part clean and avoid infection—with decreased circulation, healing is slow with a tendency toward infection.
3. An individually prescribed program of rest, exercise, and proper posture improves both arterial filling and venous return.
4. Avoid anything that constricts circulation—patients should not wear tight clothing, and elastic stockings should be fitted properly.
5. If necessary, a weight-reduction diet may be prescribed—overweight is an added burden to an already poor circulation.
6. Smoking is contraindicated because nicotine causes peripheral vasoconstriction.
7. Drugs such as vasodilators and anticoagulants may be prescribed to increase collateral blood flow and decrease the tendency of the blood to clot.

Summary

Pain in cardiovascular disorders is nature's signal of underlying disease that needs effective therapy to maintain optimal functional status of the patient. The nurse's role in assessment of the pain syndromes and the management of pain is an important one. Care is aimed not only toward providing relief of the pain, as with analgesics, but also toward prevention of pain associated with the underlying disease process. Whether pain is cardiac or vascular in origin, care is aimed at treating the total patient with an underlying disorder and not just at the presenting pain.

References

1. Alderman, E. L. Analgesics in the acute phase of myocardial infarction. *JAMA* 229(12):1646, 1974.
2. Altschule, M. D. Physiology of acute MI. *Med. Clin. North Am.* 58(2):399, 1974.
3. Applefield, M. M., and Ronon, J. A., Jr. Prinzmetal's angina with extensive spasm of the right coronary artery. *Chest* 66(6):721, 1974.

4. Ayulo, J. A. Hiatus hernia: A review. *Am. J. Gastroenterol.* 58(6):578, 1972.
5. Bentinoglio, L. G., Ablaza, S. G., and Greenberg, L. F. Bypass surgery for Prinzmetal's angina. *Arch. Intern. Med.* 134(2):313, 1974.
6. Bergan, J., and Yao, J. S. T. Modern management of abdominal aortic aneurisms. *Surg. Clin. North Am.* 54(1):175, 1974.
7. Betrui, A., Selegnac, A., and Boursassa, M. G. The variant form of angina: Diagnostic and therapeutic implications. *Am. Heart J.* 87(3):272, 1974.
8. Bomrah, V. S., Bahler, R., and Raketa, L. Hemodynamic response to supine exercise in patients with chest pain and normal coronary arteriograms. *Am. Heart J.* 87(2):147, 1974.
9. Burrell, L., and Burrell, Z. Chapter 11, Vascular surgery. In *Intensive Nursing Care*, 2d ed. St. Louis: C. V. Mosby Company, 1973. Pp. 98–102.
10. Carleton, R. Anginal subsets. *Chest* 66(6):609, 1974.
11. Clark, N. Pump failure. *Nurs. Clin. North Am.* 7:529, 1972.
12. Denzler, T., Fuller, E. W., and Eliot, R. Angina pectoris and myocardial infarction in the presence of patent coronary arteries—A review. *Heart and Lung* 3(4):646, 1974.
13. DeWolfe, V. G. Peripheral vascular disease. *Geriatrics* 28(9):57, 1973.
14. Elliot, W., and Gorlin, R. The coronary circulation, myocardial ischemia and angina pectoris. *Mod. Concepts Cardiovasc. Dis.* 10:114, 1966.
15. Epstein, S., et al. Angina pectoris: Patho-physiology, evaluation and treatment. *Ann. Intern. Med.* 75:263, 1971.
16. Epstein, S., et al. Effects of a reduction in environmental temperature on the circulatory response to exercise in man. *N. Engl. J. Med.* 280(1):7, 1969.
17. Frank, P. I. Some historical aspects of chest pain. *Practitioner* 211:96, 1973.
18. Frau, G., and Arose, G. Coronary disease and cervical arthrosis. *Cardiol. Prat.* 25(4):419, 1973.
19. Friedberg, C. K. *Disease of the Heart*, 3d ed. Philadelphia: W. B. Saunders Company, 1966.
20. Gettes, L. S. Painless myocardial ischemia. *Chest* 66(6):612, 1974.
21. Gey, G., et al. Exertional arrhythmias and nitroglycerine. *JAMA* 266(3):287, 1973.
22. Glick, S. Sufficient treatment for pain. *Ann. Intern. Med.* 78(6):974, 1973.
23. Goosch, W. H., et al. Surgical management of Prinzmetal's variant angina. *Chest* 66(6):614, 1974.
24. Guyton, A. C. *Textbook of Medical Physiology*, 4th ed. Philadelphia: W. B. Saunders Company, 1966. P. 577.
25. Horwitz, L. D. The diagnostic significance of anginal symptoms. *JAMA* 229(9):1196, 1974.
26. Hurst, J., and Logue, R. B. *The Heart, Arteries and Veins*, 2d ed. New York: McGraw-Hill Book Company, Inc., 1966. Pp. 142, 1468, 1490.
27. Kerr, F., and Donald, K. W. Analgesia in myocardial infarction. *Br. Heart J.* 36(2):117, 1974.
28. Kossowasky, W., et al. Further variant patterns within Prinzmetal's angina pectoris. *Chest* 66:622, 1974.
29. Lichstein, E., and Seckler, S. G. Evaluation of acute chest pain. *Med. Clin. North Am.* 57(6):1481, 1972.
30. Loop, F., et al. Cardiac aneurism often resectable. *Mod. Med.* 42(7), 1974.
31. MacAlpin, R. Prinzmetal's variant angina. *Circulation* 50(3):639, 1974.
32. MacAlpin, R. Who will benefit from coronary artery bypass surgery. *Chest* 66:610, 1974.
33. McMasters, R. A clinical approach to pain. *South. Med. J.* 67:173, 1974.

34. Mitchell, J., et al. Performance of the left ventricle. *Am. J. Med.* 53:481, 1972.
35. Nevens, M., and Lyon, L. Treatment of acute MI. *Med. Clin. North Am.* 58(2):435, 1974.
36. Oliva, P. B. Transient myocardial ischemia, normal coronary arteries and spasm in Prinzmetal's angina. *Adv. Cardiol.* 11:170, 1974.
37. Orchard, R. T., Yates, D. B., and Taylor, D. J. E. Acute precordial chest pain. *Practitioner* 213:212, 1974.
38. O'Rourke, R., and Ross, J. Ambulatory EKG monitor to detect ischemic heart disease. *Ann. Intern. Med.* 81(5):695, 1974.
39. Riseman, J. E. Diagnosis of angina pectoris at the present time. *Med. Clin. North Am.* 58(2):429, 1974.
40. Rosing, D., Reichek, N., and Perloff, J. The exercise test as a diagnostic and therapeutic aid. *Am. Heart J.* 87(5):584, 1974.
41. Scherf, D., and Cohen, J. Variant angina pectoris. *Circulation* 49:787, 1974.
42. Shealy, C. N. The pain patient. *Am. Fam. Physician* 9:130, 1974.
43. Silverman, M., and Flamm, M. D. Variant angina pectoris—Anatomic findings and prognostic implications. *Ann. Intern. Med.* 75(3):339, 1971.
44. Smith, R., and Pain, R. Chapter 8, Thoracic pain. In MacBryde, C. N., ed., *Signs and Symptoms.* Philadelphia: J. B. Lippincott Company. Pp. 154–178.
45. Smithen, C., et al. Variant angina pectoris. *Am. Heart J.* 89(1):87, 1975.
46. Troup, W. J. Establishing the diagnosis in patients with acute chest pain. *Can. Med. Assoc. J.* 108(9):1156, 1973.
47. Vinsant, M., Spence, M., and Capell, D. *A Commonsense Approach to Coronary Care: A Program.* St. Louis: C. V. Mosby Company, 1972. P. 73.
48. Weil, M., and Shubin, H. Shock following myocardial infarction. *Prog. Cardiovasc. Dis.* 11:1, 1968.
49. Williams, R., Wagner, G., and Peter, R. ST segment alterans in Prinzmetal's angina. *Ann. Intern. Med.* 81:51, 1974.
50. Yasue, H., et al. Role of autonomic nervous system in the pathogenesis of Prinzmetal's variant form of angina. *Circulation* 50(3):534, 1974.
51. Zohmon, L. *Exercise Your Way to Fitness and Heart Health* (Pamphlet). CPC International Inc., 1974.

20

Relief of Pain in Labor

Peggy-Anne Field

Although the physician is responsible for ordering the drugs a patient receives during labor, it is the nurse who observes the mother's progress
and who must decide whether the order is adequate. Therefore, the
nurse's judgment is vital; it should be based on a knowledge of the causes of
pain and on an understanding of the appropriate use of both psychological
measures and medications for the relief of pain.

Almost all women suffer some degree of pain in labor, varying from discomfort to an unbearable sensation. It is the nurse who normally assesses the
degree of pain experienced by the patient and who decides whether the patient is able to cope, or whether intervention is needed.

To intervene effectively, the nurse must understand the pathways of pain,
the psychological aspects, and the use and selection of drugs in labor. It is
to these dimensions that we now turn.

Pathways of Pain

It is probable that the pain of the first stage of labor is primarily due to the
dilatation of the cervix and the stretching of the lower uterine segment, and
that the contraction of the body of the uterus plays only a minor part in the
production of pain. The impulses generated by the stretching and contractions are transmitted to the hypogastric plexus and along the sympathetic
nerve fibers to the posterior roots of the eleventh and twelfth thoracic
nerves. Sensations may also be conveyed by the pelvic parasympathetic
nerves that enter the spinal cord at the second, third, and fourth sacral
segments.

Pain in the second stage of labor is mainly attributable to the distension of
the lower birth canal, the vulva, and the perineum. The sensations travel directly from the pudendal nerve along sensory pathways to the spinal cord.

In the third stage of labor, pain is due to the dilatation of the cervix by the
placenta and the contractions of the uterus. At this point, there is no pain in
the perineal region unless an episiotomy has been done.

Reprinted from *The Canadian Nurse*, December, 1974, by permission.

All methods of analgesia or anesthesia block the transmission of pain impulses at some point in the normal pathway. In addition, some distort the perception of pain. A basic knowledge of the mechanisms by which pain is transmitted is necessary to understand in what way psychological support or medications can alleviate the patient's pain.

Psychological Aspects of Pain

The fear-pain-tension syndrome was first described by Grantly Dick-Read in 1933. He believed that most women approach labor with fear and anxiety because of ignorance, prejudice, and misinformation. The result is mental tension which, in turn, leads to tension in muscles, including those of the lower uterine segment. Tension in these muscles can prevent normal cervical dilatation, can cause pain, and can delay labor.

Pain intensifiers during labor include fatigue (anemia with a hemoglobin below 70% from 33 to 34 weeks on), depression, disappointment, and fear. The amount of pain may also be modified by the individual's previous experiences, prenatal education, emotional stability, parity, fetal size and position, and the emotional support provided the woman by those attending her in labor.

Fear may provide a protective mechanism; however, if allowed to progress unchecked, fear-pain-tension may have a marked negative effect on labor.

Psychological Analgesia

Over the last 20 to 30 years, health personnel and patients alike have begun to realize the importance of psychological preparation for labor. Today, a variety of classes for psycho-physical preparation of the mother is available.

In these classes, the mother is helped to understand the process of pregnancy and labor in an effort to dispel fear. Operant conditioning is used in many types of preparation to increase the pain threshold, and an explanation is given on the methods of pain relief available during labor.

Relaxation and breathing exercises are taught, which help relieve muscular tension. Such tension could impede the descent of the fetus, delaying labor and prolonging the stretching of the lower segment and dilatation of the cervix, so increasing discomfort.

Today, the husband is being included more and more frequently, and his presence during labor is encouraged. He can provide psychological support and encouragement, helping to relieve the tension and loneliness produced by a new and strange environment.

Prenatal preparation has evolved mainly from two psychophysical methods, natural childbirth and psychoprophylaxis. Although the approaches differ, they have the same basic rationale: to reduce fear and tension, therefore reducing pain. Two other techniques that may be classified as psychological analgesia are hypnosis and abdominal decompression.

The positive attitude of the nurses, and the support given by them to mothers in the labor room who have been prepared by psychoprophylactic methods, are essential for success. Nursing care and support are still the key factors in reducing the need for analgesia in labor.

The nurse must make judgments if and when a prepared patient needs medication. Although no woman should be forced to have sedation, the nurse must be able to interpret to the patient the advantages of any analgesic when it is needed to help her progress in labor.

Use of Drugs in Labor

Although the length and severity of labors differ, most women need some form of analgesic during labor. Each labor should be evaluated individually, and decisions must be made on the use of systemic medications, regional or block analgesia or anesthesia, and inhalational analgesia or anesthesia.

There is no technique or agent that is always better than any other, and the best results are invariably obtained by using a combination of drugs and techniques. The prime consideration when choosing a drug for pain relief at any stage of labor must always be the safety of the mother and the fetus.

The "pain threshold" is the point at which an individual's senses recognize pain. The aim of the management of pain in labor is to raise the patient's pain threshold to a level where pain and discomfort are acceptable. This level of tolerance should be maintained in labor, bearing in mind that pain increases as labor progresses.

If pain is inadequately controlled, the patient will lose confidence in both the drug and the nurse. Her mental stress and anxiety level will rise, thus lowering her pain threshold. This means that a drug dosage that would have been adequate earlier may no longer be effective. *Giving too small a dose of a drug, or giving it too late, are the most common causes of unsatisfactory analgesia.*

At all times, the efficiency of drugs in raising the pain threshold must be weighed against the undesirable side effects they may produce in the mother and fetus or on the progress of labor. In the mother, preexisting conditions (such as heart disease or diabetes) or complications of pregnancy (such as bleeding or toxemia) may affect the drugs she can have or the fetal tolerance to drugs.

The fetus itself will be affected by drugs if labor is premature, if there is placental insufficiency, rhesus incompatibility, or any other condition that may already create a risk of fetal hypoxia. The nurse must always consider these factors when assessing the sedation she will give and when judging the most appropriate time for medications to be given.

Selection of Drugs

Early First Stage

Frequently, the patient arrives at the hospital early in the first stage of labor. The cervix may be thick and may be dilated only 1 cm. The patient's need at this time may be for rest to avoid fatigue before the onset of the active phase of labor. Sleep may be the major need in the middle of the day as well as during the night, and a sedative may be necessary to ensure this.

The tense, anxious patient may need a mild tranquilizer to help her relax. Some examples will help illustrate this:

Mrs. G. Gravida I, Para 0, is admitted at 7:00 a.m. Her membranes ruptured at 4:00 a.m. and she is having irregular contractions every 7 to 10 minutes. On examination, her cervix is thick and 1 cm. dilated. She appears relaxed but tired.

At this point, Seconal 100 mg. or Nembutal 200 mg. would be suitable, as her major need is for rest before labor becomes well established.

B.R., Gravida II, Para I, is admitted at 7:00 a.m. Her membranes are intact. On examination, her cervix is effaced, multips os. Contractions are moderate, every 5 to 7 minutes, and are not distressing her. She is breathing well but holds her hands tight and is somewhat anxious. She states, "I had a very rapid labor last time."

As B.R. has a history of rapid labor last time, sedation is not appropriate as her labor is likely to proceed rapidly again. She is assessed as being tense, although at this point she is managing with her breathing. Consideration should be given in one's assessment to the administration of Sparine 25–50 mg., or Largactil 25–50 mg., or a similar tranquilizer.

Middle First Stage

From a cervical dilatation of 4 cm. to 8 cm., the patient is considered to be in the active phase of labor. Contractions will be stronger and more frequent, cervical dilatation normally more rapid, and labor is established.

Tranquilizers should not be used alone in this stage of labor. If they are, the patient can become restless, confused, and uncooperative. However, the pain threshold can be raised and the dose of narcotic analgesic reduced by administering a tranquilizer *with* a narcotic analgesic.

D.R., Gravida I, Para 0, has been in labor for three hours. She has become very restless and seems to have difficulty coping with her contractions. On examination, the cervix is thin and 4 cm. dilated. Contractions are q. 4 mins. every 50 secs. The fetal heart is regular, 124.

Here, Demerol 100 mg. could be used, or a combination of Demerol 50–100 mg. and Sparine 25–50 mg. One must assess the patient's body size when determining the dose of a narcotic. What is sufficient to secure pain relief for a 95-pound patient will generally be inadequate for a 200-pound woman. ✓ Demerol takes approximately 20 minutes to be effective. For effective medication, one must estimate patient discomfort and administer the drug before distress and loss of control become evident.

P.D., Gravida III, Para II, is admitted in strong labor. Her contractions are q. 3 mins. × 45–60 secs. She is grasping the bed with each contraction and moaning. On examination, her cervix is 5 cm. dilated. The fetal heart is regular, 130.

Here we have a patient in advancing labor. She needs immediate sedation before any further examinations. Nisentil 30–60 mg. would be the drug of choice. It works rapidly and lasts 1½ to 2½ hours. Although it is more likely to cause fetal depression than Demerol if given in repeated doses, for this patient a single dose of analgesic would seem to be all that will be needed.

Last First Stage

If we return to the patient P.D., we find that an hour after receiving the Nisentil, she has feelings of rectal pressure. On examination, her cervix is found to be a rim. The fetal heart remains regular. P.D. has difficulty in restraining herself from pushing as the presenting part is low.

Inhalational analgesia, such as Entonox (premixed nitrous oxide, 50%, and oxygen, 50%), Trilene, or nitrous oxide and oxygen, may be given. All inhalational analgesics should be self-administered by the patient, using a hand-held apparatus. The patient's hand will drop before the level of anesthetic is reached and she will not become unconscious.

The nurse needs to make sure that the mother understands how to use the inhalational analgesic. Inhalation must start at the onset of the contraction if blood levels of nitrous oxide are to be maximal at the peak of a contraction. By keeping her hand on the fundus, the nurse can tell the mother when she should start using "the gas." At no time should the nurse hold the mask in place, and it must *never* be strapped on the patient's face. The concentration of nitrous oxide to oxygen should not exceed 60% : 40%.

As P.D. had Nisentil 60 mg. an hour previously, a narcotic antagonist, such as Nalorphine 5–10 mg., or Levallorphan 0.5–1 mg., should be considered to counteract any depressant effect the Nisentil may have had on the fetus.

Second Stage of Labor

In the second stage of labor, when the patient must push with her contractions, her perception of pain will frequently decrease, as she has another focus. The pain experienced now is mainly attributable to the distension of the lower birth canal and is transmitted by the pudendal nerve. At this time, an inhalational analgesic may be used during contractions.

If an episiotomy is to be performed, local infiltration of the perineum with 10 cc. of 1 or 2% Xylocaine may be carried out by the physician. If any operative procedure, such as mid or low forceps, is anticipated, a pudendal block is the most common form of anesthesia. This knocks out the pudendal nerves, relaxes the pelvic floor, and allows greater ease in manipulation of the fetus.

Some hospitals use general anesthetics for operative procedures, but in such cases the risk to both mother and fetus is increased.

R.S., Gravida II, para I, has been transferred to the delivery room. Her cervix is fully dilated and the anus is pouting, but the presenting part cannot be seen. She has not received analgesics during her rather rapid labor but is now saying, "Nurse, please give me something."

It is too late to give this patient narcotic analgesics. Entonox, or a similar inhalational analgesic, would be appropriate.

R.S. does not progress in the second stage. The doctor examines her and states that the fetal head is in a transverse position, and forceps will have to be used to rotate it.

Here, the probable anesthesia of choice would be a pudendal block, using 20 cc. of 1% Xylocaine or Carbocaine, depending on the physician's preferences.

B.D., Gravida I, Para 0, received Demerol 100 mg. 3 hours before her cervix reached full dilatation. In the case room she pushes well and the presenting part descends, but the perineum is tight and an episiotomy may be needed.

When the perineum is thinned out, it can be cut without pain and, therefore, analgesia may not be needed. Normally, however, a local anesthetic, such as 10 cc. of Xylocaine 1%, is injected fanwise into the tissue. The area is then anesthetized for suturing.

Alternative Forms of Analgesia

Paracervical Block

When a multigravida is pushing prematurely, or if the patient's cervix is rigid, the doctor may use a paracervical block. This is the infiltration of a local analgesic into the nerve plexus at the junction of the cervix and the vagina. It is not a popular method as the Xylocaine may be absorbed by the fetus and can cause bradycardia.

Epidural Anesthesia

This is the introduction of an anesthetic into the extradural space surrounding the spinal cord. It knocks out sensory impulses without inhibiting motor nerve activity. This is an excellent form of pain relief in any patient where labor is prolonged or is causing the individual excessive pain.

Because of the difficulty of the technique, it needs an expert to administer the anesthetic, and so can usually be given only in centers with resident anesthetists. Severe hypotension can occur with subsequent interference with the placental blood flow and the risk of fetal anoxia.

Spinal Anesthesia

This is usually indicated only for caesarian sections, as it interferes with the motor nerves, and the patient will need forceps delivery if spinal anesthesia is used. When operative delivery is necessary, it will not cause fetal depression and is, therefore, preferable to inhalational anesthesia.

Drug Idiosyncracies

Trilene is decreasing in favor as an inhalational analgesic, but is still used almost exclusively in some hospitals. If it is used within two hours of Demerol, fetal tachycardia may result. Trilene must *never* be used in an anesthetic apparatus where it may flow over soda lime, as it undergoes chemical changes that can harm the patient.

Nallorphine and Levallorphan should not be administered to a newborn when the mother has had a general anesthetic. They will cause further depression, even if the mother has had a narcotic drug in labor, if administered under these circumstances.

If an epidural anesthetic seems indicated by the patient's condition, it is inadvisable to administer a standing order for tranquilizers until the patient has been assessed by the obstetrician. Tranquilizers may cause hypotension, and this can be aggravated by epidural anesthesia and the anesthesia may have to be delayed.

The effect of diazepam (Valium) on the fetus is also under study. It is highly cumulative in cord blood and may cause cardiac and respiratory depression in the newborn.

Summary

By keeping the mother informed of her progress during labor and by encouraging her to take the medication ordered, the nurse can reduce the need for analgesics. Although it is the physician who orders the drugs a patient is to receive in labor, it is the nurse who observes the mother's progress and who must decide whether the order is adequate.

"Standing orders" may not always be appropriate, and the physician must be contacted and given evidence of the need for alternative medication. The nurse's judgment is vital; it is enhanced when based on a knowledge of the causes of pain and an understanding of the appropriate use of both psychological measures and medications for the relief of pain in labor.

434

References

1. Bonica. J. J. *Principles and Practices of Obstetric Analgesia and Anesthesia.* Philadelphia: F. A. Davis Company, 1964.
2. Bowes, W. A. *The Effects of Obstetrical Medication on Fetus and Infant.* Chicago: University of Chicago Press, for the Society for Research in Child Development, 1970.
3. Burnett, C. W. F. *The Anatomy and Physiology of Obstetrics: A Short Textbook for Students and Midwives.* London: Faber and Faber, 1953.
4. Dasser, C., and O'Connor, J. Continuous epidural block for obstetrical anesthesia. *Am. J. Nurs.* 60:1296, 1960.
5. McCaffery, M. *Nursing Management of the Patient With Pain.* Philadelphia: J. B. Lippincott Company, 1972.
6. Plantevin, O. M. *Analgesia and Anaesthesia in Obstetrics.* London: Butterworth, 1963.
7. Read, G. D. *Childbirth Without Fear,* 2d ed. New York: Harper's, 1953.
8. Riffel, H. D., et al. Effects of meperidine and promethazine during labor. *Obstet. Gynecol.* 42:738, 1973.
9. Thiery, M., and Vroman, S. Paracervical block analgesia during labor. *Am. J. Obstet. Gynecol.* 113:933, 1973.

21

Pain Associated with Orthopaedic Conditions

Kathleen C. Buckwalter and Joseph A. Buckwalter

The practice of orthopaedics includes the diagnosis and treatment of diseases, afflictions, and injuries of the musculoskeletal system. The musculoskeletal system consists of the bones and associated muscles, tendons, nerves, and vessels. The bones provide a supportive, protective framework for the body, store calcium and phosphorus, and contain marrow which manufactures red blood cells, white cells, and platelets. Evidence of orthopaedic problems remains from prehistoric times. Skeletons unearthed from caves and burial grounds throughout Europe, Asia, and Africa show evidence of the same types of bone pathology that plague mankind today. Ancient victims of orthopaedic disorders carried on until their lesions healed or until pain and disability made them unable to pursue food or incapable of defense [5].

Pain is an important clinical symptom and the chief presenting complaint of orthopaedic patients. Low back pain is perhaps the most common and baffling orthopaedic problem and its etiology, treatment, and psychological aspects will be discussed in this chapter. Pain is also commonly associated with traumatic injuries, infections of bone, and neoplasms. These conditions, their medical treatment, and nursing management will also be considered in this chapter. Joint pain associated with arthritis and other rheumatic disorders, and neurological conditions such as phantom-limb pain, are discussed in Chapters 14 and 16.

The basic goals of orthopaedic treatment are to restore function, to correct or prevent deformities, and to relieve pain. Pain frequently causes loss of function in patients with orthopaedic problems. The quality of their life deteriorates, and many patients suffer economic hardships because of inability to work.

Type and quality of pain often give valuable information as to the origin of pain, especially when it occurs before other clinical signs make their appearance. Pain can be differentiated by quality, duration, intensity, and distribution.

Careful analysis of the characteristics of a patient's complaint of pain may help identify tissue origin and significance. The nurse should consider the following seven dimensions of pain:

1. Bodily location—Where is the pain located? Is it localized, does it radiate?
2. Quality—What is the pain like?
3. Quantity—How intense is it?
4. Chronology—When did the pain begin and what course has it followed?
5. Setting—Under what circumstances does the pain take place?
6. Aggravating and alleviating factors—What makes the pain better or worse?
7. Associated manifestations—What other symptoms or phenomena are associated with the pain? [18].

The extent of physical impairment produced by the pain should be ascertained, as well as the character and the results of previous treatment.

Orthopaedic pain is variable, and should be analyzed in conjunction with the patient's psychological state and pain tolerance levels. Sharp pain may indicate bone injury with muscle spasm, or pressure on a nerve from a herniated intervertebral disk. A dull boring pain usually indicates a deep-seated lesion, usually of the bone, or increased tension of the soft tissues as in a growing tumor. Increase in intraosseous pressure is characterized by dull pounding pain with nocturnal exacerbations, as in Paget's disease, osteomyelitis, Brodie's abscess, or neoplasms of bone. A burning pain with paresthesia suggests a peripheral nerve irritation including sympathetic fibers. Causalgia and Sudeck's posttraumatic osteoporosis are examples of this. Increasing pain may indicate progression of an infectious process or malignant tumor. Pain that becomes worse during daytime activity may indicate joint strain, and radiating pain may be caused by the rupture of an intervertebral disk and pressure on a nerve root.

In many skeletal system disorders, periosteal pain is the presenting symptom; however, there is also pain indigenous to bone itself. The periosteum is highly sensitive to irritations of an inflammatory, circulatory, or toxic nature, as well as to pressure and tension.

Pain may also be differentiated by mode of production.

Pain Occurring Spontaneously

This may result from the direct irritation of spinal nerves and it is also observed in inflammatory conditions of soft tissue and bone, as well as in growing tumors.

Pain Produced by External Pressure

Pressure over injured bone or soft tissue, neoplasms, or infections may cause pain. Trigger points are circumscribed areas in which pressure produces a sudden, sharp pain. They are a valuable sign for locating the origin of the pain and identifying painful structures, especially in cutaneous and subcutaneous lesions.

Pain Produced by Motion

Pain produced by passive movement is a sign that either the joint or its surrounding structures, the capsule and ligaments (or muscles acting across the joint), are involved.

Pain Produced by Gravitational Strain

Pain produced by strained tissues is not isolated to specific structures. All structures engaged to provide body equilibrium—the articular and para-articular structures and musculature—are involved, and the result is pressure and tension stress.

Pain Produced by Immobilization

Immobilization is a powerful aid in the control of pain, but it can also produce pain. Stasis produced in the muscle by its reflex contracture is often responsible for a dull ache and a feeling of stiffness. It is relieved by heat, mobilization, and traction [24].

Nurses have a significant role in the prevention and relief of pain and should also be alert to the conditions causing pain that require further treatment. Nursing intervention is planned to relieve pain and to create a state of health. It is based on taking care of the total person, not just a disease or condition. The patient's reaction to pain is influenced by his past experiences, his tolerance, the duration of his pain, its cause, and the fear of its etiology. Pain interferes with thought, disturbs sleep, impairs appetite, deflates morale, and can also interfere with the function of many body parts.

Orthopaedic patients may experience increased anxiety levels because of the threat of their disorder, the presence of pain, and the fear of future painful episodes. Research has demonstrated that the discrepancy between expected and experienced physical sensations during a threatening experience will result in distress. Johnson et al [12] showed that a preparatory message that describes the sensations children experience during cast removal will result in reduced distress during the procedure.

Orthopaedic patients may experience feelings of deviance and stigmatization, depending upon the degree of visibility and permanence of their conditions. This can generate anxiety in face-to-face interactions with strangers. Nurses can help patients with orthopaedic injuries to realize that uncomfortable social situations may arise and that they may be labeled as deviant by some persons. Jones notes that "if we structure our interactions with the goal of relieving anxiety, any deviance can become almost irrelevant" [13]. The nurse caring for patients with orthopaedic problems must be cognizant of and interpret these variables of pain perception. Careful observations and assessment of the effectiveness of relief measures are an important part of nursing care. Prompt administration of analgesics, careful explanations of unavoidably painful procedures, and a gentle bedside manner communicate to the patient that the nurse cares about him and will not allow him to suffer unnecessarily.

Some specific conditions will be considered next. They are among the more common causes of pain in the musculoskeletal system.

Pain Associated with Traumatic Injuries

In traumatic injuries the pain is usually acute and directly related to the injury, although it may be exacerbated by a variety of associated conditions such as muscle spasm, reactive hyperemia, and edema. Traumatic injuries will be considered according to the type of tissue involved and include fractures, joint injuries, and injuries of the muscles and tendons.

Fractures

A fracture is a break in the continuity of the bone. Bones weakened by lesions such as tumors, osteomyelitis, and cysts may fracture more easily than normal. When this occurs it is called a pathological fracture. All fractures give rise to pain, although the intensity may vary considerably. With fractures, pain is immediate, intense, and is produced by the tear and stretching of the periosteum as the fragments become displaced. Fractures with little or no displacement are comparatively painless and may permit weight bearing until they become disimpacted. Function is lost due to pain and loss of support. The goal of fracture treatment is recovery of function of the injured part. This is accomplished by reduction of the fracture with acceptable restoration of rotation, alignment, and length of the bony fragments, followed by immobilization of the fracture to allow healing. Reduction is accomplished through manipulation, traction, or surgery; immobilization is attained through the use of traction, casts, and splints externally or nails and screws internally, or a combination of both; and restoration of function is achieved through muscle reeducation exercises. Faced with a patient complaining of increased pain after adequate reduction and immobilization of a fracture, the nurse should consider the following possible causes:

1. Compartment syndrome, with swelling and neurovasular impairment due to an associated arterial injury or venous congestion
2. Inadequate immobilization with movement at the fracture site
3. Tight cast syndrome, with pressure secondary to swelling in a rigid cast
4. Migration of traction pin with motion at insertion site
5. Venous thrombosis
6. Pressure sores under the cast
7. Infection of the pin tract
8. Infection of the fracture site

The nurse is in an excellent position to detect and evaluate early the causes of pain in the patient with fractures, and to take appropriate action once a determination has been made. See below, and Table 21-1, for the characteristic signs and symptoms of these sources of pain and appropriate relief measures.

In compartment syndrome (increased pressure within fascial compartment), the patient may complain of increased pain, especially with passive motion of the limb, numbness, weakness, and loss of sensation. There may be tenseness or firmness of the compartment involved. Progressive neurological deficit can be detected with the two-point discrimination test (the patient's ability to distinguish between two distinct points on the skin) and evaluation of blanching or capillary refill time. Blanching tests the blood supply to distal areas of the affected limb and is accomplished by sharply compressing the thumbnail or great toenail. Upon release of pressure, the capillaries should fill immediately. Compartment syndrome may develop in the presence of normal sensation, pulses, and capillary refill. If you suspect a compartment syndrome, the limb should be elevated until it can be evaluated by a doctor to determine if a fasciotomy is necessary.

With inadequate immobilization and movement at the fracture site, the patient may complain of pain with motion, or tell you he feels a "grating" sensation at the fracture site. The nurse who observes a loose-fitting cast or improper traction should see to it that the cast is changed or adjustments of the traction device are made.

The signs and symptoms of pressure secondary to swelling in a cast are similar to those found in compartment syndrome. Pain is the first and most constant complaint of the patient with a tight cast. Since all fractures are accompanied by some degree of pain and swelling, the nurse must check closely for other signs of circulatory impairment such as coldness, pallor, cyanosis, a change in distal pulses, and decreased motion of the fingers and toes. Even when peripheral circulation appears unimpaired, if severe discomfort persists, it may be best to split or bivalve the cast. Pain medication is essential to the comfort of the patient.

Ischemic muscle necrosis and contractures, called Volkmann's contracture ischemia, is one of the worst complications of a limb injury, and may result from compartment syndrome. Pain is perhaps the most important sign of this complication, and is characterized as deep, unremitting, and poorly localized. It is difficult to control with analgesics. In upper-extremity fractures, passive finger extension causes an exacerbation of the pain, and is an early physical finding.

With migration of the traction pin, the patient may complain of pain at the site of pin insertion, and the nurse may notice movement of the pin upon examination and tenting (stretching of the skin) at the pin site. She should immediately notify the physician, who can then remove and replace the pin. With venous thrombosis, the patient may complain of diffuse pain. The nurse should look for swelling of the limb, tenderness to palpation, engorged veins, and increased warmth of the affected limb. She should elevate the affected area and notify the physician, who may order a venogram or Doppler examination to determine if a thrombus does exist, in which case anticoagulant therapy may be initiated.

Pressure sores under the cast are characterized by sharply localized pain of a burning character at the pressure point. Relief of pressure, usually by windowing the cast over the sore, is indicated, and the nurse should initiate a routine of good skin care.

Infections of the fracture site and pin tract can be identified by gradually increasing dull pain, tenderness, fever, erythema, increased purulent drainage, and possibly a foul smell. The wound should be cultured, and appropriate antibiotic therapy begun. The nurse should notify the doctor who may remove, and if possible replace, the pin with another immobilization device.

Special consideration must be given to the nursing care of the patient in skeletal traction. Although only the affected limb is immobilized, the patient is usually not permitted to turn, and that may cause considerable discomfort in the back and shoulder regions. Support for the low back region and frequent alcohol rubs of these areas will help eliminate discomfort, and provide the nurse with an opportunity to inspect bony prominences for pressure points.

There is an extended healing period associated with many fractures. The nurse should therefore anticipate psychosocial and economic problems associated with prolonged hospitalization, disability, and possible fear of deformity and immobilization.

Studies have shown that perceptual and motor changes can be caused by immobilization. The amount and type of sensory information available to the patient are reduced, as is his ability to interact with his environment. Immobilization plays a part in numerous physical complications and also affects the patients' attitudes and confidence in their role as functioning human beings. A patient's inability to control his environment may produce psychological reactions such as apathy, frustration, anger, and a sense of worthlessness. His own emotions may become exaggerated as his sense of helplessness and uselessness increases.

The immobilized patient may be separated from his family and from familiar stimuli. He may also be experiencing disturbances in body image, alterations in social and economic status, and a fear of the unknown in his new immobilized role. Anxiety is a major cause of restlessness and the nurse should continually communicate with the immobilized patient to provide reassurance and to help him understand and adjust to his situation.

Nurses should be as empathetic and as gentle in their care as possible. This is particularly true for the elderly patient who has suffered a fractured hip. The pain and the shock of the injury itself may produce confusion, and the prospect of prolonged inactivity and doubtful recovery often creates significant depression in these patients. Clocks, calendars, and other reality reminders may be useful in maintaining orientation.

The nurse is part of the rehabilitation team, and as such should promote

Table 21-1 Causes, symptoms, and relief measures of pain after reduction and immobilization of fractures

Cause	Symptoms	Action
A. Compartment syndrome	1. Increased pain with passive motion of fingers and toes 2. Numbness, loss of sensation 3. Firmness, tenseness of compartment 4. Progressive neurological deficit	1. 2-point discrimination test 2. Capillary refill time test 3. Elevate limb 4. Notify physician to determine need for fasciotomy
B. Inadequate immobilization	1. Patient complains of grating sensation, pain with motion 2. Cast appears loose fitting, traction improper	1. Advise doctor a change in immobilization device is necessary
C. Tight cast syndrome	1. Pain 2. Signs of circulatory impairment (coldness, pallor, cyanosis, a change in distal pulses, and decreased range of motion in fingers and toes)	*1. Split or bivalve cast
D. Migration of traction pin	1. Patient complains of pain at site of pin insertion 2. Tenting (stretching of skin at pin site)	1. Notify physician who will remove and replace pin
E. Venous thrombosis	1. Diffuse pain 2. Swelling of limb 3. Tenderness to palpation 4. Engorged veins 5. Increased warmth of affected limb	1. Elevate affected area and notify physician who may order venogram or Doppler exam
F. Pressure sores under the cast	1. Sharply localized pain of a burning character at pressure point	*1. Relieve pressure—window cast over sore 2. Good skin care routine
G. Infection of pin tract and fracture site	1. Gradually increasing dull pain 2. Tenderness 3. Fever 4. Erythema 5. Increased purulent drainage 6. Foul smell	*1. Culture wound 2. Notify physician, so appropriate antibiotic therapy can be initiated, and if possible, pin replaced 3. Care of wound after surgical debridement

* Denotes tasks within the realm of nursing care, although commonly performed by other personnel, such as technicians.

Source: Reprinted by permission from *Clinical Symposia,* by H. A. Klein, illustrated by F. H. Netter. © Copyright 1973 CIBA-GEIGY Corporation.

active and passive exercises, and encourage the isolated, immobilized orthopaedic patient to be as active and involved with bedside projects as possible.

Patients of a similar age group who may share the same interests should be moved together. Nurses need to plan for diversified activity, and not rely on television alone. Diversions such as music, crafts, and reading may help take the patient's mind off his pain. By keeping the patient active, the nurse will also minimize boredom and dependency, and aid recovery.

Rapid rehabilitation is as important as good medical care in preventing pain and limitation, and nurses should help patients become involved with their own care and progress as early as possible.

Joint Injuries—Sprains and Strains

Whether the cause of the disorder of the joint is mechanical, inflammatory, or otherwise, the pain response comes almost exclusively from the synovial membrane, the fibrous capsule, and its ligaments. Pain arises from the stimulation from the sensory nerve endings in these structures, and is conducted by somatic sensory nerves.

Every joint is protected by ligaments. The fibrous capsule and the articular ligaments are richly supplied with sensory fibers. The pain responses of injured ligaments are always sharp and strictly localized. The origin and insertion of the ligaments are often the points of greatest tenderness.

A sprain is a tear in the ligaments and capsule fibers. Sprains are clinically classified according to the number of fibers torn, and range from the separation of only a few fibers to complete disruption of the ligament. Common examples of this type of injury are ankle sprains and cervical strains.

The occupant of an automobile struck from the rear often sustains a cervical strain. Some patients have immediate neck pain, although others have none for up to 36 hours. Patients complain of diffuse pain over the posterior surface of the neck and head. Protective muscle contraction decreases neck motion in an attempt to prevent pain. At times the patient may develop sore muscles, stiff neck, severe pain, vertigo, nausea, headache, and paresthesias. Symptoms may be intermittent or may persist for months, but eventually subside in most cases. Analgesics, heat, rest, and mild head-halter traction often relieve most acute symptoms.

Sprained ankles are often caused when the foot is forcibly inverted. The lateral ligament of the ankle is a dense, fibrous structure that becomes taut and stops further inversion of the foot. If the force is greater than the strength of the ligament, the ligament will tear, resulting in a sprained ankle. Treatment of most sprains includes support and protection of the ligament until healing. The area may be elevated and cooled to reduce swelling.

Dislocation

A dislocation is complete disruption of a joint so that the articular surfaces are no longer in contact. Dislocations damage joint capsules and ligaments. During a dislocation, articular surfaces of opposing bones are completely separated. Dislocations are associated with pain that may be severe and persist until the joint is relocated. Usually, an anesthetic is required to relax muscles that hold bones in a dislocated position while they are in spasm. Traction will reduce most dislocations; however, surgical intervention is occasionally necessary. Following reduction, the affected part is immobilized so that ligaments can heal properly.

Intra-articular Injuries

Joint trauma may produce intra-articular injuries as well as extra-articular injuries. The joint surfaces themselves may be fractured or the cartilage disrupted from an injury. In joints like the knee, with an intra-articular cartilaginous body such as the meniscus, this intra-articular cartilage may be torn or injured. Likewise, intra-articular ligaments, such as the cruciate ligaments in the knee, may be torn or ruptured, and joints may also be injured by a direct or indirect blow that contuses the synovium producing a painful knee effusion.

Injuries of Muscles and Tendons

Myalgias can be produced by traumatic, inflammatory, metabolic, or circulatory disturbances. None of these stimulants involves only the muscle to the exclusion of other tissues. The pain syndrome is thus a composite of responses of all tissues affected. Myalgic pain is often an early and premonitory sign of a generalized disease.

Muscles and tendons may also be injured by severe stress from muscle contraction as well as direct contusion or laceration. Under severe stress muscles and tendons may rupture, tearing the tendons from the bone, or rupturing the tendon or muscle itself. These injuries can be exceedingly painful, and are usually accompanied by swelling and ecchymosis as well as refusal of the patient to contract the involved muscle-tendon unit. Pain is most intense when the rupture occurs at the tendon of origin or insertion, less at the musculotendinous junction, and least in tears of the muscle belly itself. The initial treatment of these injuries includes immobilization, elevation, and analgesia. Severe injuries to critical muscle-tendon units may require surgical repair. Direct blows to muscles may produce hemorrhage into the muscle and tendon sheaths resulting in severe pain and swelling. This injury likewise will decrease the patient's ability to use the muscle-tendon unit.

Protective muscle spasm in response to a painful sensory stimulus is a common occurrence in orthopaedic conditions, and it is assumed that the reason for this spasm is suppression of pain. Although these injuries may seem minor, they may produce residual scarring within the muscle, and should be treated at least initially with elevation and possibly application of cold. Muscles and tendons may likewise be lacerated and these injuries at a minimum require thorough cleansing; in certain cases, surgical repair may be required.

Posttraumatic Osteoporosis

Posttraumatic osteoporosis, or Sudeck's atrophy, is a pathological condition following strain, sprain, or fracture. The final stage of this condition is characterized by atrophy, edema, fibrosis, and contractures, and is irreversible. Cardinal symptoms are pain and swelling. The pain is a posttraumatic reflex syndrome mediated from the peripheral somatic nerves to the vasomotor nervous system. The objective of treatment in Sudeck's osteoporosis is restoration of the autonomic equilibrium.

Active exercise to increase the stagnant blood flow must be handled with extreme gentleness and care. When these measures fail, blocks of the sympathetic nervous system by regional anesthesia or surgery may be indicated.

Pain Associated with Infection in the Musculoskeletal System

The pain associated with infections often develops insidiously, although in the case of arthritis or osteomylitis, it may develop quite suddenly. Infections may involve the bones, the soft tissues, or joints, and can cause extensive destruction as well as extend to other tissues and the blood stream resulting in severe systemic illness and possibly death. Infectious diseases are caused by various types of agents: protozoa, fungi, bacteria, rickettsia, and viruses. The clinical manifestations and pathological changes of infections of the bone differ according to alterations in cell metabolisms, resulting in a reaction between the multiplying organism and the defense mechanisms of the host.

Acute musculoskeletal infections require immediate medical care with attempts to identify the responsible organism and initiate appropriate antibiotic therapy. Elevation and immobilization of the involved limb may well decrease swelling, and partially relieve discomfort. Surgical care may be required to drain collections of purulent material. Surgery may also be required to relieve severe swelling in a limb that may eventually compromise neurovascular function.

The nurse caring for a patient with an infection of the neuromusculoskeletal system deals with an individual, his infectious condition, his fear, and his interpretation of the illness. In addition to experiencing the symptoms of pain, high fever, and malaise, he may be apprehensive and anxious about involvement of body parts, residual handicap, or death.

Osteomyelitis

Osteomyelitis is infection of bone. It is an inflammatory process that may produce necrosis of the bone. In most acute infections the onset is abrupt and is accompanied by pain, redness and swelling, and tenderness over the affected bone. Fever, rapid respirations and pulse, chills, toxemia, malaise, headache, and dry hot skin are other symptoms. Treatment with antibacterial agents may modify the course of the infection. Prognosis depends on early and adequate treatment and the following are important factors to note in caring for the patient with osteomyelitis:

1. Maintenance of fluid balance and good nutritional status
2. Adequate antibiotic therapy to combat infection
3. Complete rest of the involved area, possibly splinting
4. Draining of any abscesses that may form
5. Need for good position, rest, and support, and understanding of the patient's reaction to his condition and its implications [29]

Pain Associated with Neoplastic Conditions

A neoplasm is an abnormal proliferation of cells that may be benign or malignant. Bone neoplasms may develop in bone or metastasize to bone from other sites.

Pain phenomena depend first on the site of the tumor and its relation to sensitive structures such as periosteum, capsular tissue, and ligaments, and second on rate of growth. There are two probable sources of bone pain in tumors: intramedullary passive hyperemia with edema (venous congestion), and mechanical stress on the periosteum (stretch of periosteum from expansion of tumor).

The musculoskeletal pain in patients with neoplasms usually has an insidious onset and becomes progressively severe. In the case of extensive malignant neoplastic disease, the pain may be incapacitating for the patient. Obviously, neoplasms and neoplasticlike diseases of the musculoskeletal system require systematic medical and surgical treatment. Radiation therapy is often temporarily helpful, although amputation is usually necessary. The prognosis for patients with malignant tumors is poor. However, the nurse can be of great help to patients with these problems in providing adequate analgesia and supportive care both physically and psychologically. The patient may look deceptively well upon admission, but as the malignancy progresses and his condition deteriorates, he and his family will need help in understanding and adjusting to necessary surgical procedures and facing the likelihood of death. In patients with neoplastic diseases of the bones, it is also important to be alert to the possibility of acute increase in pain secondary to pathological fracture.

Miscellaneous Orthopaedic Conditions

There are a wide variety of painful problems of the musculoskeletal system that do not easily fit into the previously mentioned categories. Important examples of these include aseptic necrosis of bone, slipped epiphysis, and Paget's disease. Aseptic necrosis may develop idiopathically, or may be secondary to a systemic disorder such as sickle cell anemia, or it may follow trauma in the area of the epiphysis. In this condition, the epiphyseal cells undergo degeneration and necrosis probably secondary to severe ischemia. The necrosis itself is painless and remains so until the sensitive synovial tissue becomes involved; then the condition can be quite painful. Initial care should involve protection of the involved epiphysis from stress.

Another cause of orthopaedic pain is slipping of the capital femoral epiphysis in children, usually between the ages of eight and sixteen. The cause of this problem is uncertain but it involves migration of the femoral epiphysis from its usual location on the femoral neck. It can prove extremely painful, and requires immediate orthopaedic attention, so that appropriate therapy can be instituted to prevent further slipping and severe residual joint disease.

This condition usually occurs during a period of physical, social, and emotional development. Unfortunately, weight-bearing activities must be limited and the nurse should be concerned with ways to help avoid psychological and physical developmental trauma.

Paget's disease (osteitis deformans) is a chronic, progressive disturbance of bone metabolism that increases in frequency with increasing age. Although it may be asymptomatic, the disease is usually manifested by persistent pain in the affected bone, swelling, and muscle spasms. The pain is most often dull and boring, but can become sharp and radiating as in inflammatory conditions. It is commonly accompanied by headache from involvement of the cranium. There is no definite medical cure for Paget's disease, and in some cases prolonged use of analgesics has been required. Although the prognosis for life is good, deformities may lead to invalidism. Rehabilitation measures to overcome deficits in function can increase both functional ability and independence for patients suffering from Paget's disease.

Low Back Pain

Low back discomfort is one of the most common afflictions seen by the physician and nurse, and one of the most difficult to understand and treat. It affects people of all ages, races, and socioeconomic classes, and both sexes. Patients with complaints of low back pain comprise an estimated 70 percent of the referrals to pain clinics [24] and many of these patients have undergone surgery that failed to relieve their symptoms. Because low back pain affects primarily adults in their most productive years, it causes considerable loss of working days as well as an increasing volume of disability payments to patients.

This section will consider the following aspects of this important orthopaedic problem: the basic anatomy of the back, common causes of low back pain, the psychological components of low back pain, and treatment and nursing care of the patient with back pain.

Anatomy of a Backache

The spinal column is a chain of 33 vertebrae held together by ligaments and interposed cartilages. Low back pain usually stems from conditions affecting the lumbar vertebrae and the sacrum. The nerves, periosteum, periosteal tendon insertions, spinal ligaments, articulations, and muscles of the low back are all endowed with sensory fibers and cause pain in response to mechanical or inflammatory irritation. Certain portions of these tissues, where recurrent nerves return through the foramen and innervate the posterior longitudinal ligament, are the most pain-sensitive. Nerve roots transmit pain when these tissues are irritated. (See Fig. 21-1.)

Causes of Low Back Pain

There are a wide variety of causes of back pain: congenital disorders, neoplastic conditions, traumatic injuries, inflammatory diseases, circulatory dis-

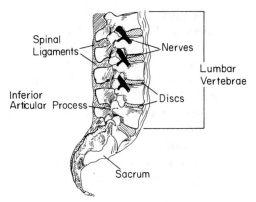

Figure 21-1   The lumbosacral spine. (Steve Hall.)

orders, degenerative diseases, metabolic disorders, infections of the spine, extrinsic and intrinsic mechanical causes, and psychogenic problems.

The nurse should be aware that the patient who complains of low back pain may be suffering from a lesion in another organ such as a kidney infection, aortic aneurism, bowel obstruction, or uterine fibroids.

She should also consider that elderly persons are especially vulnerable to back problems. With aging, the intervertebral disks dehydrate, diminishing flexibility, and the apophyseal joints may develop degenerative changes.

Narrowing of the spinal canal may cause vascular impairment of the cord, resulting in a condition known as *pseudoclaudication*. Symptoms are pain and paresthesia in the lower extremities after prolonged standing and walking. Cessation of activity and a change of posture are necessary to relieve symptoms. Postmenopausal women are especially prone to osteoporosis (a decrease in bone mass per unit volume of bone) and compression fractures can occur with relatively minor trauma, such as coughing. Metastatic disease is also more prevalent in the aged, and should be suspected when chronic low back pain persists despite treatment [8].

Trauma and strain are among the most frequent causes of back pain, and the lumbar spine is particularly vulnerable to mechanical stress. Back strain is especially common among people who are obese, or who have weak abdominal and back muscles.

Lumbar strain can be classified as acute or chronic. Acute backache is often due to a herniated intervertebral disk, and may be associated with pain radiating from the back to the lower extremities. If sacral roots are affected by the herniation, bowel or bladder incontinence may result. This is a serious development and requires immediate medical attention. If low back pain presumed to be caused by lumbar strain is not relieved by complete bed rest, one may suspect a neoplasm, spinal infection, or psychogenic cause. In patients with low back pain of long duration, many factors must be considered.

Psychological Aspects of Low Back Pain

Among the most important factors for the nurse caring for chronic back-pain patients is the psychological component of this disorder. Two psycho-neurotic problems commonly associated with low back pain are hysteria and malingering. Hysteria, though rare, may produce back pain of subconscious origin. It arises when an individual's psychological defense mechanisms are inadequate to control tension and anxiety. Although the hysteric actually suffers from pain, it is seldom caused by spinal pathology. The focus of treatment is therefore on alleviation of the patient's anxiety [13].

The malingerer, on the other hand, does not experience discomfort, but may feign symptoms of low back pain for secondary gain, often in an attempt to collect compensation following a work-related or automobile accident.

Many clinicians consider chronic low back pain to be a psychophysiological disorder. Research evidence supports the association of back pain with depression, neuroticism, a life-style of invalidism, and manipulative doctor-patient relationships [24, 29]. Sternbach refers to these patients as "low back pain losers" [25].

As part of her assessment, the nurse should endeavor to determine the importance of psychological and social factors to the back-pain patient. She should note changes in the patient's mood and should ask, in an accepting manner, about the effect of pain on his emotional state. Somatic symptoms of depression, such as disturbances in sleep and appetite, should also be noted. The nurse can become better aware of the social effects of back pain by inquiring if the patient's disorder has created problems with his family or at work, and by providing the patient with an opportunity to discuss these difficulties.

Weiner has elucidated problems of ambiguity that may arise in the treatment of low back pain when patient and staff assessment of the degree of pain differs, and the patient fails to legitimate his pain. She notes "the importance for pain work lies in the relationship between the way the staff reads the signs and the resultant assessment and relief, and in the fact that any tension produced by conflicting perspectives further tightens muscles and increases pain" [28]. The ambiguity surrounding low back pain has to do with its uncertain etiology, visibility, relief procedures, and unpredictable duration. Nurses must attend not only to the management of the pain but also to their own personal reactions to the patient's pain.

Nursing Care

The treatment and nursing care of the patient with low back pain generally consists in:

1. Local applications of radiant heat, hot tubs, or moist packs to remove muscle spasm. Paradoxically, ice wrapped in a towel or cooling aerosol sprays may also provide comfort.

2. Use of a hard bed with pillows placed to fit and support the contour of spine and legs, avoiding bony prominences.
3. Medications, including relaxants, salicylates, narcotics, and sedatives, to relieve pain and muscle spasm. To minimize the problems that often arise in analgesic therapy for chronic pain, the nurse should work to establish a good relationship with the patient. His confidence in the staff's desire to help him and willingness to comply with instructions will enhance treatment and lower chances for drug abuse.
4. After resolution of acute pain, extension exercises, diaphragmatic breathing, lifting head and shoulders from the bed, and flattening the lumbar spine by active contraction of the abdominal and gluteal muscles. The nurse should be familiar with these basic exercises and teach them to the patient [13, pp. 29 and 185].
5. Teaching correct posture and proper body mechanics, especially when lifting heavy objects [14, pp. 23 to 32].
6. If increased gravitational stress on the spinal column is due to obesity, the nurse, together with a dietitian, can initiate a program of weight reduction, and encourage a sensible, regular exercise program compatible with age and physique.
7. Immobilization by a corset or brace to maintain good alignment of the trunk and support the contour of the back when the patient is getting back on his feet. The corset should be long enough to control the gluteal muscles in back and support the abdomen in front, avoiding pressure on the pubic bone or the iliac crest.
8. As noted in the previous section, the emotional tone of the patient may be as important as his muscle tone, and consideration of emotional factors, especially depression, is an important part of evaluation and treatment. Psychiatric consultation may be necessary. Staff members need to be able to discuss their feelings about low-back-pain patients openly. This leads to better understanding of patients' needs as well as their own emotional responses to a difficult patient group.
9. Patients who engage in heavy labor may be unable to return to work. The nurse can consult with the social worker and vocational rehabilitation specialist regarding the availability of retraining programs. With this knowledge she may realistically support the discouraged patient.
10. With patients who fail to respond to these conservative treatment measures, or who have repeated attacks of sciatica, the physician may order a myelogram, a procedure where contrast media is injected into the dural sac surrounding the spinal cord in an attempt to demonstrate protruding intervertebral disk or other direct mechanical causes of pain. If a lesion is evident, surgical repair, such as lumbar disk excision, may be necessary. If there is clinical evidence that pain is due to spinal instability, then a surgical fusion to make the spine stiff may be indicated.

Low back pain is one of the most common and unpredictable orthopedic conditions. There are a wide variety of infectious, neoplastic, metabolic, and traumatic causes of back pain; however, many patients who present with low-back discomfort suffer from psychological problems as well. Nursing care of the back-pain patient consists in providing rest, relief measures such as heat and analgesics, and education concerning exercises and proper body mechanics.

Summary

Pain in the musculoskeletal system is one of the most common presenting complaints of patients seen in health-care centers. Being alert to the possible causes of these discomforts and the initial appropriate care, as well as to the nursing measures that help patients to deal with the discomfort and attendant psychosocial problems, is a critical part of nursing care for the orthopaedic patient. While the literature contains good general references to the care of patients with orthopaedic problems, much thought and research need to be devoted to the identification of more specific ways whereby nurses can alleviate discomfort and maintain emotional stability in this population.

References

1. Aegerter, E., and Kirkpatrick, J. A. *Orthopedic Diseases,* 4th ed. Philadelphia: W. B. Saunders Company, 1975.
2. American Orthopaedic Association. *Manual of Orthopaedic Surgery.* 1972.
3. Barrett, J., and Golding, D. N. The management of low back pain and sciatica. *Practitioner* 208 (243):118, 1972.
4. Bawher, J. H., and Ledbetter, C. A. Low back pain. *Am. Fam. Physician,* October, 1974.
5. Bick, E. M. *Source Book of Orthopaedics.* New York: Hafner Publishing Co., 1968.
6. Brown, S. Easing the burden of traction and casts. *R. N.* 38:36, 1975.
7. Cailliet, R. Evaluation and management of lumbar discogenic disease. *Md. State Med. J.* 51–52, May, 1974.
8. Cailliet, R. Lumbar discogenic disease: Why the elderly are more vulnerable. *Geriatrics,* 73–76, January, 1975.
9. Dahlin, D. C. *Bone Tumors,* 2d ed. Springfield, Ill.: Charles C Thomas, 1967.
10. Effects on psychosocial equilibrium. *Am. J. Nurs.* 75:794, 1967.
11. Golding, D. N. Acute backache. *Nurs. Times,* February, 1974, pp. 184–5.
12. Johnson, J., Kirchhoff, K., and Endress, P. Altering children's stress behavior during orthopedic cast removal. *Nurs. Res.* 24(6):404, November–December, 1975.
13. Jones, S. L. Orthopedic injuries: Illness as deviance. *Am. J. Nurs.* 75(11):2030–2033, November, 1975.
14. Klein, H. A. *Low Back Pain.* CIBA Clinical Symposia, 25(3), 1973.
15. Larson, C. B., and Gould, M. *Orthopedic Nursing,* 8th ed. St. Louis: C. V. Mosby Company, 1974.
16. Levine, M. E. Depression, back pain, and disc protrusion. *Dis. Nerv. Syst.,* January, 1971. Pp. 41–45.

17. Liechty, R. D., and Soper, R. T. *Synopsis of Surgery.* St. Louis: C. V. Mosby Company, 1972.
18. Morgan, W. L., and Engel, G. L. *The Clinical Approach to the Patient.* Philadelphia: W. B. Saunders Company, 1969.
19. Morris, R. Planning the care of the orthopedic patient. *Nurs. Care* 8:18, 1975.
20. The challenge of relieving chronic pain. *Nurs. Update* 3(11):2–8, 1972.
21. Raney, R. B., and Brasheur, H. R. *Shand's Handbook of Orthopaedic Surgery,* 8th ed. St. Louis: C. V. Mosby Company, 1971.
22. Rockwood, C. A., and Green, D. P. *Fractures* (Vol. 1). Philadelphia: J. B. Lippincott Company, 1975.
23. Schultz, R. J. *The Language of Fractures.* Baltimore: The Williams & Wilkins Company, 1972.
24. Steindler, A. *Lectures on the Interpretation of Pain in Orthopedic Practice.* Springfield, Ill.: Charles C Thomas, 1959.
25. Sternbach, R. A., Wolf, S., Murphy, R. W., and Akeson, W. H. Aspects of chronic low back pain. *Psychosomatics* 14:52, 1973.
26. Sternbach, R. A., Wolf, S., Murphy, R. W., and Akeson, W. H. Traits of pain patients: The low-back "loser." *Psychosomatics* 14:226, July–August, 1973.
27. Twedt, B. Control of pain in orthopedic patients. *R. N.* 38:39, 1975.
28. Weiner, C. L. Pain assessment on an orthopedic ward. *Nurs. Outlook* 23:508, 1975.
29. Wiebe, A. M. *Orthopedics in Nursing.* Philadelphia: W. B. Saunders Company, 1961.
30. Wolkind, S. N. Psychiatric aspects of low back pain. *Physiotherapy* 60(3): 75, 1974.
31. Young, Sr. C. Exercise: How to use it to decrease complications in immobilized patients. *Nursing 75* 5:81, 1975.

22

The Experience of Pain in Children

Joann M. Eland and Jane E. Anderson

The impact of disease, hospitalization, and traumatic medical procedures on children has been the object of study for years by people responsible for their care. There are many sensitive descriptions in the literature of the hospitalization experience and the effects of long-term illness and short-term trauma on children, and interest in these experiences has generated much important research. We wish to focus our attention on one particular aspect of illness in children—the experience of pain.

The literature in pediatric nursing and medicine is notable for its lack of specific information on the experience of pain in children. In standard pediatric texts, such as Nelson [17] and Barnett [2], pain is mentioned in few places, and then only with regard to the diagnosis of a particular disease. One might expect more information on the assessment of or intervention for pain in nursing textbooks, but pediatric nursing texts by Marlow [14] and Blake, Wright, and Waechter [3] have little more to offer than do medical texts. The few sentences included deal only with pain associated with specific disease conditions and not with the assessment of the intensity of pain, how children react to pain, or how they communicate about pain with others.

Nursing books on emotional care of hospitalized children by Petrillo and Sanger [19], Plank [20], and Haller [9] give excellent ideas on general management, but they give no suggestions about the assessment of, communication about, or management of pain. McCaffery [15], an experienced pediatric nurse, has offered a number of suggestions for assessing and responding to children's pain. She acknowledges that her ideas are merely suggestions, and she laments the lack of systematic research on the subject.

A thorough search of medical literature from January, 1970, to August, 1975, produced 1,380 articles on pain; only 33 dealt with pediatric pain. Of the 33 articles, 19 were on recurrent abdominal pain, eight on children's headaches, and six on miscellaneous topics. Thirty-two of the 33 articles were medical in orientation and dealt with differential diagnosis or specific

453

diagnostic examinations to be done; they contained little or no data on children's pain behaviors, their assessment, or methods of intervention other than from a strict medical model.

In the only nursing article dealing with pain in children, Schultz [22] reported the findings of a nursing study conducted on a population of 74 ten- and eleven-year-old physically well school children. One of the instructions Schultz gave was, "Underline no more than *two* of the following: When I have pain I feel afraid, brave, nervous, like crying but I don't, like crying and I do." Twenty-one of 38 boys interviewed answered *brave*, a finding that Schultz thought reflected the cultural expectation of males being strong, assertive, and courageous. Only eight out of 74 said that when they wanted to cry, they did. All of the 36 girls admitted to being *afraid* or *nervous* and only four responded as *brave*.

Schultz also reported that fear increases pain. In answer to the question, "What does pain mean to you?" fear of bodily harm and death were prominent in children's responses. For example, children said,

"It hurts. It hurts inside."
"I feel like screaming."
"The doctor."
"I think I'm going to die."
"Getting shots. Getting injections."
"It hurts so much it kills ya'."
"Like a hammer beating into me."

The children were given the words, "Pain is . . . ," and asked to complete the sentence. Their responses also illustrate the fear component in children's pain.

"Being nervous."
"Not growing up healthy."
"Being afraid."
"When you scream for help and nobody comes."
"When something hurts and you can't get help."

Anxiety was also evident in some of the responses.

"Something you have no control of."
"You think it will never end."
"Something that hurts and you can't stop it."
"When you get nervous, you sweat, and feel tense; moaning. . . ."

Schultz's findings are meaningful for the ten- and eleven-year-old well child, but what about the young child, the seriously ill child, or the child who cannot verbally express himself so well?

Schultz's study currently stands alone as the one contribution from nurs-

Table 22-1   Ages and diagnoses of children receiving no pain medication
(N = 13)

Age	Diagnosis
4	Traumatic amputation of right foot, extensive nerve damage to left leg from mower accident
	Eye irrigation and aspiration from steel splinters
	Palatoplasty, bilateral myringotomy and tube placement
5	Palatoplasty
	Myringoplasty
	Cataract
	Excision of a malignant neck mass
6	Meatotomy, urethral dilation for hypospadias
	Cystoplasty for intersex abnormalities
	Squint
	Heminephrectomy for hydronephrosis
7	Atrial septal defect repair
	Skull fracture, fractured femur with insertion of Steinman pin

ing research to the literature dealing with pain in children. The subjects for her study were well children who were not under the stress of physical illness and thus not employing the predictable defensive maneuvers children use to cope with illness and pain. Schultz has presented us with a starting point for research into the pain experience of children, research which nurses are uniquely qualified to conduct.

Does this lack of literature and meaningful research reflect a denial of our effectiveness in dealing with children's pain, the frustration of trying to assess and intervene in painful situations, or a superficial handling of children's pain? The answer is a complex one.

What happens to the hospitalized child who is in pain? One of us [6] evaluated the hospital experience of 25 children between the ages of five and eight who were hospitalized for surgery in a large Midwestern teaching hospital. In all 25 cases, surgery was performed under general anesthesia. A remarkable finding was that 13 of the 25 children *never* were given any medication for pain relief during their entire hospitalizations (the ages and the diagnoses of the children are presented in Table 22-1). For 21 of the 25 children, orders had been written for the administration of analgesics, either for narcotic or nonnarcotic medication, or a combination of the two.

During an interview, the mother of the six-year-old boy with intersex abnormalities told the investigator that her son had received only one dose of medication for pain during 13 hospitalizations. The child had undergone 13 separate surgical procedures, nine of which occurred after the age of four. A review of the child's medical record validated the mother's information.

Twelve children did receive pain medication. The types of medication, number of doses administered during their entire hospitalizations, and diagnoses are presented in Table 22-2.

Table 22-2 Type and frequency of dosage of pain medication according to diagnosis (N = 12)

Type of medication	Number of doses	Diagnosis
Noonan's*	1	Nephrectomy
Noonan's	1	Hypospadias repair
Noonan's	3	Ileal conduit
Talwin	1	Burn 40% of body, 2nd-degree
Morphine	1	Spinal fusion
Aspirin	2	
Morphine	2	Ureteroneocystomy
Acetaminophen	1	
Codeine	2	Fractured femur, multiple lacerations,
Aspirin	3	surgical amputation of left lower leg
Aspirin	1	Burn 70% of body, 2nd- and 3rd-degree
Aspirin	2	Spinal fusion
Aspirin	2	Ulnar nerve repair from grain auger accident
Acetaminophen	1	Burn 65% of body, 2nd- and 3rd-degree
Acetaminophen	1	Hypospadias repair

* Noonan's solution contains 25 mg of meperidine, 6.25 mg of chlorpromazine, and 6.25 mg of promethazine per cubic centimeter.

The dosages for 21 children with orders for pain medication were all within normal dosage limits for children, according to the American Pharmaceutical Association [23], with one exception. One dosage of morphine for a child who had hypospadias repair was 0.2 mg. The recommended morphine dosage is 0.1 to 0.2 mg per kilogram of body weight per dose. For a child weighing 18 kg, the appropriate dosage is between 1.8 and 3.6 mg; thus, the prescribed dosage of 0.2 mg was woefully inadequate.

Twelve children had orders written in their charts for a narcotic and a nonnarcotic pain medication, but only three received both during their hospitalizations. The narcotics and nonnarcotics ordered for the 21 children with orders for analgesics are contained in Table 22-3.

Why is there such a discrepancy between orders written and medication actually administered to children? It appears that nursing personnel were reluctant to exercise their prerogative to give medication ordered on a prn basis. What factors contributed to their decisions not to administer the medications? Is this discrepancy due to some outmoded attitudes and misconceptions on the part of nurses?

A matched-pair study of adults with identical diagnoses matched 18 of the 25 subjects only by diagnosis. The 18 adults received 372 narcotic analgesics and 299 nonnarcotics, making the total number of doses 671! The 25 children in this study [6] received a total of 24 doses of analgesics. An interesting point is that many of the children and adults were patients in the same hospital area, categorized by medical specialty, with the same nursing and medical staff.

Table 22-3 Medications ordered for pain

	Narcotic				Non-narcotic (acetaminophen or aspirin)
	Morphine	Codeine	Noonan's*	Talwin	
Number of children for whom medication was ordered	8	3	5	2	15
Number of children who actually received the medication	2	1	3	1	8
Total number of doses given to all children	3	2	5	1	13

* Noonan's solution contains 25 mg of meperidine, 6.25 mg of chlorpromazine, and 6.25 mg of promethazine per cubic centimeter.

Old Nurses' Tales

Giving credit where credit is due, the authors think that several "old nurses' tales," myths about dealing with pain in children, have passed from instructor to student over the years in both academic and clinical settings, with the result that they have become institutionalized axioms. We would like to raise questions about each "tale" or misconception with the goal of encouraging nurses to reexamine critically their current practices in the light of new data.

1. *Because their nervous systems are immature, children do not experience pain with the intensity that adults do.*
In the past, this statement has been one of the primary rationalizations for not intervening with children who are in pain. Swafford and Allen [24] address this problem.

   Although variation exists, it seems reasonable to believe that the infant's perception of pain is determined by the degree of cortical development. The concept is no longer held that complete myelinization is required for the function of nerve tracts; however, for full development of function, myelinization is necessary. Although myelinization is only partially completed at birth, the process proceeds rapidly when the tracts are utilized in their physiological tasks. Since myelinization proceeds at different rates among infants, the theory that the newborn does not perceive pain at one week of age is open to question.

Anyone who has seen the restraint needed for an alert newborn undergoing simple operative procedures such as circumcision without general anesthesia has little doubt about the infant's ability to perceive pain.

Very little research has been done on the relationship between age and the perception of pain. Haslam [10] determined pain thresholds in children from five to eighteen years of age by using a pressure algometer, a metal box with a spring attached to a plunger, which applied pressure to the tibia until the child said that it hurt or was painful. Haslam found that pain thresholds increased with age, that is, the younger the child, the more susceptible he was to pain.

Although more research is needed to validate this finding, it appears that small children are quite capable of perceiving pain at lower thresholds than adults, and thus are entitled to relief from pain with appropriate intervention. Rather than experiencing *less* pain than adults with comparable medical diagnoses, children may well experience *more* pain than adults under similar circumstances.

2. Children recover quickly.

This statement is another justification medical personnel sometimes use when evaluating a pediatric patient's need for pain-relief measures. Earlier, it was stated that children are neurologically capable of receiving painful stimuli, and, in many cases, the source of pain is the same in a child as in an adult, but the evaluation of the patient's pain differs.

For example, let us say an adult and a child of seven have undergone comparable open-heart surgical procedures for the repair of atrial septal defects. The type of incision and tissue manipulation will have been similar. During the child's postoperative course, it is probable that he will be ambulatory earlier than the adult and may appear to be recovering quicker. Is the earlier ambulation due to a child's ability to recover more quickly?

Primm [21], in an unpublished master's thesis, attempted to use the Ohio Pain Rating Scale which was developed for use with adults in 1964 and found to be both reliable and valid. The Ohio Pain Rating Scale utilized six criteria in the pain rating scale: attention, anxiety, verbal response, skeletal-muscle response, respiration, and perspiration. Primm found the Pain Rating Scale very difficult to use in the assessment of pain in children. In particular, the variables of verbalization and skeletal-muscle response were found to need expansion or redefinition.

Perhaps the real question is whether or not children's pain is being evaluated within an adult conceptual framework. Because a child is on his feet quicker than his adult counterpart does not mean that the pain he has experienced has been less severe. Physical activity has long been recognized as one coping technique children use to distract themselves from unpleasant stimuli.

3. It is unsafe to administer a narcotic pain medication to a child because he may become addicted.

The "addiction" rationalization has been with the nursing profession a long time. Horrendous fantasies of little children hooked for life on powerful narcotics may irrationally govern a nurse's decision not to administer narcotic pain-killers to a child, when, under similar circumstances, she would not hesitate to provide the same medication for an adult in pain.

Addiction results from prolonged use of a narcotic medication. The time period during which a child may be in acute pain following an operative procedure is usually fairly short, i.e., from the time he awakens from an anesthetic until 48 to 72 hours later. Dosages can be diminished gradually and the child withdrawn completely from narcotic medication by the time he is ambulatory. Nonnarcotic medication to take the edge off pain can be substituted once the child is alert and coping.

The question of addiction may become irrelevant for nurses caring for a dying child. In terminal situations, where death is inevitable and a child is in pain, the administration of narcotics can help him relax and be comfortable. Withholding of such medication causes the child unnecessary physical suffering and only adds to the anguish of grief-stricken family members and nursing staff.

An eight-year-old boy who was dying from a lymphoma did not have long to live. The nurses on the unit were expressing guilt because the boy was addicted to narcotics. When the whole situation was explored with several team members, they all agreed that the boy was in severe pain that could not be alleviated by anything less potent than narcotics. They also had consulted with the medical staff who confirmed that the boy was terminal and agreed with the nurses' estimation of the pain's severity. Even with medical support, the support of their peers, and their knowledge of the severity of pain and the terminal situation of the child, the nurses still felt guilty. The investigator then asked what would have happened if they had not given the analgesics on a regular basis. Their response was that the boy would have been in continuous severe pain, which is why the nurses had given the medication. It would be reasonable to assume that the nurses involved were also experiencing guilt over their own inability to prevent the child's death and the guilt expressed over his addiction to narcotics was transference of these feelings of helplessness.

4. *Narcotics always depress respiration in children.*

Another reason frequently given for the infrequent administration of pain medication is that potent narcotics depress respiration in children as well as in adults. With specific neurological conditions, respiratory depression will always be a possibility, and the authors are not questioning the rationale behind the withholding of narcotics when these conditions are present. We do question whether the threat of respiratory depression is being used as a rationalization for withholding pain medication from children with a wide variety of diagnoses when the pathological contraindications to narcotics are not present.

When dosages of these medications are calculated on a milligram-per-kilogram-of-body-weight basis, they usually represent no more danger to the patient than the administration of any other medication. An adverse reaction to any medication is always a possibility, but the benefit or necessity (or both) of its administration may outweigh (or is at least equal to) the danger of not administering the medication.

There are many potential benefits if children are given appropriate pain medication. If a small child is free from pain after a surgical procedure, he is more likely to comply with the requests of the nursing staff to turn, cough, and breathe deeply, thus reducing the effects of immobilization and its sequelae, such as pneumonia. An analgesic may reduce the fear and anxiety accompanying pain reactions that can contribute along with pain to hypoxia, acid-base imbalance, ischemia, or shock. Probably equally important is the potential that analgesics have for lessening the overall emotional trauma accompanying a child's hospitalization.

Eland's study [6] demonstrates in a dramatic way the errors of omission that occur when orders are written for prn pain medication and nurses are reluctant to administer them. This reluctance was repeatedly observed in situations where the probability of the occurrence of depressed respiration was quite low.

It is unfair to a child not to administer pain medication when a nurse's own good sense tells her that the child is suffering. It is sometimes difficult to tell where or how much a child hurts; guidelines for the assessment of pain and pain-equivalent behaviors are presented later in the chapter. Her own good sense may also tell the nurse that she would normally administer pain medication to an adult who had undergone the same operative procedure or was suffering from a similar illness. Few adults with second- or third-degree burns over substantial portions of their bodies would have to suffer without pain medication; yet, in Eland's sample, three badly burned children obtained a total of three doses of analgesics throughout their hospitalization.

Virginia Jarrett [11] best describes the relationship between nurses and the administration of prn medications:

The very nature of the PRN order means that the nurse will administer a certain drug "as needed" by a certain patient. To give anything as needed the nurse must know what the drug does, when the patient needs it, and if it has the desired effect. In no area of nursing practice is there more opportunity for independent action based on sound application of knowledge then in discovering the patient's particular needs for pain relief, in revealing the measures that work best for him and in solving the problem of pain.

5. *Children cannot tell you where they hurt.*

Swafford and Allen [24] recognized that infants do have the necessary neurological capacity to receive painful stimuli at birth but concluded that they lacked the ability to localize pain or to identify the source of pain. The authors state that "pediatric patients [age unspecified] seldom need medication for the relief of pain after general surgery. They tolerate discomfort well. The child will say he is uncomfortable or wants his parents but often he will not relate this unhappiness to pain." The implication seems to be that unless the child is able accurately to identify and label his source of discomfort, it is nonexistent, or at least it need not be relieved.

A study by Eland [7] in progress will hopefully lay this misconception to rest. One hundred seventy-two hospitalized children between the ages of four and ten were asked to place an x on a body outline to show where they hurt. One hundred sixty-eight out of 172 children correctly placed an x on a body outline and told the investigator why that specific area hurt. The placement of the x coincided with the child's pathology, surgical procedure, or painful events that occurred during the course of his hospitalization. The children were even cautious enough to place the x correctly with regard to left or right sides of the body. It would appear that some children can indeed localize the source of their discomfort even though they may be unable to verbalize how bad they feel.

One situation involving a four-year-old who was hospitalized with an immune deficiency is particularly illustrative:

The child had been hospitalized for eight weeks for an infection that involved his left leg, had gone home for two weeks, and returned with what apparently was a thrombus in the saphenous vein behind his right knee. At the time of his first interview, he placed numerous x's along his left leg and told the investigator that he only hurt at night when his leg was placed in a plaster splint which was being used to prevent a flexion contracture in his left knee. The following day he placed x's along the left leg in the same area as the previous day, and in addition, placed several x's in the region of the lower abdomen. On the third day, the patient was diagnosed as having a partial bowel obstruction. He again placed x's on the left leg and abdomen, and then colored brown the whole lower portion of right leg between his knee and ankle. Two days after the child had colored his right lower leg brown, a purulent yellow-brown material began to drain from his leg in the area of his right ankle. In reality, the child did not have a thrombus in the saphenous vein but a severe infection caused by seven specific bacteria. It was necessary to incise and drain the area, and the child endured an extended hospital stay. Ironically, the child had graphically depicted his pain and pathological condition several days prior to clinically measurable signs and symptoms or the physician's discovery of it.

An important lesson may be that a child can communicate by graphic means information he cannot communicate verbally, especially when the interrogator is the one hundred forty-first person that day to ask, "How are you feeling?" A child told the investigator at 5 P.M. one day that there had been 141 people in his room during that day and that every one of them had asked "How are you feeling?" When the investigator voiced her doubts about 141 people, the child presented a piece of paper on which he had actually kept track, and his mother confirmed the accuracy of his figures.

6. The nurse who wields the needle gets the negative feedback.

In most hospital settings, one of the primary responsibilities of the registered nurse is giving medications, sometimes to the exclusion of all other duties.

While the nurse is involved in this activity, other personnel are attending to the physical needs of each child—bathing, helping with feeding, and performing activities that are usually pleasant or, at least, not aversive to most children.

By virtue of her role as the giver of medication on the child-care team, the nurse can quickly become an emotional Typhoid Mary in the child's eyes. The nurse becomes the living personification of all that is painful to the child. He may project upon her the fears and anxieties about his hospitalization with an intensity all out of proportion to the nurse's actual role.

There is no avoiding the fact that an injection hurts. A needle arouses a predictable array of responses from most children, most of them negative. An injection is often regarded by a child as an attack, an intrusion, a threat to his body integrity, something that hurts. It is not surprising that most nurses, people who have entered their profession because of concern for others, find themselves very uncomfortable when they have to hurt another person, especially a sick, helpless child. The statement "This will hurt me more than it hurts you" may accurately describe a nurse's feelings when she administers an injection. These same feelings about hurting the child and setting herself up as an enemy may feed into the child's fears about receiving an injection; a vicious cycle can result with the child being terrified, and the nurse feeling guilty and anxious with her hesitancy only reinforcing his fears.

Nurses facing such an apparent no-win situation must guard against resorting to rationalizations that may prevent them from giving a child needed medication via injection: "the upheaval around giving the injection will do him more harm than the actual pain he is experiencing"; "he doesn't need it anyway"; "his crying will upset the whole unit"; "he's just restless"; "he wants his mother."

The nurse can be very helpful to a child if she looks upon her role as helping him to gain mastery over a threatening situation. Accurate information, presented in language he can understand, about the time lapse between the moment of injection and the diminution of pain, can help him gain some control over circumstances in which he feels helpless. The time periods for the onset of effectiveness of pain medication are known and can be told to the child.

Children who can tell time can use a watch to note the passage of the approximate number of minutes that have to elapse before he feels better. A younger child can watch the movement of a kitchen-type timer set for a specific time and then associate the ringing of a bell with the cessation of pain, a powerful reinforcer. Even if he is not entirely free from pain at that time, the use of suggestion can be almost as effective as the medication itself.

The nurse should plan to return at the time when she expects the medication to take effect so she can reinforce the benefits of having had the medication, and most important, talk about the cessation of pain in cause-and-effect terms—"You are feeling better now because the medicine from your shot is working." If the child is asleep, as often happens when pain medications take effect, the nurse can talk with the child when he is awake about the relationship between the short-term discomfort of the injection and the long-term relief from pain. If the nurse finds a child still in extreme discomfort after the time when the medication is expected to take effect, this information is valuable in the care of the child who may require an increase in dosage or a change in medication for pain relief.

Injections are not pleasant for the giver or for the receiver. In the study previously cited of hospitalized children between the ages of four and ten [7], the following question was asked: "Of all the things that have ever happened to you, what hurt you the worst?" Sixty-five of 119 children replied "a shot" or "a needle." The replies of 14 children were related to surgical procedures, the answers of nine children reflected medical treatment, and the replies of 31 were related to traumatic experiences outside of the hospital setting. It would appear that in this sample of hospitalized children, receiving a needle or shot is perceived by 55 percent of them as more painful than the events leading to their hospitalization.

The response of a four-year-old boy who had his right foot amputated after a lawn-mower accident that extensively damaged nerves in his left foot illustrates a young child's fear of injections. At the time of the interview, he was six hours postoperative and had just been asked if he hurt.

Patient   No!
Nurse   Are you fibbing to me?
Patient   Yup.
Nurse   How come?
Patient   Because if I tell you the truth, you'll go get me a shot!

This dialogue is in contrast to a discussion that took place between the investigator and an older child, an eight-year-old who had surgery for removal of a spinal cord tumor. She told the investigator that she did not like shots, but they made the pain in her back go away and shots only hurt for a little while and were "worth it." The beneficial effects of pain medication had been explained to this child, and she was able to use the information and asked for her pain medication when she needed it.

Young children cannot be expected to understand on an adult level a complex explanation about the necessity for injections, but they can be given one which is appropriate for their developmental level. Unfortunately, it is sometimes easier for a busy nurse to give no explanation than to try to help a child make sense out of a mysterious, often frightening experience.

A twelve-year-old boy asked the investigator (Eland) if she liked to give shots. She replied, "No, but in order to make people well, they are sometimes necessary." His next question was, "Well, why can't all medicines be given by pills or liquids?" After hearing her explanation, he asked, "How come no one ever told me that before?"

In making a decision to give an analgesic injection, a nurse must first assess the child's need. If a decision is made to give the injection, the nurse will probably come into disfavor with the child and may feel guilty because of the pain she will inflict in administering the medication. Research is needed to determine if guilt feelings prevent nurses from giving pain medication or prevent them from returning to the child's room and reinforcing the beneficial effects of medication.

Rather than feeling bad about her role, a medication nurse may wish to enhance her role as a "bad nurse" and have a colleague, the "good nurse," assist her with evaluating the necessity for pain medication and reinforcing its positive effects.

7. The best way to administer analgesics is by injection.

One obvious solution to the problem of injections would be to give intravenous analgesics to children who already have IVs running. In some pediatric intensive care units, giving IV pain medication is standard practice. If a narcotic is given intravenously, its maximum effectiveness will be reached in 20 minutes; if it is given subcutaneously, a child may begin to feel its effects in 20 minutes, but its maximal effectiveness is not reached until 50 to 90 minutes from the time of injection. "In some situations intravenous administration of a narcotic is preferred because of its rapid onset of action as well as greater degree of dosage control" [1].

Certainly there are more dangers associated with the administration of medication intravenously than by injection, but with intravenous antibiotics and other classifications of medication, nurses have already taken on the added responsibility. It could become an acceptable practice to administer IV analgesics until the child is able to tolerate solid food. At that time, he could be switched to oral analgesics; this procedure would eliminate entirely the need for painful injections.

Helping the Child to Cope with Pain

Before medical personnel can intervene effectively with a child in pain, they must determine how much pain he is experiencing and how he is attempting to deal with it. Until recently, a cookbook approach for the assessment of pain has frequently been used with persons of all ages. If a person had clenched fists, was perspiring, was splinting his pain, had a rapid pulse, and complained about his discomfort, medical personnel assumed that the person was experiencing pain. If the person did not demonstrate most of these behaviors, he was judged as having little or no discomfort. It is now known that adult patients with chronic pain problems may not exhibit any of these behaviors, and yet they may be experiencing pain to an almost overwhelming degree. The elusive and changing nature of pain makes assessment difficult in adults. Assessment of the pain experience in children is even more challenging, given the fact that a child is always physically, emotionally, and cognitively in a state of flux.

A child is not a miniature adult; criteria for assessing pain in adults cannot be applied uniformly to all children. It is not appropriate to talk about the pain experience of children in a global way. Infants, toddlers, preschoolers, and younger and older school-age children all respond differently to the experience of pain. Age, intellectual and developmental level, prior experience with pain, advance preparation about painful procedures, birth order, and the sex of the child are some of the factors that determine how a given child will respond to hospitalization in general and to the experience of pain in particular.

Nurses must remember this fact: a child brings his own unique interpretation to a given event. A procedure may, in reality, not be painful at all; however, it may be interpreted by a child as extremely painful or aversive because of the psychosocial context in which it occurs. The experience itself, with all of its painful properties, may not influence the child as much as the interpretation the child gives it. The following example illustrates what can happen when a child's misinterpretation colors his perception of reality.

A seven-year-old boy came to a developmental evaluation clinic in the pediatrics department of a teaching hospital. His referral problems included reading difficulties in school and hyperactive behavior at home. Despite efforts of the staff, including a pediatrician, a social worker, a public health nurse, clinical and educational psychologists, and a speech pathologist, all experienced in working with children, this little boy remained terrified and unresponsive throughout most of the day. He would not separate from his parents and communicated his fright to everyone. Even with a parent in the testing room, he scored in the range of moderate mental retardation on a standard intelligence test, a finding quite inconsistent with prior evaluations. At 4 P.M., the child quietly asked, "When am I going to die?" Gentle probing revealed that he was afraid of dying in the same hospital where his older brother had died two years before of cancer. Imagining a sword of Damocles over his head, he believed that it was only a matter of time before he, too, would die. In reality, he had nothing to fear, but his interpretation of events, unmitigated by the professionals who had spent the day with him, led him to believe that his own death was imminent.

Although knowing about the intensity of pain, the severity of illness, and the drastic nature of medical procedures is essential, the single most important task for the nurse is to understand how a child interprets what is happening to him, how the pain he is experiencing is woven into the ongoing fabric of his life.

Some Variables Influencing the Child's Interpretation of the Pain Experience

What variables would a nurse consider as she tried to make judgments about a child's pain experience? The research literature is minimally helpful in evaluating the effects of prior pain experience, advance preparation, birth order, and sex role on a child's interpretation of his pain experience.

Prior Pain Experience

Clinicians operate on the general assumption that prior experience with painful stimuli will adversely affect a child's responses to subsequent painful situations. One of the early studies on inoculation [13] suggests that after the age of six months, a young child will recall certain signal qualities of the inoculation situation—a needle, a white coat, restraint—and will tend to respond fearfully. Very little is known about what characteristics of prior painful situations are salient for children in subsequent encounters with painful stimuli. Discussing differences in responses to pain, Anna Freud [8] states: "the analytic study of such behavior reveals as different not the actual bodily experiences of pain but the degree to which the pain is charged with psychic meaning." She speculates that "the meaning of a painful experience to a child does not depend upon the type or seriousness of the operation which has actually been performed, but on the type and depth of the fantasies aroused by it."

One study with adults tried to assess the effects of painful experiences in childhood on responses to painful stimuli in adulthood. Collins [4], in a retrospective correlational study, administered the Childhood History Questionnaire to soldiers. The soldiers then received gradually increasing amounts of shock to second and fourth fingers of their right hands and were asked to report the onset of sensation, when the sensation was first perceived as painful, and when the sensation became intolerable. Pain threshold and pain tolerance were positively related to the Protection score and negatively related to the Independence score on the questionnaire. Although it was difficult to determine just how Collins related the questionnaire items to the early experience of pain, he concluded that "pain (experimental and clinical) is more likely to be perceived as significant and threatening by those having greater childhood experience with pain and suffering."

Data from retrospective studies like this one are misleading; there are countless clinical examples of children with histories of multiple pain experiences who are stoically unresponsive in pain situations, whereas many children with no significant prior history are terrified in the face of pain and exhibit low pain thresholds. The complex relationships between prior experience and current response are in need of further intensive study in research designs that do not rely on arbitrary choice of variables and the naive assumption that a person's response on a questionnaire, with all the distortions of recall, will accurately reflect his fantasies and feelings about experiences distant in time. The time of the experience of pain, the context in which it occurred, the child's cognitive understanding of what happened to him and why—these are only a few of the variables that must be explored carefully in order to understand the long-term effects of painful experiences.

In the absence of good research data, the two best sources of information for the concerned nurse are the parents and the child himself. A short interview can generate much information about how he has interpreted painful experiences in the past and what he expects to happen now. These impressions, along with an accurate medical history, can give the nurse a starting point for her interventions with a child.

Advance Preparation

No one likes to tell a child that he is going to be hurt by a procedure or will have to experience pain because of disease. However, it is logical that giving a child explanations in advance will enable him to mobilize his coping skills in preparation for the actual painful experience. Surprising the child with a traumatic or painful procedure without explanation may at times make the task easier for medical personnel, but such an approach does not give the child the opportunity to anticipate, to rehearse, to get ready for the procedure so that he will not be flooded with feelings of helplessness and anger. Such an approach, with little consideration of a child's feelings, makes him much more distrustful and suspicious of the next adult who has to care for him.

An eight-year-old who had been hospitalized for three weeks was scheduled for surgery. Since admission to the hospital, he had experienced several IVs, enemas, x-ray examinations, the passing of nasogastric tubes, insertion of a subclavian catheter, and a sigmoidoscopy, in addition to numerous venipunctures. He had been given an explanation prior to each procedure so he knew what to expect, and he was cooperative with nurses and doctors in every instance. On the evening before surgery, within a fifteen-minute period, he was subjected to the removal of one IV and the insertion of an intravenous catheter, an intramuscular injection, and an IV antibiotic, all procedures done without preparation. The child grew frightened, protested, and fought the physicians and nurses.

The strategy of realistic preparation of children for a subsequent inoculation experience receives support in a study by Vernon [25]. Thirty children, ages four to nine, were observed as they received injections during hospitalization for relatively minor surgical procedures such as myringotomies. Thirty-six hours prior to their own preoperative injections, one group observed an unrealistic film of children receiving injections—"a shot to go to sleep"; the children in the film did not express any indication of pain, fear, or emotional behavior. Another group saw a more realistic film depicting children responding with moderate pain of short duration and emotion, and a third group saw no films. Children observing the unrealistic film experienced the most pain when they received their own injections. In contrast, those who viewed the realistic film experienced the least pain. The author concludes that "modeling that conveys accurate information about the nature and/or timing of a painful stimulus can ameliorate pain, while modeling that conveys inaccurate information can increase pain."

Birth Order

Some studies [5, 25] have suggested that the first-born or only child is more likely than his later-born counterpart to experience anxiety in anticipation of potentially painful situations. In the study by Vernon [25] quoted above, the behavior of children was rated five minutes prior to injection. Early-born children became more upset than later-born children at the threat of injection, but they did not respond in a more upset fashion to the impact of the injections per se. Perhaps because of lack of experience, early-born children have not had the opportunity to rehearse their responses or to integrate and learn from the experience of someone else such as a sibling.

In a study of pain in a dental situation, DeFee and Himelstein [5] found that first-borns were rated as significantly more sensitive to pain than were later-born children.

A nurse responsible for helping to prepare a child for a painful procedure should determine the child's birth order in his family and anticipate that the first-born or only child may require some additional input to help reduce anticipatory anxiety.

Sex Differences

The few research studies in the literature reveal no sex differences in children's sensitivity to pain as assessed by standardized techniques. Nurses, like everybody else, will tend to react to children on the basis of their own ideas of sex-role stereotyping, beginning with differential treatment of infant boys and girls in the newborn nursery. There may be some short-term gain in treating boys as "little men who do not cry" to get over bad moments, but nurses who use this tactic run the risk of setting up unrealistic sex-role expectations for a child.

Although the research literature reveals no sex differences in a child's sensitivity to pain, sex-role expectations and differences are evident in a child's responses to painful experiences.

A six-year-old boy received a skull fracture, a fractured femur, and multiple lacerations and contusions when struck by a car. Interviewed in the presence of his father after five days in the hospital, the boy denied having experienced any pain. The child was again interviewed the following day, this time when his aunt was in the room. When asked about pain, he broke into tears. He was able to say in front of his aunt that he was currently experiencing pain and had been in pain on many occasions since the time of the accident.

It is not inappropriate for a boy to cry or for a girl to become aggressive under great stress, and it may be much better in the long run for the child to express his feelings rather than hold them back.

Children's Strategies for Coping with Pain

Lois Murphy [16], who has spent most of her professional lifetime studying coping strategies in children, defines coping as "a process, involving effort, on the way toward solution of a problem." According to Murphy, coping involves "struggles, trials, persistent focused energy directed toward a goal."

Lazarus et al [12] distinguish two modes of expression with regard to coping, modes that are relevant in discussing children and pain: direct actions and intrapsychic processes. Direct actions are motoric modes of eliminating danger or achieving relief from pain—in short, doing something. A child coping with overwhelming pain can become aggressive and verbally or physically attack medical personnel or family members. Another direct action, avoidance-withdrawal, is often upsetting to others but very adaptive for a child flooded with pain because it enables him to conserve energy by becoming absorbed in himself and his body.

Intrapsychic processes deal with discomfort by cognitive means. Nurses who use the technique of distraction with younger children are attempting to have the child "think about something else" for a while so he will not be preoccupied by his own discomfort.

The development of understanding through intellectual means is an important intrapsychic process for a child trying to master a painful situation, one in which he fears loss of control. Cardiac catheterization will never be a comfortable procedure for a child, but he will probably endure it with less disruption and fewer emotional sequelae if he has a chance to learn what will happen to him from someone who takes time to answer his questions. The use of realistic dolls and medical paraphernalia scaled to size in explanations to a child can help him achieve intellectual mastery over a potentially painful procedure.

Defense mechanisms such as regression and denial are intrapsychic processes that provide constructive help for a child facing the possibility of being overwhelmed by pain. Nurses are familiar with regression as a coping technique; a child who regresses usually returns to earlier patterns and behaviors that he had previously abandoned. Enuresis, demands to be fed or held, the use of baby talk, and inability to separate from parents are regressive coping behaviors.

Denial is the refusal to acknowledge displeasure or discomfort. Severely burned children can use denial effectively to cope; children who accurately perceive the threat to their lives caused by their burns may be overwhelmed by this knowledge. Nover [18], describes the pain experience of a burned child in this way: "the pain has the quality of being overwhelming, flooding, and irresistible, leading to a feeling of profound helplessness on the child's part." Denial may temporarily be the only defense available to a child in such desperate condition.

Overreliance on such defense mechanisms is sometimes seen by mental health professionals as disruptive to the psychological growth of a child. However, Murphy [16] notes, "defense mechanisms become pathological or contribute to pathology only when they interfere with progress in coping." A child's comfort and recovery may depend upon the ability of the nurse to identify and enhance the effects of all these coping devices.

Coping Strategies for Nurses

The strategies presented in this chapter are intended to help the nurse enable the child in pain to achieve mastery or control over what is happening to him. Where does the nurse start? An appropriate first step is for the nurse to ask herself these questions: How would I feel if I were this child? How would I interpret the external and internal events that are happening to me? What would help me to cope? What would make me feel less enraged, helpless, or afraid? Once the nurse can answer these questions, she is ready to help the child master his pain.

The second step in helping the child in pain is to look at the pathology involved and the diagnostic and surgical procedures that have been carried out and try to determine from a physiological viewpoint how much pain you can expect a child to have. Physicians can be very helpful to nurses in describing what a child may feel, especially if a surgical procedure has been performed. There are guidelines about what kind of pain to expect when certain neural pathways are severed in the course of surgery or when certain disease processes invade specific organs.

A third step is to spend a few minutes talking with the child's parents about his typical behavior prior to his illness or accident. If he is having elective surgery, parents will have up-to-date information about eating, sleeping, and toilet habits so that any regression will be quite apparent. It is important to learn about a child's previous hospitalizations and previous reactions to pain. The nurse can find out if the child is a first-born or only child, since research data show that birth order is related to response to pain. If the child has been injured, find out how it happened. Try to determine the child's understanding about how and why the injury occurred. Determine what his parents told him about it. Parents may need help in providing their child with a rational, age-appropriate explanation about what is going to happen to him in the hospital. The fifteen minutes it takes to gather such information and to inform parents and gain their cooperation will be time well spent if the information enables the nurse to reduce substantially the pain experiences of the child.

Children, especially young children, are experts at magical thinking, which is the attribution of cause-and-effect relationships to events that are correlated in time. A common mistake made by sick children is to assume that their pain is punishment for some bad thought or misdeed. A child may have to be told directly that his pain is not the consequence of being naughty or angry. Children who have been burned are especially susceptible to psychological distress resulting from magical thinking, since their careless behavior with matches may have caused the fire that burned them. It is easy for such a child to assume that his pain is punishment for his misdeed as well as a consequence of it.

Fourth, the nurse should talk with the child, and, more important, listen to him as he tells her how he feels. If a child uses a word she does not understand, she should ask him to explain what he means.

A six-year-old who had previously had polio came home from swimming and complained to his mother that his affected leg felt like a "lemon." His mother, a registered nurse, questioned him about this and discovered he was experiencing a "shriveled-up" feeling similar to the feeling when one sucks on a lemon drop for a long period of time. The mother's persistent questioning uncovered the use of a perfectly logical analogy.

Mothers can also be helpful because they usually know their children well enough to distinguish between behavior that is indicative of anger, restlessness, and withdrawal, and behavior expressing the fact that the child is really hurting.

It is helpful to know how children talk about pain. Our research experience indicates that children from four through ten rarely know the meaning of the word "pain" before the age of six, and most of them use the words "hurt" or "owie" instead. A nurse's question, "Are you having pain or discomfort?" may well fall on uncomprehending ears. Frequently, children are not given the credit they deserve for being able to communicate about or describe their pain.

A six-year-old hospitalized for burns engaged in this dialogue:

Nurse   What is pain?
Patient   Pain is stinging.
Nurse   Do your legs sting now?
Patient   No.
Nurse   When do your legs sting?
Patient   When I go to the whirlpool, it stings a whole bunch. But stinging means it's getting better.
Nurse   Does it sting all the time in the whirlpool?
Patient   It stings a whole bunch at first, but then after I'm in for a long time, it gets better.
Nurse   Does the stinging stop after you're in for a long time?
Patient   No, it stings all the time; it's not as bad after a while. The sting means it's getting better. When I get out of the whirlpool, I shiver and get cold (giggle).
Nurse   When you're up walking in the hall or moving in bed, does it sting?
Patient   No.

This conversation illustrates that the six-year-old could talk about his "stinging" and the circumstances under which the stinging became worse. The word "stinging" was probably synonymous with pain, and it could be used by the investigator to talk to the boy about his pain. He had also integrated the important cause-and-effect relationship between the stinging sensations and the process of healing, knowledge that could help him cope. This boy was in the hospital for three weeks and during that time received only one dosage of pain medication (Talwin) to relieve the pain of second degree burns over 40 percent of his body.

An eight-year-old girl with a spinal cord tumor described her pain as being like a "jolt" or "like an electric shock." She, too, was able to explain under what circumstances she hurt and knew that, at times, she had pain for no apparent reason.

The four-year-old boy in Eland's study [6] who suffered the traumatic amputation of one foot provides a good example of a child's ability to communicate a phenomenon rarely described in children, phantom-limb pain.

During an interview with the child, he told the investigator that his right foot (the amputated one) had hurt earlier in the day. His mother interrupted the child and reminded him that his foot could not hurt anymore because it was gone. The investigator took the mother aside and explained that her son might be experiencing phantom-limb pain. The mother was asked to keep a list of any other comments her son made regarding his amputated foot. Over several days, the child made numerous comments related to the amputated foot hurting, itching, or the sensation of a shoe being on too tight.

The investigator is aware of one reference in the pain literature referring to phantom-limb pain in children.

Whether or not children can localize the source of their pain is a question that also needs further investigation. Preliminary evidence indicates that even a four-year-old can locate the source of his pain when he is asked in a manner he understands. When more is understood about the ability of children to localize pain, this information will be invaluable in the assessment process.

The overall intent of this chapter is to sensitize nurses to the variables involved in the care of children in pain. Nurses have to examine their motives, mistakes, and misconceptions in order to help children through painful experiences with a minimum of emotional trauma and long-range negative effects. There are many research questions that need answering. When nurses have the answers to some of these questions, they will have begun to solve the riddles of pediatric pain.

References

1. *AMA Drug Evaluations.* Chicago: American Medical Association, 1971.
2. Barnett, H. L. *Pediatrics.* New York: Appleton-Century-Crofts, 1972.
3. Blake, F. G., Wright, F. H., and Waechter, E. H. *Nursing Care of Children,* 8th ed. Philadelphia: J. B. Lippincott Company, 1970.
4. Collins, L. G. Pain sensitivity and ratings of childhood experience. *Percept. Mot. Skills* 21:349, 1965.
5. DeFee, J. F., Jr., and Himelstein, P. Children's fear in a dental situation as a function of birth order. *J. Genet. Psychol.* 115:253, 1969.
6. Eland, J. M. Children's communication of pain. Unpublished Master's thesis, University of Iowa, 1974.
7. Eland, J. M. Children's experience of pain: A descriptive study. Unpublished data.
8. Freud, A. The role of bodily illness in the mental life of children. *Psychoanal. Study Child* 7:69, 1952.
9. Haller, J. A. *The Hospitalized Child and His Family.* Baltimore: The Johns Hopkins University Press, 1967.
10. Haslam, D. R. Age and the perception of pain. *Psychonomic Sci.* 15:86, 1969.

11. Jarrett, V.   The keeper of the keys. *Am. J. Nurs.* 65:68, 1965.
12. Lazarus, R. S., Averill, J. R., and Opton, E. M., Jr.   The psychology of coping: Issues of research and assessment. In Coelho, G. V., Hamburg, D. A., and Adams, J. E., eds., *Coping and Adaptation*. New York: Basic Books, Inc., Publishers, 1974.
13. Levy, D. M.   The infant's earliest memory of inoculation: A contribution to public health procedures. *J. Genet. Psychol.* 96:3, 1960.
14. Marlow, M.   *Textbook of Pediatric Nursing*. Philadelphia: W. B. Saunders Company, 1969.
15. McCaffery, M.   Brief episodes of pain in children. In Bergerson, B., ed., *Current Concepts of Clinical Nursing*. St. Louis: C. V. Mosby Company, 1969.
16. Murphy, L. B.   Coping, vulnerability, and resilience in childhood. In Coelho, G. V., Hamburg, D. A., and Adams, J. E., eds., *Coping and Adaptation*. New York: Basic Books, Inc., Publishers, 1974.
17. Nelson, W. E.   *Textbook of Pediatrics*. Philadelphia: W. B. Saunders Company, 1964.
18. Nover, R. A.   Pain and the burned child. *J. Am. Acad. Child Psychiatry* 12: 499, 1973.
19. Petrillo, M., and Sanger, S.   *Emotional Care of Hospitalized Children*. Philadelphia: J. B. Lippincott Company, 1972.
20. Plank, E.   *Working with Children in Hospitals*. Cleveland: Press of Case Western Reserve University, 1971.
21. Primm, P.   Identification of criteria used by nurses in the assessment of pain in children. Unpublished Master's thesis, University of Iowa, 1971.
22. Schultz, N.   How children perceive pain. *Nurs. Outlook* 19:670, 1971.
23. Shirkey, H. C.   *Pediatric Dosage Handbook*. Washington, D.C.: American Pharmaceutical Association, 1970.
24. Swafford, L. I., and Allen, D.   Pain relief in the pediatric patient. *Med. Clin. North Am.* 48(4):131, 1968.
25. Vernon, D. T. A.   Modeling and birth order in responses to painful stimuli. *J. Pers. Soc. Psychol.* 29:794, 1974.

IV

Annotated Bibliography
of Pain Literature

Annotated Bibliography of
Pain Literature

Kathleen C. Buckwalter, Joann W. Rains, and Jessie S. Daniels

The purposes of this annotated bibliography are to give detailed information about the articles found most useful by the authors in their respective chapters, and to supplement the text in those areas not covered in the book. The bibliography demonstrates the diversity of the pain literature in the articles selected from various professional fields, and also reflects the paucity of pain literature in some fields, including nursing.

To enable the reader to use the bibliography easily, articles are organized into fourteen major sections following the format of the book. These sections are: general; physiology; psychosocial; measurement and assessment; treatment approaches; neurology; surgical; bone and joint; cancer; burns; chest and cardiovascular; obstetrics and gynecology; pediatrics; and other. The last section is a list of books.

Articles related to more than one topic are cross-referenced and the psychosocial literature is subdivided under the headings of sociocultural, psychological, and pain tolerance–sensitivity. The final section of the bibliography presents books essential for the understanding of pain. We excluded articles excerpted from books in favor of annotating the book itself. All annotations are presented alphabetically by author.

The most important criterion for inclusion in the bibliography was that the publication's major emphasis be human pain. The literature surveyed included articles and books written in English and published between 1969 and 1975. Books and articles published before 1969 were included if the authors felt they presented "classics" or dealt with subjects not described in the more recent literature.

We attempted to select those items that make a maximum contribution to the literature; here we acknowledge the bias of a nursing perspective. Although we strived for the broadest cross section of pain literature, our value judgments for inclusion favor the nursing profession.

Elaboration of the inclusion criteria will clarify this perspective. Articles dealing exclusively with highly technical neurosurgical treatments and procedures, pharmacology, or a complex diagnostic process were excluded. Others were eliminated to minimize repetition. For practical considerations, no theses or dissertations were included.

Citations in the bibliography were derived from an extensive review of the following reference sources:

1. *Med-Line Search*
2. *Cumulative Index to Nursing Literature*
3. *International Nursing Index*
4. *Index Medicus*
5. *Psychological Abstracts*
6. University of Iowa library card catalog

Each annotation will

1. describe the theoretical perspective of the article
2. describe the article's approach: whether it is a research study, a patient case study, or nonresearch-based
3. include salient points of the article
4. describe the unique contribution this article makes to the pain literature
5. mention whether it describes clinical interventions
6. state whether a basic knowledge of anatomy, chemistry, research, and so forth is needed

In the past five years over 2,400 articles and books related to pain have been published. This annotated bibliography reflects our effort to select from this wealth of material the literature most useful for nurses and other health professionals.

General

1. A new approach to pain. *Emergency Med.* March 1974, pp. 241–254.

This article provides a good overview of the history, experimentation, and use of electrical neural stimulation. The work of three neurosurgeons is the focus of the article—Dr. C. Norman Shealy, director of the Pain Rehabilitation Center, LaCross; Dr. Charles V. Burton, Associate Professor of Neurosurgery at Philadelphia's Temple University Health Sciences Center; and Dr. Donlin M. Long, Professor and Chairman of Neurosurgery at Johns Hopkins Hospital. Melzack and Wall's gate control theory is used as a basis for the effectiveness of neuromodulation. The article refers to both acute and chronic pain. Also, dorsal column stimulators and transcutaneous neural stimulation are explained and explored.

2. Beecher, Henry K. Pain in Men Wounded in Battle. *Ann. Surg.*, January, 1946, pp. 96–105.

This study of 225 wounded soldiers is considered to be a classic piece in the pain literature. Besides a lengthy discussion on the use of morphine for pain in these soldiers, other conclusions have been drawn that seem important. It was found that severe wounds often produce little pain. This was attributed to the fact that strong emotions can block the perception of pain. Also, behaviors that were attributed to pain could instead be a reaction to mental distress and could be relieved by barbiturate sedation. Men in shock seemed to complain more of thirst than of pain.

3. Bowman, M. P. Pain. *Nurs. Mirror*, January 5, 1973, pp. 28–29.

   This brief article discusses the concept of pain, along with definitions and types of pain. The idea of "psychogenic" or "emotional" pain is presented with emphasis placed on how individuals vary in their attitude toward pain. Individualized care of the patient is necessary in appropriate and effective pain relief. Progressive relaxation is mentioned as a means of intervention.

4. Char, Walter T. Pain: The many faces of this universal phenomenon. *Med. Insight*, December, 1972, pp. 16–21.

   The subject of pain is briefly discussed according to several disciplines—biology, theology, philosophy, social anthropology, neurophysiology, medicine, psychiatry, and research. No clinical interventions are proposed. The article focuses on the idea that about two million Americans suffer from chronic pain each year, and that a great deal of research still needs to be done to find out what causes pain and how it can be controlled. Both the classic theory of pain and the newer gate control theory are cited in this good overview article, which is easy to understand.

5. *Clinical Medicine*, May 1975.

   This issue focuses on the topic of chronic pain. Eight original articles on general management concepts, psychiatric components, use of electrical stimulation, cultural aspects, the chronic pain syndrome, and central pains provide a helpful overview and concentrated resource of information on chronic pain. The backgrounds of the contributing authors include nursing, medicine, and various behavioral sciences.

6. Hackett, Thomas P. Pain and prejudice: Why do we doubt that the patient is in pain? *Med. Times*, 99(2):130–141, 1971.

   This article, written by a medical doctor, encourages the health professions to look at the patient with chronic pain in a more objective manner. Some of the common prejudices evident in the area of pain management are discussed, such as placebos, addiction, and malingering. It is reiterated that the treatment of a chronic patient should not be jeopardized by the prejudices of those trying to care for him.

7. Hardy, James S. The nature of pain. *J. Chron. Dis.* 4(1): 22–51, 1956.

   In this lengthy article, several aspects of the concept of pain are presented. Philosophical notations on pain are discussed, bringing in both physiological and psychological considerations. The term *pain experience* is differentiated from *pain sensation* and defined as all of the associated sensations, emotional reactions, and affective states as well as the physical sensations that an individual experiences. The main text of the article discusses the study of pain sensation using the thermal-radiation method and pressure. The conclusion drawn, from the studies listed, views pain as "an indication of the rate at which tissue is being damaged rather than upon the amount or the seriousness of the damage." The author ends his article with a discussion of the mode of action of analgesic drugs, and the differences between "experimental" and "pathological" pain.

8. Lenburg, C. B., Glass, H. P., and Davitz, L. J. Inferences of physical pain and psychological distress. II: In relation to the stage of the patient's illness and occupation of the perceiver. *Nurs. Res.* 19(5):392–398, 1970.

   This article describes a research study devised to investigate the inferences of pain and psychological distress made by teachers, nuns, physicians, and nurses. A second question asked is whether inferences of pain and psychological distress change with the stages of illness. Results indicate that all occupations infer greater psychological distress than physical pain regardless of the stage of illness. There are noted discrepancies between the responses of the health and non–health professionals to both questions asked. Ideas for further research are given. No clinical interventions are suggested.

9. Lenburg, C. B., Burnside, H., and Davitz, L. J.   Inferences of physical pain and psychological distress. III: In relation to length of time in the nursing education program. *Nurs. Res.* 19(5):399–401, 1970.

This article is the third of a three-part series dealing with inferences of physical pain and psychological distress. The authors explore the question "Is length of time in nursing education program related to perceptions of physical pain and psychological distress?" Results showed that first-year students inferred greater physical pain, whereas second-year students placed greater emphasis on psychological distress. Authors indicated that these results were based on courses taught over a one- or two-year time span.

10. LeShan, Lawrence   The world of the patient in severe pain. *J. Chron. Dis.* 17(2):119–126, 1964.

Although the health professional cannot entirely identify with the world of a person who has endured pain over a period of time, he can become aware of the commonalities of a chronic severe pain experience and therefore render himself more therapeutic. This article discusses the person in pain and presents some guidelines for the therapist. These guidelines lend themselves to clinical interventions of a psychosocial nature. All health professionals dealing with patients of long-term pain will benefit from this article.

11. Management of pain. *Postgraduate Medicine* 53(6), 1973.

This entire issue is devoted to the study of pain, with Dr. Bonica as the guest editor. Those articles included are by authors who have done considerable work in their respective fields. The emphasis is placed on understanding the chronic pain state and methods of treatment for the person who is involved. The pains of several disease conditions are discussed, namely, low back pain, causalgia, myofascial pain, pain due to nontraumatic joint disease, headache, cancer pain, visceral pain, and neuralgia. Each article contains a number of useful references.

12. McMasters, Robert   A clinical approach to pain. *South. Med. J.* 67:173–176, 1974.

This clinical approach is helpful to the nurse caring for any patient with pain. It identifies the complex subjective nature of pain affected by physiological, cultural, psychological, and theological factors. The parameters of pain are delineated. Treatment may involve drugs, surgery, psychology, physical medicine, and rehabilitation; however, it will only be effective when directed toward correction of pain at its origin.

13. Pain and suffering: A special supplement. *Am. J. Nurs.* 74(3):491–520, 1974.

This supplement includes a number of articles written by various health professionals on the concept of pain. The intent of these articles is to offer "basic information on the elements of the pain experience and the latest techniques being used to relieve it." Topics discussed include: the gate control theory, biofeedback, acupuncture, electrical stimulation, counterirritants, drugs, and chemical and surgical intervention. In the area of psychogenic pain, the use of hypnotic suggestion and operant conditioning are briefly discussed. Selected references are included after the respective articles.

14. Sternbach, Richard A.   *Pain Patients: Traits and Treatments.* New York: Academic Press, Inc., 1974.

This second book written by Sternbach compiles and discusses the literature written on "pain patients." Common features found in those patients suffering from chronic pain are emphasized, with discussion including psychogenic pain and acute pain states. Case studies are included to "heighten awareness of doctor-patient transactions so that diagnosis is improved." In addition to a discussion of treatment methods and evaluation, a chapter is devoted to special issues that may arise in the establishment of a pain clinic or treatment program.

15. Strauss, A., Fagerhaugh, S. Y., and Glaser, B.   Pain: An organizational-work-interactional perspective. *Nurs. Outlook* 22(9):560–566, 1974.

A new approach to the management of pain is introduced in this article. Instead of basing pain management only on physiological or pharmacological research, clinical practice, and psychological and psychiatric studies of pain, the authors are looking at the organizational setting in which the patient is being cared for. This article is the introduction to a research study done on a burn unit.

Primary emphasis is placed on three factors: (1) the type of unit that the patient is on, i.e., obstetrics, surgical, etc., (2) the type of work in which the staff is engaged, i.e., minimizing or preventing pain, enduring pain, and so forth, and (3) the nature of the interaction between the staff and patient and among the staff members themselves. A belief is expressed that unless the staff become accountable for their pain work, patient care will not be improved.

Physiology

16. Becker, Donald P., Gluck, Henry, Nulsen, Frank E., and Jane, John A.   An inquiry into the neurophysiological basis for pain. *J. Neurosurg.* 30:1–13, 1969.

This research study addresses two questions: does pain involve special pathways and is pain characterized by a unique pattern of neuronal activity. The medial mesencephalon was the anatomical site for investigation. In addition to neurophysiological information, this article includes a discussion of the difficulty of studying pain as a specific modality. A background of neurophysiology is important in the appreciation of this research.

17. Evans, R. J.   Acid-base changes in patients with intractable pain and malignancy. *Can. J. Surg.* 15:27–42, 1972.

These research findings indicate a positive correlation between the degree of metabolic alkalosis and the severity of pain, implying that acid-base changes could be important in the management of intractable pain. Chronic base excess may induce changes at a cellular level, namely an alteration of "neurocellular integrity, enzymatic function and ion exchanges." This speaks to the cellular mechanism of pain production. Strong in research and theory, this article requires a good basic science background. No clinical interventions are included.

18. Lim, Robert   Pain, and somesthetic chemoreceptors. In Kenshalo, Dan R., ed., *The Skin Senses*. Springfield, Illinois: Charles C Thomas, Publisher, 1968, pp. 458–465.

This article concentrates on somatesthesis as a means of regulating homeostatic function. It briefly discusses the research done to support the idea that there are somatesthetic receptors in the body that are chemosensitive to pain-producing substances. Injuries or nociception are cited as potential stimuli for pain. Differences between cutaneous and visceral pain are accounted for at the chemoreceptor terminals. Cutaneous chemoreceptors lie in the intercellular spaces of the epidermis, and visceral receptors can be found near the capillaries in the connective tissue space. These differences could account for the effectiveness of drugs to relieve pain of various origins.

19. Lim, Robert K.   Pain. *Annu. Rev. Physiol.* 32:269–288, 1970.

This writing reviews the physiology of the nature of pain, with a section devoted to three types of receptors—thermosensitive, mechanosensitive, and chemosensitive—that are postulated as being specific for pain. Another major section deals with a detailed presentation of the structural aspects of the neuron. The author concludes his writing with a discussion of analgesics and their sites of action, including research studies where appropriate. A basis in chemistry and physiology would be helpful in understanding this chapter.

20. Pearson, Anthony A.   Role of gelatinous substance of spinal cord in conduction of pain. *A.M.A. Arch. Neurol. Psychiatry* 68:515–529, 1952.

The translucent gray matter situated at the apex of the spinal cord dorsal horn, the gelatinous substance, is described histologically, grossly, functionally, and physiologically. This information comprises an explanation of neurological conduction of painful sensations. This article is an excellent presentation of the neural activity involved in transmission of pain stimuli; a background in neuroanatomy and physiology is assumed.

21. Werle, E.   On endogenous pain-producing substances with particular references to plasmakinins. In Janzen, Rudolph, Keidel, Wolf D., Herz, Albert, and Steichel, Carl, eds., *Pain: Basic Principles, Pharmacology, Therapy* (International Symposium on Pain, Rotisch-Egern, 1969). Baltimore: The Williams & Wilkins Company, 1972.

Beginning with the premise that "pain is a sign of a disturbance in the integrity of body tissue," this article describes mechanisms of pain as cellular responses to endogenous substances. K^+ ions, H^+ ions, acetylcholine, serotonin, histamine, and plasma kinins are presented as examples of chemicals capable of producing pain. These and other substances are normally bound by cellular membranes or stored in an inactive form; their release, as a result of detrimental influences, produces pain. This framework of cellular physiology makes this a valuable article for professionals whose background includes biochemistry. No clinical interventions or case studies included.

Psychosocial

Sociocultural

22. Drew, Francis L., and Shapiro, Alvin P.   Sociological determinants of drug utilization in a university hospital. *J. Chron. Dis.* 17:983–990, 1964.

This was a preliminary study of records done to explore possible determinants of drug administration such as race, sex and socioeconomic status. Drugs were classified as "specifics" or "supportives." Results of the study analyzed overall drug-use patterns, with particular emphasis on the population distribution of those patients receiving no supportive drugs, or supportive drugs only, and the use of postpartum analgesics. Findings suggest a need to investigate further the sociological parameter in drug utilization. The nurse-patient relationship is seen as playing a role more important in drug regulation than that of the physician. Although an older article, it is one of the few systematic studies with a sociological perspective.

23. Winsberg, B., and Greenlick, M.   Pain response in Negro and white obstetrical patients. *J. Health Soc. Behav.* 8:222–228, 1967.

This study investigated the influence of cultural factors on differential pain responses of black and white obstetrical patients, and also looked at the evaluation of pain by different health personnel. The results indicate no differences between pain reaction patterns of the two racial groups studied, suggesting that factors that determine pain expression are similar. Age and parity were rated as significant factors influencing pain response. Patients rated their pain as greater than did the medical staff. Physicians, nurses, and paramedical personnel evaluated patients' responses in a highly consistent manner, indicating that staff share a common frame of reference with respect to the evaluation of pain.

24. Wolff, B. Berthold, and Langley, Sarah   Cultural factors and the response to pain—A review. *Am. Anthropologist* 70(3):494–501, 1968.

This article emphasizes the need to study pain from a cultural anthropology perspective, since cultural factors exert a significant influence on pain perception. A brief historical review of the research on pain is included, but the focus is on those few papers discussing ethnic or cultural factors, among them Zborowski's work [see Number 186].

25. Zola, Irving K.   Culture and symptoms—An analysis of patient's presenting complaints. *Am. Sociol. Rev.* 31:615–630, 1966.

This classic article presents evidence that labeling and defining a bodily condition as a symptom or problem is part of a social process. It suggests that focusing entirely on etiology and ignoring what the individual and society feel are deviations, obscures understanding of the treatment of illness.

The article points out that the decision to seek aid may be unrelated to objective seriousness and discomfort. Zola suggests that socially conditioned selective processes operate to determine what is brought in for treatment. A study of these selective processes in the differing complaints of Italian and Irish patients with identical disorders is reported. In addition, this article discusses the conception of disease, the interplay of culture and symptoms, and sociocultural communication.

Psychological

26. Ball, Thomas S., and Vogler, Roger E.   Uncertain pain and the pain of uncertainty. *Percept. Mot. Skills* 33:1195–1203, 1971.

This study employed behavioral measures of the aversiveness of shocks in human subjects to explore strategies for the management of pain. Subjects preferred shocking themselves to passively awaiting a random, preprogrammed shock. This is consistent with previous research findings indicating that predictable pain is greatly preferred to nonpredictable. Interestingly, four subjects accepted double shocks in order to avoid administering shocks to themselves. An interesting discussion of phenomenological interpretations follows the experimental results.

27. Bond, Michael   Personality studies in patients with pain secondary to organic disease. *J. Psychosom. Res.* 17:257–263, 1973.

The work reported in this article was designed to demonstrate relationships that exist between pain as experienced in organic disease and personality dimensions as defined by Eysenck (extraversion/introversion and neuroticism/stability). Two studies are presented. The first deals with patients who have a potentially painful illness (carcinoma of the cervix). The connection between awareness of pain, complaint behavior, and personality structure is in this population examined. The second study explores personality changes that occur in patients with intractable pain relieved by surgical means. The significance of the results is discussed in terms of underlying neurophysiological mechanisms.

28. McCranie, E. James   Conversion pain. *Psychiatr. Q.* 47:246–257, 1973.

This paper presents a conceptual model of conversion pain that allows for acceptance of the validity of pain "as a positive expression of an underlying psychodynamic process." Case material is presented under three headings: (1) the symptom, (2) the pain-prone personality, and (3) developmental background. Dynamic formulations, emphasizing conversion pain and depression, are presented with implications for treatment. Knowledge of basic psychodynamic concepts is helpful in understanding mechanism of symptom formation as displacement of psychic pain to the soma. The article is relevant for all health professionals.

29. Murray, John B. Psychology of the pain experience. *J. Psychol.* 78:193–206, 1971.

Psychological factors of the pain experience are considered in this paper, which provides an excellent overview and many references on pain. Included are major sections on the cognitive and affective aspects of pain, which highlight theories on anxiety, the placebo effect, hypnosis, and audioanalgesia as used in medical research. A good background reference for all health professionals.

30. Rosillo, Ronald H., and Fagel, Max Z. Pain affects and progress in physical rehabilitation. *J. Psychosom. Res.* 17:21–28, 1973.

This article examines the relationship between pain and progress in physical rehabilitation. Pain is considered to act as a drive mobilizer, or drive state itself. Sex differences are also discussed. Psychological tests of affect are correlated with pain ratings. The findings are interpreted in the context of conditioning experiences and cultural expectations. Knowledge of research methodology would be helpful. The article is most applicable to the care of physically disabled patients.

31. Spear, G. G. Pain in psychiatric patients. *J. Psychosom. Res.* 11:187–193, 1967.

This paper summarizes investigations into various aspects of pain, a common symptom in psychiatric patients. Factors in the genesis of pain, its association with other somatic symptoms, social characteristics, and general characteristics of pain in psychiatric patients are discussed. Pain as a diagnostic and prognostic symptom is reviewed, and the author suggests that successful treatment of mental illness may resolve pain problems in these patients. Understanding of research methodology is assumed.

32. Wilson, W. P., and Nashold, B. S. Pain and emotions. *Postgrad. Med.* May 1970, pp. 183–187.

The authors develop the idea that pain not only is a sensation, but also can be recognized as an emotion. Some discussion of "central pain" is presented. An understanding of neuroanatomy would be helpful. Psychogenic pain is also discussed with the focus that emotional concomitants of pain are also present in affective disorders. Pain can occur in neurosis and schizophrenia. No clinical interventions are cited.

33. Yakimovich, Dorothy, and Sultz, Eli Helping behavior: The cry for help. *Psychonomic Sci.* 23:427–428, 1971.

This research study suggests that the critical variable that determines helping behavior is *not* degree of distress, but rather verbal control by the victim over helping behavior. An injured person calling out for help received assistance from significantly more subjects than victims (under identical conditions) who simply groaned and writhed in pain. Situational variables are more crucial than personality variables in determining helping behavior. The study results have important implications for nurses and all health professionals caring for patients expressing pain.

Pain Tolerance—Sensitivity

34. Barber, Theodore X., and Cooper, Barbara J. Effects on pain of experimentally induced and spontaneous distraction. *Psychol. Rep.* 31:647–651, 1972.

This study was conducted to evaluate the pain-reducing effects of three distraction mechanisms: listening to a story, adding aloud, and counting aloud. The first two distractors were effective in reducing pain only for one-minute duration of the stimulus. Postexperimental interviews with subjects revealed they used their own methods to distract themselves from the pain stimulus, and in painful stimulations lasting more than one minute, distractions appear ineffective.

35. Blitz, Bernard, and Dinnerstein, Albert J.   Role of attentional focus in pain perception: Manipulation of response to noxious stimulation by instruction. *J. Abnorm. Psychol.* 77(1):42–45, 1971.

This study was conducted on the role of instructions and suggestion in pain perception (induced by cold). Three groups of subjects were used— the first group was instructed to dissociate their experience of cold and pain and focus on the cold. The second group also focused on the cold, but was asked to interpret it as pleasant and the third group acted as control subjects. Both pain threshold and quit point were measured, with a significant elevation in the former found in both instruction groups. These results have clinical implications for the technique of restructuring of pain perception in cases where complete distraction cannot be achieved.

36. Bobey, Marie J., and Davidson, P. O.   Psychological factors affecting pain tolerance. *J. Psychosom. Res.* 14:371–376, 1970.

This article reports on a study designed to explore the role of cognitive factors in a person's ability to tolerate repeated exposures to experimental pain. It also includes a brief but valuable review of current theories about psychological factors, especially anxiety.

The study concludes that relaxation techniques are the most effective methods for dealing with a painful stressor. Experimental and clinical implications of the results are discussed.

37. Clark, W. Crawford   Pain sensitivity and the report of pain: An introduction to sensory decision theory. *Anesthesiology* 40(3):272–287, 1974.

This article presents the sensory decision theory, also known as signal detection theory, and discusses its usefulness for measuring experimental pain. The importance of this theory lies in its two-component division of the traditional pain threshold. Clark states that, "Sensory decision theory emphasizes the distinction between the pain experience itself and an individual's criterion for reporting pain."

Using this theory as the framework, an experimental study is presented, along with a discussion of the mathematics involved and method of data analysis. A major contention is the newness of this theory and the fact that it has not been widely used, especially in the area of clinical pain.

38. Clark, W. Crawford, and Mehl, Louis   Thermal pain: A sensory decision theory analysis of the effect of age and sex on d', various response criteria, and 50% pain threshold. *J. Abnorm. Psychol.* 78:202–212, 1971.

This article begins with a review of research on the attitudinal and sensory components of pain thresholds, with emphasis on signal-detection theory as applied to pain perception. An experiment was conducted that demonstrated response pain as a function of a variety of sensory and nonsensory variables. The advantage of signal-detection theory, which can monitor both components, over traditional psychophysical procedures is stressed. Interestingly, at noxious intensities, older men and women endure greater pain before reporting it, and the article concludes that age and sex differences in pain thresholds are caused by variation in the criterion for pain rather than differences in sensitivity. Knowledge of research methodology is essential to understanding this complex but valuable article.

39. Craig, Kenneth, and Weiss, Stephen   Vicarious influences on pain-threshold determinations. *J. Pers. Soc. Psychol.* 19(1):53–59, 1971.

This article focuses on the role that modeling plays on a person's responses to pain tolerance. Different subjects and a constant confederate were placed in an area and received increasing voltage of electric shocks. Both the subject and the confederate were to respond to the shock by a signal light, with the subject responding first. The confederate's responses were based on the subject's responses. In a postexperimental questionnaire, the subjects stated that the model had no influence on their ratings, but they had more influence on the confederate's rating. The conclusions drawn from the findings indicate that "verbal reports of pain are not linearly related to electric shock intensity but represent complex reactions to physiological, experimental, and social cues." These factors interact to determine a person's behavioral response.

40. Geer, James H., Davison, Gerald C., and Gatchell, Robert I.   Reduction of stress in humans through nonveridical perceived control of aversive stimulation. *J. Pers. Soc. Psychol.* 16(4):731–738, 1970.

The results of this research indicate that the perception of control over experimentally induced pain, even if it is not actual control, can affect the autonomic response of the subject. The implications of the finding are discussed in relation to similar research findings and their applicability to clinical settings. The theoretical framework involves perceived control over the stressful aversive stimuli. A psychology background would be helpful in the appreciation of this article, but all professionals involved in clinical interventions would find it useful.

41. Greene, Robert J., and Reyher, Joseph   Pain tolerance in hypnotic analgesia and imagination states. *J. Abnorm. Psychol.* 79(1):29–38, 1972.

This study was designed to investigate the effectiveness of hypnotically suggested analgesia and pleasant imagery conditions in modifying pain tolerance. The authors report a significant increase in pain tolerance for hypnosis subjects in analgesia experimental conditions, using an electrical stimulus. Pleasant imagery conditions did not produce significant group tolerance increase, although non–body-oriented images were most effective. The relationship between anxiety levels and tolerance was also examined. State anxiety was not related to tolerance, and there was a negative correlation between trait anxiety and tolerance changes.

42. Hilgard, Ernest R.   A neodissociation interpretation of pain reduction in hypnosis. *Psychol. Rev.* 80(5):396–411, 1973.

This article reports on the paradoxical findings of clinical experiments using hypnotically suggested analgesia to reduce cold pressor pain. It reveals that at some cognitive level subjects experience and can report cold intensity, even though suffering is significantly reduced. The theoretical problems generated by these clinical findings are discussed in terms of neodissociation theory and then compared with psychoanalytic ego theory and role theory interpretations. The neodissociation theory and experimental findings using hypnosis are also explained in relation to Melzack-Wall's gate control theory of pain. A theoretical background in psychiatry would be helpful.

43. Hilgard, Ernest R., Morgan, Arlene H., Lange, Arthur F., Lenox, John R., MacDonald, Hugh, Marshall, Gary D., and Sachs, Levis B.   Heart rate changes in pain and hypnosis. *Psychophysiology* 11(6):692–702, 1974.

This report analyzes heart rate changes as functions of change in water temperature, of the hypnotizability of the subject, and in four experimental conditions, including hallucinated pain. It determines that the motivational-emotional aspects of pain are more labile than the sensory-discriminative aspects. Heart rate rise is seen as a function of *felt* pain, not just a consequence of physiological stress. Experimental evidence is interpreted in accordance with Melzack-Wall's gate control theory. Understanding of research methodology would be helpful.

44. Neufeld, Richard W. J.   The effect of experimentally altered cognitive appraisal on pain tolerance. *Psychonomic Sci.* 20(2):101–107, 1970.

This article reports on an experimental study of tolerance to radiant heat as measured under three forms of cognitive appraisal. Additionally, subjects were informed that each form of appraisal was endorsed by a different source. Results indicate that denial is the form of cognitive appraisal best able to raise pain tolerance; however, the effects of the different appraisals varied in relation to sources of endorsement. The paper presents a brief discussion of the experimental results, based on the effects of cognitive appraisal on pain tolerance as compared to the effects on tolerance of experimental threat. This study has important clinical implications.

45. Schalling, D.   Personality and tolerance for experimentally induced pain. A review. *Report on Psychological Habits*, University of Stockholm, 1970, No. 305.

This manuscript discusses the relations between personality and the ways of experimentally inducing pain. Specificity theory and the gate control theory were briefly presented in discussing the differences between sensation and reaction. A listing of the studies done with thermal, pressure, and electrical stimulation and various personality characteristics are reviewed. Findings from the review show that sex, age, race, and motivation play a role in a person's responses to noxious stimuli. A lengthy bibliography is included.

46. Staub, Ervin, Tursky, Bernard, and Schwartz, Gary   Self-control and predictability: Their effects on reactions to aversive stimulation. *J. Pers. Soc. Psychol.* 18(2):157–162, 1971.

The influence of control and predictability on aversive stimulation is experimentally tested in this research study with the use of electric shock. Results showed that those subjects who had predictability and control over the administration of shock could tolerate a more intense shock. Their cardiac responses also differed from those subjects who had no control or predictability. The latter exhibited large heart-rate responses at all levels of intensity. It has been suggested that control and predictability can function in reducing the threat and impact of an aversive stimuli.

47. Staub, Ervin, and Kellet, Deborah   Increasing pain tolerance by information about aversive stimuli. *J. Pers. Soc. Psychol.* 21(2):198–203, 1972.

Several factors that affect the reactions to experimentally induced aversive stimuli were presented in this research report. Subjects were divided into four groups: control group, apparatus information group, sensation information group, and apparatus-plus-sensation information group. Subjects received electric shocks in increasing intensities, and were asked to report when they could tolerate no more shocks. The results showed that those who received both types of information could endure more shocks, and noted more intense shocks as painful. The two types of information were considered interactive, such that one enhanced the other and vice versa. The results from this experiment were found to add support to the idea that cognitive factors can influence reactions to aversive stimuli.

48. Tursky, Bernard   Physical, physiological and psychological factors that affect pain reaction to electric shock. *Psychophysiology* 11(2):95–112, 1974.

This article deals with the broad topic of factors that affect pain responses to electrical shock in the research laboratory. Several years of research are reviewed, and many factors that contribute to the pain responses are analyzed. This is a valuable summary article with a lengthy bibliography included. No clinical interventions are reviewed. This article addresses an audience that is interested in the research aspect of pain.

[See also Numbers 72, 77, 81, 91, 92, 95, 97, 98, 99, 110, 130, 140, 167, 175]

Measurement and Assessment

49. Baer, Eva, Sauitz, Lois Jean, and Lieh, Renee Inferences of physical pain and psychological distress: 1. In relation to verbal and nonverbal patient communication. *Nurs. Res.* 19(5):388–392, 1970.

Seventy-four practitioners volunteered to complete an instrument that consisted of 16 paired vignettes describing a variety of patients. The results showed that social workers inferred the greatest pain, and nurses and doctors inferred the least pain. All three groups inferred the greatest amount of pain from verbal communications. All groups also inferred greater psychological distress from nonverbal communications. The results of this research bring up questions about the *effectiveness* of staff-patient communications.

50. Davidson, P. O., and Neufeld, R. W. J. Response to pain and stress: A multivariate analysis. *J. Psychosom. Res.* 18:25–32, 1974.

The need to explore the multidimensional aspects of pain and stress prompted this investigation. These psychologists experimentally created a situation inducing pain and stress in a number of subjects. The behavioral, physiological, and psychological responses to each stimulus were measured and analyzed. Results showed that it is possible to discriminate pain from other stressors using the appropriate measures. It was found that in the pain group, there was a significant increase in frontalis muscle tension and respiration rate.

51. Drew, Francis L., Moriarty, Richard W., and Shapiro, Alvin P. An approach to the measurement of the pain and anxiety responses of surgical patients. *Psychosom. Med.* 30(6):826–836, 1968.

This article reports on a two-phase research study conducted on supportive drug use postoperatively. It concluded that examination of drug-usage patterns of surgical patients can indicate the degree of anxiety or pain experienced by the patient, and that this is largely predictable by observation of recovery-room responses. This measurement, however, cannot be used as a method to differentiate between pain and anxiety. Knowledge of research methodology is helpful in reading this article.

52. Graffam, Shirley Ruth Nurse response to the patient in distress: Development of an instrument. *Nurs. Res.* 19(4):331–336, 1970.

The purpose of this research study was to develop a reliable tool for the study of a nurse's response to adult patients' complaints of distress. Findings from the study showed that nurses' responses were often automatic, impersonal, and limited. The leading cause of distress complaints were those conditions causing pain, comprising 62 percent of the total. Emotional distress comprises another 15 percent of distress complaints.

53. Lipowski, F. J. Physical illness, the individual and the coping processes. *Psychiatry Med.* 1:91–102, 1970.

Although the topic of pain is not specifically addressed in this article, it is a classic piece central to the assessment of pain. The psychosocial components of physical illness are discussed in terms of coping with the stress of illness. Methods of coping are expressed in behavior and are pertinent determinants of illness outcome. This is valuable information for any professional involved in the assessment of pain or who is interested in understanding patient behavior in a more complete way.

54. Melzack, R., and Torgerson, W. S.   On the language of pain. *Anesthesiology* 34(1):50–59, 1971.

These investigators have found that there exists a need to describe the qualities and dimensions of pain as well as the intensities of pain. Two studies are presented that strive to increase information about pain qualities.

A list of 102 words to describe pain were compiled in the first study. These words were then categorized into 3 major classes: (1) words that describe sensory qualities, (2) words that describe affective qualities, and (3) evaluative words that describe one's subjective experience with the pain phenomena. The second study was involved with rating each of the descriptive words on a scale from least to most pain. Data from the cited studies show that there is considerable agreement in the categorization of words that describe pain, and on how much pain each word represents, across a variety of cultural socioeconomic and educational backgrounds.

55. Melzack, Ronald   The McGill Pain Questionnaire: Major properties and scoring methods. *Pain* 1:277–299, 1975.

This article discusses the usefulness of the McGill Pain Questionnaire as a sensitive instrument in the measurement of clinical pain. The questionnaire consists of various sections that are described and discussed in the article, along with directions for administration. A report of a study done using the questionnaire with 297 patients, exhibiting a variety of pain categories, is presented. At this time, the questionnaire has been found useful for detecting differences among methods of pain relief and provides data that can be statistically treated.

56. Merskey, H.   The perception and measurement of pain. *J. Psychosom. Res.* 17:251–255.

Pain is considered a subjective experience, and, therefore, measurement of this sensation has to be approached indirectly. Several methods of assessing pain are briefly discussed: "the threshold of pain complaint, the point of maximum tolerance, the difference between threshold and maximum tolerance, the response to a noxious stimulus of fixed size, the dol scale of just noticeable differences, rating scales: (a) verbal, (b) visual, (c) auditory, and the measurement of drug dosage needed to abate pain." These particular techniques are reviewed because of the writer's familiarity or interest in them; the article does not provide an exhaustive listing of available techniques.

57. Peck, Robert E.   A precise technique for the measurement of pain. *Headache*, January, 1967, pp. 189–194.

The development of a technique for measuring pain is presented in this article. The technique has been named *Thymometry*, and the instrument used is a *Thymometer*, which can be substituted for an audiometer. The process of measurement involves having a person manipulate the intensity of the tone to what he feels matches his intensity of pain. A number of trials can be done and the median taken if it appears that there is considerable variability among responses. Several clinical examples of the use of this technique have been cited. The value of this instrument is that it is simple, quick, and easy to use.

58. Storlie, Francis   Pain: Describing it more accurately. *Nursing '72*, June, pp. 15–16.

This short article on the assessment of pain highlights six basic facts about pain that can be elicited from the patient. The emphasis is for the nurse to probe for what the experience of pain means to the patient. Specific questions are mentioned that may get at this information. No specific clinical interventions for relieving pain are cited.

59. Wolff, B. Berthold Factor analysis of human pain responses: Pain endurance as a specific pain factor. *J. Abnorm. Psychol.* 78(3):292–298, 1971.

Experimentally induced pain with chronic arthritis patients was measured and responses were subjected to factor analysis. This research identified the factor of pain endurance, the interval between pain tolerance and threshold, to be the specific behavioral pain factor. A discussion includes the clinical application of these experimental findings. A research background is helpful in the appreciation of this article.

[See also Numbers 99, 151]

Treatment Approaches

60. Billars, Karen S. You have pain? I think this will help. *Am. J. Nurs.* 70(10): 2143–2145, 1970.

This article emphasizes that there are other means of nursing intervention for pain relief, in addition to the administration of medication. The author briefly cites a few research studies focusing on the idea of suggestion as a means of pain relief. She describes her own research involving repositioning and suggestion as a means of pain relief in patients who have undergone gallbladder, gastric, or intestinal surgery. A brief discussion of the theoretical framework of pain according to Melzack, Beecher, and Sternbach is included.

61. Diers, D., Schmidt, R. L., McBride, M. A., and Davis, B. L. The effect of nursing interaction on patients in pain. *Nurs. Res.* 21(5):419–428, 1972.

This article describes a five-year nursing study of the effect of nursing approaches on the relief of pain. The nursing approaches were divided into three categories using the *Nurse Orientation System*, which is an interaction analysis scheme. Pain is the dependent variable and there are three treatment areas defined, based on the various pain theories being viewed. A knowledge of research methodology is essential. A good bibliography is included.

62. Howitt, Jack W., and Stricker, George Objective evaluation of audio analgesia effects. *J. Am. Dent. Assoc.* 73(4):874–877, 1966.

This study identified clinical effects of audio analgesia in six experimental groups of children, and investigated possible sources for the effects. It concluded that the basis for the clinically demonstrable effect of audio analgesia is suggestion, and that this effect is mediated by psychological rather than physiological factors.

63. Luna, Herminigilda Q. The effects of varied types of nursing approach on pain behavior after surgery. *The ANPHT Papers*, July-December, 1971, pp. 7–31.

This article reports on a research study done in a clinical setting by nurses, who are seen as the people most likely to come into contact with patients before and after surgery. Patients undergoing emergency appendectomies were the subjects. Combinations of six types of nursing approaches were utilized: (1) with preoperative support, (2) without preoperative support, (3) with postoperative reinforcement, (4) without postoperative reinforcement, (5) five nurse visits, (6) one nurse visit. The dependent variable was the amount of pain that a patient exhibited after surgery through verbal or nonverbal cues, and medication usage. Results showed that adequate preparatory communication, postoperative reinforcement, and postoperative visits by the nurse seem to play an important role in a patient's use of adaptive mechanisms. Good operational definitions of the above factors are included in the text of the article.

64. Markham, M. M.   The relief of pain. *Nurs. Times* 66:1579–1581, 1971.

The article focuses on a brief description of a pain clinic in England at Hope Hospital. Admitting criteria are cited and the process of admission is reviewed. Types of treatments that are discussed include intrathecal or extradural injection and peripheral nerve blocks. The goal of the treatments is to provide some relief of a patient's pain.

65. McBride, Mary Angela B.   Session 5: Scientific bases for therapeutic nursing practice—Evaluation of nursing action: "Pain" and effective nursing practice. *ANA Clinical Sessions*, 1968, pp. 75–82.

This article describes a research study done to investigate the effects of three nursing approaches on complaints of pain by general surgical patients. The orientations of the three approaches are: (1) Experimental approach was oriented to the physical, intellectual, and emotional aspects of the patient. (2) Control Nursing I was oriented toward the physical and intellectual aspects of the patient, and (3) Control II emphasized the physical component. These approaches are defined according to *Diers' Nurse Orientation System*. Results showed that 86 percent of the patients nursed experimentally experienced some pain relief, and this group were the only ones who had decreased pulse and respiration rates both immediately and long-range. The author emphasizes the fact that means other than administration of medication can be used by the nurse to relieve pain. She uses a holistic approach in defining the concept of pain. A good bibliography is included.

66. McGlashan, Thomas H., Evans, Frederick J., and Orne, Martin T.   The nature of hypnotic analgesia and placebo response to experimental pain. *Psychosom. Med.* 31(3):227–246, 1969.

This research study focuses on experimentally induced muscle pain and the subject's expectations regarding treatments to reduce the pain intensity. The two interventions were hypnosis and placebo analgesia. The findings indicate hypnotic analgesia has two components, one being a placebo effect and the other a distortion of perception. This article can be appreciated by someone with a knowledge of research or someone interested in utilizing hypnosis as a mode of pain reduction.

67. Sharp, Robert, and Meyer, Victor   Modification of "cognitive sexual pain" by the spouse under supervision. *Behav. Therapy* 4:285–287, 1973.

This is a case study of an otherwise healthy young male with unbearable pain in his glans penis during intercourse. Because of particular childhood circumstances, it was determined that the patient had a conditioned painful response. Four variables were involved in the experience of pain, and treatment included the manipulation of one of those variables, attention. The patient's spouse was an active participant in treatment program, using distraction technique. The article emphasizes the usefulness of a good client history and of conceptualizing pain cognitively as well as physiologically.

68. Wiley, Loy   Intractable pain: How nursing care can help. *Nursing '74* September, pp. 55–59.

This article presents a patient case study of a woman who was experiencing pain from leg ulcers. It discusses the process that the nursing staff employed to alleviate this woman's pain. The article mentions a few clinical interventions such as giving the patient a sense of control, regimen of medication administration, and distraction.

[See also Numbers 103, 107, 109, 157, 162, 166, 171]

Neurology

69. Frazier, Shervert H., and Kolb, Lawrence C. Psychiatric aspects of pain and the phantom limb. *Orthop. Clin. North Am.* 1(2):481–495, 1970.

   The topic of phantom pain is well developed from the psychiatric perspective. This discussion's framework places emphasis on the interpretation of the pain, the meaning one attaches to the pain experience, and the particular socialization for the pain expression. The physiology and psychology of the phantom phenomenon are discussed. No case studies or research findings are included, but a section dealing with treatment covers possible interventions.

70. Greenhoot, J. H. The management of intractable pain: Present status and future expectations. *Va. Med. Mon.* 97:117–120, 1970.

   Greenhoot presents pain as "an adaptive phenomenon, but when no longer useful as a warning, it is disintegrative and requires relief by whatever means are available." Several surgical methods of pain relief are briefly discussed; rhizotomy, cordotomy, and percutaneous cordotomy. Rhizotomy appears to be of most benefit in pain due to benign diseases, and percutaneous cordotomy has been effective in most malignant pain states. A brief reference to electrical stimulation as a future method of pain relief concludes the article.

71. Melzack, Ronald Phantom limb pain: Implications for treatment of pathologic pain. *Anesthesiology* 35(4):409–419, 1971.

   Discussion of phantom-limb pain is divided into general characteristics of the phenomenon and the search for causal mechanisms. A new model for the cause of phantom-limb pain has been formulated that appears to be consistent with the gate control theory. This model is the concept of a central biasing mechanism with the brainstem reticular formation playing a key role "by exerting a tonic inhibitory influence, or bias, on transmission at all synaptic levels of the somatic projection system." Implications of the model for pain management and (unanswerable) questions are presented. A bibliography of 49 references is included.

72. Melzack, Ronald How acupuncture works—A sophisticated western theory takes the mystery out. *Psychology Today*, June, 1973, pp. 28–38.

   The effects and advantages of acupuncture analgesia are explored, and this ancient Chinese treatment analyzed in terms of current theories of pain. Melzack and Wall's gate control theory of pain is offered as the best explanation of how acupuncture works. The traditional Chinese Yin-Yang explanation is briefly outlined also. The article is not highly technical, but provides a fairly thorough explanation of central biasing/gate closing mechanisms as related to acupuncture. Basic anatomical knowledge is assumed.

73. Sinha, R. P., Ducker, T. B., and Perot, P. L. Stopping pain. *J. SC Med. Assoc.*, October, 1971, pp. 428–434.

   A brief discussion of pain mechanisms sets up the framework for the presentation of several neurosurgical treatment modalities being employed in the clinical area. These neurosurgical procedures are presented under four classifications, those involving peripheral nerves, spinal nerve roots, the spinal cord, and brain and cranial nerves. The relative effectiveness of each procedure is mentioned, along with documentation for its use. This article provides a brief overview of neurosurgical procedures available for the alleviation of intractable pain.

74. Swanson, August G., Buchen, George C., and Alvord, Ellsworth C. Anatomic changes in congenital insensitivity to pain. *Arch. Neurol.* 12:13–18, 1965.

   This article discusses the rare phenomenon of congenital insensitivity or indifference to pain. A case study of two male siblings with pain and temperature sensation defects is presented. At age 12, one of the brothers died following a brief febrile illness. This article includes neuropathological analysis of autopsy findings, as well as figures of stained cross sections. The abnormal pain and temperature sensations are viewed as developmental defects occurring early in embryogenesis, and due to the absence of primary sensory neurons. Results of the autopsy support the doctrine of specific energies—that pain and temperature are conducted over specific neurons in the peripheral nervous system. Knowledge of neuroanatomy is helpful in understanding this report.

75. Urban, Bruno J.   The current use of nerve blocks in the management of chronic pain. *Clin. Med.* 82(5):27–30, 1975.

   This article discusses the rationale for use of nerve blocks as a diagnostic tool in chronic pain syndromes, and as an effective treatment modality. Nerve blocks intercept the perception of pain and concomitant reflex mechanisms. A section is devoted to various agents used in the administration of blocks—local anesthetics, neurolytic agents, and unrelated compounds to increase effectiveness. Concentration levels are mentioned. A large portion of the paper is concerned with procedures of regional anesthesia. Specifically noted are the following blocks: spinal, epidural, peripheral, paravertebral, sympathetic ganglion, and local infiltration. Application of this treatment is based on the concept that the experience of pain must have a neurophysiological substrate.

76. Wilson, M. E.   The neurological mechanisms of pain. *Anesthesia* 29:407–421, 1974.

   The discussion of pain is centered on the neuroanatomy and neurophysiology of the structures involved. A review of the classic theory of pain and the gate control theory is presented. Several methods of pain relief are suggested, along with a brief discussion of some clinical causes of pain. A lengthy bibliography of 49 references concludes the article.

   [See also Numbers 14, 156, 177, 184, 185]

Surgical

77. Bruegel, Mary Ann   Relationship of preoperative anxiety to perception of postoperative pain. *Nurs. Res.* 20(1):26–31, 1971.

   This article reports on a descriptive nursing study that was done with patients undergoing intra-abdominal surgery. The question studied was "Are postoperative perceptions of pain associated with preoperative levels of anxiety?" Tools employed were the IPAT Anxiety Scale, administered the night before surgery, and the Chambers-Price modified pain scale, completed approximately 32 hours postoperatively. Results showed that there was no relationship between anxiety and pain perception, but that marital status, occupation, and surgical variables did influence the pain perception, as shown by the pain ratings and analgesic medication records. A base in research methodology would be useful in reading this research study. No clinical interventions were advocated, but a good bibliography was included.

78. Gildea, James   The relief of postoperative pain. *Med. Clin. North Am.* 52 (1):81–90, 1968.

   A brief history of pain relief through drugs begins this article. The author systematically discusses various influences on the nature of postoperative pain, both from a psychological and physiological perspective. Under the section dealing with treatment of pain, several methods are discussed: use of narcotics, nonnarcotic analgesics, local anesthetics, inhalational analgesia, and hypnosis. Stress is placed on knowing the nature of pain and surrounding circumstances, plus observation and evaluation to satisfy a patient's individual needs during the postoperative period.

79. Hackett, Thomas P. The surgeon and the difficult pain problem. *Int. Psychiatr. Clin.* 4(2):179–188, 1967.

This author addresses the topic of long-standing chronic pain. A problem case is one that presents persistent pain despite medical or surgical interventions, may carry an emotional rather than a physical etiology, or discomforts the physician managing the case. Dr. Hackett elaborates on misconceptions that interfere with chronic pain evaluation, speaks to the nature of chronic pain, and considers the possibility that all pain should not be cured. A case history is included; no research is reported nor are interventions described. This is beneficial background knowledge for any health professional involved in pain assessment and management.

80. Johnson, Jean E. Altering patient's responses to threatening events—Surgical study. Paper presented at NLN Convention 1975, New Orleans, May 21, 1975.

This paper reports on a research study done with patients undergoing elective cholecystectomy to see how preparatory information would affect their postoperative course. Type of preparatory information was classified as procedural, sensation, and exercise information. These were tried alone and in combinations on the selected population.

Results showed that patients who were given exercise instruction and sensory information had a shorter postoperative hospital stay. Suggestions for nursing intervention are briefly discussed.

81. Johnson, Jean E., Dabbs, James M., and Leventhal, Howard Psychosocial factors in the welfare of surgical patients. *Nurs. Res.* 19(1):18–29, 1970.

This article reports on an investigation done with surgical patients. Using emotional drive theory, the researchers tested whether or not level of fear preoperatively would affect emotional adjustment postoperatively. Several variables in addition to level of fear that were examined were focus of control, mood, physiological response, and birth order. Data suggested that a patient's instrumental responses may be independent of emotional drive. The significance of this study was geared toward the theoretical understanding of patients' responses and not to specific clinical care. A knowledge of research methodology would be helpful to the reader.

82. Keats, Arthur S. Postoperative pain: Research and treatment. *J. Chronic Dis.* 4(1):72–83, 1956.

A systematic look at the nature of postoperative pain is presented in this 1956 article. Several characteristics involved in postoperative pain are briefly discussed. Included are: incidence of pain from various types of surgery, occurrence of the use of narcotics, pain and other symptoms of discomfort, duration of pain from surgery, patient characteristics of those experiencing pain, and response to placebo and suggestion.

The second part of this article focuses on the research done in the treatment of postoperative pain, with emphasis placed on the use of analgesic drugs. Studies done to determine the effectiveness of various analgesics (oral and parenteral) and placebos are mentioned.

The article ends with several suggestions for the treatment of postoperative pain: drugs and doses used, relief of other symptoms besides pain, and good nursing care.

83. Peng, Alfred T. C., Yoshiaski, Omura, Cheng, Huan Chen, and Blancato, Louis S. Acupuncture for relief of chronic pain and surgical analgesia. *Am. Surg.* January 1974, pp. 50–53.

The mechanism of acupuncture's pain relief is speculated to be a function of both neural mechanisms (including the Melzack-Wall gate control theory) and cellular biochemical and physiological changes. The background of acupuncture is summarized in this article. Four terminal cancer patients are described. No nursing interventions for pain are included. The merit of the article is a hint of the link between cellular explanations of pain and the gate control mechanism of pain. Acupuncture is explained by the speculation that "many physiochemical factors, including release of many enzymes and chemical substances from cell membranes penetrated by acupuncture needles, might mediate or initiate certain physiological changes" (p. 52).

84. Quimby, Charles W., Jr.   Preoperative prophylaxis of postoperative pain. *Med. Clin. North Am.* 52(1):73–80, 1968.

This article emphasizes the important role that the internist, surgeon, and anesthesiologist play in the patient's postoperative period. The more information that can be obtained from the patient preoperatively concerning his prior experience with pain, and his methods of coping with pain, the better able the physicians would be able to manage the patient's pain postoperatively. The idea of rapport and support on the part of the physician is important.

Suggestions to improve the postoperative period include: (1) advanced information about site, intensity, and duration of pain, (2) realistic explanation of surgery and course of treatment, and (3) appraisal of anxiety and denial, and use of these mechanisms to help the patients postoperative course.

[See also Number 51]

Bone and Joint

85. Barrett, J., and Golding, D. N.   The management of low back pain and sciatica. *Practitioner* 208:118–124, 1972.

The main point stressed in this article is the view that the etiology of low back pain and sciatica is still an unsolved mystery to the physician. Treatment is based on the presenting symptoms of the individual. The writers have reviewed groups of clinical cases and modes of treatment based on roentgenological examination and degree of mobility exhibited by the patient. The basic groups discussed were those patients with acute lumbar pain, acute sciatica, chronic lumbar pain, and chronic sciatica.

86. Bradley, K. C.   The anatomy of backache. *Aust. NZ J. Surg.* 44(3):227–232, 1974.

The anatomy of backache is discussed and illustrated in this article with special emphasis placed on the pain sensations arising from the posterior primary rami of the spinal nerves. The innervation of a posterior vertebral joint is described, and also the arrangement of nerves on the posterior aspect of the sacrum. This knowledge of the anatomical system of the back would be helpful in the treatment of backache.

87. Cailliet, René   Lumbar discogenic disease: Why the elderly are more vulnerable. *Geriatrics,* January 1975, pp. 73–76.

This article begins with a brief review of the normal vertebral column as a contrast to the changes that may occur through aging. Several common disorders are discussed, such as, spinal stenosis, metastatic disease, osteoporosis, disk infection with osteomyelitis, and Paget's disease. Several general methods of treatment are briefly reviewed, with a conservative approach being advocated.

88. Hart, F. Dudley, and Hustisson, E. C. Pain patterns in the rheumatic disorders. *Br. Med. J.* 4:213–216, 1972.

This informative presentation differentiates the sensation patterns in gout, osteoarthrosis, ankylosing spondylitis, rheumatoid arthritis, prolapsed intervertebral disk and others. They state that if "pain is made up of the totality of the sensations and reactions provoked by a nociceptive stimulus, then suffering appears as the consciousness of these sensations and reactions" (p. 213). Suggestions for interventions stem from the premise that "an occupied mind suffers less than the unoccupied one" (p. 216). This article displays a sensitivity to psychosocial needs of people experiencing these pain patterns and an awareness of realities of the clinical setting, and a commitment that each pain pattern calls for a different therapeutic approach.

89. Hart, F. Dudley Control of pain at night. *Nurs. Times,* May 3, 1973, pp. 559–562.

Emphasis in this article is placed on how the nurse can help patients get a comfortable night's sleep. Those patients suffering from rheumatoid arthritis and chronic osteoarthritis are the main population studied. In addition to the alterations of physical factors to promote sleep, the discriminate use of drugs is discussed. The advantages of certain classifications of drugs to relieve pain are enumerated; these include anti-inflammatory agents, analgesics without anti-inflammatory effects, potentially addictive drugs, hypnotics, and antidepressants.

90. Keim, Hugo A. Low back pain. *Ciba* 25(3), 1973.

This clinical symposium provides a comprehensive discussion of low back pain, with detailed discussions of anatomical, physiological, and psychological aspects of the disorder. Multiple etiologies of low back pain—metabolic, degenerative, circulatory, and congenital disorders; trauma and mechanical causes; tumors; toxicity; and psychoneurotic problems—are examined. Frank Netter's detailed illustrations of the lumbosacral spine and examination of the patient augment the text. A section devoted to principles of treatment concludes this informative chapter on low back pain.

91. Levine, Mathew E. Depression, back pain and disk protrusion. *Dis. Nerv. Syst.* 32:41–45, 1971.

This article examines the complex interrelationships between low back pain and depression. Research on the pathophysiology of depression and stress is reviewed. Two case histories are presented, which illustrate the pitfalls of attempting to attribute all symptoms in low back pain patients to either disk protrusion or depression alone, although depression appears to be significant in the pathogenesis. The author concludes that a combination of conservative management (bed rest) and psychiatric treatment may be most useful with low back pain patients.

92. Levit, Herbert I. Depression, back pain and hypnosis. *Brief Clin. Rep.* p. 266–267.

This article presents a case study of a young man with a history of severe back pain. The emotional aspects of back pain, particularly depression and anger, are highlighted, and the use of hypnosis for relief of pain examined.

93. Lidström, Anders, and Zachnisson, Marianne Physical therapy on low back pain and sciatica. *Scand. J. Rehabil. Med.* 2:37–42, 1970.

The authors discuss physical therapy for the person who has low back pain and sciatica. A research study is presented that compares two treatment modalities for their effectiveness. The first group receives the conventional treatment (hot packs, massage, and spine exercises), the second group receives the alternative treatment (intermittent traction, psoas-relaxing position, and isometric exercises), and the control group receives only hot packs and rest. Findings show that the alternative treatment causes a significantly greater improvement than the conservative treatment. Interpretations of findings have to allow for the difficulty in evaluating effectiveness of treatments and the undeterminable etiology of the disease conditions.

94. Moldofsky, H., and Chester, W. J. Pain and mood patterns in patients with rheumatoid arthritis: A prospective study. *Psychosom. Med.* 32(3): 309–318, 1970.

This article reports on a longitudinal psychosomatic study done with RA patients during hospitalization. A total of 21 separate studies were carried out over a two-year period. Two pain-mood patterns (a synchronous state and a paradoxical state) emerged. These patterns relate mood states to joint tenderness (articular pain). A follow-up study 1 to 2 years later found the paradoxical group had a less favorable outcome. This has implications for the prognostic significance of the pain-mood patterns of interest to anyone working with arthritis patients.

95. Robinson, Harry, Kirk, Robert F., Frye, Roland F., and Robertson, James T. A psychological study of patients with rheumatoid arthritis and other painful diseases. *J. Psychosom. Res.* 16(1):53–56, 1972.

This study was conducted to determine if personality traits labeled "characteristic of rheumatoid arthritis" are disease functional. Newly diagnosed and "older" RA patients' profiles were compared with other chronic pain sufferers, and it was hypothesized that all patient groups would show personality profile similarities, especially in the areas of anxiety and depression. Study results partially supported this hypothesis, and the authors concluded, "observed personality traits of individuals and groups represent attempts on their part to adjust and cope with the stresses encountered in their environment." Implications for further study in this area are discussed.

96. Rose, Donald L. The decompensated back. *Arch. Phys. Med. Rehabil.* 56: 51–58, 1975.

The term *decompensated back* is defined by the writer as "the clinical state resulting from inability of the back musculature to meet the functional demands imposed on it." The discussion is centered on the clinical presentation of a person who has a decompensated back and some of the functional characteristics peculiar to the back. The gate control theory by Melzack-Wall and its relation to back pain is included in the article which concludes with several factors that are important in the treatment of the individual with back pain.

97. Sternbach, R. A., Wolf, Sanford R., Murphy, R. W., and Akeson, W. H. Aspects of chronic low back pain. *Psychosomatics* 14:52–56, 1973.

Based on experience at their own pain clinic, the authors present evidence that chronic low back pain is associated with "disturbances of affects, with a skewed self-concept and life style, and with a peculiar way of relating to physicians." They recommend treatment similar to other psychophysiological disorders, and psychiatric consultation viewing low back pain as a convenient focus for patient's depression, invalidism, and passive-aggressive "pain games." Knowledge of psychological terminology and testing is helpful. Findings from orthopedic low-back clinics can be generalized to clinical settings treating chronic pain disorders and are of interest to all health professionals.

98. Sternbach, R. A., Wolf, S. R., Murphy, R. W., and Akeson, W. H. Traits of pain patients: The low-back "loser." *Psychosomatics* 14:226–229, 1973.

This study examines personality characteristics (MMPI profile) of chronic low back pain patients, an impressively large category of disabled persons who consume billions of dollars of health care annually. The personality profile highlights differences between males and females, and acute versus chronic patients. Physical findings and the effect of pending compensation are also discussed. Two major conclusions are drawn: (1) the chronic low back patient has a psychophysiological musculoskeletal disorder, with depression that should be treated, and (2) the attempt to distinguish between "organic" or "functional" low back pain is useless.

99. Weiner, Carolyn L. Pain assessment on an orthopedic ward. *Nurs. Outlook* 23(8):508–516, 1975.

The concept of pain work, discussed previously by Strauss, Fagerhaugh, and Glaser, is presented here in relation to the pain problems exhibited on an orthopedic ward. The study centers on problems of pain assessment by staff and the need for patient legitimization of pain. Because the etiology of back pain is ambiguous, there is a greater need for accurate pain assessment, with particular attention given to the interactional and experiential factors that are involved in the process of assessment. The emphasis, in this report, has been placed on the staff's difficulty in assessing pain and how this can cause an undesirable change in patient behavior that could further complicate pain assessment and account for inadequate relief. It was suggested that "if the staff does not think organizationally and interactionally about their pain work . . . they will continue to be less understanding of patient behavior and to rely on the simplification provided by stereotyping."

100. Wilfling, F. J., Klonoff, H., and Kokan, P. Psychological, demographic and orthopaedic factors associated with prediction of outcome of spinal fusion. *Clin. Orthop.* 90:153–160, 1973.

This article focuses on the need for more objective data to support the psychological factors that have been attributed to the patient who suffers from low back symptoms. In this study, information was gathered from a number of subjects who had undergone lumbar invertebral fusions from 2 to 9 years previously. Several psychological tests were administered and these scores were analyzed in relation to the success or failure of the spinal fusions and to the number of operative procedures experienced. Findings support the idea that generalizations about the psychological constitutions of people with low back syndrome can be made.

Cancer

101. Bader, Madelaine Personalizing the management of pain for the terminally ill patient. In Goldberg, Ivan, Molitz, Sidney, and Kutscher, Austin, eds., *Psychopharmacological Agents for the Terminally Ill and Bereaved.* New York: The Foundation of Thanatology, Columbia University Press, 1973, pp. 202–211.

A case study of a 61-year-old woman suffering with a terminal illness was presented by the author to show the importance of an individualized medication regime. The goal of therapy is to enable the patient to be as pain-free as possible, yet to maintain mental alertness. Every person is given the opportunity to be an active participant in the process of pain management by recording such factors as type of drug, time drug received, effectiveness, and speed of relief. Based on the preceding information, the most effective drug can be determined.

102. Heusinkveld, Karen Billars Cues to communication with the terminal cancer patient. *Nurs. Forum* 11(1):105–113, 1972.

This interesting article discusses some of the psychological mechanisms that can play a role in aiding the nurse, or other health professionals, in relating to the cancer patient. Emphasis is placed on giving the patient realistic cues to help him in coping with his condition. The concept of realistic cues has been defined by the author in the text of this article. Evaluation of the effectiveness of these cues is necessary to the communication process existing between the patient and the nurse. Conversations dealing with death and dying are discussed with emphasis on the giving of realistic cues.

103. Matthews, George J., Zarro, Vincent, and Osterholm, Jewell L. Cancer pain and its treatment. *Semin. Drug Treat.* 3(1):45–53, 1973.

This is a succinct, inclusive review of a vast topic, presented with a sensitivity that reveals clinical expertise. The various causes of pain (primary lesions, recurrence, metastasis, and scarring) serve as the framework for the discussion of early, intermediate, and late-stage cancer pain. Clinical interventions are the focus of this article. No case studies or research findings are included. This is valuable information for any health professional interested in cancer, and care of the cancer patient. The bibliography includes 24 references on pharmacology, general theory, psychosocial aspects and neurosurgical interventions with cancer patients.

104. Nelson, Kenneth M., Hewett, William J., Chuang, Facog, and Chuang, Justin T. Neural manifestations of para-aortic node metastasis in carcinoma of the cervix. *Obstet. Gynecol.* 40(1):45–49, 1972.

Four case reports demonstrate that the presence of anterior thigh pain in advanced cervical carcinoma indicates retroperitoneal metastasis. The anatomy of the pelvic nerves and nodes provides the framework for the informative discussion. Interventions may arise from this knowledge; for example, "pain increases when the affected nerve is stretched by hip extension and may be relieved by flexion." This is important anatomy for nurses working with gynecological oncology patients.

105. Parker, Robert G. Selective use of radiation therapy for the cancer patient with pain. In Bonica, J. J., ed., *Advances in Neurology*, Volume 4. New York: Raven Press, 1974, pp. 491–494.

Pain produced by some offending tumors can be reduced by irradiating the tumor. Parker states that pain relief can be "frequent, long lasting, and without serious treatment-produced morbidity." In addition to pain relief, successful radiation therapy can result in preserving anatomical structure and function.

106. Pilowsky, I., and Bond, M. R. Pain and its management in malignant disease. *Psychosom. Med.* 31(5):400–404, 1969.

The authors reported on a research study done to explore staff-patient interaction on the management of pain in patients suffering from malignancy. Assessment of pain was subjective, by the patient completing a scale. A record of medication administration was kept by the nursing staff. Three results emerged from the study: (1) patients who viewed themselves as ill asked for pain relief more frequently and received less powerful analgesics from the staff, (2) with female patients, the staff would give powerful analgesics without waiting for patient request, and (3) older patients tended to receive less powerful analgesics and the staff would wait for the patient's request. Findings stress the need for an active interactional process between staff and patient to promote effective pain management.

107. Saunders, Cicely The treatment of intractable pain in terminal cancer. *Proc. R. Soc. Med.* 56(3):195–197, 1963.

This article is based on clinical experience with cancer patients at St. Joseph's Hospital. The discussion centers on the use of analgesics for pain. The idea of addiction is commented on. Recognizing the type of medication that does relieve a patient's pain, and the most opportune schedule of administering this medication is of utmost importance in the control of the pain.

108. Senescu, Robert A. The development of emotional complications in the patient with cancer. *J. Chronic Dis.* 16:813–832, 1963.

This article is primarily geared to the physician and his contact with patients having cancer, but the content can also be valuable to other health professionals. Several fundamental reactions to disease are discussed, namely, fear, the feeling of damage and reduction of self-esteem, dependency, guilt, anger, and loss of gratification and pleasure. These emotional components are discussed in terms of how they affect a person's acceptance of his illness and ability to continue living. Hints for clinical interventions are included, and a good bibliography completes the article.

109. Twycross, R. G. Principles and practice of the relief of pain in terminal cancer. *Update,* July 1972.

The author relates eleven principles of practice that he has found helpful in working with patients who have terminal cancer. These principles concern various aspects of care, ranging from the benefits and side effects of diamorphine to the relationships developed with the patient and his family. Additional measures of analgesia are mentioned besides medication. The article is primarily geared to the physician, but the principles are applicable to all health professionals working with the patient with intractable pain.

[See also Numbers 17, 83, 176]

Burns

110. Andreason, N. J. C., Noyes, Russell, Hartford, C. E., Brodeard, Gene, and Proctor, Shirlee Management of Emotional Reactions in Seriously Burned Adults. *N. Engl. J. Med.* 206(2):65–69, 1972.

This article details emotional and management problems of seriously burned adults—including shock, deformity fears, depression, regression, delirium, and pain. It emphasizes the individuality of the pain experience for burn victims, noting increase during dressing changes and debridement, and effects of anxiety on thresholds. Case studies accompany each problem discussed. Adequate provision of pain medications is stressed. Clinical management information is primarily aimed at physicians. Findings from psychiatric evaluation and multidisciplinary team follow-up provide insight into the nature and causes of reactions of burned patients relevant for all health professionals.

111. Fagarhaugh, Shizuko Y. Pain expression and control on a burn care unit. *Nurs. Outlook* 22(10):645–650, 1974.

The interorganizational-work-interactional perspective of pain is applied to an intensive burn unit. Because pain cannot be eliminated, the work of pain management includes endurance and control of pain expression. Burn pain is described in phases: initial acute phase, secondary intense pain from treatments and donor skin-graft sites, and a final dull chronic phase of nerve regeneration. Case studies and implications for patient care are included to give this article a strong clinical base.

112. Fox, Charles L. Evaluation of the burn. *Mod. Treatment* 4:1196–1198, 1967.

A two-paragraph section entitled "Relief of Pain" speaks of the excruciating nature of a burn pain. Immediate relief of pain is paramount, and the intervention outlined is cold soaks over the exposed regions very quickly. Mechanism of pain from thermal trauma is explained on a cellular level, the first part of a chain reaction being proteolytic enzyme release. No research or case studies are included in this brief section; its merit lies in cellular explanations of a pertinent pain intervention. A knowledge of cellular physiology is assumed.

113. Hamburg, David A., Hamburg, Beatrix, and de Goza, Sydney   Adaptive problems and mechanisms in severely burned patients. *Psychiatry* 16:1–18, 1953.

This classic study of 12 severely burned patients reports their major adaptive problems and the consequent adaptive mechanisms. The former include the threat of the injury itself, separation from home and family, specific circumstances associated with the accident, the threat of interference with previously important activities, dependence, sexual problems, and others. Mechanisms of adaptation during the one-year follow-up include first those of emergency defenses, then recovery mechanisms, and finally those of convalescence. Recovery includes mobilization of hope, and restoration of relationships and self-esteem. The major concept of the research is adaptation; many clinical examples are cited. Although it does not include interventions for pain it lends insight to the complexity of burned patients' needs. This article assumes psychology background.

114. Hamburg, D. A., et al.   Clinical importance of emotional problems in the care of patients with burns. *N. Engl. J. Med.* 248(9):355–359, 1953.

This article translates the classic research described in the previous annotation into clinical applicability. Pain and prolonged discomfort are cited as primary problems; elaboration states "emotionally induced pain is a much more serious problem than is generally recognized" (p. 357). Relief of fear and anxiety needs to accompany relief of pain. Interventions develop from the framework of encouraging adaptive mechanisms. This article assumes psychology background.
[See also Numbers 136, 138]

Chest and Cardiovascular

115. Bomrah, V., Bohler, R., and Rakita, L.   Hemodynamic response to supine exercise in patients with chest pain and normal coronary arteriograms. *Am. Heart J.* 87(2):147–157, 1974.

The purpose of this research study is to identify more definitive diagnostic tests that will better establish functional status and underlying coronary pathology for patients with chest pain who have normal coronary arteries. It identifies the diagnostic dilemma and subsequent intervention for the patient with pain from nonocclusive artery disease. In assessing the cause of chest pain, the true etiology may be missed because of inadequate or as yet unresearched diagnostic criteria.

116. Burrell, Lenetta, and Burrell, Zeb   Vascular surgery. In *Intensive Nursing Care.* St. Louis: The C. V. Mosby Company, 1973, pp. 98–105.

This chapter identifies some of the pathophysiology, symptomatology, and therapeutic management of vascular problems amenable to surgery. Pertinent information for the clinical application of nursing care of the postsurgical vascular patient is included. The role of pain as a part of the symptoms evaluated by the nurse is elaborated on.

117. Crozier, Robert E., Gregg, James A., and Garabedian, Mamigon   Obscure chest pain as a symptom of reflex esophagitis. *Med. Clin. North Am.* 56(3): 771–780, 1972.

The merit of this article for nursing lies in its presentation of pathophysiology, symptoms, and a discussion of reflex esophagitis. Symptoms include regurgitation, heartburn, dysphagia, and chest pain; the latter may be chronic and severe and difficult to distinguish from coronary artery disease. Eleven patients are presented to demonstrate these symptoms and the resultant diagnosis. No clinical interventions are described. Anatomy and physiology of the GI tract are helpful in understanding this article. The unspoken statement regarding pain in this article is the elusive nature it may assume in the clinical presentation of pathology.

118. Denzler, T., Fuller, E. W., and Eliot, R.   Angina pectoris and myocardial infarction in the presence of patent coronary arteries—A review. *Heart and Lung* 3(4):646–653, 1974.

This article is a review of current concepts and supporting research about angina and myocardial infarction in the absence of occlusive disease. This information is useful for physicians and nurses in identifying pathophysiology and theoretical etiologies for these conditions. Pain is a unique presenting symptom in both conditions and an understanding of the etiology is important for proper management.

119. Epstein, Stephen, et al   Angina pectoris—Pathophysiology, evaluation and treatment. *Ann. Intern. Med.* 75:263–296, 1971.

This is a classic article identifying therapeutic interventions based on evaluation of the underlying pathology causing angina. The information provides implications for nursing intervention, but none are specifically outlined. The clinical approach identified in terms of drug therapy, avoidance of precipitating factors, and exercise is based on research.

120. Frank, P. I.   Some historical aspects of chest pain. *Practitioner* 211:96–104, 1973.

With an increase in diagnosed coronary artery disease and lung cancer, and improved methods of diagnosing pathology of the gastrointestinal tract, there has been renewed interest in the phenomenon of chest pain. This symptom is traced from a historical perspective through the Greco-Roman Era, which focused on cardiac and esophageal disease, the eighteenth century when angina pectoris was described, and the present century, which describes myocardial infarction, an "effort syndrome," and esophageal reflux. This historical presentation includes no case studies, research findings, or clinical interventions, but offers an interesting perspective on the evolution of thought regarding chest pain.

121. Kerr, F., and Donald, K. W.   Analgesia in myocardial infarction. *Br. Heart J.* 36(2):117–121, 1974.

This is a presentation of old and still-valuable interventions for pain and the use of proper analgesics. The hemodynamic effects of analgesics in the patient with a myocardial infarct is discussed in relation to the importance of prompt relief. The degree of pain and the amount of infarcted tissue as evidenced by the extent of electrocardiogram and enzyme changes supports the nurse's responsibility for prompt medication of the infarct patient with chest pain.

122. MacAlpin, Rex   Who will benefit from coronary bypass surgery. *Chest* 66(6):610–611, 1974.

This clinical review of research studies on the functional status of patients with angina after bypass provides important background information for nurses. The purpose of the presentation is to clarify various therapeutic approaches in light of prevailing controversy over the benefit of surgery for the pain patient. It elaborates on the differences in results for the angina patient with occlusive and nonocclusive vessel disease and states that the best results are achieved with the patient with classic angina.

123. Orchard, R. T., Yates, D. B., and Taylor, D. J. E.   Acute precordial chest pain. *Practitioner* 213:212–217, 1974.

   This is a medical research study whose sample was 200 patients admitted with symptoms of chest pain. The purpose was to classify this population according to diagnosis and defined assessment criteria; findings are helpful for nurses in their assessment role. It was determined that 43 percent of the population had myocardial infarcts, 40 percent had ischemic heart disease without myocardial infarct, 11 percent had gastrointestinal problems, and the remainder had miscellaneous disorders.

124. Troup, Wallace J.   Establishing the diagnosis in patients with acute chest pain. *CMA Journal* 108:1156, 1973.

   This discussion is presented for the practicing clinician, including physicians and nurses. It reviews some of the more common causes of chest pain and their associated symptomatology. The following is identified as the clinician's role in dealing with chest pain: (1) allay fear and anxiety, (2) assess etiology, (3) medicate to relieve pain, (4) treat underlying pathological cause.

125. Vinsont, Marielle, et al   *A Commonplace Approach to Coronary Case: A Program.* St. Louis: C. V. Mosby Company, 1972, pp. 71–73.

   A basic and practical approach is outlined for nursing. Nursing care plans and responsibilities with the patient experiencing chest pain are presented with clinical applicability. Included are assessment criteria and the nurse's role in chest pain management when cardiac disease is suspected.

Obstetrics and Gynecology

126. Anstico, Elizabeth   Ask any woman. *Nurs. Times,* November 30, 1972, pp. 1516–1517.

   This article centers on the topic of dysmenorrhea, discussing two different types, "spasmodic" and "congestive." Means of obtaining relief are mentioned. The premenstrual syndrome is cited as having effects on the behavior of women during the paramenstruum. Emphasis is placed on the need to understand that this may be a cause for some women's monthly mood change. This article would be of value to the general public. No theoretical framework.

127. Castelnuovo-Tedesco, Pietro, and Krout, Boyd M.   Psychosomatic aspects of chronic pelvic pain. *Psychiatry Med.* 1(2):109–126, 1970.

   Data gathered on three groups of women some with and some without chronic pelvic pain, revealed a consistent relationship between pain of this nature and psychiatric disturbance, primarily character disorders; organic pelvic pathology was not consistently related to chronic pelvic pain. The literature review sites the classic research of H. C. Taylor; he "regards pelvic congestion as one of the chief physiologic mechanisms by which pain occurs under the influence of adverse emotional factors . . . [for] vaginal blood flow [is] increased greatly during discussion of personal problems" (p. 110). This article presents the thesis that these patients choose their reproductive system as the site of their stress and suffering. This is a provocative presentation of interest to professionals or laymen dealing with gynecological patients. Substantial research supports the thesis; no clinical interventions are included.

128. Crawford, J. S.   Analgesia and anaesthesia in labour. *Practitioner* 212:677–688, 1974.

   This article reviews the appropriate analgesic for premonitory labor, first- and second-stage delivery, and caesarean section. Three generalizations are considered: powerful analgesics may retard progress early in labor: the halted gastrointestinal absorption during labor eliminates the oral route as an effective one; and lastly, all drugs that act directly on the central nervous system will reach the fetus via the placenta. No nursing interventions are included. The merit of this article lies in the comprehensive coverage of the topic of analgesia and anesthesia in labor.

129. Davenport-Slack, Barbara, and Bowlan, Claire Hamblin Psychological correlates of childbirth pain. *Psychosom. Med.* 36(3):215–223, 1974.

This research intended to standardize the report of the childbirth experience that appears to vary so greatly. The childbirth outcome is most importantly affected by training, attitudes toward childbirth, reactions to pain in general, medication expectation, and desire for husband's presence. Other factors were reported as correlates of importance. The underlying factor of most importance in a positive childbirth experience is the woman's desire to be an active participant in the experience. This report lends understanding to the important variables influencing the experience and, hence, supplies background for clinical interventions.

130. Guerriero, W. F., Guerriero, C. P., Edward, R. D., and Stuart, J. A. Pelvic pain, gynecic and nongynecic: Interpretation and management. *South. Med. J.* 64(9):1043–1048, 1971.

This article evolves from a succinct discussion of pelvic neuroanatomy and neurohistology as a framework for pelvic pain. Also discussed as factors influencing pelvic pain are cortical projection of pain patterns, emotional and physical status, and nature of the pain (direct, referred, or both). Interpretation of the pain depends on its location, quality, severity, and duration. Nongynecic causes include pain referred from bladder, bowel, rectum, or connective tissue; infection; overdistention; or adhesions. Gynecic causes include pain referred from the cervix, uterine fundus, fallopian tubes, or ovaries. No patients are presented and no interventions are cited. Information is essential background knowledge for nurses working with gynecological patients.

131. Huttel, F. A., Mitchell, I., Fischer, W. M., and Meyer, A. E. A quantitative evaluation of psycho-prophylaxis in childbirth. *J. Psychosom. Res.* 16(2):81–92, 1972.

This research is intended to justify the use of psychoprophylaxis in childbirth. The prepared women who were accompanied by their husbands demonstrated more self-control and requested less medication. The obstetric nurse and gynecologist could benefit from this substantiation.

132. Klusman, Lawrence E. Reduction of pain in childbirth by the alleviation of anxiety during pregnancy. *J. Consult. Clin. Psychol.* 43(2):162–165, 1975.

Forty-two primigravidas in their last trimester of pregnancy were given courses in childbirth education and child care, and this research indicated that fear and anxiety can be reduced by group classes. Informational instruction and support from other pregnant women in the group contributed positively to the experience. The hypothesis that high anxiety enhances pain perception was confirmed. This finding has implications for nurses in the areas of teaching and support.

133. Kopp, Lois M. Ordeal or ideal—The second stage of labor. *Am. J. Nurs.* 71(6):1140–1143, 1971.

This sensitive article describes the second stage of labor from the perspective of the delivering woman's needs and urges. Nursing interventions that promote the safety of the delivery and enhance the satisfaction of the experience are described. (This nursing focus makes the article most pertinent for a nursing audience.) No research or case studies are included.

134. Lennans, K. Jean, and Lennans, R. John Alleged psychogenic disorders in

women—A possible manifestation of sexual prejudice. *N. Engl. J. Med.* 288(6):288–292, 1973.

Organic etiologic factors and physiology explaining the pain phenomena in dysmenorrhea, nausea of pregnancy, pain in labor, and infantile behavior are presented; the authors contend that ascribing only a psychogenic origin to the pain in these conditions is an erroneous assumption and a subtle form of sexual prejudice against women. This is a somewhat controversial article of interest to any woman, or any person dealing with women. The article is based on physiology; no case studies are included.

135. Rowbotham, C. J. F.   Obstetric pain. *Physiotherapy* 60(4):103–106, 1974.

This brief article presents the anatomy and physiology of obstetric pain and a review of the management possibilities for both labor and delivery. Rather than including research findings or patient case studies, this presentation focuses on commonalities of the obstetric experience. It can be appreciated by health professionals with some pharmacology background. The value of this piece lies in the succinct style and inclusive format.

[See also Numbers 150, 160]

Pediatrics

136. Loomis, W. G.   Management of children's emotional reactions to severe body damage (burns). *Clin. Pediatr.* 9(6):362–367, 1970.

Hamburg's (114) research identified pain and discomfort as the paramount problems for patients with burns. This article utilizes knowledge gleaned from adult burn patients and applies it to the unique situation of children. Pain becomes instrumental in the psychodynamics of their response; it was often viewed as a punishment for a misdeed. Overwhelmed by the magnitude of the pain and the entire illness, regression to more infantile levels of psychosocial development is seen. Pain is one of the factors that may augment withdrawal by superimposing delirium on the stress and demands of the burn experience. Intervention termed mother-substitute approach is described as a corrective emotional experience. Three case studies are included. The framework and the background assumed is psychology, specifically of children.

137. McCaffery, Margo   Brief episodes of pain in children. In Bergersen, Anderson, Duffey, M., Lohr, M., and Rose, M., eds., *Current Concepts in Clinical Nursing*. St. Louis: C. V. Mosby Company, 1969, pp. 178–191.

This chapter provides the nurse with some basic knowledge in helping children who are experiencing brief episodes of pain. Various factors that influence the child's behavioral responses to pain in a situation are discussed. Several suggestions for nursing interventions during anticipation, experience, and aftermath of pain are also presented. Those children twelve years and younger are the focus of this discussion.

138. Nover, Robert A.   Pain and the burned child. *J. Am. Acad. Child Psychiatry* 12(3):409–505, 1973.

Pain is viewed as a contributing factor to a child's emotional reaction to the situation of having been burned. It serves as one of the variants that appears to play an important role in the hospital management of these children. A case study of a five-year-old burned boy is presented. It is included in the article to illustrate how the role of pain influences the responses of the child, his family, and the hospital staff.

139. Rich, Eugene C., Marchall, Richard E., and Volpe, Joseph J.   The normal neonatal response to pin-prick. *Dev. Med. Child Neurol.* 4:432–434, 1974.

This brief article reports on a research study that was designed to study a neonate's responses to a pinprick. The results showed that the normal response to this type of stimuli is movement of the upper and lower limbs accompanied by crying or grimacing, or both. It was proposed by the authors that these results can be useful in searching for disturbances in the central nervous system of a neonate during neurological examinations.

140. Saub, Lawrence I., and Biglan, Anthony Operant treatment of a case of recurrent abdominal pain in a 10 year old boy. *Behav. Therapy* 5:667–681, 1974.

This is a case study of a child with a 2½-year history of recurrent abdominal pain. The treatment program is based on a Skinnerian operant conditioning model, including a token system designed to decrease reported levels of pain, increase school attendance, and end severe pain attacks. New behaviors were then maintained at a high performance rate through the use of a variable reinforcement schedule. This is a unique approach to treatment of pain that can be implemented by a variety of health professionals.

141. Schultz, Nancy V. How children perceive pain. *Nurs. Outlook* 19(10): 670–673, 1971.

The basic focus of this article is the influence of the stages of normal growth and interaction development in a child's perception of pain. Schultz has studied 10- and 11-year-old children, to discover "how" they view pain through a list of questions. From the answers obtained, Schultz discusses the nurse's responsibility in the clinical area while working with these children. She emphasizes that the nurse must take into account the child's constantly changing nature and his interaction with the environment, and how these factors can influence his view of pain and reactions to it.

Other

142. Earlam, Richard Epigastric pain. *Nurs. Mirror*, March 16, 1973, pp. 30–32.

Dyspepsia is a common complaint of many people who seek medical help; the most common cause of dyspepsia is from duodenal ulcers. This article focuses on some of the recent research that has been done reproducing duodenal ulcer pain. The author concluded that epigastric pain that occurs with this illness could be due to gastroesophageal reflux. Based on this assumption, clinical means for the management of epigastric pain are discussed.

143. Fosnat, Harold, ed. Tracking the cause of facial pain. *Patient Care*, September 15, 1972, pp. 20–77.

A round-table discussion of various etiologies of facial pain was presented by six doctors and one dentist. Case studies are presented throughout the article in relation to certain disease processes. Four questions represented the framework of the discussion: (1) Where does it hurt? (2) When does it hurt? (3) How much does it hurt? (4) Do you have other complaints?

Good diagnosis, charts, and illustrations of areas of pain aided in making the article useful for the practitioner. Basic knowledge of facial anatomy would be helpful.

144. Glozis, George G. Evaluation of patients with maxillofacial pain. *Dent. Clin. North Am.* 17(3):379–389, 1973.

This review of facial pain is approached from a dental perspective but remains pertinent for other health professionals who deal with patients experiencing maxillofacial pain. The preliminary question is whether the origin is odontogenic or nonodontogenic. The following entities are discussed and differentiated as possible diagnoses: trigeminal neuralgia, glossopharyngeal neuralgia, ayptical facial pain, cluster headaches, temporal arteritis, carotid pain, myofascial pain, dysfunction syndrome, temporomandibular joint arthritis, pathology of salivary glands, and maxillary sinusitis. Each entity is described as to the nature of sensation. No case studies or interventions are included. This dental presentation is didactic, using clinical pathology as a framework.

145. Kudrow, Lee   Systemic causes of headache. *Postgrad. Med.* 56(3):105–112, 1974.

Headache is discussed as a symptom of a systemic disorder. The most frequent causes of headaches are cerebrovascular strictures and cranial artery injury. Several case summaries are reviewed to support the idea of careful evaluation of headache complaints with history and physical examinations. It is the writer's opinion that several blood tests are also important in the evaluation of a primary headache complaint.

146. Robins, Ashley H.   Functional abdominal pain. *S. Afr. Med. J.* 47:832–834, 1973.

"Functional" is descriptive of symptomatology for which there is no structural lesion; "psychogenic" differs from this classification in that psychiatric disorder or psychogenesis must be present. To preface the discussion of the etiology of abdominal pain, it is said "that the gut is the mirror of the mind." Included under the general heading of functional abdominal pain are psychogenic exaggerations of pain due to actual physical disease, hallucinatory and delusional pain, psychophysiological mechanisms in pain production, hysterical conversion, and simulation of abdominal pain. Several studies are reported and included in a 26-item reference list. No case studies or interventions, but it includes a helpful general coverage of the topic.

147. Simmons, Sandra, and Given, Barbara   Acute pancreatitis. *Am. J. Nurs.* May 1971, pp. 934–939.

This article discusses the pancreas from functional and anatomical perspectives. Recommendations for nursing care are made. Various medical and surgical treatments are mentioned. The article also discusses the cause of pain and nursing pain management of a patient experiencing acute pancreatitis.

148. Thiele, George H.   Anorectal pain. *AFPI* 6(2):55–62, 1972.

The location and type of pain occurring in the anorectal area will usually, unlike other areas of medicine, suggest symptoms leading to a correct diagnosis. The innervation of this area assists with clarification of the pathology; anorectal pain always indicates disease at or below the anorectal line, for this line delimits the innervation of autonomic and cerebrospinal nerves. The article includes a helpful presentation of anatomy, and tables categorizing characteristics of pain-producing lesions. The pain patterns of the following diseases are discussed: anal fissure, anal cryptitis, gonorrheal cryptitis, chancroid, anal stenosis, hemorrhoidal disease, abscesses, and cancer. This is a readable, comprehensive coverage of the topic of anorectal pain, enlarged from an anatomy background. No case studies are presented. Medical treatment of pathology is included but no interventions specific to pain.

149. White, Thomas Taylor   Visceral pain. *Postgrad. Med.* 53(6):199–202, 1973.

The patient who presents with chronic or recurrent abdominal visceral pain may pose a difficulty in diagnosis or management. Five broad groups of pathology to consider with this pain are biliary disease, duodenal ulcer, pancreatic disease, diseases of the colon, or diseases of the spinal column. The pain patterns included are briefly described. A detailed history and physical examination including a psychological evaluation precedes any diagnosis. This article has a highly diagnostic focus that may be of more benefit to independent practitioners. There appears to be a paucity of literature on abdominal visceral pain per se that addresses a nursing audience.

Books

150. Bean, Constance A. *Methods of Childbirth*. Garden City, New York: Doubleday and Company, Inc., 1974.

    This book is a summary of childbirth classes and maternity care helpful for nurses, physicians, and interested nonprofessionals. It includes the physical experiences of the birth process and the changing societal attitudes toward this process.

151. Beecher, Henry K. *Measurement of Subjective Responses: Quantitative Effects of Drugs*. New York: Oxford University Press, 1959.

    Considered a classic in the literature, this book focuses on quantitative effects of drugs on subjective responses in man. The book is divided into two sections, the first dealing exclusively with the measurement of pain, and the second with various subjective states and how they are influenced by drugs. Methods of measuring pain are developed, and research on pain, both experimentally induced and pathologically present, are cited. Both human and animal studies are reviewed. Beecher incorporates most of the work done on pain before 1959 in the text of his writing. An extensive bibliography consisting of 1,063 references is included in the book.

152. Bonica, John J. *The Management of Pain: With Special Emphasis on the Use of Analgesic Block in Diagnosis, Prognosis, and Therapy*. Philadelphia: Lea & Febiger, 1954.

    This is to be considered a classic in the pain literature. It is intended to be a comprehensive treatise of the fundamental aspects of pain, methods of management, and pathology producing pain. Included in these 1,500 pages are bibliographies of most important references. In keeping with the goal of completeness this volume is of working value to a variety of health professionals. This publication is a fine contribution to the literature on pain.

153. Bonica, John J., ed. *Advances in Neurology*. Volume 4: International Symposium on Pain. New York: Raven Press, 1974.

    The proceedings of the International Symposium on Pain held in May, 1973, in Washington were the basis for this book. Reports by numerous professionals have been systematically compiled into two major sections: namely, recent investigations, and diagnosis and therapy. This book exceeds others in the thorough coverage of the vast area of multidisciplinary practice in the field of pain study.

154. Bonica, John J., Procacci, Paolo, and Pagni, Carlo A., eds. *Recent Advances On Pain: Pathophysiology and Clinical Aspects*. Springfield, Illinois: Charles C Thomas, Publisher, 1974. 373 pages, 334 to text.

    From the proceedings at the International Symposium on Recent Progress on Pain Pathophysiology and Clinics held in Florence, Italy, in 1972, a composite of papers, on both the basic aspects of pain and clinical implications for practice, were compiled for this book. Information on the recent work in drug action, nerve blocks, operant conditioning, neurosurgical operations and psychotherapy is available.

    Pain is presented as both a symptom and a disease, with emphasis placed on chronic pain. Towards the end of the book, Bonica discusses the organization and management of a pain clinic, which proves to be very informative.

155. Cailliet, René *Neck and Arm Pain*. Philadelphia: F. A. Davis Company, 1964.

To acquire an understanding of pain mechanisms of the neck and arm, the author acknowledges the need to understand the musculoskeletal system both statically and kinetically. Many drawings and sketches complement the text. The contents are organized according to the following chapters: functional anatomy, neck pain originating in soft tissues, cervical disk disease, subluxations of the cervical spine (including "whiplash"), diagnosis of neck pain, and differential diagnosis. The author's expertise in physical medicine produces an interesting approach to neck and arm pain. This 100-page text is quite easy to understand.

156. Cassenari, Valentino, and Pagni, Carlo *Central Pain: A Neurosurgical Survey*. Cambridge, Massachusetts: Harvard University Press, 1969.

This book presents the concept of "central pain" with a discussion of the anatomy, physiology, and pathology involved in this pain state. Various theories postulating on the cause of central pain are briefly introduced. The authors have emphasized surgical operations that can contribute to the onset of central pain, and on those surgical procedures performed in hopes of alleviating the pain.

157. Crowley, Dorothy M. *Pain and Its Alleviation*. Los Angeles: U.C.L.A. College of Nursing, 1962.

This brief book was written as an exposition to a film, "Pain and Its Alleviation," that was developed by faculty to serve as a teaching guide in caring for the patient with pain. The book covers two broad areas: the nature of pain, and the management of pain. The emphasis in the section dealing with pain management is primarily geared to the nurse. Three phases are identified: (1) assessment of the situation, (2) active intervention, and (3) evaluation. This book offers some up-to-date clinical interventions and also has a good bibliography.

158. Crue, Benjamin L. *Pain and Suffering: Selected Aspects*. Springfield, Illinois: Charles C Thomas, Publisher, 1970.

This book is a composite of research that was presented at the Symposium on Pain and Suffering at the City of Hope National Medical Center in Tuante, California on May 10, 1969. A basis in neurophysiology would be helpful in understanding some of the technical approaches to the problem of intractable pain presented. In the 204 pages, the primary emphasis is on neurosurgical procedures, both clinically applicable and experimentally tried. A section on medicolegal aspects of pain and suffering is also presented.

159. Crue, Benjamin L., ed. *Pain: Research and Treatment*. New York: Academic Press, Inc., 1975. 417 pages.

The writings in this book have been compiled from those contributors who participated in a symposium at the City of Hope. Theories based on neurophysiology, treatment modalities, and research studies dealing with various aspects of the pain experience have been presented. Each inclusive article provides a lengthy bibliography and illustrations to aid the reader.

160. Dick-Read, Grantly *Childbirth Without Fear*. New York: Harper and Row, 1972.

The major thesis of this book is that the natural process of labor and delivery, uninterrupted by needless interventions, is the method of least danger for both mother and child. Pain is discussed in reference to the history and development of the species. This classic book was written before the concept of natural and pain-free childbirth was a viable subject, and has weathered the years to remain as a major work for layman and health professionals.

161. Finneson, Bernard E. *Diagnosis and Management of Pain Syndromes*. 2d ed. Philadelphia: W. B. Saunders Company, 1969. 337 pages.

This neurosurgeon bases his writings on his clinical experience with various painful conditions and his therapeutic mode of treatment. Two sections, dealing with the use of drugs in pain relief and management of musculoskeletal pain were written by guest physicians, Grallman and Meltzer, respectively. In the discussions of painful conditions, symptoms and pathophysiology are presented, in addition to the management of pain. The text of the book is supplemented with numerous useful illustrations.

162. Freese, Arthur S. *Pain: The New Help For Your Pain.* New York: G. P. Putnam's Sons, 1974. 235 pages.

Both the general concept of pain and a number of interventions to relieve pain have been discussed in this book by Dr. Freese, a specialist in the field of head and facial pain. His writing is geared to the layman, and his discussion of forms of therapy includes several new treatments such as electronic relief of pain, hypnosis, acupuncture, and biofeedback. A lengthy discussion of the concept of pain clinics and pain doctors is presented, with special reference to the clinic in Seattle.

163. Friedman, Arnold P., and Merritt, H. Houston *Headache: Diagnosis and Treatment.* Philadelphia: F. A. Davis Company, 1959.

The vast topic of headache is covered very thoroughly in this classic piece. The basic diagnostic and management information make this book practical for clinicians. The following are individually considered as sources of headache: eye; ear, nose, and throat; allergy; systemic disease; intracranial disorders; tension; psychogenic factors; and cervical spine. Although the contributing authors are medical doctors and the intended audience of the book is practicing physicians, it contains basic and useful information for other health professionals interested in headache.

164. Friedman, Arnold P., and Frazier, Shervert H. *The Headache Book.* New York: Dodd, Mead & Company, 1973.

That "a headache is a pain in the head" introduces laymen and health professionals to a readable book covering the extensive topic of headache. Included in this 173-page text are some sources of headache pain in current society, for example hangover, hunger, and tension. Several variations of chronic headache are addressed. Even a section on the anatomy of headache is understandable by laymen. Current theories in headache therapy present information on intervention.

165. Frieger, Norman *Pain Control.* Chicago: Buck-und Zeitsckriften-Verlag "Die Quintessenz," 1974. 143 pages.

Pain control in the field of dentistry is the basic slant of this book. Emphasis is placed on how the individuality of a person is of prime importance in the management of pain. There is a need for dentists and dental schools to broaden their spectrum of thought in regard to pain beyond the need of "local" or "general" anesthesia. The care of the patient is divided into three phases: pretreatment patient evaluation, intraoperative methods, and postoperative management. Illustrations are used to supplement the text. A basic understanding of pharmacology would be advantageous to the reader.

166. Hart, F. Dudley, ed. *The Treatment of Chronic Pain.* Lancaster, England: Medical and Technical Publishing, 1974. 180 pages.

Six authors who have attempted long-term control of chronic pain have collaborated in this publication. The authors come from a variety of backgrounds—from surgery to anesthesia to psychiatry—and have each presented their own treatment methods. E. C. Huskisson presents pain mechanisms and measurement, T. S. Szasz speaks from a psychiatric perspective, F. D. Hart on rheumatic disorders, G. Westbury on incurable malignancies, J. C. White on neuralgias of nonmalignant etiology, and S. A. Feldman on chemical neurolysis. The result of this collaboration is interesting and the varied approaches juxtaposed in a very readable 180-page text.

167. Jacox, Ada, and Stewart, Mary *Psychosocial Contingencies of the Pain Experience.* Iowa City: University of Iowa Press, 1973.

This monograph reports on a descriptive study of pain. A sound basis in statistics would be helpful in understanding the material presented. The purpose of the study was "to contribute to the knowledge of the pain experience by exploring relationships among factors that influence how persons interpret and respond to pain." A biopsychosocial approach to the study of pain, following Sternbach, has been developed in the conceptual framework. Factors such as personality characteristics, health self-concept, past experience with pain, sex, and age were analyzed and reported. Implications of the results for clinical practice and for research are discussed.

168. Janzen, Rudolph, *Pain Analysis: A Guide to Diagnosis.* Bristol, England: John Wright and Sons, Ltd., 1970.

This book of 87 pages is a very succinct and concentrated collection of writings. Case studies and literature reviews are eliminated, thereby making it less of a reference book: the purpose of the book is to present a synopsis of salient principles. The editor's expertise in clinical neurosurgery becomes evident in the strong clinical emphasis. Following the general chapters on morphology of receptors, superficial and deep pain, elucidation of terms, and principles of clinical pain analysis; the specific anatomical areas of head, trunk, extremities, thorax, upper and lower abdominal, cardiac, and vascular pain are included. The final chapter deals with pain analysis in childhood. This book is heavy reading due to its concentrated form.

169. Keele, K. D. *Anatomies of Pain.* Springfield, Illinois: Charles C Thomas, Publisher, 1957.

These 200 pages present the evolution of ideas regarding the concept of pain, spanning time from ancient medicine to the present. This background is presented not as a conclusive historical document but rather as a survey of the anatomical and physiological concepts that have evolved as the framework for current theories. The thesis of this historical review is that in order for ideas to survive they must be produced in a time in which there is "sufficient contextual background to support them." This book offers an interesting approach to the concept of pain in a readable manner.

170. Macbryde, Cyril M., and Blacklow, Robert S., eds. *Signs and Symptoms: Applied Pathologic Physiology and Clinical Interpretations.* 5th ed. Philadelphia: J. B. Lippincott Company, 1970.

This text attempts to synthesize relevant pathophysiology, normal physiology, clinical manifestations of disease, and the thought process that culminates in a clinical diagnosis. Although the entire text is not devoted to the topic of pain, 11 of the 40 chapters address the phenomenon of pain in a variety of anatomical locations. Head, eye, ear, mouth, thorax, abdomen, urinary tract, back, joints, and extremities are the focus of individual chapters. Pain is approached from the perspective of understanding the processes that result in its clinical manifestations. This book is very readable.

171. McCaffery, Margo *Nursing Management of the Patient with Pain.* Philadelphia: J. B. Lippincott Company, 1972. 248 pages. 137-reference bibliography.

The subject of pain and its management has been presented here in a problem-solving framework. One of the goals has been to provide the nurse with a variety of interventions that can be incorporated into the patient's care for the relief of pain and attainment of comfort. The reader is exposed to the concept of pain by progressing through the steps of nursing assessment, nursing diagnosis, nursing intervention, and evaluation of nursing intervention. Case studies are presented throughout the chapters to provide examples of problems that may arise, as well as suggestions on resolving them. In addition to discussing a number of interventions applicable to clinical practice, the author has made good use of references.

172. Mehta, Mark *Major Problems in Anaesthesia*, Volume 2 of the series. William W. Mushin, consulting ed. Philadelphia: W. B. Saunders Company, 1973.

The emphasis of this book is practicality; it is addressed to those professionals who face in their daily work patients with intractable pain. The author, an anesthetist, intends for this book to encourage other anesthetists to develop interest in the treatment of pain. This 300-page book contains three parts: the first focuses on the nature of intractable pain, basic mechanisms, pharmacology, clinical assessment and psychological aspects. The second speaks of conditions giving rise to intractable pain. Part three deals exclusively with technique and procedures of treatment. Although the slant of this book is anesthesiology, the contribution it makes to the nursing literature is the readable and pertinent presentations of intractable pain mechanisms and related pathology. An understanding of treatment procedures, although not performed by the nurse, enhances the readers' insight for care of the total patient.

173. Mines, Samuel *The Conquest of Pain*. New York: Grosset & Dunlap, Inc., 1974.

In this 203-page book, the author has briefly mentioned the current therapies used in the treatment of chronic pain and the people who are responsible for initiating these treatments. Pain was traced back to the witch doctors, spiritualists, mystics and faith healers. Information was included throughout the text on the pain clinics that are developing in this country. The book has merit in that it is easy for the layman to read and understand. An appendix is included in the book that lists the research entries and credentials of the people who presented their work at the first International Symposium on Pain, held in Seattle, Washington in May, 1973.

174. Melzack, Ronald *The Puzzle of Pain*. New York: Basic Books, Inc., Publishers, 1973.

Melzack's stated goal in writing this book is to introduce both the health professional and layman to the problem of pain. The book is divided into two sections: the first section deals with the psychology, physiology, and clinical aspects of pain. The second section discusses the major theories of pain, with a lengthy discussion of the controversial gate control theory of pain that was developed by Melzack and Wall in 1965. Added features are a glossary of basic medical terms used and an extensive list of references.

175. Merskey, H., and Spear, F. G. *Pain: Psychological and Psychiatric Aspects*. London: Bailliere, Lindall and Cassell, 1967. 219 pages.

The theoretical framework of this book is drawn heavily from the area of psychology. Various research works are interspersed as they apply to either the clinical setting or experimental psychology. The authors themselves have done research with the pain experience. A theory of pain is proposed that is derived basically from Szasz's hypothesis of pain, which views pain as a psychological phenomenon, but allows for explanation of a variety of types of pain. A good bibliography is presented.

176. Naylor, Vera, and Michaels, David *The Sufferings of the Cancer Patient*. London: Hutchinson Benham, 1967.

This book, written by a social worker, relates her conversations with various cancer patients. She has found several factors that most patients speak of:

bereavements, accidents, and personal sorrows. Mention is also made of diversional therapy that Naylor has used with the cancer patients receiving treatments, namely, playing card games and puzzles. A second part of the book, by Michaels, attempts to analyze the cases presented by Naylor and also the letters received in response to an earlier book, *Emotional Problems of Cancer Patients.*

177. Noordenbos, W.   *Pain.* New York: Elsevier Publishing Co., 1959.

Pain is approached by this neurosurgeon as a symptom to be treated surgically. Of primary concern are the neurological nature and the physiological transmission of those afferent impulses that are interpreted as pain. This book reports the common neurophysiological findings in patients who complain of pain, so as to explain the general mechanism of pain. This inclusive coverage of the fundamental features of a variety of painful conditions requires a background in neuroanatomy and neurophysiology.

178. Sergeant, Richard   *The Spectrum of Pain.* London: Rupert, Hart-Davis, 1969.

Alliteration that begins with the word pain is expanded to supply the organizing framework for this book, namely, pathways of pain, purposes, problems and penalties, prevention and relief, and the paradox of pain. The great complexity of the topic of pain is acknowledged, and is therefore presented from a variety of perspectives. This multidisciplinary approach includes opinions and theories from philosophy, psychology, religion, sociology, and anatomy. The contribution made by this publication is the presentation of debatable opinions on certain aspects of pain, which, according to the author, produces "some hard constructive thinking." This is a provocative 175-page book.

179. Sternbach, Richard A.   *Pain: A Psychophysiological Analysis.* New York: Academic Press, Inc., 1968. 185 pages.

This book is written with a multidisciplinary approach to pain. Emphasis is placed on both the physical and mental nature of pain as interrelated dimensions in a person's pain experience. The book is divided into three areas: (1) a review of current literature (as of 1968) on pain from the anatomical, psychological, and sociological aspects, (2) discussion of research on the differentiation between clinical pain and experimentally induced pain, and (3) discussion of common concepts of the pain mechanisms, along with three "paradoxes" of pain—insensitivity to pain, phantom pain, and hypnotic and placebo effects.

The content of this book has more relevance for the management of chronic or intractable pain. The author includes a 262-item bibliography.

180. Swerdlow, Mark, ed.   *Relief of Intractable Pain.* New York: Excerpta Medica, 1974. In *Monographs in Anaesthesiology* Vol. 1. Editor-in-Chief: A. R. Hunter.

The topic of intractable pain is handled in a concise and comprehensive manner, making this book a valuable reference; it is addressed to a wide variety of health professionals who deal with patients in chronic pain. Included in this book are the neurophysiology of pain, psychological aspects of pain relief, descriptions of pain clinics, and several chapters on a variety of pain-alleviation modalities.

181. Szasz, Thomas S.   *Pain and Pleasure.* 2d ed. New York: Basic Books, Inc., Publishers, 1975.

This book is a study of bodily feelings. It explores the mind-body problem from both philosophical and psychological perspectives and examines elements of pain and pleasure.

First published in 1957, the 1975 revised edition contains an additional chapter "Pain in a New Perspective, 1975." Here Szasz details his concern with pain experience and communication, refuting the commonly made distinction between organic and psychogenic pain. The author presents a dramaturgic-existential approach to pain that borrows from psychiatry, sociology, and philosophy. He proposes that the treatment and control of pain in certain situations is unlike that encountered in standard medical practice. Szasz explores pain as a "career" and discusses the important role of the physician in the mastery of pain, emphasizing the confusion and deception that flourished in contemporary medical practice. He also conceptualizes a model of the "painful person," which makes this book an excellent basic reference.

182. Trigg, Roger *Pain and Emotion.* Oxford: Clarendon Press, 1970. 187 pages.

This book emphasizes the philosophical perspective of pain. It discusses a basic question, "Is pain a sensation, an emotion, etc.?" The distinction between "nonpainful pain" and "pleasant pain" is presented with comments on the concept of suffering. The book closes with a case of insensitivity to pain and suggests how similar cases can add to our knowledge of the concept of pain quality.

183. Weisenberg, Matisyohu, ed. *Pain: Clinical and Experimental Perspectives.* St. Louis: The C. V. Mosby Company, 1975. 385 pages.

A multidisciplinary composite of reprinted articles dealing with various aspects of pain are incorporated into this book. Readings deal with both experimental research and clinical studies that would be useful for all practitioners and educators. In addition to theoretical discussions of variables in the pain experience, selected disease conditions are discussed with ideas presented on some means of pain control. A 24-page annotated bibliography of selected articles from 1965 to 1972 is also featured.

184. White, James C., and Sweet, William H. *Pain and the Neurosurgeon: A Forty-Year Experience.* Springfield, Illinois: Charles C Thomas, Publisher, 1969.

This is a second of two extensive volumes on the topic of pain written by these two neurosurgeons. The first, *Pain: Its Mechanisms and Neurosurgical Control,* was published in 1955 and includes fundamental aspects of pain perception and techniques for intervention. The later volume is designed to avoid repetition of the first volume and to provide an update. Included are clinical presentations of intractable pain and the most effective methods for surgical intervention. The 900-page text and 60-page bibliography attest to its inclusiveness. The authors' wealth of clinical experience and knowledge render this a valuable resource.

185. Wolff, Harold G. *Headache and Other Head Pain.* 2d ed. New York: Oxford University Press, 1963.

Wolff is a neurologist who incorporated a holistic approach to patients; the following statement attests to this: "essential though his awareness must be of the physical and chemical processes and procedures pertinent to the symptom, ultimately the physician's therapeutic effectiveness depends upon his genuine interest in human troubles and his appreciation of the many and complex factors in man's experience that can result in headache" (quoted from preface). This publication is intended to unify the fragmented topic of headache by presenting historical information and theories on mechanisms that lend themselves to pain prevention or relief. A 1,095-item bibliography and a 710-page text indicate the completeness of this publication.

186. Zborowski, Mark *People In Pain.* San Francisco: Jossey-Bass, Inc., Publishers, 1969. 274 pages.

This book is a qualitative study of responsive patterns to pain. It suggests that cultural background determines ways in which people tolerate and express pain. Differences among four national groups, and similarities among individuals within each group, are examined. Research techniques used by anthropologist Zborowski include participant observation and interviews, excerpts of which are reported in text. Findings heighten professional awareness of cultural components of pain, and provide implications for practical use by anyone dealing with "people in pain."

Index

Index